TEXTBOOK OF PEDIATRICS

VOLUME 2

SUBSPECIALTIES, COMPLEX DISORDERS, AND CRITICAL CARE

Dr. Maruf Tinsae

ALLIED HEALTH PRESS

Textbook of Pediatrics Volume 2

Subspecialties, Complex Disorders, and Critical Care

Author: **Dr. Maruf Tinsae**

Allied Health Press
4164 Lakeshore Road
Burlington ON L7L 1A4
Canada
www.alliedhealthpress.com
Email: orders@arclereducation.com

ISBN: 978-1-77956-845-8

ABOUT THE AUTHOR

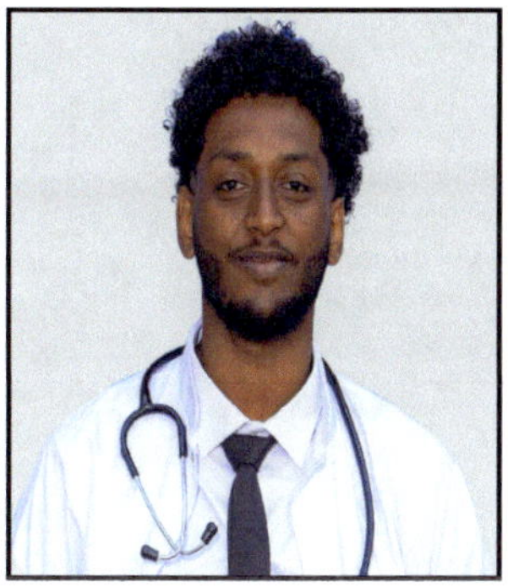

Dr. Maruf Tinsae is a Medical Doctor and current Internal Medicine Resident with over fi ve years of clinical experience. He obtained his Doctor of Medicine degree from Hawassa University,Ethiopia in 2020. His professional journey includes roles as a physician at Black Lion Hospital, HUSCH, and Panesiya General Hospital, where he has been actively involved in patient care, medical training, and academic contributions.

His areas of expertise include clinical assessment, diagnosis, and management of diverse medical conditions. In addition, he is deeply engaged in medical writing, journal and book reviews, authorship, and research. He is one of the writers of the MedStar Book Series, one of the largest and most recognized medical short guide collections in Ethiopia, contributing to accessible and practical medical knowledge for healthcare professionals.

Brief Table of Contents

Getting Started with This Book

Chapter Openers

A list of Chapter Outline is presented providing a brief Introduction to what will be covered in the chapter.

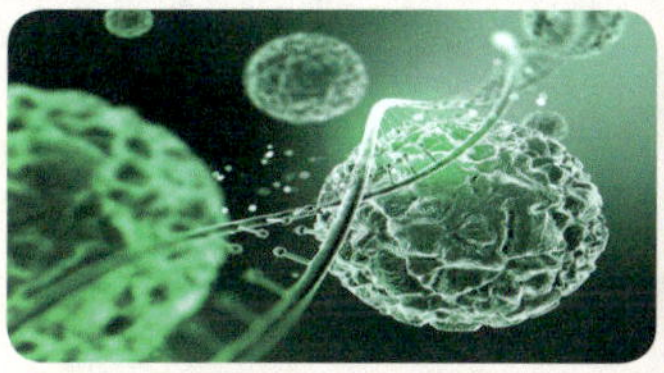

LEARNING OBJECTIVES

After studying this chapter, you will be able to:

1. Discuss the scientific method in biology;
2. Explain the cell theory;
3. Discuss the genetics and heredity;
4. Evolution and natural selection;
5. Focus on ecology and ecosystems;
6. Learn about human biology;
7. Evaluate the plant biology;
8. Explain the microbiology;
9. Focus on current trends in biology.

Introduction

Often referred to as the science of life, biology is a broad field of study aimed at comprehending the several kinds of life on Earth, from tiny creatures to sophisticated multicellular entities. Comprising several subfields, including molecular biology, ecology, and evolutionary biology, each of which advances our knowledge of living systems, this field clarifies the mechanisms controlling life events, including development, reproduction, and interaction with the surroundings, which is the central goal of biology. Moreover, biology fills in the void between the natural sciences and medicine by offering a necessary understanding of health, illness, and the interactions between organisms and their environments. Dealing with urgent global issues such as climate change, biodiversity loss, and new diseases depends on an awareness of these complex biological interactions, therefore highlighting the critical part biology plays in modern civilization. Fundamentally, biology explores and tests ideas about the living world using the scientific method. Through methodical observation and experimentation,

1.1. The Scientific Method in Biology

Learning Outcome

1. Describe the steps of the scientific method;
2. Focus on hypothesis formation;
3. Learn about experimental design.

Learning Outcomes

The beginning of each section of every chapter contains a set of Learning Outcomes that inform students of concepts they should understand. These outcomes help students understand what they should be able to do if they have mastered the material in that section.

Test Your Knowledge

Throughout each chapter, Test Your Knowledge cues you to note which topics have been covered and to self-test your understanding of the material presented.

Test Your Knowledge

1. Explain why correlation does not imply causation in scientific experiments.
2. How does the scientific method help reduce the influence of personal opinions in research?

Chapter Summary

The Summary Section appear at the end of each chapter and summarize main concepts covered throughout the chapter. These points provide key concepts in an engaging and meaningful way.

Summary

The investigation of biological principles highlights the importance of a comprehensive view of life by reflecting the intricate interactions that occur within living systems. The complexity of biology goes beyond individual species or systems, as this essay highlights; it also includes the interactions that mold ecosystems and affect biodiversity. Researchers can conduct in-depth analyses of metabolomic data using sophisticated technologies like MetaboAnalyst, which offer insights into the molecular mechanisms underlying these interactions. As demonstrated by the developments in MetaboAnalyst, for example, the integration of diverse omics data promotes a thorough understanding of metabolic pathways and helps identify important biological markers necessary for research on development and disease (Chong et al., 2018). Additionally, the phenomenon of ecological invasions is a key component of biological research and a vital field of study. The introduction of non-native species into unfamiliar habitats has significant ramifications and calls for multidisciplinary management strategies. Examining the origins and effects of these biological incursions, invasion science has become a crucial field that highlights the need to comprehend ecological dynamics and community interactions. As interest in biological invasions increases, new findings are emerging that put conventional ecological theories and practices to the test. The importance of incorporating various scientific viewpoints is shown by this developing discipline, which also highlights how invasive species shape ecosystems and advances our knowledge of ecological resilience (David et al., 2013). When taken as a whole, these discoveries from invasion science and metabolomics highlight the value of multidisciplinary biology research. Fostering cross-disciplinary collaboration and utilizing technological breakthroughs to improve our comprehension of intricate biological interactions are crucial as we look to the future of biological research. In addition to deepening our understanding of the complexities of life, this method lays the groundwork for tackling urgent environmental issues. Future studies can ensure the continued relevance of biology in a world that is constantly changing by acknowledging the interconnection of biological systems and opening the door to creative solutions that support sustainability and biodiversity conservation. We might imagine a thorough comprehension of life that serves both academia and society at large through ongoing investigation and integration of scientific knowledge.

Knowledge Assessment

The chapter includes material designed to review and reinforce each content. It includes Critical Thinking Questions to help test of your understanding of information presented in the chapter and Short answer Questions to review your understanding of the key concepts presented in the chapter.

Critical Thinking Questions

1. **Who is known as the "Father of Modern Biology"?**
   a. Aristotle
   b. Charles Darwin
   c. Gregor Mendel
   d. Louis Pasteur
2. **What is the basic unit of life?**
   a. Atom
   b. Molecule
   c. Cell
   d. Organism
3. **Which branch of biology studies the interaction of organisms with their environment?**
   a. Genetics
   b. Ecology
   c. Physiology
   d. Botany
4. **Which macromolecule is the main source of energy for living organisms?**
   a. Proteins
   b. Lipids
   c. Carbohydrates
   d. Nucleic acids
5. **DNA is primarily responsible for which function in living organisms?**
   a. Energy production
   b. Protein synthesis
   c. Storing genetic information
   d. Regulating body temperature

Short Answer Questions

1. What is biology, and why is it important to study biology?
2. What are the three main domains of life, and how are they different from one another?
3. Define homeostasis and give an example of how it works in living organisms.
4. What is the cell theory, and why is it fundamental to biology?
5. How do autotrophs and heterotrophs differ in the way they obtain energy?
6. What is the scientific method, and how is it applied in biological research?
7. Discuss how biology helps address global challenges such as climate change, disease, and food security.
8. Explain the levels of biological organization from the smallest unit to the largest. Provide examples at each level.
9. Describe the relationship between structure and function in biology, giving specific examples from cells or organs.
10. How has the discovery of genetics shaped our understanding of inheritance and variation among organisms?

Supplementary Materials

Key Terms: A list of key terms is given for quick reference

KEY TERMS FROM THIS CHAPTER

Annotation enrichment analysis	Biological structure	Cell
Cell theory	Cellular structure	Ecology
Ecosystems	Genetics	Human biology
Microbiology	Natural selection	Organism
Plant biology		

Further Resources: Recommendations for additional readings, websites, and multimedia resources.

References

1. Argelaguet, R., Velten, B., Arnol, D., Dietrich, S., Zenz, T., Marioni, J. C., Buettner, F., et al. (2018). Multi-omics factor analysis—A framework for unsupervised integration of multi-omics data sets. *Molecular Systems Biology, 14*. https://doi.org/10.15252/msb.20178124.
2. Bacher, S., Blackburn, T. M., Essl, F., & Genovesi, P. (2017). *Socio-Economic Impact Classification of Alien Taxa (SEICAT)*. https://core.ac.uk/download/286567949.pdf (accessed on 8th March 2025).
3. Barnett, R., Brace, S., Cucchi, T., & Dobney, K. (2013). *Divergent Evolutionary Processes Associated with Colonization of Offshore Islands*. https://core.ac.uk/download/20664364.pdf (accessed on 8th March 2025).

Detailed Table of Contents

CHAPTER 7

Common Pediatric Psychiatric Disorders 187

CHAPTER 8

Vaccine-Preventable Pediatric Diseases 221

LIST OF FIGURES

PREFACE

As children progress to later stages of development, they present with a spectrum of health issues that require sophisticated expertise. Pediatric professionals integrate knowledge of normal development patterns with expertise in rare diseases and multisystem chronic illnesses. The rheumatologic, renal, dermatologic, endocrine, and nervous systems each present unique challenges to diagnosis in children, typically with unique presentations compared to adults. Early treatment and diagnosis have a profound impact on long-term outcomes, and therefore, advanced training and familiarity with new pediatric subspecialty therapies are essential.

Pediatric critical care demands rapid assessment and precision in resuscitative measures. From acute decompensation to long-term monitoring, clinicians must adjust for smaller airways, varied pharmacokinetics, and psychological requirements of children and families. Similarly, the management of mental illness and behavioral disorders requires attention to the setting of development, home life, and stigma that may preclude care. With advancements in vaccine technology, delivering full immunization coverage to prevent vaccine-preventable diseases is a cornerstone of children's public health. Surgical and palliative care aspects also illustrate the range of pediatric practice, ranging from simple procedures to end-of-life care responsive to both clinical needs and parental preferences.

This book, *Textbook of Pediatrics: Volume 2,* continues the principles of its companion book by providing in-depth coverage of subspecialty subjects and high-impact interventions. Each chapter provides comprehensive summaries, diagnostic strategies, and management recommendations tailored for students and practitioners seeking to enhance their skills in advanced pediatric practice.

Chapter 1 presents pediatric rheumatology, describing mechanisms of juvenile idiopathic arthritis, systemic lupus erythematosus, and vasculitic disorders. It discusses clinical presentation, laboratory evaluation, and current treatment plans involving biological agents. Chapter 2 covers pediatric nephrology, describing congenital and acquired kidney diseases, proteinuria and hematuria management, and principles of fluid and electrolyte management. Chapter 3 covers pediatric dermatology, including the evaluation of skin dermatitis, psoriasis, and inherited skin diseases, as well as instruction on topical and systemic therapies. Chapter 4 deals with endocrine diseases in children, including growth disorders, thyroid disease, and puberty disorders, as well as diagnostic testing and hormone replacement therapy. Chapter 5 talks about assessment and monitoring, presenting techniques, such as pulse oximetry, growth charting, pain scales, and developmental screening tests. Chapter 6 covers pediatric emergencies and critical care, including airway management, pediatric advanced life support, and the management of shock and sepsis. Chapter 7 discusses the most common pediatric psychiatric conditions, including attention-deficit/hyperactivity disorder, mood disorders, and anxiety disorders, with an emphasis on diagnostic features and treatment options. Chapter 8 describes vaccine-preventable conditions, reviewing epidemiology, immunologic principles, and public health interventions to achieve herd immunity. Chapter 9 addresses pediatric surgery, outlining typical procedures , such as hernia repair, appendectomy, and the management of surgical emergencies. Chapter 10 outlines pediatric pulmonology, addressing asthma, cystic fibrosis, and bronchopulmonary dysplasia, including imaging and long-term management. Chapter 11 addresses pediatric psychiatry and behavioral health, addressing autism spectrum disorder, behavioral treatment, and collaborative care models. Chapter 12 concludes the discussion by addressing pediatric palliative and end-of-life care, including pain management, psychosocial support, and ethical considerations in advanced illness.

This is suitable for a broad readership. Pediatric fellows and residents will have detailed guidance on subspecialty rotations, and general pediatricians will be able to refresh their practice know-how of complex conditions. Critical care nurses, respiratory therapists, and clinical pharmacists will welcome protocols tailored to pediatric patients. Mental health clinicians, social workers, and educators may also find the chapters on psychiatric and behavioral health useful for collaborative practice. Combining the latest available research with clinical experience, this text is designed to equip all healthcare professionals dedicated to improving the well-being of children with a diverse range of health problems.

PEDIATRIC RHEUMATOLOGY

1

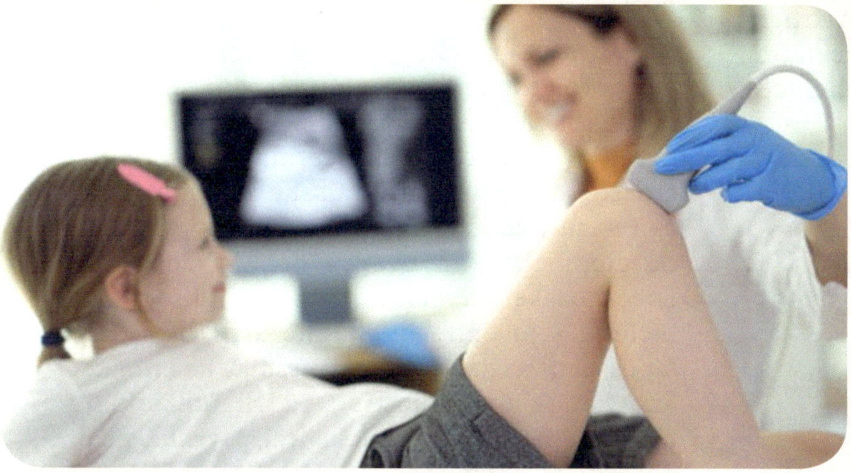

LEARNING OBJECTIVES

After studying this chapter, you will be able to:

1. Discuss common pediatric rheumatic diseases
2. Point out symptoms and diagnosis
3. Gain knowledge of treatment and management
4. Identify challenges for pediatric rheumatology
5. Gain knowledge of research and advances in pediatric rheumatology
6. Discuss the case studies and clinical examples

Introduction

Pediatric rheumatology is a medical specialty that specializes in the diagnosis and treatment of rheumatic diseases of children. Rheumatic diseases, encompassing a wide range of inflammatory and autoimmune conditions, can present early in life and cause enormous morbidity if not diagnosed and treated early. Pediatric rheumatologists are uniquely trained to value the subtle presentation and highly variable symptoms that might be very different from adults. Early treatment is essential in these patients since it cane long-term prognosis, such as, such as function and quality of life. It is crucial to be familiar with the general differences between adult and pediatric rheumatic ir proper treatment inasmuch assince etiologic determinants and therapeutic effects may or may not be proportionate to established paradigms in adults. As technology continues to influence the many medical specialties, pediatric rheumatology is not exempt. The addition of artificial intelligence (AI) to practice means pediatric rheumatology has the potential to revolutionize the diagnostic and management process. Machine learning (ML) algorithms are increasingly used to screen and read large datasets, which can be utilized to classify patients, identify disease subtypes, and discover new biomarkers for application in pediatric rheumatic disease. With their capacity for managing vast amounts of lab data, these solutions enhance decision-making by providing more accurate and timely information to caregivers. This new procedure has the potential not only to ease the diagnostic process but also to complement the principles of precision medicine, tailoring interventions that meet the individualized needs of children with rheumatic diseases (Galozzi et al., 2023).

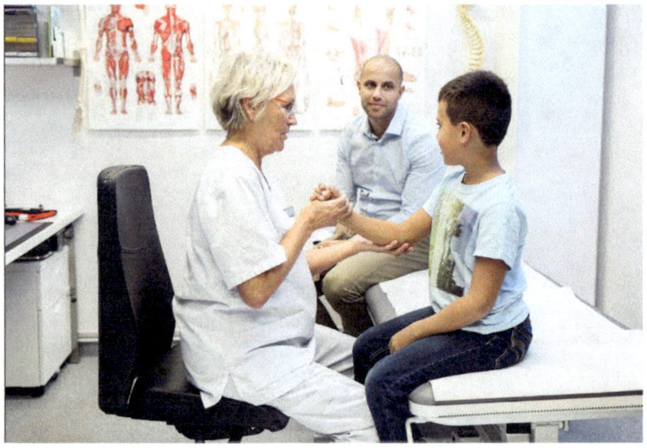

Figure 1.1. The field of pediatric rheumatology.

Source: https://dam.northwell.edu/m/10287fe655cd71c5/Drupal-Web_GettyImages-551423805.jpg.

Also, the deployment of AI technologies is set to promote cross-functional working among multidisciplinary teams in managing complex cases of pediatrics. Integrating AI into clinical workflows can enhance patient outcomes and treatment planning through advanced data visualization and predictive modeling. In pediatric rheumatology, this fusion of technology and clinical practice promises improved treatment strategies and results.. These developments can also lead to further investigation of the pathophysiology and treatment of rheumatic disease in children, adding to the greater body of knowledge in this important area of healthcare. As development in these areas advances, monitoring adherence to ethical guidelines and patient-focused care will also be of critical concern, so that technological advances are reflected in tangible gains in the lives of child rheudisease patients (Keser & Pekineret al., 2023) (Figure 1.1).

Definition and Scope of Pediatric Rheumatology

Pediatric rheumatology is a medical subspecialty that involves the diagnosis and management of rheumatic diseases in children. Such diseases, most frequently manifesting with joint, muscle, and connective tissue inflammation, can significantly impact a child's physical development and overall health. The field encompasses a wide range of disorders, including juvenile idiopathic arthritis (JIA), lupus, and vasculitis, that necessitate an intimate knowledge of pediatric and rheumatologic principles. The unique biological, psychological, and social needs of children with rheumatic conditions necessitate tailored therapeutic approaches that are unlike those commonly applied in adults. Sophisticated diagnostic techniques and therapeutic approaches have been specifically designed to address the needs of the complexity of children's disorders and therefore strengthened the profession by integrating evidence-based practice with the specific needs of child care. Pediatric rheumatology is not merely confined to the simple identification and management of rheumatic diseases but rather includes multidisciplinary collaboration to provide holistic care. Effective treatment of these disorders requires cooperation among several healthcare practitioners, including pediatricians, rheumatologists, physical therapists, and psychologists. This is necessary because pediatric rheumatology often intersects with other specialties, since most rheumatologic illnesses have implications that transcend only the musculoskeletal system. Additionally, the incorporation of evidence-based care into treatment protocols is mandatory. A classic example in this context is the Health-e-Child project, which seeks to systematically investigate and integrate biomedical knowledge regarding diseases like JIA to optimize clinical performance through improved data management and analysis (Anjum et al., 2007). The project is a good classic representation of the ever-changing nature of pediatric rheumatology, which reiterates the necessity of a data-driven approach in the provision of optimal care.

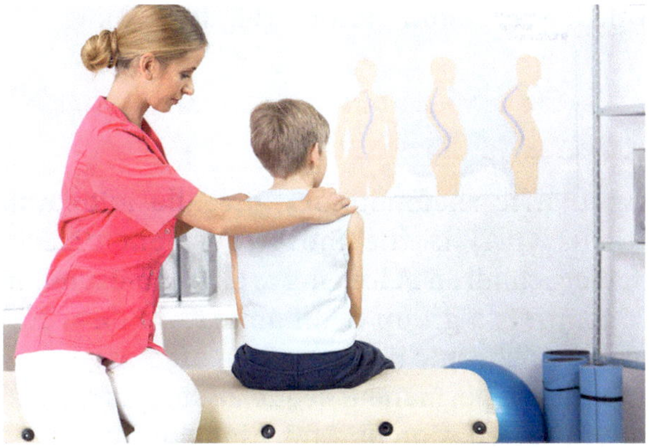

Figure 1.2. Pediatric rheumatology is a specialized branch of medicine that focuses on the diagnosis and management of rheumatic diseases in children.

Source: https://static.bookinghealth.com/uploads/clinics/gallery/m/9470-6143-1503500467_otr_shutterstock_464420933-1.jpg.

The transition of adolescents with chronic diseases from pediatric healthcare systems is especially problematic, such as, such as in pediatric rheumatology. Effectively pransition processes must be imented so that ongoing chien grow into adulthood get and receive the best care of for their ongoing rheumatic ailments. Optimal transitions require evidence suggesting that age-related education in self-management, communication between pediatric and adult clinicians, and patient and family involvement are integral (Bagnall et al., 2013). The approaches not only empower young patients but also mitigate possible health decline associated with transitions. With the advancement of pediatric rheumatology, understanding the intricacy of these transitions becomes more and more critical to healthcare systems aiming to provide quality and long-term care to adolescents with chronic medical conditions (Figure 1.2).

Importance of Early Diagnosis and Treatment

Early identification and management of pediatric rheumatic diseases are critical for improving patient outcomes and reducing long-term morbidity. Conditions such as juvenile idiopathic arthritis (JIA) can significantly affect physical and mental health if not treated promptly. Delayed detection often leads to irreversible joint damage, increased pain, and impaired quality of life. Furthermore, early treatment has been shown to lessen the socioeconomic burden of chronic diseases like JIA. The efficacy of newer treatments relies on the ability to detect and treat early signs, again underlining the critical role of healthcare professionals in detecting early signs. Thus, increased awareness and aetiologically oriented educational programs of the initial presentations of pediatric rheumatic illnesses will significantly enhance diagnostic aic responsiveness in everyday clinical practice, contributing therebythereby contributing to optimal treatment of such children from the earliest possible moment. It irtant to diagnose rheumatic diseases early enough for the purposes of both symptom control and prevention. Studies have shown that the majority of MAS cases are seen in the first presentation of related rheumatic diseases, namely systemic juvenile idiopathic arthritis (sJIA) (Huang et al., 2024). The clinical significance of this finding underscores the need for health practitioners to be alert while assessing pediatric patients for manns of rheumatic disease. Effective biomarkers for predicting MAS, such as, such as ferritin levels and platelet count, may be used to enable early diagnosis for interventions in a timely manner. The linkage between early diagnosis and positive clinical outcome is likewise attested by evidence that early treatment wards off dangerous complications. Consequently, the use of stringent diagnostic guidelines and educational campaigns can exert a major influence on both prognosis in individuals and overall public health. Second, early intervention not only cures acute health problems but also encourages better long-term outcomes in children with rheumatologic conditions. As noted by current research, the long-term effects of not treating JIA can seriously impact mental, social, and physical well-being (Deborah et al., 2024).

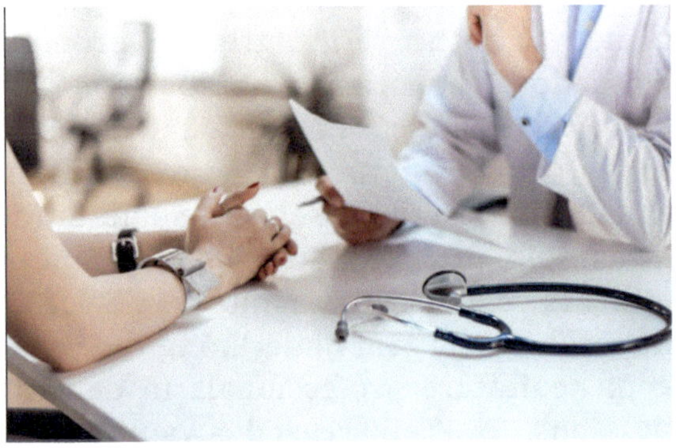

Figure 1.3. Physician discussing medical results with a patient, highlighting the importance of communication in healthcare.

Source: https://cdn.prod.website-files.com/62c99da818 58a07cad2e713c/668d35dc1177f368503a342d_AD_4nXfOKukrBFOVWUe9WNP5q- lPbOpk1bf9dlnTChQ7_kOIPDznSJ9YQDiSXI9zcYKw28fzMRchwAmvpJciP8F83G_yTxAeZA16qOYdpJMb0n5J9crsjdczaVZv_fEdbljx06Fx9Zkl0e_Hgqp4hFxWhxxK0TPu.png.

Parents of children with these conditions are stressed and anxious in managing advanced healthcare systems, thus emphasizing the need for intervention at an early stage in limiting psychological and social effects. Multimodal models that engage patients, families, and clinicians are essential in constructing a comprehensive image of the multifaceted impact of these diseases. Initiatives like the PAVE project engage in co-constructing patient-centered models that target these issues and prioritize appropriate resource allocation. Ultimatelhancing early diagnosis and treatment models is most critical to enable that children can succeed despite their diagnoses, and equipping them with an integrated approach to pediatric rheumatology (Figure 1.3).

1.1.1 Overview of Common Pediatric Rheumatic Diseases

In pediatric rheumatology, juvenile idiopathic arthriis (JIA) is the most prevalent disease affecting children belonging to all socio-economic group. JIA is a group of inflammatory disorders charad by chronic inflammation of joints, which can result in permanent sequelae such as, such as growth retardation and functional impairment. The subtypes of JIA, including systemic onset JIA (SOJIA) and polyarticular JIA, have different clinical presentations and prognoses. It has been observed that SOJIA appears at a younger age and is associated with systemic manifestations, making the diagnostic process more complex and resulting in the delay of starting treatment. Polyarticular JIA, on the other hand, appears later and is associated with a greater number of joints, which frequently leads to more severe limitations in growth and development than in healthy controls, highlighting the need for early and qualified medical treatment for such patients. Another serious pediatric rheumatic disorder is systemic lupus erythematosus (SLE), which, even though less common than JIA, poses considerable management difficulties due to its multisystem involvement and potential for severe complications. SLE affects a variety of organs, including the skin, kidneys, and central nervous system and produces an extensive array of clinical manifestations. Children with SLE are likely to have a more prolonged disease course before diagnosis compared to JIA patients and might also be at higher risk of increased morbidity, along with psychosocial difficulties, including growth restriction and delayed puberty. The multifaceted nature of SLE demands an overall approach towards treatment that not only addresses the physical symptoms but also provides vital support for the emotional well-being of the patients (Konte et al., 2024). The efficacy and safety of treatment mes are also a matter of utmost concern when treating pediatric rheumatic diseases such as, such as JIA and SLE. Another interleukin-1β inhibitor, canakinumab, has also gained prominence due to its long-term safety profile in children. In a nine-year retrospective observational study, canakinumab's need for continuous monitoring of adverse effects in patients was introduced, showing that the rate of severe side effects was not appreciably higher with cumulative dosing. These findings underscore the importance of taking the utmost care in juggling the benefits and potential risks associated with pediatric rheumatological illnesses, so that therapeutic interventions do not compromise the general well-being and growth of affected young people (Konte et al., 2024). With thoroughly informed treatment strategies, healthcare providers are better positioned to offset the impact of such diseases and achieve positive health outcomes.

1.1. Common Pediatric Rheumatic Diseases

Learning Outcome

1. Juvenile Idiopathic Arthritis (JIA)
2. Systemic Lupus Erythematosus (SLE)
3. Juvenile Dermatomyositis (JDM)

Among pediatric rheumatology, juvenile idiopathic arthritis (JIA) is the most common rheumatic condition among children worldwide. JIA is a heterogeneous group of inflammatory forms of arthritis, leading to swelling and pain of the joints that can severely damage growth and development. Among its various subtypes, SOJIA has been specifically linked with an early age of onset and severe systemic manifestations, which might complicate diagnosis and treatment. Interestingly, research has highlighted that JIA-diagnosed children usually have lower height and weight compared to their age-matched peers, reporting the need for early treatment to improve growth parameters and quality of life in JIA-affected children. Therefore, understanding JIA is also important for pediatric rheumatologists since it constitutes a large percentage of their practice. Systemic lupus erythematosus (SLE) is another prevalent condition in pediatric rheumatology that emphasizes the subtleties of managing chronic inflammatory disorders in children. While historically SLE has been thought to be an autoimmune disease that overwhelmingly affects females, pediatric SLE presents unique challenges, including a longer duration of illness before diagnosis. Children with SLE have been demonstrated to experience a considerable delay in being appropriately diagnosed and treated, often resulting in more severe disease at presentation for treatment (Konte et al., 2024). As complex as the condition is, SLE requires an expert response that attends not just to the medical care of inflammation but also to psychosocial repercussions that may impact long-term outcomes in affected children. Amidst the spectrum of pediatric rheumatologic disorders, it is impto identify the potential side effects of therapeutic modalities, most notably biologic drugs such as, such as canaThis interleukin-1β inhibitor has successfully been employed to manage inflammatory diseases, such as, such as JIA and periodic fever syndromes, but with risks of its own. One such study documented multiple side effects in the patients over the years and indicated that respiratory infections were among the most common complications observed (Konte et al., 2024). The findings further illustrated that even though there were severe adverse events noted, no increased side effect with increased doses of the drug was seen, revealing that, with careful monitoring, canakinumab could be safely administered to decrease the burden of these chronic illnesses. These results are significant in guiding clinical practice in pediatric rheumatology and establishing that the risk is outweighed by the benefits of therapy in children (Figure 1.4).

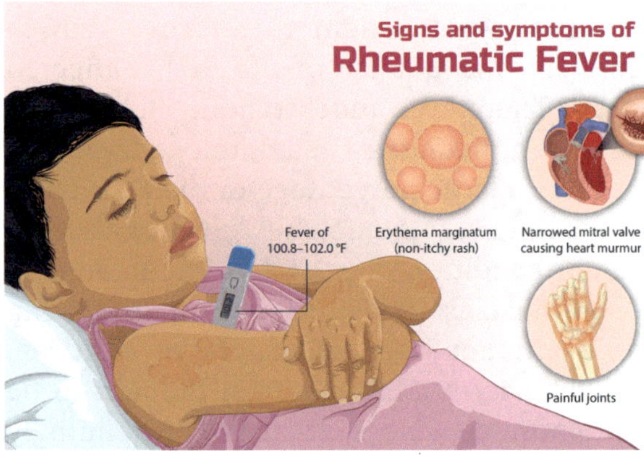

Figure 1.4. Common pediatric rheumatic diseases.

Source: https://www.physio-pedia.com/images/thumb/e/e5/Rheumatic_Fever.png/300px-Rheumatic_Fever.png.. ***Juvenile Idiopathic Arthritis (JIA)***

JIA is the most prevalent rheumatologic disorder in childrenthat is, characterized by frequent joint inflammation, having continuous effects on physical, social, and emotional growth. The condition occurs in various forms, and one of the most common subtypes is polyarticular JIA, which in most situations necessitates unique treatment modalities due to the individual demands of children. Traditionally, treatment recommendations for JIA have been largely based on research involving non-African patients, but recent efforts have begun to try making region-specific recommendations that consider the myriad difficulties of the environments in African healthcare settings. Current recommendations mention the importance of one that utilizes treatment to target and tries to achieve functionally meaningful results for patients while considering the resource limitations of these settings (Abu-Zaid et al., 2025). In addition, sJIA also poses special diagnostic and management difficulties, warranting regular professional education of physicians. In a Chinese national survey, many doctors reported encountering suspected sJIA cases, describing the prevalence and resultant diagnostic challenge. While most doctors utilize consensus guidelines that have been agreed on for diagnosis, the variable adherence to diagnostic criteria indicates the need for superior educational materials and training. Incorporation of more extensive education programs can also enhance physicians' diagnostic abilities, leading to improved, timely management of patients and potentially better outcomes for participating children. The survey also indicated the pressing issue of cost of treatment, discovering that while treatments like glucocorticoids and IL-6 receptor monoclonal antibodies are promising, lack of availability is a major disincentive to best treatment (Tan et al., 2024). The inclusion of evidence-based clinical practice guidelines is crucial to ensure optimal management in children with JIA. New developments in the pathophysiology of JIAs underscore the need for individual patient factors in the customization of the treatment regimens. Physicians are being increasingly encouraged to embrace collaborative decision-making with the family in order to ensure improved adherence to treatment and shared understanding of the disease process. This combination of scientific advances and patient-centered care can potentially significantly reduce disease activity and improve quality of life in children with JIA. In pursuing these objectives, there is a requirement for continued research and clinical practice to remain in concert with the evolving nature of JIA management to ensure that all professionals concerned with the management of children with JIA are skilled with the most up-to-date knowledge and techniques to address this complex condition.

1.1.2. Systemic Lupus Erythematosus (SLE)

The atypical presentation of systemic lupus erythematosus (SLE) poses significant challenges in pediatric rheumatology. Its variable clinical course and diverse manifestations complicate diagnosis and management. Compared to adults, children with SLE often exhibit distinct clinical features and a more severe disease course. Early diagnosis is essential to initiate appropriatey and prevent permanent organ damage. Furthermore, psychosocial effects of a chronic illness like SLE can spread exacerbate the already compounding symptoms of children, leading to higher rates of depression and anxiety. Determination of these issues of mental health is crucial, as they can have significant effects on treatment adherence and quality of life, calling for an integrative care approach that addresses physical and psychological aspects of disease (Gerdes et al., 2014). Both depression and anxiety have been identified to be prevalent among adolescent patients diagnosed with SLE, emphasizing the greatest importance of multidisciplinary treatment strategies. In a comparison study, SLE patients were revealed to have a substantially increased percentage of symptoms of depression when compared to normal subjects, with a remarkable proportion also having proof of suicidal ideation (Gerdes et al., 2014). This underscores the necessity of having healthcare professionals actively screen for mental health symptoms in routine visits. Of particular alarm is the fact that within those with such a high prevalence of such symptoms, a high percentage had not previously received mental health care. Care practice would involve routine screening for mental health and referral when appropriate to facilitate improved health outcomes, keeping in mind the interdependence of physical and psychological health in populations of children.

In addition to addressing the psychological health issue, the regulation of vitamin D status in child patients with SLE is also an issue of primary concern. Emerging evidence suggests that children withtoimmune conditions, including SLE, have an increased risk of vitamin D deficiency, which may have implications on for immune modulation and health. Given that the therapeutic value of vitamin D is to enhance the immune system, information on the status of vitamin D in these patients is becoming increasingly relevant. However, caution should be taken with supplementation, since additional studies must be performed to confirm that dosing regimens are effective and safe in this vulnerable group. Adding nutritional assessments and supplementation to the treatment protocols of pediatric SLE patients can offer additional spport in disease management and improving health outcomes, ultimately supporting the development of a whole-persons approach to pediatric rheumatology (Figure 1.5).

Systemic Lupus Erythematosus
(SLE)

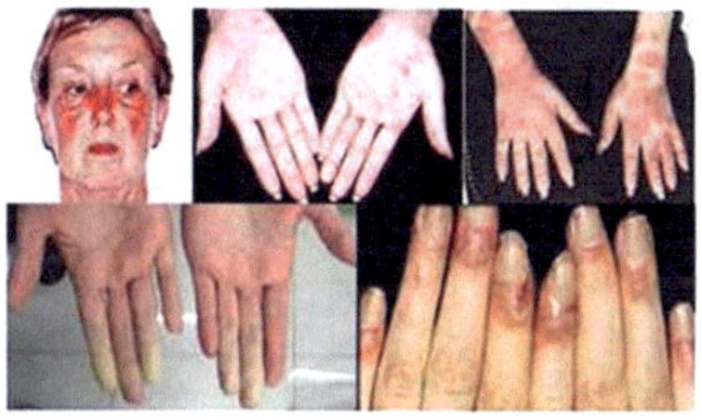

Figure 1.5. The multifaceted nature of systemic lupus erythematosus (SLE) presents significant challenges in pediatric rheumatology.

Source: https://drshrutibajad.com/images/services/Systemic-Lupus-Erythematosus.jpg.

1.1.3. Juvenile Dermatomyositis (JDM)

JDM is a complex and multidimensional condition within pediatric rheumatology with autoimmune inflammation affecting both the skin and proximal muscles. JDM is mostly found in children with specific cutaneous and muscular manifestations that can have the potential to highly affect on the quality of life in a child. The diagnosis of the diseases largely relies on clinical experience since evidence-based guidelines were not consistently applied in all regions, including Egypt. One of the recent endeavors by the Egyptian College of Pediatric Rheumatol was an attempt to create comprehensive clinical practice guidelines encompassing diagnostic and management strategies to for JDM based on the Delphi technique. It sought to emphasize the importance of standardization of treatment to enhance outcomes as well as the overall quality of life of the affected children (Miedany et al., 2022). The evolving pattern of JDM management both reflects progress in therapeutic options and perpetuates issues t cases. The traditional management methods involve corticosteroids and immunosuppressive agents, with the goal of managingto manage inflammation and reducing symptoms. Certain patients, however, end up with refractory disease, wquires new therapeutic interventions. Existing literature has also explored the efficacy of Janus kinase inhibitors such as, such as tofacitinib, which target novel pathways suspected to be implicated in JDM pathology. A pilot trial demonstrated favorable outcomes in three cases of steroid-refractory JDM because patients with tofacitinib improved dramatically in muscle strength, cutaneous lesions, and overall life quality with successful tapering of corticosteroids. This trend demands additional randomized controlled trials to further establish the magnitude and effectiveness of these treatments in pediatric patients (Yu et al., 2020). Finally, an understanding of the multifaceted relationship between clinical signs, diagnostic criteria, and therapeutic approaches is essential to optimize outcomes in JDM therapy. The clinical setting for JDM is characterized by varying levels of disease activity that may have a profound impact on patient prognosis and therapeutic response. Imperative suggestions from the consensus views highlight taking into account the status of disease activity and risk stratification of high-risk patients to make corresponding modifications in treatment strategies. Implementation of core sets for determining clinical improvement has also maximized follow-up for response to interventions. With advancing pediatric rheumatology, the syncretism of diversified treatment modalities combined with evidence-based recommendations will be pivotal in giving children with JDM high-quality and individualized treatment (Miedany et al., 2022).

Test Your Knowledge

1. What are the major clinical subtypes of Juvenile Idiopathic Arthritis (JIA), and how do they differ in presentation?
2. Which organ systems are most commonly affected in pediatric Systemic Lupus Erythematosus (SLE)?

1.2. Symptoms and Diagnosis

Learning Outcome

1. Common symptoms in pediatric patients
2. Diagnostic criteria and tools
3. Role of imaging and laboratory tests

Symptom recognition in pediatric rheumatology is significant, as it has the potential to affect disease diagnosis and treatment significan as, such as for juvenile idiopathic arthritis (JIA). Children's presentations can range from a wide range of nonspecific sympth as, such as pain, swelling, and stiffness in joints. These can extend beyond the musculoskeletal system in certain presentations to involve systemic sympth as, such as fever, rash, or lethargy. Early detection of these symptoms will lead to early referral to specialized services, and these are essential in enhancing patient outcomes. Literature has proven that children with an earlier diagnosis of JIA are more likely to exhibit special demographic featch as, such as younger age and being female, pointing towards the need for awareness of these symptoms by healthcare professionals to facilitate early diagnosis (Marino et al., 2024). Accurate diagnosis of pediatric rheumatological conditions is dependent upon clinical assessment and appropriate diagnostic tests. The classic physical examination, in the form of the pediatric gait, arms, legs, and spine (pGALS) examination, offers a formal method of assessing musculoskeletal function in children. One recent study used a video version of pGALS (v-pGALS) for precise remote assessment, with sensitivity and specificity of 92.6% and 100%, respectively, in diagnosing musculoskeletal abnormalities (Balik et al., 2024). These tools are very important in distinguishing JIA from other illnesses because incorrect diagnosis leads to inappropriate management and prolonged morbidity. Thus, extensive training in these evaluation tools is essential for pediatricians and allied health professionals who are also the first line of contact for such patients. Also hindering the path to a correct diagnosis in child rheumatology is diagnostic delay. In the majority of instances, children must wait for protracted durations before receiving a definitive diagnosis, primarily due to the nonspecific nature of their symptoms and the complexity of the rheumatological setting. Evidence has proven that patients with JIA waited considerably longer to see a pediatric rheumatologist following their initial healthcare contact, with waiting times playing a significant role in when diagnosis and, consequently, treatment were initiated (Marino et al., 2024). These delays are worse given the chronic progressive nature of JIA and the potential for permanent joint damage. Increased awareness and early clinical response to presenting symptoms are therefore essential in offering children timely diagnoses, reducing the duration of morbidity associated with untreated rheumatological disease (Figure 1.6).

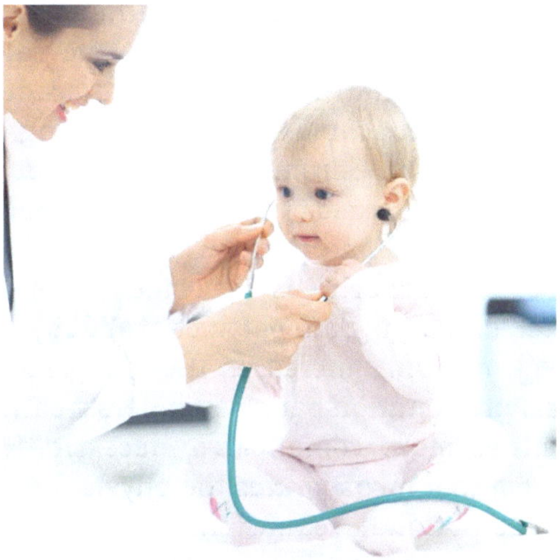

Figure 1.6. Pediatrician playfully engaging with a child during a check-up, emphasizing a gentle approach in pediatric care.

Source: https://gainesvillepediatricgi.com/wp-content/uploads/2024/07/Spotting_Pediatric_GERD_Symptoms_and_Diagnosis_in_Children.webp.

1.2.1. Common Symptoms in Pediatric Patients

In pediatric rheumatology, it is crucial to identify typical symptoms in children to make the correct diagnosis and treat them accordingly. One of the most frequently seen symptoms is diffuse musculoskeletal pain, which occconditions such as, such as juvenile primary fibromyalgia syndrome (JPFS). A study highlighted that up to 91% of their cohort patients had the symptom, along with excessive fatigue (84%) and disrupted sleep (82%) (Boneparth et al., 2019). These presentations not only disrupt daily life but also lead to substantial psychological distress, affecting the child's quality of life. Detection of these signs at an early stage allows timely intervention, which is very crucial in the prevention of long-term complications of musculoskeletal conditions in children. Fatigue, yet another prevailing characteristic of pediatric rheumatology, is most commonly found in connection with conditions such as, such as juvenile idiopathic arthritis (JIA). Here, it is possible that fatigue can be overwhelming and affects a child's academic performance at school, social functioning, and physical activity. Chronic pain syndromes like JPFS are characterized by the complex interaction between fatigue and pain, where moderate to severe pain severity is reported among the affected children (Boneparth et al., 2019). Such synergy not only increases the complexity of clinical presentation but also renders treatment modalities more complicated, necessitating a care plan that incorporates the physical as well as the emotional realms. An understanding of the implications of chronic fatigue is essential because it has direct consequences on compliance with treatment and overall patient well-being. Furthermore, comorbidity frequency in pediatric rheumatology prompts the need for an integrative model of symptom control. For instance, the connection between chronic uveitis and allergic disorders is found in juvenile idiopathic arthritis, which indicates that children's symptoms are correlated. Children with JIA and allergies are said to have much increased rates of chronic uveitis, hence making their clinical presentation more complex. This interrelation requires a multidisciplinary care strategy, with rheumatologists conferring with allergists and other experts to consider the entire range of the child's health. Identification of these symptoms early on can contribute to improved long-term management, making it crucial for a detailed and anticipatory management plan to be employed in pediatric rheumatology.

1.2.2. Diagnostic Criteria and Tools

Pediatric Rheumatology diagnostic criteria and instrumentation are of the highest significance due to the varied physiological and developmental stages of children compared to adults. This necessitates personalized criteria and diagnostic procedures that adequately address the unique onset of rheumatic diseases among children. In the past, numerous criteria have been based on adult definitions, and this has made it difficult to properly diagnose conditions like juvenile idiopathic arthritis and systemic lupus erythematosus in children. Misapplication of improper diagnostic standards can lead to underdiagnosis or misdiagnosis of these conditions, making care and management cumbersome. Therefore, a constant redefinition and calibratievices in accordance withfollowing age, gender, and effect of puberty are needed to improve clinical outcome in children with rheumatic diseases, as has been the case in the case of pediatric metabolic syndrome (Soliman et al., 2025). Technologies have encouraged the development of new diagnostic devices in pediatric rheumatology. Artificial intelligence-based machine learning models are beginning to be helpful tools in this field. They help in the identification of the most significant biomarkers and improve patient stratification based on disease course and presentation. They also improve diagnostic accuracy through the application of artificial intelligence-based imaging and noninvasive diagnostic modalities. By studying big data, such technologies can identify patterns that may never be seen in run-of-the-mill clinical assessments, and this leads to more precise diagnoses and tailored treatment approaches for children. The importance of relying on such advanced techniques ct be overstated, given how their capacity to revolutionize diagnostic practices by providing timely and sufficient interventions for rheumatic diseases (Bella et al., 2025). Yet, new diagnostic criteria and instruments entering clinical practice should be adopted cautiously. Ethical considerations and the requirement for complete validation remain of utmost importance. With increasing involvement of artificial intelligence and machine learning in diagnosing rheumatic conditions in children, it is important that their judgments are always challenged by physicians for their validity. It is this vigilant oversight that ensures context-dependent interpretation of data generated by theshisticated instruments to beis both true and useful in the case of individual patients. Ultimately, while diagnostic criteria and approaches in pediatric rheumatology developed are incredibly promising, it is crucial that these advances are utilized prudently, reinforcing diagnostic certainty without jeopardizing misuse and interpretational errors (Bella et al., 2025) (Figure 1.7).

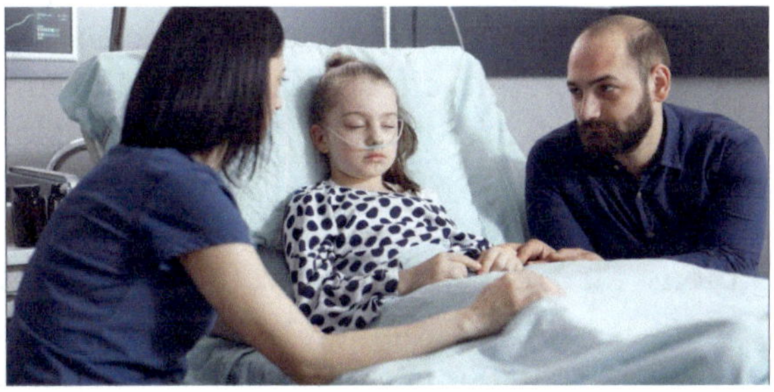

Figure 1.7. The diagnostic criteria and tools in pediatric rheumatology.

Source: https://news.cuanschutz.edu/hubfs/09.25.2024_QuickHit_SepsisCriteria.jpg.

1.2.3. Role of Imaging and Laboratory Tests

In children with rheumatology, laboratory and imaging studies play a central role in proper diagnosis and effective management of the majority of rheumatological conditions. Imaging modalities like magnetic resonance imaging (MRI) and ultrasound have become more crucial because they allow for the evaluation of joint inflammation and soft tissue damage without subjecting children to ionizing radiation. Use of musculoskeletal ultrasound is particularly helpful as it facilitates real-time assessment of inflammatory changes in the joints, tendons, and surrounding structures. This is particularly relevant in juvenile idiopathic arthritis and spondyloarthropathies, where early diagnosis of inflammation is necessary in order to achieve the maximum benefit with treatment. Moreover, imaging use assists in the assessment of the course of the disease, which is key in individualizing therapeutic strategies according to pediatric patients' evolving needs. Laboratory investigations complement imaging modalities by providing valuable information on the fundamental immunological mechanisms of rheumatic diseases. Laboratory investigations typically measure inflammatory markers, i.e., erythrocyte sedimentation rate (ESR) and C-reactive protein (CRP), that indicate the presence and magnitude of inflammation. These measures in children may not always coincide with clinical presentation or extent of disease and thus are not useful in diagnosis. Hence, while these tests can be useful in deriving a broader view of the activity of the disease, their limitations need to be approached with caution for interpretation. Furthermore, some se tests for autoantibodies, such as, such as antinuclear antibodies (ANA) and rheumatoid factor (RF), are invaluable in estab a diagnosis of conditions such as, such as systemic lupus erythematosus and juvenile idiopathic arthritis. While such laboratory exams can be extremely valuable, they must also be integrated with clinical findings and imaging reports to yield a whole picture. Lastly, the interplay between imaging and lab studies illustrates the complexity of diagnosing and treating pediatric rheumatological diseases. Thus, for instance, a systematic approach with these diagnostic tests combined can help in early identification of joint and systemic involvement, which is crucial in such cases as juvenile spondyloarthropathies, where clinical presentation can be multifaceted, from arthritis to extra-articular disease. Continuing technological developments in imaging technology, combined with improved awareness about laboratory markers, can enhance diagnostic sensitivity as well as monitoring with therapy. Furthermore, the use of standardized imaging and laboratory assessment protocols can allow for timely intervention and improve patient care. As pediatric rheumatology expands, clinicians need to remain vigilant about the role these instruments have in maximizing treatment options and improving quality of life in children with rheumatic disease.

Test Your Knowledge

1. What are the most common symptoms seen in pediatric patients with rheumatic diseases?
2. How do imaging studies and laboratory tests assist in the diagnosis and monitoring of pediatric rheumatic diseases?

1.3. Treatment Approaches

Learning Outcome

1. Pharmacological treatments
2. Non-pharmacological interventions
3. Importance of multidisciplinary care

Effective management in pediatric rheumatology relies on a thorough understanding of the unique clinical features of juvenile primary fibromyalgia syndrome (JPFS) and related rheumatologic disorders. Diagnosis and care of JPFS are primarily within the scope of pediatric rheumatologists, as evidenced by multi-site registries detailing the symptomatic and demographic profiles of affected children. Most patients were female, White/Caucasian, with a mean age of approximately 15.4 years, presenting with diffuse musculoskeletal pain, fatigue, and insomnia. Treatment is typically multidisciplinary, targeting both physical symptoms and overall functioning to improve quality of life. However, follow-up studies indicate persistent impairments and limited improvement in most patients, highlighting the need for continuous monitoring and adaptive therapeutic strategies (Boneparth et al., 2019). Addressing the complexities of pediatric rheumatology, particularly inflammatory conditions such as juvenile idiopathic arthritis (JIA), requires a spectrum of therapeutic approaches. Pharmacologic management often includes traditional disease-modifying antirheumatic drugs (DMARDs) and biologics, with biologics providing more targeted therapy and fewer systemic effects. Clinical guidelines emphasize patient education, shared decision-making, and adherence to ensure that treatment aligns with each child's individual needs. Effective regimens also necessitate careful monitoring for disease progression and adverse effects, underscoring a dynamic, patient-centered model of care (Dick et al., 2018). The psychosocial dimension of pediatric rheumatology is equally critical. Children with chronic pain frequently face emotional and psychological challenges that complicate clinical management. Integrative care involving psychologists, physical therapists, and occupational therapists addresses both symptom relief through rehabilitation and mental health support, fostering coping skills and overall well-being. Evidence suggests that holistic treatment plans incorporating psychological interventions substantially enhance quality of life. Given the persistent symptoms observed in JPFS, treatment providers must identify and address these nuances to optimize outcomes (Boneparth et al., 2019) (Figure 1.8).

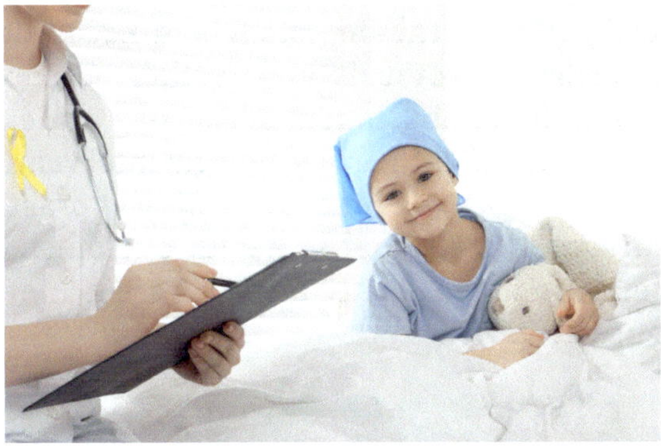

Figure 1.8. The treatment approaches in pediatric rheumatology.

Source: https://healthyturkiye.com/storage/media/4299/pediatric-oncology-treatment-option.jpg.

1.3.1. Pharmacological Treatments

The management of juvenile rheumatology has progressively relied on drug therapy to manage symptoms and improve the quality of life in children afflicted with these conditions. Nonsteroidal anti-inflammatory drugs (NSAIDs), corticosteroids, and disease-modifying antirheumatic drugs (DMARDs) are the keystone of such therapies. NSAIDs are generally the first-line treatment of choice due to their potential in managing inflammation and pain. Nonetheless, despite these drugs being largely prescribed, recent systematic reviews reveal a disconcerting deficit of evidence for their long-term efficacy and safety in the pediatric population. More specifically, trials of NSAIDs have not been shown to be superior to other treatments, leaving the adoption of a very skeptical stance toward their use in treating chronic musculoskeletal pain in children (Caes et al., 2018). Apart from NSAIDs, the advent of biologic agents has transformed therapeutic modalities in children with rheumatology. Biologics, which target specific pathways of immune response, provide other options for children who are unresponsive to standard therapies. Present guidelines highlight using these agents effectively while considering patient-specific factors and the specific rheumatologic condition being treated. Growing emphasis on individualized medicine in this field underlines the need for clinicians to closely monitor for potential side effects and treatment strategies as and when appropriate for an individual patient. Yet, the optimal timing at which biologic therapy is introduced remains the subject of ongoing research, emphasizing the need for robust evidence iion-making within pediatric settings (AcharyaDick et al., 2018). With clinical practice evolving towards interdisciplinary care, the synergy of pharmacological and non-pharmacological treatments becomes essential in the management of children with severe rheumatological disease. This demands an integrated approach where pharmacotherapy is supplemented by psychological and physical therapies. While relief of symptoms continues to be the focus of pharmacological therapy, additive therapies can help count the pervasiveness of long-term disease upon in a child's life. A recent publication has suggested that highly intensive interdisciplinary treatment programs, although not available universally, have potential for enhancing outcomes in younger patients. Without an evidence base to firmly determine the pharmacological interventions employed, continuous assessment and reassessment of treatment protocols will be crucial to addressing the diverse needs of children with rheumatologic diseases (Caes et al., 2018).

1.3.2. Non-Pharmacological Interventions

Non-pharmacologic treatments have become an integral component of pediatric rheumatology, particularly in managing juvenile arthritis and related conditions. These approaches help reduce the psychosocial burden of chronic disease and enhance children's overall sense of well-being. Physical therapy, cognitive-behavioral therapy (CBT), and mindfulness training have been reported to be promising in pain attenuation, enhancing function, and improving quality of life. By addressing both the physical and emotional components of patient experience, such therapies are of unique importance, often resulting in better compliance with drug treatment regimens. The incorporation of these approaches emphasizes the requirement for holistic models of care that include multidisciplinary teams to enable practitioners to tailor interventions to the individual needs of pediatric patients with rheumatic diseases. In addition to standard therapeutic procedures, studies suggest that non-pharmacologic treatment may involve the management of stress and anxiety, which are generally present in children with rheumatic diseases. Pain control procedures through music and relaxation techniques, for instance, have been linked to positive outcomes among child populations. Studies on dental anxiety show that music is an effective intervention in alleviating discomfort during procedures, making it usable beyond the traditional healtetting (Kong et al., 2024). Interventions such as, such as patient and family education can equip them with coping mechanisms, thus building up their resilience when managing chronic conditions. Through the integration of these varied non-pharmacological interventions, practitioners are able to develop an accommodating setting that maximizes the total treatment satisfaction of children. As encouraging as the potential of non-pharmacological interventions may seem, further investigation is necessary to establish their full capacity in the fediatric rheumatology. Existing research, such as, such as systematic reviews, emphasizes the necessity of thorough assessments of these treatments in order to identify ideal results. For instance, a systematic review of non-pharmacological treatments for pediatric delirium highlights the importance of educational and multimodal interventions in patient outcomes (Kim et al., 2024). These findings raise pertinent questions about the feasibility and applicability of such interventions across pediatric rheumatology and necessitate standardized protocols and further research. Through the establishment of a strong evidence base, optimal non-pharmacological intervention use can be achieved, improved clinical practice ensues, and finally, better health outcomes for children with rheumatic diseases are achieved (Figure 1.9).

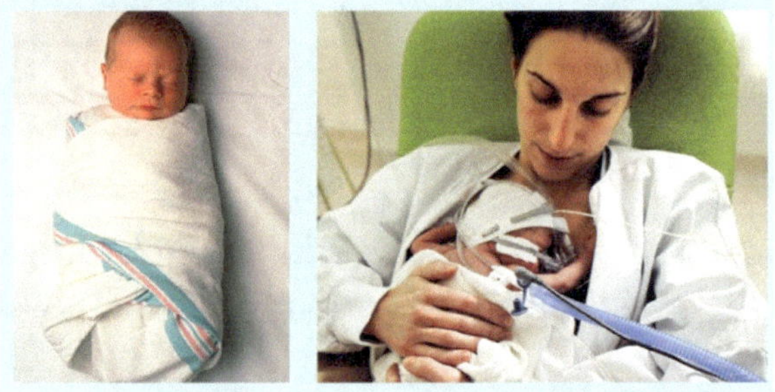

Figure 1.9. Non-pharmacological interventions.

Source: https://cdn.ps.emap.com/wp-content/uploads/sites/3/2017/05/fig-1_660.jpg.

1.3.3. Importance of Multidisciplinary Care

The pediatric rheumatology demands a multidisciplinary care model, which assumes a pivotal position in overseeing the various needs of the children. It is a system that combines specialists across various fields like rheumatology, psychology, physical therapy, and nutrition to enable comprehensive disease management of conditions like juvenile idiopathic arthritis (JIA). Such combined care not only enhances clinical outcomes but also improves the overall patient experience by minimizing communication fragmentation among providers. Effective collaboration among health providers facilitates evidence-based treatment plans that address the physical, emotional, and social dimensions of health and ultimately facilitate better long-term management of chronic diseases (Bagnall et al., 2013). Thus, the multidisciplinary team role is paramount in the management of pediatric rheumatologic disease of augmented sophistication, where heterogeneous skills can congregate to best optimize patient results. Furthermore, parents of patients with rheumatic illnesses show overwhelming preferences for multidisciplinae, and underscore its perceived value in treatment resultoutcomes. Assessments note that parents put significant value on improving their kids' ability to perform daily activities and manage pain ahead of other aspects of services, inferring that structured care significantly influences perceived health outcomes (Bernatsky et al., 2014). Notably, using more than on specialist ensures that multiple treatment components, —e.g., drug treatment, pain management modalities, and psychosocial support—are considered simultaneously. Such wholeness is not only crucial for the improvement of physical well-being but also for alleviating the emotional burden imposed by chronic illness on patients and families. The emphasis on all-around care derives from the realization that optimal pediatric rheumatologic care extends beyond strictly therapeutic interventions. In addition, multidisciplinary advice builds an enabling environment for both patients and families, working to increase treatment adherence and satisfaction. Through combining the expertise of different professionals, such teams can provide educational tools, emotional support, and seamless care transitions, thereby reducing obstacles to effective management. For instance, adolescent chronic condition transition programs show that effective multidisciplinary organization is linked to less disrupted transitions from pediatric to adult care (Bagnall et al., 2013). This consistent involvement is particularly beneficial within the field of pediatric rheumatology, where an ultimate lifelong management plan necessitates a multi-disciplinary strategy. By assigning priority to feedback from the various specialties, health systems can enable families to gain access to full-care care specifically tailored to their individual experiences, ultimately maximizing the outcomes for children affected by rheumatic disorders (Figure 1.10).

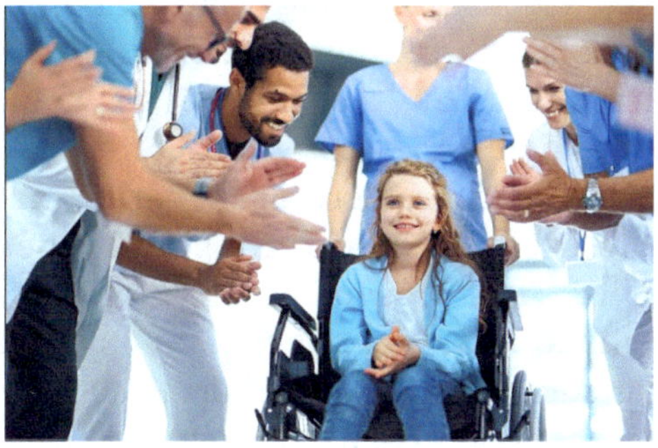

Figure 1.10. The complexities associated with pediatric rheumatology necessitate a multidisciplinary approach to care.

Source: https://static.wixstatic.com/media/58e90e_13a72d837e2740b8b264904214356a76~mv2.jpg/v1/fill/w_724,h_482,al_c,q_80,usm_0.66_1.00_0.01,enc_avif,quality_auto/58e90e_13a72d837e2740b8b264904214356a76~mv2.jpg.

Test Your Knowledge

1. What are the main pharmacological treatments used to manage pediatric rheumatic diseases?
2. How do non-pharmacological interventions, such as physical therapy and lifestyle modifications, support treatment?
3. Why is a multidisciplinary care approach important in managing children with rheumatic diseases?

1.4. Challenges in Pediatric Rheumatology

Learning Outcome

1. Variability in disease presentation
2. Psychological impact on children and families
3. Access to specialized care and resources

Pediatric rheumatology is a range of multifactorial illnesses with the potential to greatly affect children and their way of life. Insufficiency of specialized practitioners is among the key obstacles in pediatric rheumatology, particularly in regions with limited medical resources. It is revealed through research that there are insufficient trained rheumatologists to address the conditions of children with rheumatologic disease, which is limiting timely and proper diagnosis and treatment. This shortage is supplemented by the nature of pediatric rheumatologic illnesses, which often present somewhat uncharacteristically and thus are difficult even for seasoned practitioners to recognize. The upshot is that reliance on generalists and non-specialists is great to address such cases. Use of intervenuch as, such as diagnostic decision support software can be used to bridge this gap, hence enhancing diagnostic accuracy in settings where there is limited specialized treatment, as seen through enhanced clinician performance with the use of such tthreyaSegal et al., 2016). The transition of care as children mature into adults is another significant challenge that pediatric rheumatology experiences. The transition is particularly complex for patients with chronic diseases, including rheumatic diseases. For instance, adolescents undergoing a transition from pediatric to adult care can experience disruptions that affect their disease self-mnagement, and, consequently, experience complications like deteriorating health outcomes. Evidence identifies that there is a requirement for joint collaborative efforts by pediatric and adult care professionals, as well as structured transitional programs, for improving this process. Developmentally appropriate education and training in self-management become important components for flawless transfers. Through consideration of these variables, healthcare systems are better able to provide care as patients enter into the new healthcare environments, ultimately improving their quality of life and global health outcomes (Bagnall et al., 2013). Lastly, the multifactorial etiology of rheumatologic diseases of children provides intriguing but complicated diagnostic and therapeutic problems. With so many overlapping findings and such a wide differential diagnosis, prompt recognition of individual conditions can often be postponed. Additionally, the heterogeneous manifestation of such diseases complicates the treatment regimens, with therapeutic outcomes varying widely between children.

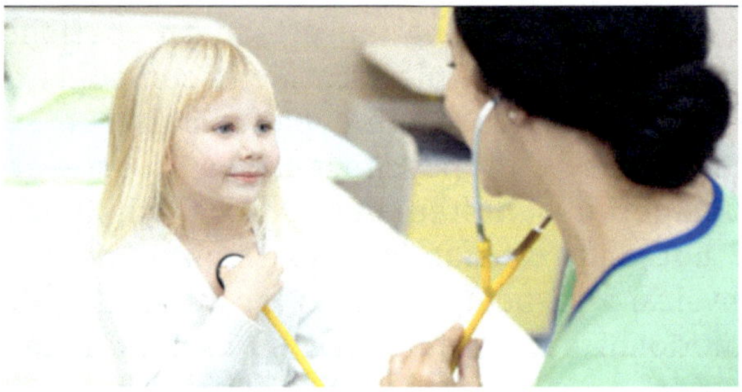

Figure 1.11. A healthcare professional engaging a child in a medical examination using a stethoscope, fostering comfort and trust during pediatric care.

Source: https://www.the-rheumatologist.org/wp-content/uploads/2017/07/NestorRizhniak_Shutterstock_GenericChild_500x270.jpg.

Not only is correct management a matter of proper diagnosis, but also an understanding of the psychosocial variables that affect the child and family. Heterogeneous variables of age, developmental stage, and support from family can lead to nonadherence and success of treatment. As pediatric rheumatology continues to evolve, resolution of these challenging issues through research, education, and utilization of innovative tools will be most essential in improving patient outcomes and managing disease (Figure 1.11).

1.4.1. Variability in Disease Presentation

Variability in disease presentation is one of the main pediatric rheumatology problems that affect diagnosis, treatment, and management of patients. For example, presentation in juvenile primary fibromyalgia syndrome (JPFS) can be fairly variable among the children involved, potentially leading to varying symptom patterns. Presentation could involve diffuse musculoskeletal pain, fatigue, sleep disturbance, and headache. Interestingly, demographic factors play a role in this heterogeneity, as the majority of patients are Caucasian/White, non-Hispanic, and female, which suggests that gender and ethnicity may influence the severity and presentation of symptoms among this population (Boneparth e, 2019). Not just only does the heterogeneity complicate diagnosis, but also calls for customized treatment regimens with consideration of patient-specific variables, further substantiating the role of a personal medical model in the treatment of pediatric rheumatology. Moreover, the heterogeneity also includes the outcomes of ongoing treatments, which can differ substantially between patients diagnosed with the same conditions. In autoinflammatory syndromes (AIDs), the expression can be severe or mild, and that is why close monitoring and adaptive management are required. Treatment can involve the administration of biologics, as for example anakinra, to relieve symptoms. However, response to medication is potentially very inconsistent in some cases, leading to periodic surprise in the challenges faced with resolving symptoms. Such inconsistency emphasizes continuous clinical monitoring and adjustment of treatment protocols to adequately address the variable presentations of AIDs. Through all attempts by pediatric rheumatologists to optimize care, appreciation of this inconsistency is crucial to ensure optimization of therapeutic response and quality of life in patients (Corsello et al., 2017). Also, an understanding of etiologies of variability in disease presentation is a gateway to more efficient intervention strategies for pediatric rheumatology. Environmental exposures, genetics, and psychosocial determinants are a few among the determinants that can be influential in determining how diseases are presented in children. For instance, men in JPFS have been found to endorse greater impairment in functioning compared to women, suggesting that gender also contributes to disease experience and treatment response (Boneparth et al., 2019). Identification of these differences not only permits individualized care but can also direct future research studies to the mechanisms behind these diseases. By focusing on variability, pediatric rheumatologists can work to develop more universal yet flexible treatment plans that address the unique requirements of the patient in order to achieve improved health outcomes.

1.4.2. Psychological Impact on Children and Families

The diagnosis of Juvenile Idiopathic Arthritis (JIA) often triggers sere psychological stresses in the affected children and their families. Cdren with JIA uso suffer not only suffer physical discomfort and pain caused by the condition but also high levels of depression and anxiety. The mental health challenges are further compounded by unpredictable episodes of the disease flares and the chronic constant nature of the treatment, which may entail multiple visits to the doctor and interventions. For the parents, the psychological cost can be equally debilitating; they can feel isolated, with a terrain of unpredictable hopes regarding their child's future. This can establish titanic psychological anguish, as parents continue to grapple with feelings of helplessness and unease regarding their own ability to help their child navigate such a challenging diagnosis. Thus, it is necessary to grasp these intricate psychological impacts in providing comprehensive care to child patients with JIA and their families (Karina et al., 2024). Parental support plays a critical role in mitigating the psychological impact of juvenile idiopathic arthritis (JIA). Research shows that parents' knowledge and attitudes significantly influence the long-term well-being of children with chronic disease. As primary caregivers navigating complex medical systems, parents often experience stress, frustration, and financial challenges. These difficulties are amplified in resource-limited settings, which can compromise their ability to provide optimal support (Silim et al., 2023). Parents, too, experience social outcomes, including strained family relationships and diminished quality of life, creating a cycle of stress for both child and caregiver. As caregivers attend to their own mental health, they become more capable of promoting resilience in children, thereby enhancing family functioning and coping capacity. Interventions that address the psychological needs of children and their families are essential in pediatric rheumatology. Interventions like the Juvenile Arthritis Support Program (JASP-1) have proven to be effective in enhancing the mental health and quality of life of the participants. Organized support through education, community, and psychological resources facilitates these programs to provide enhanced understanding of the disease, along with pathways for emotional support. The rising satisfaction recorded among JASP-1 participating families echoes a seeming correlation between structured support and improved mental health outcomes, observing the necessity of such integrative modalities in child treatment (Karina et al., 20there is recognition growinggrowing recognition that qualitative research centering on the experiences of parents will continue to elucidate the stressors families endure, adding depth to the discourse of holistic care approaches and ensuring the psychological well-being of patients as well as their families takes center stage within pediatric rheumatology clinics (Silim et al., 2023) (Figure 1.12).

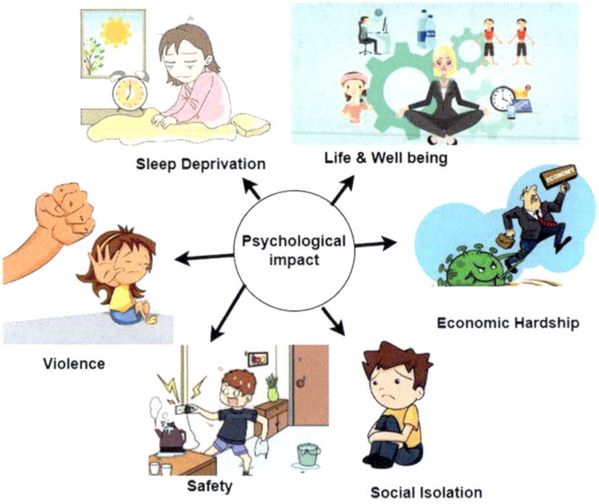

Figure 1.12. Psychological impact on children and families.

Source: https://media.springernature.com/lw1200/springer-static/image/art%3A10.1186%2Fs43045-022-00256-3/MediaObjects/43045_2022_256_Fig4_HTML.png.

1.4.3. Access to Specialized Care and Resources

Availability of specialized resources and care is a major issue in pediatric rheumatology, with far-reaching effects on patient outcome and quality of life for children with rheumatic diseases. Pediatric rheumatology subspecialists are seriously underrepresented, and many families have to travel quite considerable distances to reach specialist clinics. Approximately 31.4% of children are more than 40 miles from the closest pediatric rheumatologist, demonstrating substantial geographic disparity in access to care (Lakshminrusimha et al., 2023). This limitation is further worsened by the limited growth in pediatric subspecialty fellows over the last couple of years, particularly in outpatient-centered subspecialties, which makes it even more difficult for families to obtain required evaluations and treatments. Delayed diagnosis leads to worse health outcomes and increased long-term health costs, which underscore the value of expanded access to specialty services. Furthermore, pediatric rheumatology high-level care often extends beyond straightforward clinical visits; it is access to multidisciplinary staff that can aid with complex eeds. Rheumatic diseases children can benefit from coordination among rheumatologists, physical therapists, and mental health specialists to maximize their treatment outcomes. The current pediatric healthcare system in place is usually not geared toward such integrated care models, limiting the efficiency with which families can make use of health services. Evidence has shown that in the long run, urban cities have witnessed a concentration of specialized care, with rural communities still being underserved, further perpetuating inequities of access to health (Lakshminrusimha et al., 2023). For the families seeking comprehensive care, such service disparities can result in frustration and adverse health outcomes, which highlights the need for reformed solutions towards augmenting access to pediatric rheumatology services. Moreover, financial factors associated with pediatric treatment additionally encumber families attempting to access specialty services. With lower pay rates for pediatric rheumatologists than their adult equivalents, recruitment of new specialists into pediatric rheumatology is challenging. This is yet another financial deterrent for potential candidates from applying for pediatric rheumatology fellowships and thereby sustaining the shortage of trained specialists. With the pediatric population of people living with chronic conditions on the rise, so is the demand for universal access to the necessary care and resources needed for proper control of the conditions. The policymakers and healthcare stakeholders should therefore prioritize investment in pediatric rheumatology through increased provision of services, coordination of care, and removal of economic barriers that limit access among disadvantaged communities.

Test Your Knowledge

1. How does variability in disease presentation affect the diagnosis and management of pediatric rheumatic diseases?
2. What psychological challenges do children with rheumatic diseases and their families commonly face?
3. What barriers exist in accessing specialized care and resources for pediatric rheumatology patients?

1.5. Research and Advances in Pediatric Rheumatology

Learning Outcome

1. Current research trends and findings
2. Emerging therapies and clinical trials
3. Future directions in pediatric rheumatology

Advances in pediatric rheumatology have vastly expanded the understanding and management of auto-immune and inflammatory diseases in children. Studies have increasingly focused on early diagnosis of these diseases, as conditions like juvenile idiopathic arthritis (JIA) significantly impair the physical and psychological development of a child in the long run. All these advances are predicated on cutting-edge biomarker studies that allow clinicians to identify at-risk populations and initiate treatment protocols before existing practice would permit. Not only do these early treatments improve outcomes, but they also have the potential to change disease trajectory. Further, the greater emphasis on multidisciplinary collaborative investigations has generated a more advanced understanding of the underlying mechanisms of pediatric rheumatologic illnesses, thereby enhancing prevention and treatment modalities. Telemedicine, as has been documented in current studies, has emerged as a valuable resource within pediatric rheumatology, especially in managing chronic disease necessitating ongoing care. With the ability to take consultations to distant areas, experts are able to communicate with patients and families in real time, hence providing a more supportive and responsive health setting. Since chronic illnesses among children continue to rise, using telemedicine can ensure timely interventions that reduce the level of hospitalization and face-to-face contacts, which are typically time-consuming for families. This new approach also prevents overwhelming healthcare systems as it maximizes care management and lowers costs associated with traditional face-to-face consultations. Lastly, telemedicine not only enhances access but also promotes patient-controlled care in pediatric rheumatology with the possibility of constant monitoring and communication with healthcare providers (Antodaro et al., 2023). As pediatric rheumatology expands, adapting digital innovation is becoming more and more core to the future of patient care. Steps are being made toward the development of comprehensive telemedicine systems that integrate healthcare providers, patients, and families inclusively. These frameworks are informed by consensus reports of leading scientific bodies, which encourage high-quality telehealth services towards enhancing the management of children with rheumatologic conditions. Including patient involvement from the design stage may assist telemedicine to be maximized in fulfilling the specific needs of pediatric rheumatology so that services are effective while at the same time convenient.

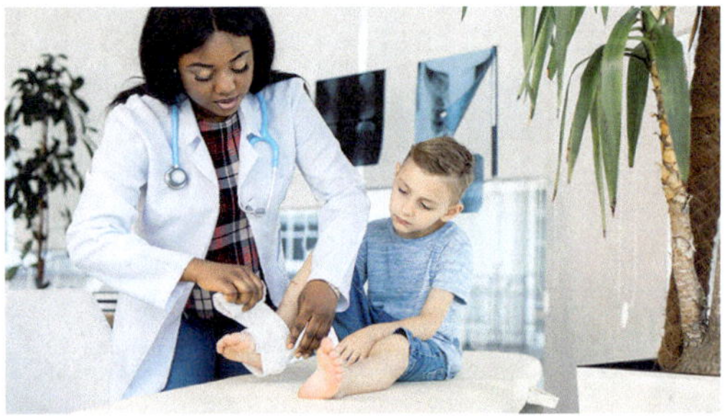

Figure 1.13. Research and advances in pediatric rheumatology.

Source: https://images.contentstack.io/v3/assets/bltee37abb6b278ab2c/bltefce32b75108c944/64b0303d82c5c67cc2c39eba/rheumatologist-pediatric-patient-ankle-wrap.jpg.

In addition, by dismantling geographic walls, such innovations can contribute to the facilitation of equitable access to high-level treatment for all children, regardless of location. The incorporation of digital solutions in this way thus constitutes a substantial advancement, as far as the broad goal of care enhancement in pediatric rheumatology is concerned (Antodaro et al., 2023) (Figure 1.13).

1.5.1. Current Research Trends and Findings

Pediatric rheumatology is also experiencing major developments, particularly insight into the molecular mechanisms of various autoimmune diseases in children. There have been recent studies reporting genetic and environmental determinants of these multifactorial diseases, with improved classificf diseases such as, such as JIA. Studies have proved that early diagnosis and treatment significantly alter the natural history of the disease, hence, timely active mant in children being is significant. In addition, advances ing modalities such as, such as ultrasound and MRI, allow for better observation of disease activity and response to treatment. The growing number of published papers indicates a rising interest in the subject area by researchers, as it leads to multidisciplinary collaborative research involving pediatric healthcare practitioners and rheumatology specialists, paving the way for more effective treatment plans and outcomes (Sk et al., 2024). The second prevailing trend in the research underway is an emphasis on interdisciplinary management of autoimmune diseases in children. One important advancement is the establishment of joint pediatric dermatology-rheumatology clinics that bring the two specialties together to address the intricacies of diseases like systemic lupus erythematosus and dermatomyositis. A recent survey at 13 North American sites reported notable benefits of torative model, such as, such as effective patient care and enhanced treatment plans considering both cutaneous and systemic features of disease (Cherepakhin et al., 2024). By capitalizing on the strengths of each discipline, healthcare teams are able to deliver holistic care that meets the diverse needs of complex rheumatic disease in young patients. Further research into the efficacy of these multidisciplinary clinics is needed to establish best practices that others can follow. Lastly, the incorporation of new treatments, including biologic agents and targeted therapies, is a significant pediatric rheumatology research trend. These novel therapies are aimed at the underlying pathophysiologic processes of the autoimmune diseases, providing new hope for improved management strategies. Active research is needed to ascertain the safety and efficacy of these therapies in the pediatric population, a group never represented in rheumatologic literature. The findings of such studies are valuable not only for the extension of treatment but also for informing practice guidelines to optimize patient outcomes. As research in the area continues to advance, personalized medicine will continue to take center stage, with the interventions tailored to each patient's profile on the basis of genetic and phenotypic parameters, with the aim of transforming the practice of pediatric rheumatology in the long term (Sk et al., 2024).

1.5.2. Emerging Therapies and Clinical Trials

The world of pediatric rheumatology is being transformed at its very foundations by innovative therapies and clinical trials aimed at optimizing patient outcomes. Traditional treatment has been founded on a restricted array of therapeutic modalities, which are not always suited to the unique needs of the pediatric patient. Innovations in the last few years, particularly with biologic agents and small molecules, are transforming therapeutic models. These novel therapies are designed to directly hit specific pathways involved in the inflammatory processes, a strategy that recent research has suggested by explaining the failure of present treatments to give lastission in diseases such as, such as ulcerative colitis. Awareness of these advances is necessary for pediatricians who practice because they are able to offer individualized and more effective treatment regimens that take into account the evolving etiology of disease in children. Moreover, clinical trials have now become a crucial component in the development of these novel therapies, including the exemplar according to which their safety and efficacy may be evaluated in different populations. These trials not only generate data but also offer insight into the pharmacodynamics of novel therapies, potentially to guide future use in pediatric rheumatology. Improvements in trial design have enabled recruitment of diverse groups, including those with uncommon rheumatologic conditions, enhancing generalizability.

The employment of artificial intelligence in such medical settings has also begun to help maximize trial protocols. As recent studies have shown, AI algorithms can be beneficial in stratifying patient groups and metreatment response, whether despite their current drawbacks in clinical significance and ethics as discussed in the present review of pediatric rheumatology literature (Koker et al., 2024). The exploration of novel administration routes and mechanisms of action is evident in the development of new therapeutic agents for chronic inflammatory diseases. Advances such as oral or subcutaneous delivery systems for tumor necrosis factor inhibitors represent significant progress, potentially improving patient compliance and treatment convenience. Additionally, emerging agents, including toll-like receptor agonists and certain phosphodiesterase inhibitors, offer promising new therapeutic options that could transform disease management. These developments highlight the importance of continued research and clinical trials in pediatric populations to expand treatment alternatives and improve outcomes in pediatric rheumatology (AlAmelel et al., 2023) (Figure 1.14).

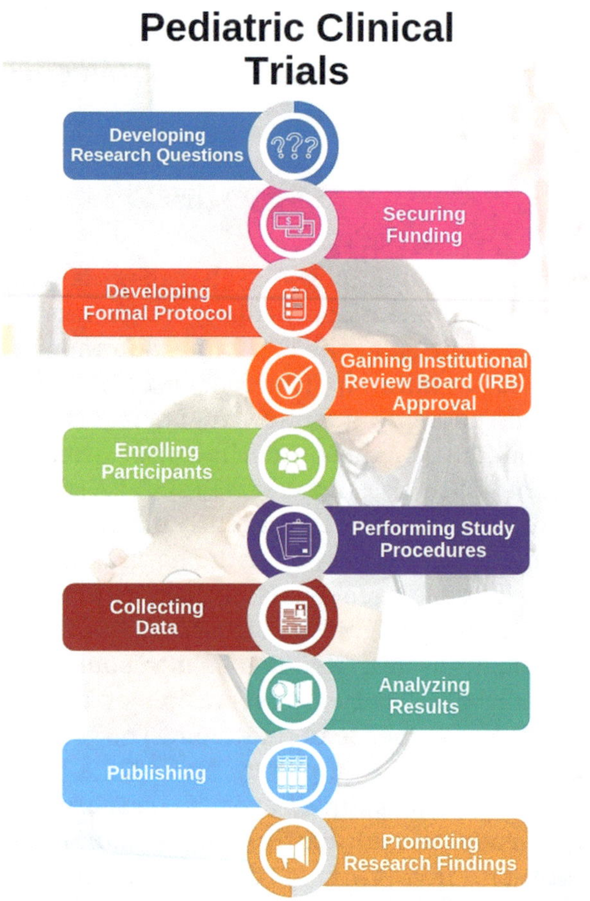

Figure 1.14. The landscape of pediatric rheumatology is undergoing significant transformation as a result of emerging therapies and clinical trials aimed at improving patient outcomes.

Source: https://pubrica.com/blog/wp-content/uploads/2019/09/Pediatric-clinical-trials.jpg.

1.5.3. Future Directions in Pediatric Rheumatology

The field of pediatric rheumatology is rapidly evolving with very rapid advances in the understanding of disease mechanisms and therapeutic technology. Emerging evidence oathophysiology of conditions such as, such as Behçet's disease directs us to the complex interplay between genetics and the environment, particularly its higher prevalence along the Silk Road countries. Understanding these factors is imperative for treatment strategy development for pediatric populations, given that children manifest different clinical symptoms and responses to therapy than adults. Thus, subsequent studies must focus on unraveling the pathophysiology of pediatric autoimmune illnesses and translating findings into useful clinical practices. This will yield a foundation for more successful individualized treatment regimens and ultimately improved patient outcomes and quality of life in children who are suffering from these challenging conditions (Lavalle et al., 2024). Another exciting area of pediatric rheumatology is the research into targeted therapies, particularly after the advent of biologic. The emergence of treatments such as, such as Bruton's tyrosine kinase (BTK) inhibitors signals the potential for targeted therapy in the treatment of autoimmune diseases. BTK inhibitors introduce a novel mechanism that may offer better efficacy and safety profiles over the currently available conventional immunosuppressive agents. Because the majority of children patients each have their own unique patterns of disease, the study must first focus on the use of these targeted therapies among the population. Moreover, the incorporation of biomarkers to predict response to these therapies may allow for personalized medicine approaches, allowing clinicians to identify which patients will benefit most from specific therapeutic approaches (Amneh et al., 2024). This shift towards precision treatment is an important benchmark in the advancement of pediatric rheumatology. The future of pediatric rheumatology will also be dependent on incorporating considerations of mental health into integrated care paradigms. Chronic rheumatologic disorders can also profoundly affect the psychological health of children, and consequently, could cause anxiety as well as depression. As more and more children receive attention for these mental illness issues, pediatric rheumatologists are faced with creating a holistic treatment philosophy that includes psychological support. This is to be achieved through teamwork with mental health specialists so that psychological care becomes part and parcel of the treatment process. Future studies need to investigate the optimal management of mental health disorders as well as physical health management in children with rheumatologic illness, ultimately culminating in global well-being for such patients. By taking a more integrated approach to care, pediatric rheumatology can maximize therapeutic results and well-being for these children and their families.

Test Your Knowledge

1. What are the current research trends and recent findings in pediatric rheumatology?
2. Which emerging therapies and clinical trials are showing promise in treating pediatric rheumatic diseases?
3. What are the key future directions and goals for advancing pediatric rheumatology care and research?

1.6. Case Studies and Clinical Examples

Learning Outcome

1. Case study of a child with JIA
2. Case study of a child with SLE
3. Lessons learnd from clinical experiences

In pediatrics rheumatology, case studies form the core of illustrating the diagnostic complexity and clinical presentation of various rheumatic diseases in children. For example, the use of diagnostic decision support software (DDSS) has exerted a significant impact on the accuracy of diagnoses offered by general practitioners. Research demonstrated that clinicians using DDSS registered a dramatic decrease in diagnostic mistakes from 28% to 15% following the integration of the tool into their practices. It is particularly noteworthy given the increasing prevalence of pediatric rheumatologic conditions and the limited specialists within the field. Thus, case studies reporting on the successful use of DDSS not only underscore its success but also illustrate the growing need for innovative approaches to bridging the expertise gap in pediatric rheumatology. These innovations have a significant potential to influence cliecision-making and patient outcomes (gal et al., 2016). Chronic diseases, such as, such as juvenile idiopathic arthritis (JIA), reflect the intricacy of pediatric rheumatologyries of JIA often reveal comorbidities, such as, such as chronic uveitis, that can have a major impact on the quality of a child's life. Research has revealed strong associations between allergic diseases and chronic uveitis in patients with JIA, rendering a complete assessment fundamental in treatment planning. By employing retrospective cohort studies, clinicians are able to track patterns and risk factors of these disabling disorders. The findings verify that clinical correlations enhance risk stratification, which allows the practitioner to anticipate and avoid the complications that are associated with JIA. The case histories not only enlighten the interconnectedness of rheumatic diseases in children but also stimulate a worldwide approach to diagnosis and treatment, hence improving pediatric rheumatology (Bauer-Mehren et al., 2013). Moreover, the use of clinical data warehouses to analyze pediatric rheumatic diseases yields rich data that enhances our understanding of these complex diseases. Through analysis of large datasets by means of validated analytical pipelines, researchers can determine salient associations and refine clinical practices. The case of discovering specific patient characteristics that correlate with chronic uveitis is a key illustration of the benefit of data-driven research at the clinic. These case studies are a valuable tool to clinicians, enabling the use of evidence-based practice tailored to individual patients' profiles. With continuing advancements in pediatric rheumatology, syntheses of technology and research evidence will be critical in improving diagnostic specificity and treatment efficacy lation carrying such disorders (Athreya et al., 2016; Bauer-Mehren et al., 2013; Segal et al., 2016) (Figure 1.15).

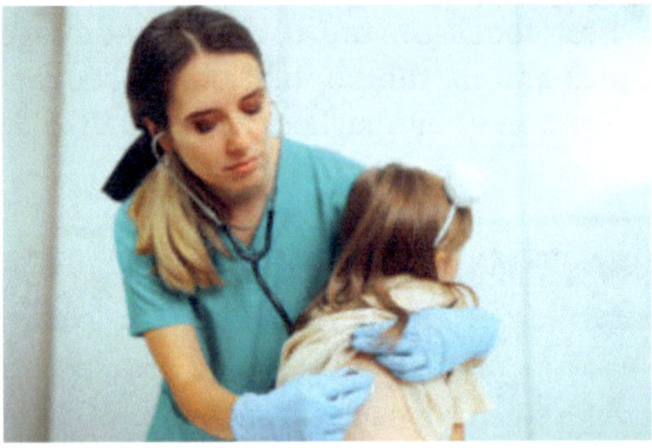

Figure 1.15. In pediatric rheumatology, case studies play a pivotal role in illustrating the diagnostic complexity and clinical manifestations of various rheumatic disorders in children.

Source: https://www.pediatricexperts.com/wp-content/uploads/2024/02/AdobeStock_722676488-Case-Study-300x200.jpeg.

1.6.1. Case Study of a Child with JIA

Presentation of a case of a child with JIA is fascinating in comprehending the complex nature and treatmentissues of this autoimmune disease in children. JIA is an heterogeneous group of diseases with chronic arthritis in children, with etiopathogenetic mechanisms yet to be studied. A case in point is a 6-year-old boy with oligoarticular JIA who was diagnosed at age 2 years. After initial treatment with glucocorticoids and non-steroidal anti-inflammatory drugs (NSAIDs), the symptoms did not abate, and the need to switch to biologic therapy arose. After the introduction of etanercept, there was remission within a period of 10 months. This case highlights the evident need for early and effective therapy to suppress symptoms and prevent chronic joint damage, highlighting the potential utility of new biologic agents in pediatric rheumatology, particularly when conventional treatment fails (Martini et al., 2024). Another relevant case is that of a boy aged 12 years with polyarticular JIA and X-linked agammaglobulinemia, illustrating the challenges of management in children with concomitant immunies. The patient experienced a poor response to a number ofmany therapies, which inNSAIDs, methotrexate, and various biological agents such as, such as anti-TNF-alpha and tocilizumab. The case presents the complexity involved in treating JIA, particularly in patients with comorbidities. A combination of sirolimus and abatacept later introduced, had a very good outcome, with the disease achieving remission within four months. This case is indicative of the position of personalized medicine in pediatric rheumatology and of the requirement for ongoing assessment and adjustment of therapy to address the unique needs oild (Martini et al., 2024). Innovation in the field, such as, such as the application of Janus kinase inhibitors (JAKi), is an effective treatment for JIA in children. JAKi are pharmaceutical small molecule inhibitors of critical signaling pathways involved in inflammation. Initial results indicate that these inhibitors can effectively cause remission in juvenile onset rheumatic disease, particularly in those with moderate to low disease activity. In a cohort of adults with a history of pediatric-onset JIA, patient outcomes indicated an encouraging rate of remission associated with JAKi therapy, particularly in oligoarticular forms of disease. This new treatment has the potential to bring additional layers of choice to practicing clinicians seeking to maximize care for kids with JIA, ultimately leading to enhanced patient results in pediatric rheumatology.

1.6.2. Case Study of a Child with SLE

The complexity of systemic lupus erythematosus (SLE) in children is reflected in case reports highlighting the diversity of clinical presentations and diagnostic and management challenges. SLE in children, while relatively rare, often accompanies severe hematologic abnormalities, including anemia, neutropenia, or thrombocytopenia, that need to be carefully evaluated and monitored. In a retrospective study of children with SLE, there was a high incidence of hematologic invol highlighting the importance of tic evaluation such as, such as autoantibody profiles such as, such as anti-dsDNA and anti-RNP (Babgi et al., 2024). In addition, prompt recognition of pediatric SLE is important because it may have an important influence on treatment and long-term prognosis, which remains a vibrant area of pediatric rheumatology. From a diagnostic standpoint, the new EULAR/ACR SLE criteria provide a contemporary approach to pediatric patient assessment. High sensitivity and specificity rates using these classification criteria relative to the older SLICC criteria were noted in a study involving a group of children with SLE. This study emphasized the nuances in diagnosing childhood-onset SLE, wherein early detection procedures can aid patient management and treatment (Babgi et al., 2024). As the disease and differential diagnoses are also complex and often clinicians are left bewildered to diagnose them, these updated criteria are particularly useful to ide in the early stages of the disease, and potentially changing change the course of disease management in such children. Pediatric SLE management is naturally complicated, requiring a multidisciplinary team of pediatric rheumatologists, hematologists, and others. Therapy must be individually tailored to address both the physical and emotional needs of children. The results of a case study shed light on the importance of serial monitoring of hematologic factors and autoantibody titers, which are related to disease activity and flares. With the largest age group being children under 12, as determined in many studies, targeted interventions need to be formulated that consider the growth and development needs of this age group (Hassan et al., 2024). Placing greater importance on patient education and family involvement will also serve to further raise rates of adherence to treatment regimens, which will ultimately lead to better control of pediatric SLE (Figure 1.16).

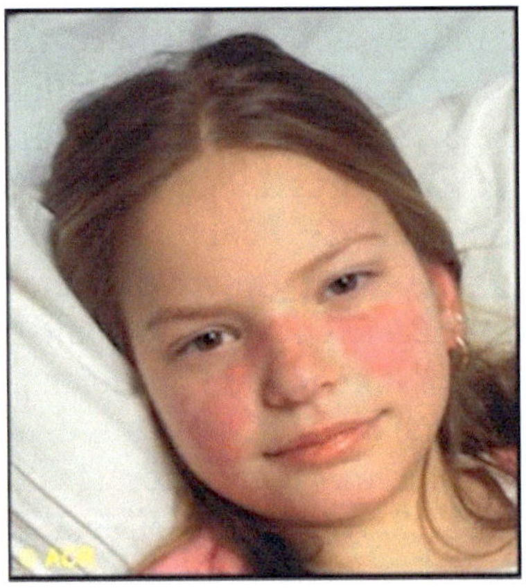

Figure 1.16. Child presenting with a classic malar rash, a characteristic clinical feature of systemic lupus erythematosus (SLE).

Source: https://www.jpeds.com/cms/10.1016/j.jpeds.2018.01.045/asset/9587e051-9427-4dcb-b709-8fe059d32e0b/main.assets/ympd9751-fig-0002_lrg.jpg.

1.6.3. Lessons Learned from Clinical Experiences

Through clinical exposure in pediatric rheumatology, providers have come to understand the top priority of engaging patients and families directly in the care process. Active engagement facilitates an atmosphere of co-operation, in which communication constitutes the fundamental in achieving the unique challenges of pediatric rheumatological patients. Through the use of evidence-based care strategies, clinicians are able to best meet the individual needs of young patients while making their families feel engaged and informed. A recent compilation of best practices emphasized that keeping the lines of communication open regarding patient and family experience has a strong influence on total patient carmes. Clinicians are nudged to promote feedback at moments such as, such as discharge that can help modify interventions and ultimately lead to the improvement of pediatric patients' quality of life. These results illuminate how effective communication can enhance treatment adherence and satisfaction, reiterating the value of teamwork in pediatric rheumatology (Hays et al., 2020). Besides, lessons learned from clinical encounters demand the use of patient research partners (PRPs) in rheumatology. The inclusion of PRPs in practice in care and research can help promote the relevance and applicability of research findings to a large extent. Partnerships offer individuals with intimate familiarity of childhood rheumatological disease conditions an uncommon perspective, hence helping to enhance the quality of treatments and studies. As observed, involving PRPs early in research has more significant effects and enhances the confidence of younger patients and their families in the treatment process. This method, however, has its limitations, concentrating chiefly on communication and support for researchers and PRPs. Establishing a supportive environment, which involves adequate training of both providers, is critical to guarantee the maximum effect of PRPs in pediatric rheumatology settings (Aouad et al., 2024). Lastly, quality improvement (QI) activities in pediatric rheumatology emphasize the need for continuous practice assessment of care. By regular collection and analysis of patient and family experience data, health care professionals are in a position to determine what needs to be corrected and effectively utilize steps to enhance care. Internal performance feedback systems, as noted in recent studies, allow open communication among hospital administrators and health care staff. These preventive steps, besides optimizing funcg processes, encourage the culture of learning and adaptation among in clinical settings. Of particular interest, the identification of empiric drivers of international care ratings encourages staff motivation and accountability, building a patient-centric system that prioritizes quality outcomes. Subsequently, practice lessons learned are used to inform an integrated approach towards improved pediatric rheumatological care by fostering continued involvement, research collaboration, and systematic quality improvement (Hays et al., 2020).

Test Your Knowledge

1. What type of dehydration is this and what is the initial management?
2. What is the most likely diagnosis?

SUMMARY

Pediatric rheumatology has developed as a necessary subspecialty, providing care to the distinctive needs of the difficulty of rheumatic disease in children. Unique pathophysiologic features and disease presentations in pediatric patients necessitate sophistiiagnostic and treatment modalities. Recognition of conditions such as, such as juvenile idiopathic arthritis (JIA) and familial Mediterranean fever (FMF) has been crucial, with scientists and clinicians working to improve patient outcomes. Current studies have also contributed to understanding significant predictors of disease outcome, as well as the importance of early intervention techniques, further supporting the need for advanced pediatric rheumatology care. Pediatric rheumatologists are in a prime position with ongoing research and collaborative care practices to continue to improve clinical practice, ultimately providing a better quality of life for affected children. Moreover, the application of evidence-based guidelines has significantly enhanced the management programs in pediatric rheumatology. The existing clinical guidelines have shown a focus on dev treat-to-target protocol, particularly for conditions like JIA, in order to formulate treatment plans more effectively and tailor them to patients. The use of Delphi methods within groups of experts has also led to increased consensus about management plans to the extent that there is a complete understanding of the pros and cons associated with a set of therapeutic options. Clinicians are therefore emboldened to make informed decisions that yield maximum treatment outcomes. The development of algorithms for JIA care, unique to the environment, highlights the multidisciplinary nature of care, contemplating the interplay of healthcare professionals in overcoming challenges of pediatric rheumatic illnesses. Ultimately, the adoption of development and the ntegration of personalized medicine into pediatric rheumatology contributes additional vaportunities for improved patient outcomes. Clinical scoring systems, sucs, such as that suggested for homozygous M694V genotype patients of FMF, is are an example of the shift towards predictive and personalized models of care. The advances, coupled with ongoing patient education and counseling, are all a part of constructing successful health trajectories. Future studies need to continue to explore new avenues of therapy and simplify existing protocols. Lastly, these mutual initiatives will ensure that pediatric rheumatology not only meets the medical requirements of the day but also proactively responds to evolving patient demands, setting itself uements in the management of childhood rheumatic disease (Tunce et al., 2025; Miedany et al., 2022; Tunce et al., 2025).

In the past couple of years, pediatric rheumatology has experienced a sea change with the advancement of artificial intelligence. Most striking is the use of machine learning models, which allow for the identification of key biomarkers essential in understanding a host of rheumatic diseases of children. With the application of supervised and unsupervised learning models, physicians can predict outcomes of treatment and easily stratify patie to individual presen and phaof disease progression. As an indicationindicated by Lavalle Bella et al. (20252024), such technological innovations lead to improved accuracy in diagnosis as well as encouraging individualized treatment approaches, which marks a significant step forward in the practice of pediatric rheumatology. Beyond machine learning technologies, the movement system (MS) paradigm is also gaining popularity within pediatric physical therapy, which overlapped with pediatric rheumatology. This movement-based approach streamlines diagnosis so that therapists can develop more effective intervention plans that are tailored to the needs of individual patients. Obviously, using a standardized nomenclature for MS diagnoses will enhance communication between providers and serve patients better. Emphasis on mobility as a critical component of children's health care is an expression of greater recognition of the interconnectedness of global health and physical function, which makes it imperative that pediatric rheumatologists consider these while making treatment plans (Cobb et al., 2025). Furthermore, ongoing development and adaptation of non-invasive imaging devices through the use of artificial intelligence are a promising prospect for pediatric rheumatology. Not only do these advanced technologies make diagnosis of inflammation aent of disease activity possible, but they also crvenues tds patient-friendlier friendly evaluation methods. According to Lavalle Bella et al. (20252024), embedding advanced imaging techniques and machine learning algorithms presents challenges to traditional diagnosis methods, providing more accurate results and more customized treatment plans. By the integration of knowledge of technology and physical therapy, pediatric rheumatologists can optimize treatment modalities and enhance the quality care for children with rheumatologic disease. Such a comprehensive approach is the best of for the future of pediatric rheumatology, the objective being comprehensive, family-centered care.

KEY TERMS FROM THIS CHAPTER

- Anxiety
- Chronic conditions
- Diagnosis
- Juvenile idiopathic arthritis (JIA)
- Macrophage activation syndrome (MAS)
- Pathophysiology
- Pediatric
- Potential health
- Artificial intelligence (AI)
- Clinical practice
- Healthcare systems
- Machine learning (ML)
- Medical management
- Patient management
- Pediatric patients
- Rheumatic diseases

CRITICAL THINKING QUESTIONS

1. **What is the definition of pediatrics?**
   a. Study of diseases in adults
   b. Study of surgical diseases in infants
   c. Branch of medicine dealing with the health and medical care of infants, children, and adolescents
   d. Study of maternal health
2. **Up to what age is a person typically considered a pediatric patient?**
   a. 12 years
   b. 16 years
   c. 18 years
   d. 21 years
3. **Who is considered the "Father of Pediatrics"?**
   a. Sigmund Freud
   b. Hippocrates
   c. Abraham Jacobi
   d. William Osler
4. **Which of the following is a primary focus of pediatric care?**
   a. Only curative treatment
   b. Adult chronic disease management
   c. Preventive health care and developmental monitoring
   d. Geriatric care
5. **Which of these vaccines is typically given at birth?**
   a. DPT
   b. BCG
   c. MMR
   d. IPV

Short Answer Questions

1. What is a growth chart and how is it used in pediatric care?
2. Why is importants immunization of in pediatrics?
3. Define low birth weight and mention its significance.
4. What is meant by anticipatory guidance in pediatrics?
5. What is the difference between preterm and term infants?

Answer to Critical Thinking Questions

1.(c); 2.(c); 3.(c); 4.(c); 5.(b)

REFERENCES

1. AlAmeel, T., Almutairdi, A., & Al-Bawardy, B. (2023). Emerging therapies for ulcerative colitis: Updates from recent clinical trials. *Clinical and Experimental Gastroenterology, 16*, 147–167. https://www.semanticscholar.org/paper/71dd9d1b7834fa37fd4e1dfb40c9f28f79ff8fae (accessed on 16th June 2025).
2. Aouad, K., Benavent, D., Bertheussen, H., de Wit, M., et al. (2024). Patient research partner involvement in rheumatology research: A systematic literature review informing the 2023 updated EULAR recommendations for the involvement of pal. (2016). Evidence-based decision support for pediatric rheumatology reduces diagnostic errors. Segal, M. M., Athreya, B., Son, M. B., Tirosh, I., Hausmann, J. S., Ang, E. Y., Zurakowski, D., Feldman, L. K., & Sundel, R. P. (2016). Evidence-based decision support for pediatric rheumatology reduces diagnostic errors. *Pediatric rheumatology online journal, 14*(1), 67. https://doi.org/10.1186/s12969-016-0127-z (accessed on 16th June 2025).
3. Bernatsky, A., Gafni, A., Tong, A., Barron, A. C., Williams, A. E., Cahill, A. M., Arthritis and Musculoskeletal Alliance (ARMA), et al. (2014). An exploration of parents' preferences for foot care in juvenile idiopathic arthritis: A possible role for the discrete choice experiment. https://core.ac.uk/download/9376072.pdf (accessed on 16th June 2025).
4. G Bilican, T Karakan, Ö Eğritaş Gürkan, H Sabhan, C Hedin, A Forss, G Petrousis, M Cindoruk, A Can, S L Haas, P0376 Advancing intestinal ultrasound for IBD in Turkey: results of a national survey, *Journal of Crohn's and Colitis*, Vo*Crohn's and Colitis.*https://www.semanticscholar.org/paper/30611e47cd0b36def50c23f1da2c6676be6ab456 (accessed on 16th June 2025).
5. Burnham, J. M., & von Scheven, E. (2011). Vitamin D supplementation in the pediatric rheumatology clinic. https://core.ac.uk/download/323072035.pdf (accessed on 16th June 2025).
6. Caes, L., Clinch, J., Eccleston, C., Fisher, E., et al. (2018). Current evidence-based interdisciplinary treatment options for pediatric musculoskeletal pain. https://core.ac.uk/download/157569796.pdf (accessed on 16th June 2025).
7. Cherepakhin, O., Ringold, S., Ronis, T., Kirkorian, A., & Brandling-Bennett, H. (2024). A survey assessment of combined pediatric dermatology–rheumatology clinics. *Pediatric Dermatology, 41*, 667–670. https://www.semanticscholar.org/paper/0ee79aa267f0330c40ffab36ef1e4de8a66ad39b (accessed on 16th June 2025).
8. Corsello, G., Cantarini, L., Maggio, M. C., Cimaz, R., & Corpora, U. (2017). Anti-IL1 in patients with low penetrance mutations for autoinflammatory diseases: Tuscany and Sicilian case series from paediatric to adult age. https://core.ac.uk/download/286077880.pdf (accessed on 16th June 2025).
9. Fares, A. A., Carracedo Uribe, C., Martinez, D., Ur Rehman, T., Silva Rondon, C., & Sandoval-Sus, J. (2024). Bruton's tyrosine kinase inhibitors: Recent updates. *International Journal of Molecular Sciences, 25*, 2208–2208. https://doi.org/10.3390/ijms25042208 (accessed on 16th June 2025).
10. Galozzi, P., Basso, D., Plebani, M., & Padoan, A. (2023). Artificial intelligence and laboratory data in rheumatic diseases. *Clinica Chimica Acta, 546*, 117388–117388. https://doi.org/10.1016/j.cca.2023.117388 (accessed on 16th June 2025).

11. Gerdes, M., Gutstein, A., Keren, R., Knight, A. M., et al. (2014). Depression and anxiety and their association with healthcare utilization in pediatric lupus and mixed connective tissue disease patients: A cross-sectional study. https://core.ac.uk/download/46954630.pdf (accessed on 16th June 2025).

12. Hays, R. D., Lerner, C., Palimaru, A., Quigley, D., et al. (2020). A review of best practices for monitoring and improving inpatient pediatric patient experiences. https://core.ac.uk/download/287622168.pdf (accessed on 16th June 2025).

13. Keser, G., & Namdar Pekiner, F. (2023). *Artificial Intelligence Applications in Dentistry.* Özgür Yayınları eBooks. https://doi.org/10.58830/ozgur.pub91.c383 (accessed on 16th June 2025).

14. Kim, K., Jeong, J. H., & Choi, E. K. (2024). Non-pharmacological interventions for delirium in the pediatric population: A systematic review with narrative synthesis. *BMC Pediatrics, 24.* https://www.semanticscholar.org/paper/887a72d6e86a37fc20c3c5e4f2ef3209b406231a (accessed on 16th June 2025).

15. Lavalle, S., Caruso, S., Foti, R., Gagliano, C., Cocuzza, S., La Via, L., Parisi, F. M., et al. (2024). Behçet's disease, pathogenesis, clinical features, and treatment approaches: A comprehensive review. *Medicina, 60*, 562–562. https://doi.org/10.3390/medicina60040562 (accessed on 16th June 2025).

16. Lazar, M. C., Man, O., Sur, L. M., Samașca, G., & Bolunduț, A. C. (2025). Juvenile spondyloarthropathies: Diagnostic and therapeutic advances—A narrative review. *Journal of Clinical Medicine, 14.* https://www.semanticscholar.org/paper/d62d9dfdf1df46ae7f44c5d523ce05105fa76b83 (accessed on 16th June 2025).

17. Mördrup, K., Jungner, J. G., Broström, E., Palmblad, K., & Bartholdson, C. (2024). Benefits of a Juvenile Arthritis Support Program (JASP-1) for children recently diagnosed with juvenile idiopathic arthritis and their parents. *BMC Rheumatology, 8.* https://www.semanticscholar.org/paper/04625860007dd4b069a343f8547332aa8bdf185e (accessed on 16th June 2025).

18. Yu, Z., Wang, L., Quan, M., Zhang, T., & Song, H. (2020). Successful management with Janus kinase inhibitor tofacitinib in refractory juvenile dermatomyositis: A pilot study and literature review. *Rheumatology.* https://www.semanticscholar.org/paper/795d781a724e16c955b59e111177fb3a9e0142bd (accessed on 16th June 2025).

PEDIATRIC NEPHROLOGY

2

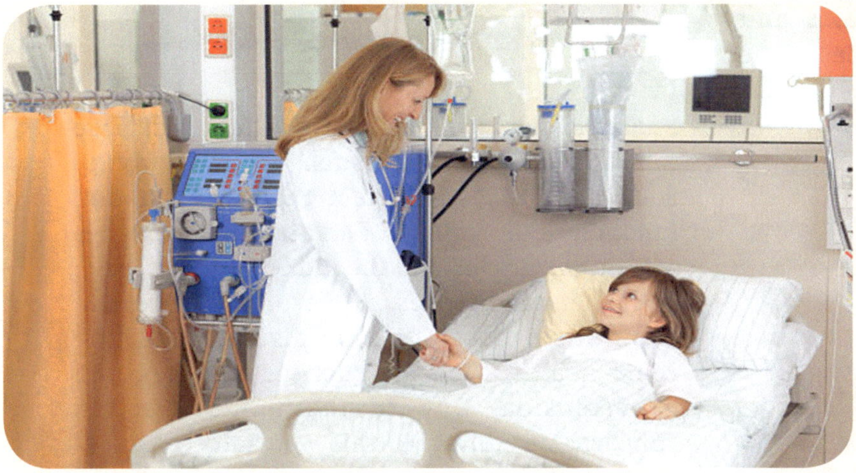

LEARNING OBJECTIVES

After studying this chapter, you will be able to:

1. Discuss pediatric kidney anatomy and physiology
2. Point out major pediatric kidney diseases
3. Describe the diagnosis in pediatric nephrology
4. Point out treatment in pediatric nephrology
5. Be mindful of long-term care and follow-up
6. Understand ongoing studies and developments in pediatric nephrology

Introduction

Pediatric nephrology is a branch of medicine that specializes in the diagnosis and management of kidney disease in children. It recognizes that renal disorders in children manifest differently than in adults, necessitating an individualized approach. Concomitant kidney disorders common in children include congenital anomalies, nephrotic syndrome, chronic kidney disease (CKD), and urinary tract infections (UTIs). Interestingly, pediatric nephrology is concerned with the long-term effects of acute kidney injuries, leading to chronic diseases in children during their old age. As research findings indicate, early identification and intervention among vulnerable groups is of high concern, as children are more responsive to interventions like kidney replacement therapyts. Therefore, it is basically important for child nephrologists to understand the individualized characteristics of these conditions and their impact on growth and development. The epidemiology of renal disease in children varies geographically, which requires thoroudies in order to ascertain their its prevalence and characteristics. For instance, research in Bangladesh has documented the patterns of renal disease in children and identified nephrotic syndrome as the most prevalent disorder encountered in inpatient and outpatient settings. In a research study involving over 6,000 children as patients, a high rate was discovered to have nephrotic syndrome was discovered, which suggests the requirement for focused management and screening among them. This population-based study shows that males are more frequently engaged than females and illustrates that pediatric nephrology has to be adjusted based on various local health care habits and socio-economic environments.

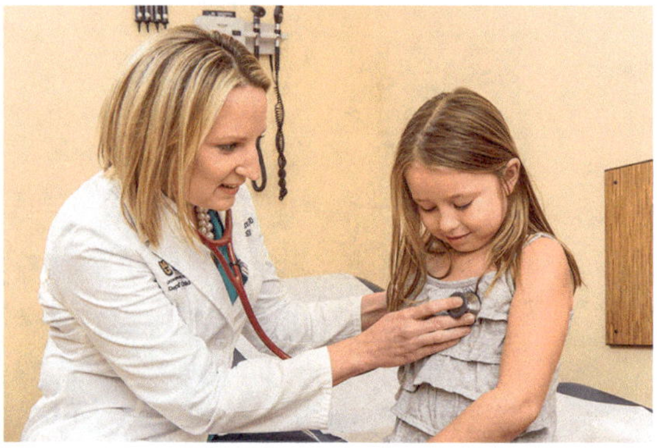

Figure 2.1. Pediatric nephrology.

Source: https://www.muhealth.org/sites/default/files/inline-images/Pediatric-Nephrology-760-compressor.png.

These results can impact policy and resource designation for pediatric nephrology care across regions. Lastly, specialization of pediatric nephrology is crucial in the administration of child kidney health, given the life-long effects of renal disorders. Pediatric nephrologists play a pivotal role not only inthe management of the current conditions, but also in screening and preventing complications in the future. The constantly changing nature of the specialty requires a multidisciplinary effort with collaborations between healthcare providers, researchers, and policymakers to ensure pediatric patients receive the optimal outcomes. Focusing on renal disorder epidemiology, diagnosis, and treatment, child nephrology hopes to improve the quality of life for children with such problems. Additionally, heightened awareness among parents and the general population about the requirements and possibilities of childhood kidney disease will lead to improved health and increased access to treatment for these children (Figure 2.1).

Definition and Scope of Pediatric Nephrology

Pediatric nephrology involves kidney disease in children, such as, such as an array of conditions that can affect the structure and function of the kidneys. Pediatric nephrologage conditions intrinsic to the kidney, such as, such as congenital diseases, glomerulonephritis, and nephrotic syndromystemic diseases affecting renal health, such as, such as diabetes and hypertension. Due to the unique growth concerns in children, this specialty requires a deep level of comprehension of growth and maturation processes. In particular, the impact of renal disease on physical and cognitive development is a central theme of pediatric nephrology that requires an interdisciplinary management strategy. Additionally, pediatric nephrologists often collaborate with other specialties like urology and endocrinology to provide the complete package of care for children with complex health conditions. The broad scope of pediatric nephrology also encompasses early detection and treatmeKI and CKD. AKI can be induced by many reasons such as, such as dehydration, infections, or genetic disorders, which are very prevalent in children. As outlined in later texts, children with specific mcies are at higher risk of AKI due to therapies such as, such as chemotherapy, and thus the need for careful monitoring and treatment needs to be noted (Benoit et al., 2016). Owing to the specific etiologies of renal disease in children versus adults, pediatric nephrology emphasizes personalized diagnosis and treatment that considers both developmental context and age. This targeted subspecialty helps to shorten the long-term outcomes of kidney disorders, ultimately enhancing children's health pathways. In addition to acute and chronic conditions, pediatric nephrology also addresses rare syndromes and disorders, giving high priority to understanding complex pathophysiology and early intervention. An example of this is atypical hemolytic uremic syndrome (aHUS), which involves extreme renal impairment accompanied by hemolytic anemia and thrombocytopenia. Advances in diagnostic criteria now allow more effective identification and treatment of aHUS (Ashida et al., 2021), which enables better outcomes for the children suffering from it. The new face of pediatric nephrology extends to advances in treatment modalities, including renal replacement therapies, that become inevitable as children transition to adulthood with kidney failure. As our knowledge of these uncommon conditions continues to grow, pediatric nephrologists are still leadin the way in enhancing diagnostic methods and promoting multi-disciplinary cooperation to further enhance patient care.

Importance of Kidney Health in Children

The significance of healthy kidneys in children cannot be exaggerated since kidneys are central to homeostasis and overall body function. Early detection and management of kidney ailments are imperative to prevent sequelae over the long term due to untreated pediatric kidney disease. Congenital illness, glomerulonephritis, and urinary tract infections could have long-term effects if not treated. The challenge is that many kidney diseases in children are asymptomatic early on, and therefore, awareness and regular screening are important. As highlighted by recent guidelines, pre-emptive interventions are required in the assessment of risk fand comorbidities that affect candidacy for procedures such as, such as transplantation, towards ultimately improving their health outcomes (Steven et al., 2020). urden of kidney disease is deplorable in light of the fact thatbecause it leads to massive morbidity and mortality on a worldwide scale. Kidney disease in global health not only affects single famiit also puts pressure on the healthcare systems. Evidences have has demonstrated that pediatric kidney health has disproportionate effects due to socioeconomic and environmental determinants. For instance, disparities in care and treatment access are apparent when low-income and high-income countries are compared. Children or resources are at higher risk of developing conditions such as, such as CKD and AKI, which can trigger a series of health complications if not managed (Deidra et al., 2019).

Therefore, it is essential to bridge such differences through equal healthcare policies, prevention strategies, and health education within the community. Lastly, integrating pediatric nephrology into child health programs is indispensable in a bid to foster peak kidney function right from childhood. The approach must be founded on preventive care, early detection of renal disorders, and effective management approaches to meet children's special physiological needs. Involvement of children and their families in educational programs has the potential to enable them to recognize warning signs and receive appropriate medical attention in a timely manner. Coordination of pediatricians, nephrologists, and allied health professionals is essential in developing a multidisciplinary model of care that addresses varied factors influencing kidney health. As the foundation for adult health, ensuring children are provided with access to quality nephrology services sets the stage for healthier adult life and reduces the long-term cost of kidney disease in populations (Steven et al., 2020) (Figure 2.2).

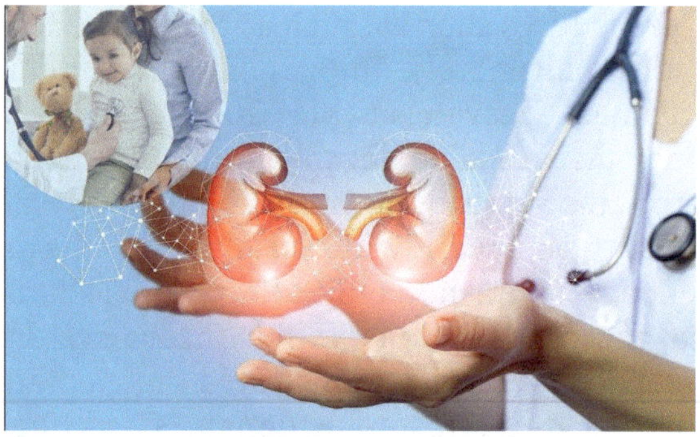

Figure 2.2. The significance of kidney health in children.

Source: https://www.vachhanihospital.com/blog/wp-content/uploads/2024/05/Pediatric-Nephrology-Understanding-Kidney-Health-in-Children-1.jpg.

Overview of Common Pediatric Kidney Disorders

Pediatric kidney diseases encompass a broad spectrum of disorders that significantly affect children's health and development. Among these, idiopathic nephrotic syndrome is particularly common, characterized by diffuse proteinuria, hypoalbuminemia, and edema. Its global incidence ranges from 1.15 to 16.9 per 100,000 children per year. Initial treatment typically involves glucocorticoids, which achieve satisfactory responses in approximately 85–90% of patients, distinguishing steroid-sensitive nephrotic syndrome (SSNS) from more resistant forms. However, frequent relapses in 70–80% of SSNS patients present substantial management challenges, necessitating long-term follow-up to minimize steroid-related side effects and ensure the child's health (Brad et al., 2024).. Lupus nephritis, a serious condition in pediatric nephrology, also needs proper evaluation and management due to its multifactorial nature as a complication of systemic lupus erythematosus. The 2024 Clinical Practice Guideline for Management of Lupus Nephritis lays emphasis on the use of evidence-based approaches both in diagnosis and therapy. More recent revisions, after following randomized controlled trials, point out the particular problems of treating lupus nephritis in children, where renal injury can lead to late morbidity and reduced kidney function. The guideline proposes individualized treatment regimens, not only on the basis of the efficacy of therapy but also their safety profile, taking into account the unique physiological features of children. Clinicians are encouraged to stay current with evolving paradigms of treatment to optimize care and outcome in young patients with this disabling illness (Brad et al., 2024). Alongside nephrotic syndrome and lupus nephritis, pediatric patients may present with any of a variety of congenital anomalies of the kidney and urinary tract (CAKUT), which, if not promptly diagnosed and treated, can lead to gross renal impairmene congenital anomalies range from obstructive uropathy to malformations such as, such as agenesis and dysplasia, and all are managed differently. Early diagnosis by routine prenatal ultrasound scans and postnatal examinations is crucial in making timely interventions. The management may be surgical repair or palliative, depending on the nature and severity of the anomaly. Furthermore, similar to other kidney diseases, the psychosocial impact on such children and families calls for models of care that are multi-dimensional in nature and address not only medical complications but also emotional and educational concerns (Trautmann et al., 2022).

2.1. Anatomy and Physiology of the Pediatric Kidney

Learning Outcome

1. Developmental differences in pediatric kidneys
2. Functions of the kidneys in children
3. Impact of age on kidney function and health

The pediatric kidney possesses a unique anatomy tailored to meet the metabolic and physiological demands of growth and development in children. The size and shape of the kidneys of infants are very different from those of adults; the pediatric kidney is more compact with reduced nephron length and different nephron patteowth, the kidneys of children pass through various developmental stages, such as, such as changes in architecture and function. The kidneys at birth possess filtration function but not the complete regulatory function of mature children and adults. This dynamic process of development is crucial since the renal system is under the challenge of providing for fluid balance and the removal of metabolic waste while adjusting to changing body composition and metabolic rates typical of growing up. A complete understanding of the physiology of the infant kidney reveals distinctive features necessary for the maintenance of homeostasis in children. The glomerular filtration rate (GFR) is much lower in neonates than in older children and adults, reflecting the immature status of renal function in the newborn period. GFR increases precipitously during the first year of an infant's life and is as high as a mature adult at 2 years of aldren's kidneys have also increased sensitivity to physiological stre such as, such as dehydration or infections and should be monitored closely. This The physiology of children points to the greater significance of certain processes to renal illness and health care, and the focus should be on understanding these developing processes in the field of pediatric nephrology. Recent research in nephrology has utilized novel methodologies to distinguish the complexity of the child's kidney. For instance, pluripotent stem cell (PSC)-derived kidney organoids and adult stem cell (ASC) tubuloids are two prospective in vitro models for kidney development and disease analysis. PSC-derived organoids recapitulate the intricate nephrogenesis processes, allowing scientists to investigate nephron structure and function at multiple stages of development. Alternatively, ASC tubuloids provide information on repair processes in the mature kidney while permitting disease modeling and drug efficacy to be investigated. Both models complement each other in advancing our understanding of hereditary, infectious, and metabolney diseases, thereby paving the way for innovation in regenerative medicine and aimed targeted therapies that are directly applicable to pediatric populations, demonstrating the shifting landscape of pediatric nephrology (Fjodor et al., 2020) (Figure 2.3).

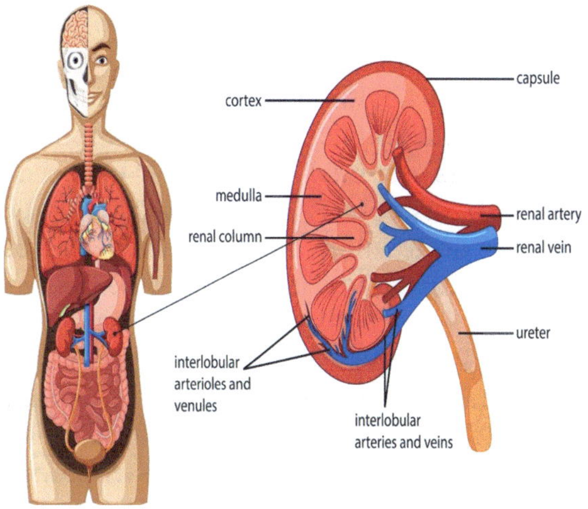

Figure 2.3. The anatomy of the pediatric kidney is uniquely adapted to meet the metabolic and physiological demands of growth and development in children.

Source: https://img.freepik.com/free-vector/human-kidney-anatomy-cartoon-style-infographic_1308-49728.jpg.

2.1.1. Developmental Differences in Pediatric Kidneys

The developmental features of pediatric kidneys are essential to the understanding of the treatment of renal pathologies in the pediatric patient. In children, renal function and structure change dramatically with age, which compels unique clinical strategies to care for the patient. Newborns possess kidneys that are smaller and functionally less mature than in adults, resulting in disparate metabolic responses and filtration capacities. This is especially so in pediatric nephrotic syndrome, which may present as steroid-resistant nephrotic syndrome (SRNS) with associated genetic mutations like those in the COQ genes. Evidence suggests that disease presentation is at a different age in individuals who have the COQ2, COQ6, and COQ8B variants with varied clinical presentations and outcomes (Drovandi et al., 2022). Consequently, practitioners must consider these developmental differences when diagnosing and managing kidney-related disorders in children, aiming for tailored interventions that promote optimal renal health. A deeper understanding of the clinical implications of developmental differences is essential, particularly concerning genetic disorders. Primary Coenzyme Q10 (CoQ10) deficiency, for instance, reveals significant variability in kidney disease onset depending on the specific genetic variant involved. Research shows that infants with COQ2 mutations commonly present with kidney disease at age one, whereas individuals with COQ8B mutations are sometimes asymptomatic until late adolescence.tion highlights the need for age-specific screening and monitoring strategies age-specific for pediatric nephrology (Drovandi et al., 2022). The occurrence of extrarenal signs, including sensorineural hearing impairment or neurologic manifestations in patients with COQ6, further reflects the multi-organ system nature of these diseases. It is clear that the pediatric patient must have integrated care management that takes into consideration not just the renal but extrarenal manifestations of genetic kidney diseases as well. The trajectory of development of pediatric kidneys also determines the choice of appropriate therapeutic modalities and outcomes. Pediatris who are candidates for kidney transplantation have distinct challenges from adults, such as, such as differing comorbidities and psychosocial issues that can impact adherence and overall health status. Pediatric nephrologists frequently have to deal with the intricacies involved in taking care of pre-existing ailments, like cardiac or metabolic disorders, that could affect transplant candidacy. Additionally, insight into how growth and development affect postoperative outcomes and graft survival in the long term is vital. The incorporation of these developmental concerns into the management of pediatric kidney disease not only improves clinical outcomes but also informs future research agendas to meet the complex needs of this vulnerable group.

2.1.2. Functions of the Kidneys in Children

The kidneys play a crucial role in maintaining homeostasis within children's bodies, a task that is essential to their development and growth. One of the primary tasks of the kidneys is to balance the fluids, which involves the filtering of blood to remove waste products and excess water. By eliminating these compounds through urination, the kidneys ensure that toxic accumulation in the body is avoided, a critical aspect of a child's metabolic health. The kidneys also assist in regulating soassium, and calcium, which are components essential to different physiological activities, such as, such as nerve transmission and muscle contraction. Thus, kidneys are not only excretory organs but also play a vital role in maintaining a stable internal environment, essential for growth and development. In kids, kidneys also exhibit functionaptations beneficial towards their ongoing growth. A case is the ability to concentrate urine that which is weaker in kids compared to adults; such a shortcoming necessitates higher fluid intake in order to prevent dehydration. The kidneys develop compensatory changes to adapt to some challenges, e.g., disease or congenital defects. A good example is a congenital solitary kidney (CSK), whereby the remaining kidney hypertrophies to compensate for the loss of function. Compensatory hypertrophy should be followed up through repeated ultrasound evaluations to ensure optimal function and to detect potential complications, e.g., hypertension or decreased glomerular filtration rate. Such adaptations point towards the dynamic aspect of kidneys and emphasize the necessity of individualized management strategies for treating kids suffering from renal anomalies (Scola et al., 2022). Along with kidney function-suppressing disorders, cildren are also susceptible to idiopathic nephrotic syndrome, which primarily occurs in pediatric ages. This condition also has significant implications for the health of a child, for example, protein loss via the urine and consequent complications like edema and predisposition to infections. Early diagnosis and management are essential to prevent long-term sequelae. Management programs for this sort of condition, like steroid-sensitive nephrotic syndrome, focus on limiting relapses and maintaining kidney function so that children can live a normal life despite having this medical condition. Evidence-based practice integration in pediatric nephrology underscores the importance of timely intervention and continuous observation, ultimately resulting in positive long-term outcomes for kidney diseased patients (Ehren et al., 2021) (Figure 2.4).

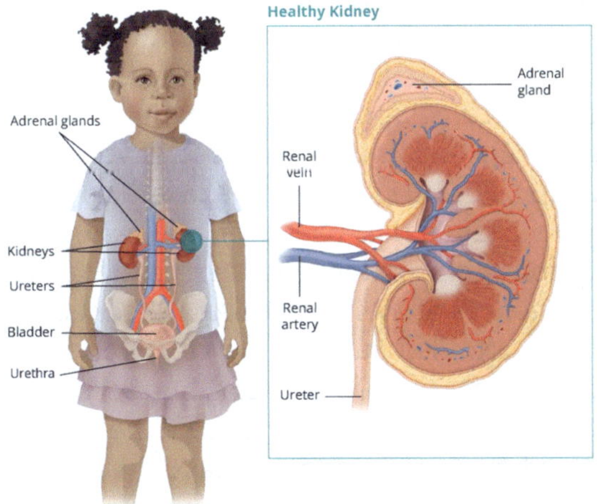

Figure 2.4. Functions of the kidneys in children.

Source: https://stjude.scene7.com/is/image/stjude/K01003-TOG-kidney-normal?fit=crop,1&fmt=png-alpha&wid=1200.

2.1.3. Impact of age on Kidney Function and Health

The relationship between age and renal function is also of specific interest in pediatric nephrology, since the kidneys develop their critical function during childhood. The renal function is still immature in early life, and this may affect the clearance of waste products and make children vulnerable to a variety of health issues. For instance, the glomerular filtration rate (GFR) in infants is considerably lower compared to adults and typically results in the accumulation of metabolites, posing a threat to health in general. Children's GFR increases slowly with rising age, particularly in the first year of life, until it equals that of adults in the adolescent period. Hence, recognition of such age-related alterations is significant for the timely interventions and management of pediatric renal health to avoid long-term sequelae of chronic kidney disease and other kidney impairments in later life. The impact of age on ealth in children is further complicated by the presence of various pediatric nephrological disorders such as, such as nephrotic syndrome (NS). Research indicates that endothelial dysfunction and oxidative stress are the key determinants of NS pathophysiology in perhaps exacerbated by their age-linked physiological response. In particular, antioxidant treatment, such as, such as dl-α-tocopherol and ascorbic acid, has been shown to be efficient in preventing oxidative stress in children with NS aged 1 to 15 years, expressing the importance of appropriate treatment for the subject age group (Mellyana et al., 2015). Hence, pediatric patient development necessitates consideration of some age-related vulnerabilities and drug effects, justifying the significant role of pediatric nephrology in renal care. Also, pediatric end-stage kidney disease patients' quality of life is often largely based on the age at diagnosis and treatment initiation, particularly when hemodialysis becomes necessary. A recent study developed the Hemodccess-Related Quality of Life measure to investigate the specific impacts that vascular access devices, such as, such as fistulas, grafts, and catheters, have on children's health-related quality of life (HRQOL) (Gage et al., 2020). Owing to the problems of having a chronic condition, things about their vascular access can change their day-to-day lives, emotional state, and social relationships. Therefore, age-based treatment planning considerations are essential to overcome the unique challenges pediatric patients face, ultimately to improve the health outcome and their quality of life.

Test Your Knowledge

1. What developmental differences distinguish pediatric kidneys from adult kidneys?
2. What are the primary functions of the kidneys in children?
3. How does age influence kidney function and overall renal health in pediatric patients?

2.2. Common Pediatric Kidney Disorders

Learning Outcome

1. Congenital anomalies of the kidney and urinary tract (CAKUT)
2. Glomerular diseases in children
3. Urinary tract infections (UTIs) and their implications

The pediatric kidney disease spectrum is characterized by a wide range of disorders, each with diagnostic and management issues unique unto itself. The most prevalent cause of chronic kidney disease (CKD) in children is congenital ano the kidney and CAKUT and accounts for approximately 30% of children with CKD. These congenital abnormalities, such as, such as renal agenesis and obstructive uropathies, demand coordinated attention between urologists and pediatric nephrologists to treat complex issues of bladder function and possible surgical intervention. As children grow up to be adults, understanding the impact of CAKUT on long-term outcomes of the kidneys becomes more essential, thus emphasizing the need for an integrated approach in clinical management. Another significant area in pediatric nephrology is the development and management of mineral and bone diseases (MBD) of chronic kidney disease. According to current clinical practice guidelines, close monitoring of calcium nutrition is essential in this population since both an excessive level and a deficient level of calcium enhance nephrocalcinosis and weaken bone strength. Recommendations involve maintaining calcium intake at an age-adjusted level of 800–1000 mg/day, closely monitoring for the risk of adverse balances, which can exacerbate renal bone disease further. Pediatric nephrologists must actively incorporate interventions for MBD not only to optimize bone but also to decrease renal-related complications as patients advance through age and enter adulthood (Evenepoel et al., 2023). Pediatric patients with kidney disease are at variable risk based on their respective condition, which influences short- and long-term consequences of their health. Apart from CAKUT, children are also susceptible to lower urinary tract obstruction (LUTOh can be the result of anatomical abnormalities and, if not treated, will lead to severe renal damage. In disorders such as, such as posterior urethral valves (PUV), prenatal imaging for early diagnaffect early intervention that is crucial for improving prognosis. Although newer modalities of fetal intervention, such as, such as vesicoamniotic shunting and endoscopic ablation, hold promise, long-term follow-up evaluation of bladder and kidney function remains necessary to prevent end-stage renal disease (ESRD) in adulthood. The appreciation of such intricate interaction between congenital anomalies and ensuing kidney function highlights the importance of comprehensive management strategies in pediatric nephrology (Rebecca et al., 2022) (Figure 2.5).

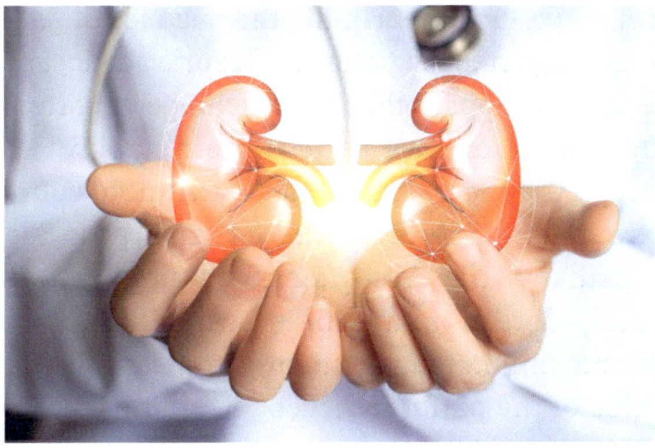

Figure 2.5. Conceptual image of kidneys held in a healthcare professional's hands, symbolizing renal care and the importance of kidney health.

Source: https://www.everccom/wp-content/uploa022/08/shutterstock_598101971-scaled.jpg.

2.2.1. Congenital Anomalies of the Kidney and Urinary tract Tract (CAKUT)

CAKUT are is a wide category of disorders that affect renal and urinary tract development, with a compromise on the quality of life and health of the children. CAKUT consists of structural defects that are detected prenatally or in early postnatal life and include renal agenesis, hydronephrosis, and posterior urethral vUV). There is a need to compreheT in pediatric nephrology since early intervention and diagnosis are achievable prior tobefore developing complications such as, such as repeated UTIs and renal insufficiency, ultimately leading to end-stage renal disease (ESRD). The value of a comprehensive definition of CAKUT as a broad term serves effective diagnosis and treatment approaches to the benefit of clinical practice in children affected (Knoers et al., 2022). Investigations have shown that CAKUT is a prevalent condition in children, with reported prevalence rates in as many as 20% of children with renal abnormalities. Curiously enough, the male-to-female ratio for CAKUT is approximately 4.4:1, which shows greater susceptibility in males. Presentation age is generally during the first year of life, and this underlines the need for thorough screening of newborns and infants. In patient cohorts examined, PUV is also one of the most frequent types of CAKUT, where most children with the condition presented with bladder and collecting system malformations (Okoronkwo et al., 2016).

These phenotypic differences not only complicate management at the clinical level but also determine genetic and environmental factors in the etiology of CAKUT (Okoronkwo et al., 2016). The relationship between CAKUT and urinary tract infection is most serious because children with these malformations are most likely to develop UTI, which will increase renal damage and lead to long-term health consequences. Findings of studies are that approximately 42% of the children with CAKUT developed a UTI, and there existed a strong correlation between bladder abnormality and the incidence of UTI. Also, the resistance of antibiotics is a significant factor in managing the infection because most of the first-line drugs become ineffective as resistant bacterial organisms multiply more frequently. This makes the application of individualized antibiotic prophylaxis necessary for high-risk patients, particularly PUV patients. There is a need for continuous monitoring and further studies to identify the effective treatment protocols and achieve the long-term impact of CAKUT on renal function and the health of children (Okoronkwo et al., 2016) (Figure 2.6).

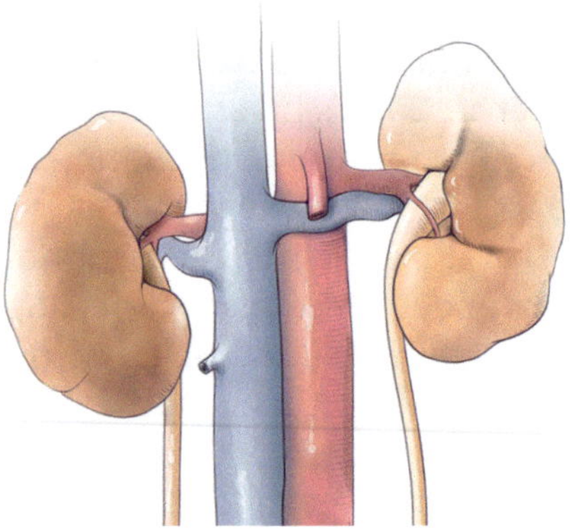

Figure 2.6. Anatomical illustration of the human urinary system, highlighting the kidneys, ureters, and associated blood vessels.

Source: https://pediatricsnationwide.org/wp-content/uploads/2021/01/Urinary-system-No-Background-kidney-header-1024x575.jpg.

2.2.2. Glomerular Diseases in Children

Glomerular diseases in children constitute a significant area of interest in pediatric nephrology, as they may lead to long-term morbidity if not properly diagnosed and treated early. Among the most prevalent glomerular diseases in children are minimal change disease (MCD) and focal segmental glomerulosclerosis (FSGS). MCD is most commonly observed in preschool-aged children and is typically characterized by edema and massive proteinuria.

Although prognosis with corticosteroid therapy is generally favorable, recurrences are common. For FSGS, however, it is more challenging due to the unpredictable course of the disease and response to treatment, some of which may result in end-stage renal disease. Pediatric nephrologists need to have an understanding of the pathophysiology and clinical presentations of these disorders to develop appropriate treatment modalities and improve patient outcomes. The long-term outcome of glomerular diseases in children is a crucial aspect in pediatric nephrology. Research has shown that survivors can experience persistent renal impairment and resultant complications like hypertension and chronic kidney disease (CKD) in adulthood.

For example, in a study of childhood sarcoma survivors, it was seen that about 10% of the survivors had features of CKD on long-term follow-up, underlining the need for ongoing monitoring in these patients. Despite advances in therapeutic approaches, a percentage of patients may still experience toxicity from nephrotoxic therapy they received during their initial course of treatment. Therefore, there is an urgent need for pediatric nephrologists to employ methods of early detection and intervention in order to offer maximum management throughout the life course of the patient, thereby avoiding possible long-term renal outcome (Andreoli et al., 2018). Advances in research have encouraged improved understanding of the distinctive aspects of glomerular disease in children, particularly with disorders like IgA nephropathy (IgAN) and IgA vasculitis (IgAV).

A recent study has illuminated clinical presentation differences between the two conditions, with children with IgAV presenting at a younger age and higher estimated glomerular filtration rates compared to those with IgAN. This has implications for treatment, with children with IgAV increasingly being treated with immunosuppressants. Distinguishing these differences lies at the heart of the pediatric nephrologist's practice, as it informs directed treatment that is responsive to each condition's specific requirements. By broadening the foundation provided by ongoing research work, an improved understanding of pediatric glomerular diseases will further elucidate the best practices in pediatric nephrology (Ambruzs et al., 2018) (Figure 2.7).

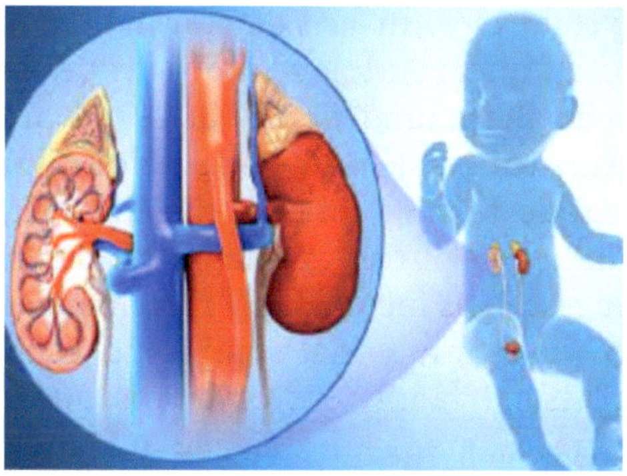

Figure 2.7. Glomerular diseases in children represent a significant area of concern within pediatric nephrology.

Source: https://encrypted-tbn0.gstatic.com/images?q=tbn:ANd9GcTpCn4-v6CJTOgclza_bqVB1fAuzxrpzMTGWLeKilungW-u3EYtwXFHy75SYR8_fAu0vuI&usqp=CAU.

2.2.3. Urinary Tract Infections (UTIs) and Their Implications

High incidence of UTIs in children warrants serious attention in pediatric nephrology. UTIs are among the most common infections that children present with, often resulting in acute illness as well as chronic complicationst adequately treated. Contributing to the fact that UTIs are common in children is the presence of anatomical abnormalities, like those which that predispose to recurring infections. The implications of such infections can be profound, ranging from scarring of the kidneys to chronic kidney disease and hypertension. More precisely, the link between recurrent UTIs and nephrological complications brings to the fore the importance of early diagnosi and effective interventions. In a bid to reduce such risks, understanding the causative determinants of UTIs is crucial for implementing multi-faceted management approaches. The relationship between urinary tract infections and other renal diseases is complex, as evidenced in new studies that reveal the immediate and distant impacts of UTInal function. UTI can present itself in children in any of several signs, from easy urinary manifestations to more perilous consequences such as, such as pyelonephritis, which ultimately lead to renal injury. When recurrent UTI patients are being considered, nephrologists must consider the susceptibility of underlying abnormalities to increase the risk of infection. Vesicoureteral reflux, for example, has the potential to contrnificantly to perpetuating UTIs and therefore increase the risk of renal damage. Besides, the relation of UTIs with metabolic conditions, such as, such as urolithiasis, makes the clinical situation even more complicated and calls for multidisciplinary treatment and management (Velásquez-Forero et al., 1978). In addition, long-term effects of urinary tract infections do not end at the acute phase but typically affect a child' of life in addition to long-term kidney function. Recurrent UTIs in pediatric patients can also give rise to psychosocial complications, such as, such as concern about repeated medical visigma due to incontinence. In addition, the potential for urinary tract infections to evolve into more serious nephrological complications, such as, such as chronic kidney disease, is a concerning issue for healthcare providers. In this respect, attention to prevention through proper hygiene education and early intervention programs is paramount. Also, ongoing research into the pathophysiologic mechanisms of UTIs can provide data that will direct site-specific treatments towards ultimately reducing the incidence of such infections and their associated renal effects (Butani et al., 2017).

Test Your Knowledge

1. What are the common glomerular diseases seen in children, and how do they typically present?
2. What are the implications of recurrent urinary tract infections (UTIs) on kidney health in pediatric patients?

2.3. Diagnostic Approaches in Pediatric Nephrology

Learning Outcome

1. Clinical evaluation and history taking
2. Laboratory tests and imaging studies
3. Role of renal biopsy in diagnosis

For pediatric nephrology, diagnostic practice for diseases like UTIs is essential to the care of children's health. Due to renal injury and subsequent complications, further testing after proven UTI is justified. However, a systematic review demonstrates that the majority of standard proposed diagnostics are useless for the prevention of recurrent infection or renal scarring. The results suggest that regular imaging will not yield much, and clinicians are mpelled to look at diagnostic protocols that have so far been applied routinely. More specifically, the study suggests that less invasive tests such as, such as ultrasound, have their limitations in ruling out upper urinary tract infection or renal scarring, and that a review of current policies and the implementation of improved, evidence-based practices are necessary in the diagnostic process (Biggi et al., 2005). A further significant aspect of pediatric nephrology's diagnostic approach is autosomal dominant polycystic kidney disease (ADPKD) in asymptomatic children at risk. The latest guidelines by an expert panel, including pediatric nephrologists and patient advocates, have suggested a convergence of continued observation and immediate diagnostic screening for the disease. Ultrasonography is the diagnostic test of preference for screening, offering a non-invasive way to detect renal cysts, the hallmark lesion of ADPKD. The shortcomings of sonography underscore the value of precise diagnostic criteria because a negative result does not entirely exclude the diagnosis in children. This complexity demands personalized surveillance methods, primarily among children with a risk factor in their family, to offer an intervention at the right time when required (Bergmann et al., 2019). Moreover, the utilization of new-generation imaging and genetic testing reflects the evolving face of pediatric nephrology diagnosis strategies. Genetic testing is increasingly recommended for infants who show initial symptoms, especially if there is no family history. This allows for better assessment of disease advancement and linical decision-making, but as more widespread treatment becomes available, practitioners must recognize the nuances of pharmacologic management, such as, such as selective and appropriate applicationopressin antagonists and statin choice. Further research into successful treatment remains necessary, including considering lifestyle modification such as, such as salt intake on renal health. Lastly, these diagnostic and treatment developments are aimed at enhancing patient outcomes and alleviating the long-term impacts of pediatric kidney conditions (Bergmann et al., 2019) (Figure 2.8).

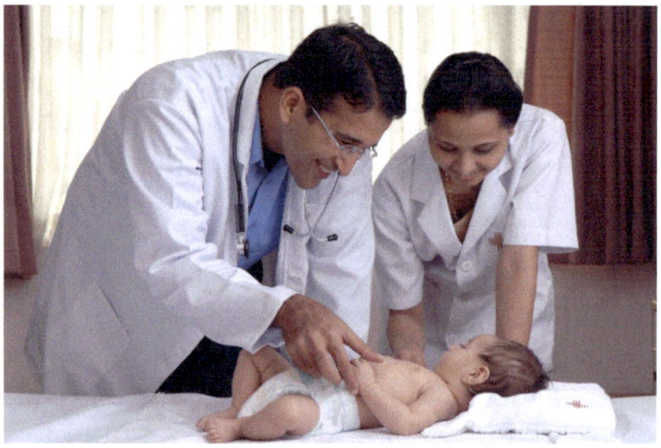

Figure 2.8. Diagnostic approaches in pediatric nephrology.

Source: https://www.sitarambhartia.org/wp-content/uploads/2017/12/DSC_5932-1024x680.jpg.

2.3.1. Clinical Evaluation and History Taking

In pediatric nephrology, history taking and clinical assessment are central components that inform diagnosis and treatment of children with kidney disease. A thorough clinical history is not just the child's medical history but also hereditary patterns of kidney disease, urinary symptoms, and co-morbid conditions that compound renal impairment. Specific inquiries should focus on the child's growth and development, diet, and fluid intake since these are crucial aspects of renal health. Clinicians can tailor their assessment and intervention accordingly based on the knowledge of a child's nuances of presentation and experience with the disease. The intertwining of this broad historical background with clinical findings forms a foundation upon which educated guesses can be made regarding potential nephrological illness and upon which further research and treatment can be aimed. Physical examination plays an equally important role in the clinical assessment of the child suspected of having renal illness. Providers must conduct a thorough examination that includes vital signs assessment, palpation of the abdomen for tenderness or masses, checking for dehydration or edema on the skin, and a genitourinary examination. The presence of hypertension, increasingly known to be an issue in children too, similarly needs to be takct throughout the clinical evaluation course, as outlined in recent guidelines for its increasing trend and importance to cardiovascular health (Agabiti-RoseiLurbe et al., 2016). Moreover, differentiation of primary renal illness from illnesses involving systemic manifestations with renal importance is necessary as well. These variations may guide management and refer to specialists if necessary to provide timely intervention in conditions like acute kidney injury or chronic kidney disease. In the case of pediatric nephrology, investigations by way of laboratory and imaging studies the immediate alternatives after history taking and initial clinical evaluation. Interpretation of urinalysis results is crucial because any variation such as, such as proteinuria or hematuria will be highly informative for kidney pathologies that may be present. Furthermore, imaging modalities, including ultrasonographic assessments, can offer non-invasive means of visualizing anatomical disorganization or obstructions that possibly may be responsible for the child's renal presentation. Notably, definitions and paradigms for the diagnosis of illnesses like acute kidney injury (AKI) and chronic kidney disease (CKD) have been made more standardized, assisting clinicians to rightly diagnose these in pediatric patients (Dewitte et al., 2017). A complete understanding of the relationship between history, physical examination, and diagnostic testing ultimately enables clinicians to properly implement management plans tailored to the unique needs of pediatric patients with renal disease.

2.3.2. Laboratory Tests and Imaging Studies

In pediatric nephrology, the evaluation of kidney disease relies heavily on laboratory investigations and imaging studies. These are essential for identifying underlying pathologies responsible for renal dysfunction. Comprehensive laboratory assessment typically includes urine and blood analyses, with emphasis on markers such as serum creatinine, blood urea nitrogen (BUN), and the urinary protein-to-creatinine ratio (UPCR). These parameters are critical for assessing glomerular filtration and proteinuria, aiding in the diagnosis of conditions such as nephrotic syndrome. For example, elevated urinary protein excretion is characteristic of minimal change disease (MCD) and focal segmental glomerulosclerosis (FSGS), two prominent pediatric glomerular disorders (Mariani et al., 2022). Accurate interpretation of these results is imperative to guide clinical management and therapeutic decisions. Imaging studies further support the diagnostic process by enabling visualization of renal anatomy and pathology. Ultrasound is usually the first-line modality because it is non-invasive, readily available, and effective for evaluating kidney size, structure, obstruction, and cystic disease. Doppler ultrasound additionally provides information on renal blood flow, aiding in the detection of vascular abnormalities such as renal artery stenosis. Advanced imaging techniques, particularly magnetic resonance imaging (MRI), offer superior resolution for renal tissue assessment and can detect subtle pathology not evident on ultrasound. MRI is particularly valuable in complex cases and in pre-surgical planning (Bryan et al., 2021).

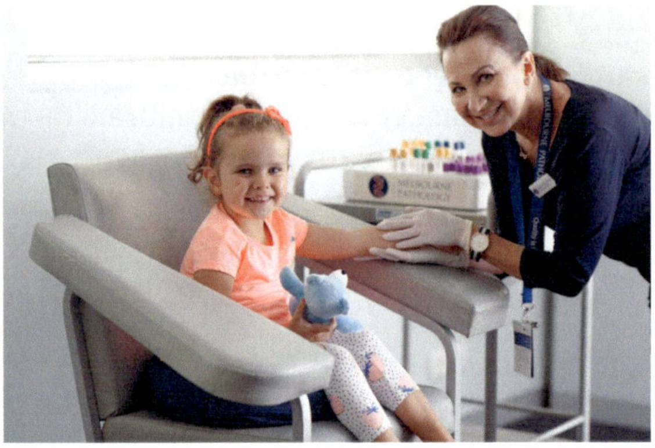

Figure 2.9. In pediatric nephrology, the evaluation of kidney conditions is fundamentally reliant on laboratory tests and imaging studies.

Source: https://www.mps.com.au/media/7210/chloe-and-donna-to-camera.jpg.

The integration of imaging tests contributes to worldwide understanding of a child's renal condition and is significant in guiding treatment. Additionally, integration of imaging tests and laboratory testing is also significant in advancing individualized treatment plans for children with nephrology. For instance, correlation between specific laboratory markers and imaging findings can facilitate the establishment of molecular profiles that are predictive of disease outcome and response apy. Recent studies have also identified key molecular pathways shared in children with MCD and FSGS, suggesting potential biomarkers for outcome prediction such as, such as activation of the tumor necrosis factor (TNF) pathway (Mariani et al., 2022). Future investigation utilizing integrated approaches will likely enhance individualized therapy in these conditions, designing interventions based on each patient's profile. Therefore, continuing development and application of laboratory tests and imaging techniques will remain central to the improvement of outcomes and management of pediatric nephrology (Figure 2.9).

2.3.3. Role of Renal Biopsy in Diagnosis

In pediatric nephrology, the diagnostic value of renal biopsy is valuable in offering profound insight into various renal patho This technique allows for direct visualization of kidney tissue, which allows clinicians to establiexact etiology of kidney disease. In challenging cases such as, such as nephrotic syndrome or acute interstitial nephritis, often non-invasive diagnostic methods such as, such as imaging and urinalysis may not yield sufient information. The precise histological evaluation offered by renal biopsy not only enables correct diagnosis but also facilitates appropriate treatment strategies to for the specific pathology identified. Hence, kidney biopsy has emerged as a critical diagnostic tool in pediatric nephrology, providing direct histopathological insight into renal tissue. It plays a pivotal role in distinguishing between different glomerular diseases, assessing the extent of chronic damage, and guiding therapeutic decisions. By correlating biopsy findings with clinical and laboratory data, pediatric nephrologists can determine prognosis, tailor individualized treatment plans, and monitor disease progression more effectively. Moreover, renal biopsy can be critical to the differential diagnosis between acute and chronic kidney disease, which require very different management. For instance, in acute kidney injury (AKI), discrimination between pre-renal, intrinsic, and post-renal etiologies often requires histopathological confirmation. Renal biopsike a diagnosis of glomerular diseases, interstitial nephritis, or vascular diseases, thus settling on the treatment options. Recent advances in molecular diagnostics, such as, such as the identification of specific patterns of gene expression associated with rejection, refer the evolving role of renal biopsy in contemporary nephrology. Studies have determined that a subset of biomarkers of expression in allograft biopsies can provide insights on into the presence of acute rejection, further solidifying the biopsy's role in diagnostic and prognostic applications (Bestard et al., 2019). In children, where kidney disease is different from that in adults, the function of renal biopsy is extended to cover not only diagnostic needs but also long-term care and follow-up. By establishing pathology, clinicians can more effectively track disease progression and treatment response. Similarly, as with recent studies, some gene expressions associated with rejection correspond strongly to histological markers of graft injury. This interconnectivity provides room for innovative methods for the care of pediatric patients post-transplant, delineating the kidney's flexibility as well as the need for precise tracking. The becoming norm of renal biopsies within clinical practice directs to their inherent function, not only for initial diagnosis but also for ongoing follow-up and treatment of pediatric renal diseases (Butler et al., 2017).

Test Your Knowledge

1. Why are detailed clinical evaluation and history taking essential in diagnosing pediatric kidney disorders?
2. How do laboratory tests and imaging studies assist in identifying and monitoring kidney diseases in children?
3. What is the role of renal biopsy in confirming the diagnosis of pediatric nephrological conditions?

2.4. Treatment Modalities in Pediatric Nephrology

Learning Outcome

1. Pharmacological interventions
2. Dietary management and lifestyle modifications
3. Surgical options for kidney disorders

The pediatric nephrology treatment modalities are diverse and encompass the entire spectrum oities used to treat a wide variety of renal afflictions in children. Among the most common issues treated are UTIs, which, if not treated, can lead to severe consequences such as, such as renal scarring. Current studies indicate that the benefit of standard imaging in children with proven UTIs may not reduce the risk of repeat infection or kidney damage significantlnderlines the need for a particular strategy to further management and investigation with an emphasis on patient outcomes, and on consideration of new imaging techniques, such as, such as contrast-enhanced ultrasound, that offer benefits without exposing young patients to ionizing radiation (Biggi et al., 2005). The refinement ofotocols for UTIs thus requires further study, particularly in determining the most suitable investigation strategies. In acute kidney injury (AKI) patients, therapy most often isis most often dictated by the etiology and the general condition of the child. Children are particularly vulnerable to AKI due to dehydration, infection, and renal toxic drugs. The presence of a malignancy makes it even more complicated, with patients of pediatric oncology having frequent development of AKI secondary to both the disease process and treatment regimes. Current literature suggests that the pathogenesis of AKI in children is similar to that in adults, with a focus mainly on prerenal pathology and acute tubular necrosis. However, specific aspects of pediatric nephrology place a distinctive clinical approach, most importantly, the potential for developing chronic kidney disease after AKI. Completeness of care involves awareness of these underlying risks in addition to the application of effective renal replacement treatments when required, thus creating the optimal possible path towards recovery for such at-risk patients (Benoit et al., 2016). Multidisciplinary care models are also applicable in pediatric nephrology.

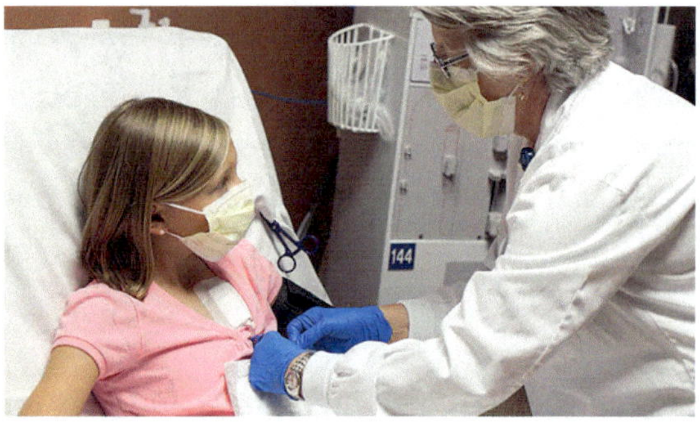

Figure 2.10. Treatment modalities in pediatric nephrology.

Source: https://www.mayoclinic.org/-/media/kcms/gbs/patient-consumer/images/2019/07/09/17/59/nephrology-dept-8col-3202981-0014.jpg.

The treatment modalities extend beyond pharmacologic intervention and can include nutritional management, psychosocial care, and ongoing education of families. For instance, for chronic kidney disease, dietary modifications and adherence to medications prescribed are critical elements that may have a significant bearing on the severity of disease and quality of life. The psychological toll of children with chronic renal disease also requires multi-dimensional support systems to address their emotional and developmental issues. As clinicians and rers navigate the ever-changing field of pediatric nephrology, continued attention to treatment modalities, including the utilization of less invasive diagnostic methods and new therapytherapies, will serve to improve overall patient care and outcomes. Treatment modality should be individualized to the specific clinical and developmental requirements of the pediatric patient (Figure 2.10).

2.4.1. Pharmacological Interventions

Pharmacotherapy of pediatric nephrology is at the core of the management of many kidney diseases, and more importantly, in the field of hypertension, which has become a major problem among children and adolescents. The increasing prevalence of hypertension in this population necessitates having an extensive plan encompassing lifestyle modification as well as pharmacologic treatment based on the physiology of children. Contemporary guidelines present an emphasis on the accuracy of blood pressure measurement and the pathophysiology of isolated systolic hypertension. This better comprehension of hypertension in teens has resulted in clinicians adopting certain pharmacologic interventions that optimize both safety and efficacy. The clinicians must be kept informed of the evolving guidelines for such treaing on the integration of clinical expertise and scientific research to inform decision-making, thereby leading to more effective management strategies forensive children (Agabiti-RoseiLurbe et al., 2016). In addition to hypertension management, pharmacological therapy plays a key role in the management of specific pediatric nephropathies such as, such as autosomal dominant polycystic kidney disease (ADPKD). The introduction of pharmacotherapy in ADPKD treatment has opened up possibilities for the betterment of long-term outcomes among children with the condition. Present recommendations indicate the requirement for observation of manifestations of disease, including blood pressure and albuminuria, among children with a confirmed family history of ADPKD. Standard vasopressin antagonists are not usually recommended, but there is leeway for their off-label usage in specific cases where the benefit would outweigh the risks. Pediatric nephrologists are thus encouraged to use these therapeutic strategies judiciously, along with encouraging lifestyle modifications, particularly restriction of dietary salt intake, for disease control. Pharmacological interventions in the form of these customized treatments underscore vigilance in managing chronic kidney disease in the pediatric population (Bergmann et al., 2019). Pharmacological management also entails newer therapies for modulating the course of disease in the various nephropathies. Literature suggests conducting clinical trials and systematic reviews to better understand the effectiveness of the potential treatments. For instance, although using mTOR inhibitors and somatostatin analogues is currently not advised, the exploration of other pharmacological interventions could be useful in the future. In the area of pediatric nephrology, the necessity exists to develop regimens of treatment that not only are scientifically sound but also consider the development age of the child population. This, therefore, is prioritized by multidisciplinary consultations among nephrologists, pediatric geneticists, and dietitians to optimize care. Such a broad strategy exemplifies a commitment to enhancing children's therapeutic benefits from renal diseases, and it shows the constantly evolving nature of pharmacotherapy in pediatric nephrology (Bergmann et al., 2019).

2.4.2. Dietary Management and Lifestyle Modifications

In pediatric nephrology, nutrition is a core component in the treatment and management of children with kidney disease. The intake of nutrients can play a dramatic role in the progression and complications of kidney disease. For instance, high sodium intake has been directly associated with the onset of hypertension, a condition that is very much on the rise among chihas been noted by recent studies, dietary approaches focusing on reduced intake of sodium are important in managing hypertension in children. In addition, fruits, vegetables, and whole grains inclusion may result in better health outcomes, thereby minimizing the dans associatd with cardiovascular diseases among the vulnerable group. The dietary recommendations suggested for management are also a cruciafor pediatric nephrologists and dietitians, hey equips families with appropriate information to be able to make improved food choices suitable to the child's individual requirements (Agabiti-RoseiLurbe et al., 2016). Lifestyle interventions such as, such as physical activity and behavior change strategies, serve the same purpose in the overall management of pediatric kidney patients. Children with metabolic syndrome and chronic kidney disease (CKD) must be encouraged to exercise regularly in order to promote cardiovascular health, weight management, and general health. The Pediatric Renal Nutrition Taskforce recommends an individualized exercise plan based on the age, stage of CKD, and personal function of the child. Physical exercise not only helps in the maintenance of optimal body weight but also synergistically interacts with dietary changes to minimize long-term kidney disease complications. Counseling and education can benefit children and families in behalf of successful behavior change, reinforcing an interactive process towards maximizing favorable health behaviors and lifestyle change (Anderson et al., 2021). These comprehensive strategies pave the way for better management and outcome. The clinical role of care providers has an important role in guiding dietetic management and lifestyle changes in pediatric nephrology. Dietitians and pediatric nephrologists must collaborate to develop individualized care plans addressing both physical activity and dietary needs. This partnership ensures that treatment regimens are informed by the latest evidence-based guidelines, which outline the risks and management choices specific to childhood obesity and metabolic syndrome and their potential effects on the kidney. Through ongoing surveillance of food consumption and lifestyle modification, significant improvements can be achieved towards kidney function restoration and the avoidance of complications. Moreover, ongoing education and support from the family work to consolidate these changes, involving them in their child's health journey. By acquiring a comprehensive, interdisciplinary approach, healthcare teams are able to effectively enhance the quality of life in children with kidney disease (Anderson et al., 2021) (Figure 2.11).

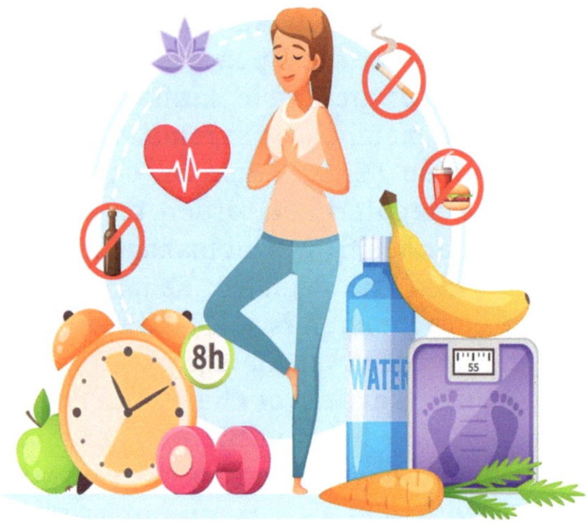

Figure 2.11. Dietary management and lifestyle modifications.

Source: https://i0.wp.com/curaadvancedphysiotherapy.in/wp-content/uploads/2023/06/screenshot-2023-06-07-4.32.50-pm.png?resize=474%2C402&ssl=1.

2.4.3. Surgical Options for Kidney Disorders

Surgical interventions for pediatric kidney disease are increasingly important to correct a variety of conditions, from congenital defects to acquired disease. These surgical interventions include nephrectomy, involving the excision of a whole kidney, and nephron-sparing operations to excise only the affected portions of the kidney while preserving as much of the normal tissue as possible. These procedures can be critical in cases of renal tumors, hydronephrosis, or sepsis. Furthermore, the therapy for diseases in children's kidneys is often tailored to prevent complications without impairing kidney function, particularly since children are establishing their own renal systems. Improvements in surgical technique, including minimal-access laparoscopy, have contributed to shorter recovery times and better results in infant and juvenile patients with kidney disease. In addition, children patients may require surgical corrections for urologic conditions affecting overall kidney function. Vesicoureteral reflux, through which urine flows back from the bladder towards the kidneys, typically will be surgically corrected to prevent recurrent urinary tract infection and subsequent kidney damage. One of the common surgeries employed to fix urinary flow is ureteral reimplantation. Another major procedure is pyeloplasty, which is to relieve renal pelvis obstruction, and this can lead to increased pressure within the kidney and potential damage. These surgical interventions are not only the key to preserving kidney function but overall long-term health of the urinary tract system within children. Increasing understanding and application of these operative techniques are in line with the g field of pediatric nephrology, focused on optimizing outcomes with emerging treatment strategies. As part of its efforts to identify superior management strategies for pediatric kidney disease, nes such as, such as the American Association for the Study of Liver Diseases direct practice. While these suggestions are largely applied to liver transplant candidacy, candidacy procedures in interventions such as, such as kidney transplantation mirror each other in assessing patient candidacy on a person's health record (Steven et al., 2020). In cases where conventional surgical intervene not available or fail, kidney transplantation can be the most viable option for end-stage renal disease patients. Transplantation requires proper evaluation, including comorbid and psychosocial evaluation, prior tobefore the transplant to ensure the success of the surgery and long-term health of the child. Combining surgical decision-making with comprehensive care can set young patients on the track toward better lives, as pediatric nephrology gets progressively better, leading to increasingly successful treatment modalities for kidney disorders.

Test Your Knowledge

1. What pharmacological interventions are commonly used to manage pediatric kidney disorders?
2. How do dietary management and lifestyle modifications contribute to kidney health in children?
3. When are surgical options indicated for treating pediatric kidney disorders?

2.5. Long-Term Management and Follow-Up

Learning Outcome

1. Importance of regular monitoring
2. Transitioning care from pediatric to adult nephrology
3. Psycholoupport for affected families

Follow-up and care of pediatric nephrology in the long term are necessary in order to gble results to children with kidney disease. Monitoring the patients on a regular basisregularly enables doctors to assess renal function, detect indicators of worsening, and make effective interventions in a timely mannerpromptly. Patients with chronic kidney disease (CKD) must be managed meticulously in order to prevent the progression of disease and eventually end-stage renal disD). Regular follow-up, targeted educational interventions, and age-specific counseling tremendously increase a child's adherence to treatment protocols. Additionally, the psychosocial management of chronic illnesses, such as, such as the reduction of anxiety and allowing family involvement, also significantly contributes to a child's long-term success in the maintenance of their renal status. In children, the interrelatedness of AKI and CKD is ever more recognized, reflecting the importance of long-term follow-up. The KDIGO guidelines are the essential blueprints for the definitions of AKI and CKD, highlighting the importance of early diagnosis and ongoing monitoring of renal function. Evolution to AKD from AKI may highlight the value of multimodal management plans, which are just in the process of evolving. These interventions need to be a synergy of medical and lifestyle so that children can manar illness effectively. Follow-up appointments enable routine modification of treatment plans based on kidney function tests, enabling normalization of renal function where possible. Furthermore, neoplastic conditions such as, such as primary renal lymphoma present the biggest challenge in long-term management of children with renal manifestations. A case of a child diagnosed with primary renal lymphoma, initially presenting with chronic kidney disease, highlights the importance of differential diagnosis in children. The child ultimately recovered well with aggressive chemotherapy, regaining renal function effectively despite residual functional impairment secondary to therapy. These experiences underscore the need for nephrologists to remain vigilant for potential underlying malignancies in children with unexplained renal issues, reinforcing the role of multi-disciplinary approaches in optimizing long-term results. Maintaining strong comprehensive follow-up protocols guarantees that treatment is not just reactive but also proactive, foreseeing complications ahead of time before they become serious issues (Figure 2.12).

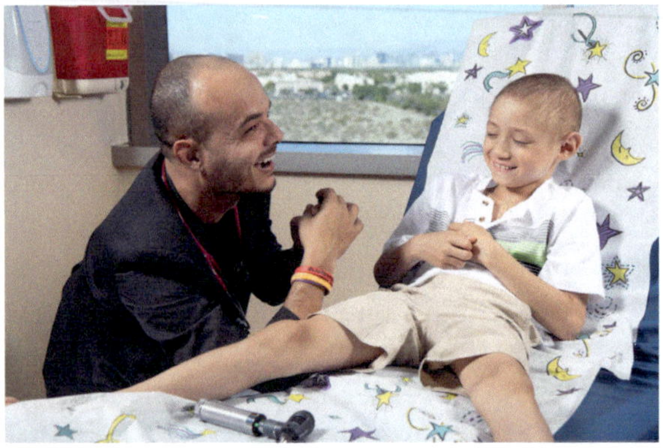

Figure 2.12. Long-term management and follow-up in pediatric nephrology.

Source: https://cure4thekids.org/wp-content/uploads/2020/02/C4K_Longterm-Followup_03-1024x683.jpg.

2.5.1. Importance of Regular Monitoring

In pediatric nephrology, frequent observation cannot be overstressed since it is critical in early intervention and treatment of renal disorders. Children, unlike adults, are susceptible to rapid changes in physiology, and thus their medical practitioners must closely observe renal function. Regular monitoring allows for early recognition of any potential abnormalities, including proteinuria or hypertension, that can lead to advanced complications if not treated. Using formalized monitoring guidelines allows for an environment where pediatric nephrologists can detect and treat these problems before they develop furtherafeguarding the long-term health outcomes and well-being of the child. Moreover, regular monitoring is also vital in staying abreast of the evolving clinical profile of childhood hypertension, a new public health problem. Increasing The increasing prevalence of hypertension among children and adolescents necessitates that physicians be attuned to the nuances of blood pressure management. Standardization of monitoring tools, including the utilization of centralized blood pressure values, allows for more accurate measurement of hypertension among youthsted by recent guidelines, the integration of systematic monitoring into practice functions to identify persons at risk and implement effective treatment interventions that are specifically tailored to the child population (Agabiti-RoseiLurbe et al., 2016). In addition to the mere prevention of short-term cardiovascular risks, such vigilance also helps reduce the risk of long-term health complications of elevated blood pressure. Lastly, integrating mentorship in pediatric nephrology enhances the value of regular monitoring thrthe imposition of a culture of continuous learning and personal development. Mentorship-mentee sessions can be key in training would-be nephrologists to prioritize regular checks, thereby reinforcing best practices in patient care (BradyVasylyeva et al., 2019). These affiliations not only provide clinical guidance but also encourage innovation in monitoring and treatment adherence strategies. Active communication through mentorship encourages youthful professionals to listen to the integral value of regular patient assessment, leading to better health outcomes for children suffering from nephrological diseases. By instilling these values early in their professional development, qualified professionals will be best placed to tackle possible health issues effectively throughout their careers.

2.5.2. Transitioning Care from Pediatric to Adult Nephrology

Transition of care from pediatric to adult nephrology is an important phase of care for adolescents who have kidney disease. Effective transition ensures continuity of care with the handling of the adolescent's unique psychosocial and medical needs. Doctors know that this transition is likely to occur at a susceptible period in the lives of adolescents, when there are high rates of non-adherence to treatment and allograft loss for transplanted kidneys. Research points out that though clinicians realize the importance of successful transitions, the use of systematic processes is sporadic, which can significantly impact outcomes. The absence of written policies that are a causative factor for this lack of consistency indicates the necessity of an even more harmonized approach that transitions care into the individual patient's context and promotes a smoother transition phase of adjustment into adult healthcare settings (Bethe et al., 2017). This conversion of pediatric to adult nephrology is not only medical in content but also involves understanding the psychological and social dynamics involved in this conversion for the adolescent. New health care providers, treatment protocols, and increased self-managed participation in their own medical care are all things that young patients have to get used to as part of this conversion. This process is particularly challenging for kidney transplant patients or those with chronic kidney disease because they might have to navigate complex treatment regimens and lifestyle modifications. Establishing an environment that supports open communication among healthcare teams and patients can greatly simplify this process. Additionally, equipping adolescents with self-management skills is critical to empowering them in their own health care, thereby inducing compliance and improving long-term outcomes (ADQI 26 workgroup et al., 2024). Furthermore, healthcare systems need to develop transitional care services that target the needs of young adult patients with kidney disease. Such services should integrate pediatric and adult nephrology services to facilitate a transition process. Recognizing that specialties may possess disparate structuractice, collaboration between pediatric and adult nephrologists, nurses, and psychosocial staff becomes a necessity. The multidisciplinary team facilitates practitioners to address matters that present during the process of transition, such as, such as mismatches in the expectation of treatment and care. Tailored interventions that recognize the richness of each patient's unique experience, as well as considering the structural variables of healthcare provision, are crucial for the achievement of successful transitions. Lastly, transitional care must become the focus of attention of the nephrology community so that the health outcomes of young adults during this critical transformation can be improved by streamlining (Bethe et al., 2017) (Figure 2.13).

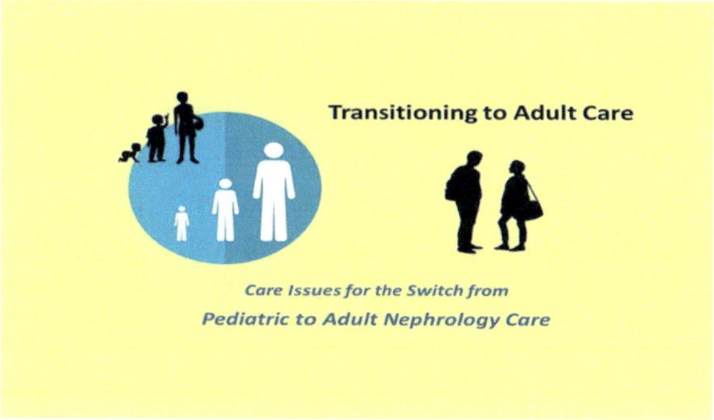

Figure 2.13. Transitioning care from pediatric to adult nephrology.

Source: https://www.ahusallianceaction.org/wp-content/uploads/2020/01/transition-border-Pedi-to-Adult-1.jpg.

2.5.3. Psychological and Social Support for Affected Families

Diseases of pediatric nephrology are likely to impose a heavy emotional and social burden on the involved families due to the chronic illness of a child. The caregiving stress could lead to isolation and helplessness among family members, including siblings who may have difficulty managing their own emotional responses to an ill sibling. Research indicates that such healthy siblings perceive their home life in a different manner than other families, sacrificing time with their peers to care for their sick sibling. This new paradigm has the power to yield rich emotional experience, which is defined by ambivalence and feelings of inadequacy when handling these new roles in the family setup (Madill et al., 2007). Thus, strong psychological support is essential for both siblings and parents to help them talk about their feelings and establish resilience by coping with their respective problems. Social support then becomes a robust factor in lessening the psychological load of families. It is sary for families to establish connections with the extended family and peer support groups, which can help shatter the feeling of loneliness and provide a sense of belongingness. Emotional and practical support from extended family members have has been known to facilitate the adaptation of family relations under difficult circumstances. Furthermore, nurses and medical institutions are most critical in connecting families with access to support services and material resources based on their specific requirements. Social work, psychology, and nephrology can collaborate to devise a whole care environment that is most effective not just for the participating child but for wholies. By open communication and peer relationship formation, healthcare teams can normalize experience and thus improve emotional well-being (Bergmann et al., 2019). When families must deal with the intricacies of chronic childhood disease such as, such as nephrology-specific conditions, psychological and social support becomes increasingly essential in the long term during the development of the child. Extended interaction with both healthcare professionals and support systems may initiate coping strategies and adaptation behaviors resulting in emotional resilience. For instance, parents who have access to planned psychological interventions report improved overall family functioning and lower levels of stress. Regular consultations, guidance, and educational workshops can also allow family members to be prepared with knowledge and skills to overcome immediate as well as future challenges related to the child's health. Moreover, there needs to be an understanding of the changing dynamics with increasing children; support must be changed to accommodate the varied needs of growing siblings and parents, too. Eventually, an appropriate support system can greatly affect the mental well-being of families with pediatric nephrology, promoting an atmosphere encouraging emotional and social adjustment (Madill et al., 2007).

Test Your Knowledge

1. Why is regular monitoring important in the long-term management of pediatric kidney diseases?
2. What challenges and considerations are involved in transitioning care from pediatric to adult nephrology?
3. How do psychological and social support systems benefit children with kidney disorders and their families?

2.6. Current Research and Advances in Pediatric Nephrology

Learning Outcome

1. Innovations in treatment and technology
2. Genetic research and its implications
3. Future directions in pediatric nephrology

Significant progress has been made in pedlogy, particularly in the management of chronic kidney disease (CKD) and renal replacement therapy, in the past few years. The direction of the latest research is to emphasize early diagnosis and intervention by maintaining renal function in an effort to avoid long-term CKD complications in children. For instance, studies have established that close collaboration with pediatric nephrologists will improve outcomes for children with CKD because the condition will significantly affect their development and growth. Advances in renal imaging tools and biomarkers have allowed for early identification of renal abnormalities, leading to timely therapeutic options that optimize patient quality of life and prognosis. With evolving developments in pediatric nephrology, multi-disciplinary management is increasingly essential to deliver the best care according to the developmental requirements of the child. Adopting standardized treatment protocols for renal replacement therapy (RRT) is another milestone development in pediatric nephrology. These are based on international guidelines that are tailored to meet the unique requirements of the pediatric patient, unlike adults. Recent research has shown significant evidence about the timing of when to initiate dialysis, with some guidelines proposing initiation by peritoneal dialysis as the best way of preserving residual kidney function in children. Furthermore, the role of the multidisciplinary team is now more robust, including psychosocial care for the family and children receiving treatment. Future research will likely further simplify these guidelines, ultimately resulting in tailored treatment based on individual patient criteria, as technology and treatment protocols improve to offer increasingly more precise and efficient methods of managing renal failure in children (Watanabe et al., 2015). Moreover, pediatric nephrology is also witnessing advances in the transplantation practice, since this has become a primary treatment modality for end-stage renal disease (ESRD) in children. Current studies have considered the long-term outcomes of kidney transplant in children, emphasizing the importance of post-transplantation care and adherence to immunosuppression therapy.

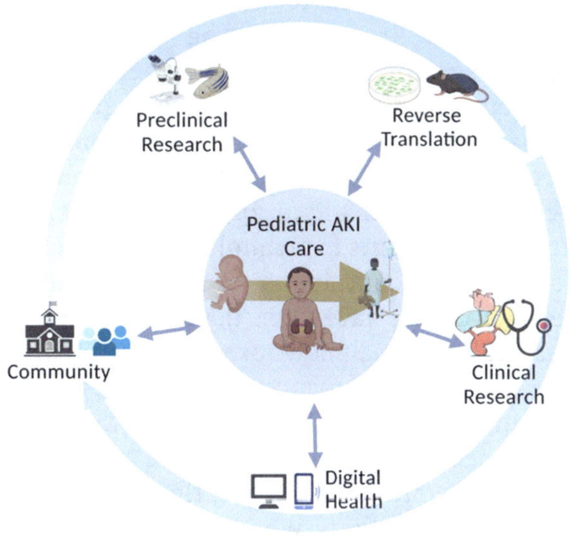

Figure 2.14. Current research and advances in pediatric nephrology.

Source: https://media.springernature.com/lw685/springer-static/image/art%3A10.1007%2Fs00467-023-06154-y/MediaObjects/467_2023_6154_Fig1_HTML.png.

New immunosuppressants have been developed that are designed specifically for use in pediatric patients, with a focus on reducing side effects while optimizing graft function. Research into the psychosocial dimension of transplantation also plays a significant role in addressing outcomes, as mental health and family function both have a direct impact on treatment adherence. As pediatric nephrology continues to advance, it is most critical that these new trends are embraced so that children with renal disease are afforded holistic and empathic care, tailored to their physiological and psychological needs (Kotanko et al., 2019) (Figure 2.14).

2.6.1. Innovations in Treatment and Technology

Over the last few years, pediatric nephrology has focused intensely on improving modalities of treatment of acute kidney injury (AKI) in children. Specifically, the evolution of neonate-specific extracorporeal therapies has changed the treatment for this age group dramatically. In the past, dialysis methods were borrowed from adults and proved less effective and difficult to apply to infants. Yet, with advancements in technology, machines like the dedicated continuous kidney replacement therapy (CKRT) have been developed, catering specifically to small newborns. These machines have a smaller extracorporeal volume, which prevents complications arising from the use of larger machines. This is reflective of a wider scientific revolution involving the treatment of neonates and infants who need acute kidney support, leading eventually to better outcomes and the overall quality of care provided to this group. Technology is essential in this discipline to address the unusual clinical challenges the pediatric nephrologists face during the contemporary period. Furthermore, advances in peritoneal dialysis and hemodialysis techniques contribute significantly to creating effective kidney replacement therapy for children. Peritoneal dialysis is well accepted as a first-line treatment since it can be applied even in the youngest patient due to its simplicity and effectiveness in the removal of excess fluid. On the other hand, HD offers rapid solute clearance but is plagued with a myriad of clinical issues in children, primarily vascular access and fluid management. The introduction of smaller catheter sizes has recently allows for better rates of blood flow without compromising safety, overcoming some previous disadvantages of HD in children. With such techniques advancing, pediatric nephrologists now have an increased capacity to individualize treatment for the individual patient, further enhancing the overall care of kidney disease in children. Additionally, studies have also paved the way for new possibilities in future pediatric nephrology developments in the shape of new biological therapies. Current investigations into the pathophysiology of kidney disease have established that additional insight can lead to new treatment regimens, particularly in relation to the management of such conditions as polycystic kidney disease. Emerging therapy modalities like gene therapy and regenerative medicine promise to provide significant therapeutic options forcongenital as well as acquired kidney diseases. For instance, as noted in manye application of new biopharmaceuticals can result in effective interventions that address the etiology of certain kidney disease rather than merely its symptoms. The future of pediatrics nephrology stands at the threshold of revolution, underlining the importance to integrateof integrating technological innovations and biological advancements tise the standard of care and enhance the outcome among patients in the field.

2.6.2. Genetic Research and Its Implications

The last few years have seen an increasing influence of the advances in genetics on the practice of pediatric nephrology, with the latter bringing to the light many congenital and hereditary diseases of the kidney. Most such diseases have a genetic basis and are reflected in the form of chronic kidney disease (CKD) during childhood. With increasing focus on precision medicine, genetic testing has become a must-have tool for doctors to detect specific mutations that lead to some renal illnesses. Genetic study, even in initial stages, not only illuminates the mechanisms of disease but also provides new avenues for targeted therapies. This research emphasizes the importance of family genetic history, especially among children, where recognizing patterinform preventive interventions and treatment plans that ultimately lead to better patient outcomes. Genetic discoveries are more than just diagnostic; they are also involved in clinical management strategies in pediatric nephrology. As an illustration, some gene mutations such as, such as the p.N215S mutation for Fabry disease, have been discovered to foretell some phenotypes and the level of disease severity. Evidence has shown that renal impairment among the p.N215S mutation patients rises with the progression of age, particularly among men, where the necessity for personal monitoring and treatment approaches considering genetic backgrounds is underscored (Brand et al., 2018). As genetic information becomes a part of the standard clinical assessment, medical practitioners can take proactive approaches to management that anticipate the prevention of future implications. This shift towards increased personalization of care not only enhances the quality of the care but also increpower of families to make decisions regarding their children's health trajectory. Genetic research also offers recommendations for public health policy aimed at early detection and intervention of pediatric kidney disease. Being aware that certain adverse early life events, such as, such as preterm birth or congenital abnormalities, predispose the development of CKD later in life, it is essential to establish top-level monitoring guidelines for risk populations (Schaefer et al., 2016). The background of genetic studies informs training programs aimed at sensitizing individuals regarding the interaction between genetic susceptibility and environmental factors influencing kidney health. By advocating for close monitoring and early intervention, public health organizations can ensure improved outcomes, allowing healthcare systems to focus their resources on the most at-risk children. Genetic science, thus, not only guides pediatric nephrology clinical practice but also takes a pivotal role in guiding broader health policy to ensure the impact of renal disease at an early age is averted (Figure 2.15).

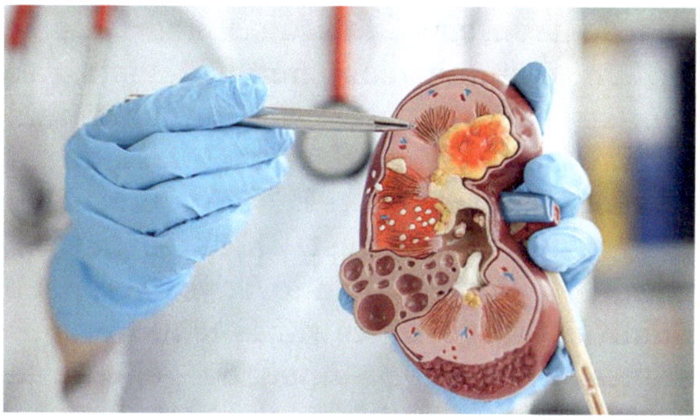

Figure 2.15. Genetic research and its implications.

Source: https://my.clevelandclinic.org/-/scassets/images/org/health/articles/24214-nephrologist.

2.6.3. Future Directions in Pediatric Nephrology

The future of pediatric nephrology is being shaped more and more by technological advancements, primarily in terms of substituting artificial intelligence (AI) anng. With the complexities of kidney diseases in children complicating diagnosis and treatment, AI supports nephrologists in reaching more accurate and timely decisions. The use of sophisticated algorithms in analyzing data can help identify risk factors, prognosis, and individualizing individualize treatment protocols. Such revolutionary technologies promise an enormous capacity to drive pediatric nephrology personalized medicine to new heights by providing therapies based on individual patient profiles. Further, AI-driven models bring prospects to make patient education and communication more efficient and effective, hence enhancing the overall quality of care. Thus, nephrologists must embrace these upcoming innovations in order to be ahead in pediatric care, triggering better patient management strategies towards improved patient experience (Miao et al., 2023). Apart from technological innovation, collaborative research initiatives are central to advancing pediatric nephrology. Interdisciplinary studies between pediatricians, nephrologists, and scientists can accelerate the understanding of kidney disease and its manifestation in children. Collaborative research is crucial not only for developing best practices but also for the development of innovative therapeutic modalities targeted towards children. For instance, knowledge gained by genetic and genomic research can form the basis for novel interventions and therapy, broadening the scope of personalized medicine in nephrology. Such a culture of collaboration paves the way for robust clinical trials that examine how new therapies work to explore and overcome the unique challenges of pediatric patients. Greater collaboration among the medical community will ultimately foster innovation and drive the future of pediatric nephrology forward (Suppadungsuk et al., 2023). Ultimately, ethical concerns around the application of cutting-edge technology and investigation n pediatric nephrology cannot be dismissed. As AI and machine learning increasingly become incorporated into clinical practice,around data privacy, algorithmic bias, and informed consent are paramount. Ensuring technology is utilized in the optimal interest of children and adolescents patients within the parameters of ethics is important. Stakeholders must have ongoing discussions to offer guidelines that are ensured designed to guarantee patient rights and protection for vulnerable populations. Moreover, the inclusion of stakeholder views, like those of patients and families, is important in ensuring that developments in pediatric nephrology adhere to ethical codes and competencies in culture. Finally, as the profession goes towards innovation and collaboration, it is still necessary to work on these aspects of ethics so that pediatric patients' well-being is always the concern in nephrology practice (Suppadungsuk et al., 2023).

Test Your Knowledge

1. What recent innovations in treatment and technology are improving outcomes in pediatric nephrology?
2. How is genetic research enhancing the understanding and management of pediatric kidney diseases?
3. What are the key future directions and goals in advancing pediatric nephrology research and care?

SUMMARY

The field of pediatric nephrology stands at the intersection that is characterized by newer treatments and evolving methods for addressing various renal abnormalities in children. The role of artificial intelligence in clinical practice has arrived with the potential of bising in the field of enhanced diagnostic capabilities and personalization of treatment. Such technology consolidations, apart from having streamlined the treatment of the patients with improved results, have reduced the workload imparted on the healthcare professionals both in regard to decision decision-making as well as data management. But as the profession continues to evolve in the use of these technological innovations, care must be taken to also watch out for the ethical issues that accompany the use of AI, particularly with respect to accuracy, informed consent, privacy, and data protection, which are of utmost importance in pediatric environments. Awareness of these complexities will facilitate a more cautious application of AI solutions in nephrology (Karalis, 2024). Moreover, understanding the intricacy of health disparities is critical in pediatric nephrology care. The race context concerning health reminds one of the necessity to address the social determinants of health that most affect diverse populations. By examining the intersectionality between race and health inequities, nephrology professionals are in an improved position to conceptualize better, culturally attuned care strategies that account for the specific concerns of complex patient groups. Such an approach aligns with the broader health equity shift wherein addressing structural inequalities takes on a paramount role in improving child health outcomes. Through the esthment of commitment to equity in nephrology, health systems are able to help dismantle barriers that lead to unequal access and outcomes, ultimately benefiting the health of all children with kidney disease (Macias et al., 2023). Finally, the future of pediatric nephrology is inextricably tied with to ongoing research, innovation, and the creation of a fostering clinical climate. Encouraging interdisciplinary collaboration among nephrologists, healthcare providers, and researchers is crucial to broaden knowledge and enhance the treatment of pediatric renal disease. Long-term investment in education, training, and community health promotion must persist to equip providers with the education required to address both clinical and societal concerns of pediatric nephrology appropriately. As the science evolves, it is important that clinicians advocate for policies that enhance access to care, support research activities, and be actively involved in dialogue regarding the appropriate ethical use of technology. Overcoming these challenges and advocating for equitable practices will not only enhance pediatric nephrology but also create a healthier future for children with kidney disease.

Pediatric nephrology addresses a broad spectrum of renal pathology in children, with increasingly focal attention to genetic and developmental factors predisposing to these diseases. Among the more significant disorders are Lowe syndrome and Dent-2 disease, which are both caused by mutations in the OCRL gene. According to studies, children with these tubulopathies typically present with progressive chronic kidney disease (CKD) with variable prognosis according to the specific disorder. For example, studies have shown that the median eGFR of Lowe syndrome is significantly lower than what has been observed in Dent-2 disease, suggesting a more severe renal impairment in affected individuals. These findings reiterate the importance of early diagnosis and intervention that will be directed at inhibiting the progression of CKD among child populations affected by genetic nephropathies and thus form a crucial aspect of pediatric nephrology. Evaluation oKD development in children suffering from genetic kidney disease needs to be evidence-based. In a patient population with Lowe syndrome and Dent-2 disease, stage II-V CKD was found in approximately 82% of the population under observation, further confirming that such mutations result in significant loss to of renal function. Of particular interest is that survival analysis demonstrated the natural history of CKD to be substantially more aggressive in patients with Lowe syndrome than in Dent-2. These results demonstrate the need for long-term monitoring and the use of customized treatment strategies based on each disorder's specific genetic etiology, ultimately improving prognosis and quality of life in children afflicted with either disorder. Full understanding of and ongoing research into potential determinants of CKD progression are thus essential in the field of pediatric nephrology. The Kidney Disease: Improving Global Outcomes (KDIGO) guideline provides a framework for the diagnosis and treatment of CKD-MBD, which is essential in children. Updated guidelines highlight the importance of addressing abnormalities of bone and mineral derangements, given that children with CKD experience unique physiological changes. Specifically, the guidelines are advocating for efficient means of maintaining calcium levels and lowering phosphate, eventually avoiding related complications. The process of systematic reviews applied in the guidelines also points out areas for more research, thus allowing healthcare providers to utilize best-evidenced practice when treating CKD-MBD in children. By abiding by such recommendations, pediatric nephrologists may enhance patient care to become healthier and even alter the path of CKD among affected children (Wheeler et al., 2017). Talking about these critical points not only teaches clinical practice but also builds a greater understanding of nephrological disease among young patients.

KEY TERMS FROM THIS CHAPTER

- Acute kidney injuries (AKI)
- Atypical hemolytic uremic syndrome (aHUS)
- Glomerular filtration rate (GFR)
- Lupus Nephritis
- Nephrotic Syndrome
- Pediatric patients
- Steroid-resistant nephrotic syndrome (SRNS)
- Adult stem cell (ASC)
- Chronic kidney disease (CKD)
- Kidney health
- Nephrology
- Optimal kidney health
- Pluripotent stem cell (PSC)
- Urinary tract infections (UTIs)

CRITICAL THINKING QUESTIONS

1. **What is the most common cause of nephrotic syndrome in children?**
   a. Focal segmental glomerulosclerosis
   b. Minimal change disease
   c. Membranous nephropathy
   d. IgA nephropathy
2. **Which of the following is NOT a classical feature of nephrotic syndrome?**
   a. Proteinuri.
   b. Hypertension
   c. Hypoalbuminemia
   d. Edema
3. **The most common cause of acute glomerulonephritis in children is:**
   a. Lupus nephritis
   b. Post-streptococcal glomerulonephritis
   c. IgA nephropathy
   d. Hemolytic uremic syndrome
4. **What is the most common organism causing urinary tract infection (UTI) in children?**
   a. Streptococcus pyogenesStreptococcus pyogenes
   b. Klebsiella pneumoniae
   c. Escherichia coli
   d. Pseudomonas aeruginosa
5. **Which of the following is a typical feature of nephritic syndrome?**
   a. Massive proteinuria
   b. Hyperlipidemia
   c. Gross hematuria
   d. Hypoalbuminemia

Short Answer Questions

1. Define nephrotic syndrome in children.
2. Differentiate between nephritic and nephrotic syndrome.
3. What is the most common cause of acute glomerulonephritis in children?
4. Describe the management of minimal change disease in nephrotic syndrome.
5. List two causes of acute kidney injury (AKI) in children.
6. What is the role of ultrasound in pediatric nephrology?

Answer to Critical Thinking Questions

1. (b); 2. (c); 3. (b); 4. (c); 5. (c)

REFERENCES

1. Afroz, S., Begum, A., Hanif, M., Hoque, M., et al. (2016). Renal diseases in children attending pediatric nephrology centers of Dhaka City. https://core.ac.uk/download/483636758.pdf (accessed on 16th June 2025).
2. Ashida, A., Fujimaru, R., Fujimura, Y., Hataya, H., et al. (2021). Clinical guides for aHUS. https://core.ac.uk/download/425282981.pdf (accessed on 16th June 2025).
3. Baron, D. A., Bergman, P. J., Bryan, J. N., Calvet, X., et al. (2016). A One Health overview, facilitating advances in comparative medicine and translational research. https://core.ac.uk/download/323068355.pdf (accessed on 16th June 2025).
4. Butani, L., & Ducore, J. (2017). Primary renal lymphoma presenting as end-stage renal disease. https://core.ac.uk/download/323069034.pdf (accessed on 16th June 2025).
5. Butler, C. L., Reed, E. F., Thomas, K. A., Valenzuela, N. M., et al. (2017). Not all antibodies are created equal: Factors that influence antibody mediated rejection. https://core.ac.uk/download/323079645.pdf (accessed on 16th June 2025).
6. Ceschia, G., Parolin, M., & Vidal, E. (2023). New perspectives in pediatric dialysis technologies: The case for neonates and infants with acute kidney injury. https://core.ac.uk/download/576928440.pdf (accessed on 16th June 2025).
7. Karalis, V. (2024). The integration of artificial intelligence into clinical practice. *Applied Biosciences, 3*, 14–44. https://doi.org/10.3390/applbiosci3010002 (accessed on 16th June 2025).
8. Knoers, N. V. A. M. (2022). The term CAKUT has outlived its usefulness: The case for the defense. https://core.ac.uk/download/543462289.pdf (accessed on 16th June 2025).
9. Kotanko, P., Rosales, L., & Ronco, C. (2019). Preface–Advances in CKD 2019. *Blood Purification, 47*, 197–198. https://doi.org/10.1159/000495158 (accessed on 16th June 2025).
10. Lombel, R. M., Brakeman, P., Sack, B. S., & Butani, L. (2022). Urologic considerations in pediatric chronic kidney disease. *Advances in Chronic Kidney Disease, 29*, 308–317. https://doi.org/10.1053/j.ackd.2022.02.006 (accessed on 16th June 2025).
11. Macias-Konstantopoulos, W., Collins, K. A., Diaz, R., Duber, H. C., Edwards, C. D., Hsu, A., Ranney, M. L., et al. (2023). Race, healthcare, and health disparities: A critical review and recommendations for advancing health equity. *Western Journal of Emergency Medicine, 24.* https://doi.org/10.5811/westjem.58408 (accessed on 16th June 2025).
12. Madill, A., Banister, P., Bluebond-Langner, M., Britton, C., Charmaz, K., Dunn, J., Glaser, B. G., et al. (2007). Amplified ambivalence: Having a sibling with juvenile idiopathic arthritis. https://core.ac.uk/download/51906.pdf (accessed on 16th June 2025).
13. Mariani, L., Eddy, S., Alakwaa, F., McCown, P. J., Harder, J. L., Nair, V., Eichinger, F., et al. (2022). Precision nephrology identified tumor necrosis factor activation variability in minimal change disease and focal segmental glomerulosclerosis. *Kidney International, 103*, 565–579. https://doi.org/10.1016/j.kint.2022.10.023 (accessed on 16th June 2025).
14. Schaefer, F., Ingelfinger, J. R., Kalantar-Zadeh, K., & null, null. (2016). Averting the legacy of kidney disease: Focus on childhood. https://core.ac.uk/download/pdf/81549064.pdf (accessed on 16th June 2025).

15. Velásquez-Forero, F., Esparza, M., Salas, A., Medeiros, F., et al. (1978). Risk factors evaluation for urolithiasis among children. https://core.ac.uk/download/pdf/82758815.pdf (accessed on 16th June 2025).

16. Watanabe, Y., Yamagata, K., Nishi, S., Hirakata, H., Hanafusa, N., Saito, C., Hattori, M., et al. (2015). Japanese Society for Dialysis Therapy clinical guideline for "hemodialysis initiation for maintenance hemodialysis." *Therapeutic Apheresis and Dialysis, 19*, 93–107. https://doi.org/10.1111/1744-9987.12293 (accessed on 16th June 2025).

PEDIATRIC DERMATOLOGY

3

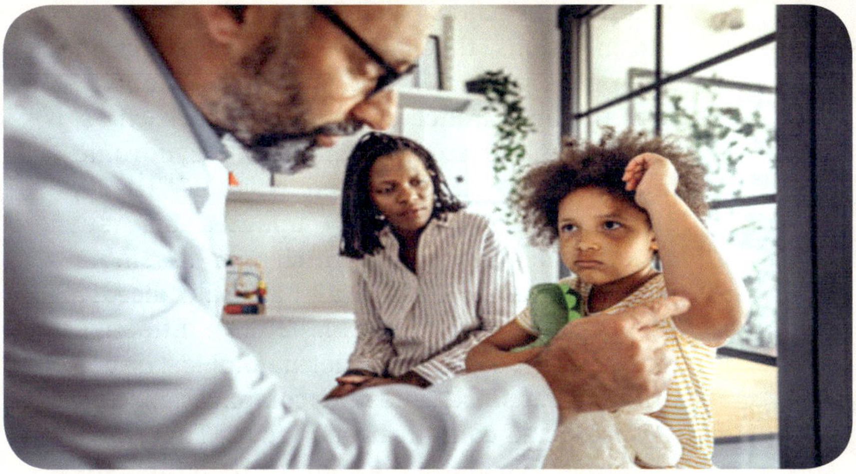

LEARNING OBJECTIVES

After studying this chapter, you will be able to:

1. Define the prevalent pediatric skin conditions
2. Describe diagnosis and treatment methods
3. Highlight psychological and social implications
4. Understand preventive care and health promotion

Introduction

The pPediatric dermatology plays a significant role in addressing the unique dermatological requirements of infants, children, and adolescents. The subspecialty addresses skin disorders that occur in younger patients, which are quite different from those experienced in adults. Not only is the skin of children more sensitive, but also constantly changing so making accurate diagnosis and treatment is very important. Pediatric dermatologists need to contend with different disorders, ranging from common diseases like eczema and psoriasis to rare genetic disorders. Additionally, the psychological impact of skin disease on pediatric patients and their families should not be overlooked, as these diseases most frequently affect self-esteem and interpersonal relationships. Thus, a fundamental knowledge of pediatric dermatology is critical for medical professionals since it enables them to offer whole-person care, which involves the physical as well as the emotional health of children's skin. This essay seeks to provide a comprehensive description of the principles and practices of the critical spec (Figure 3.1).

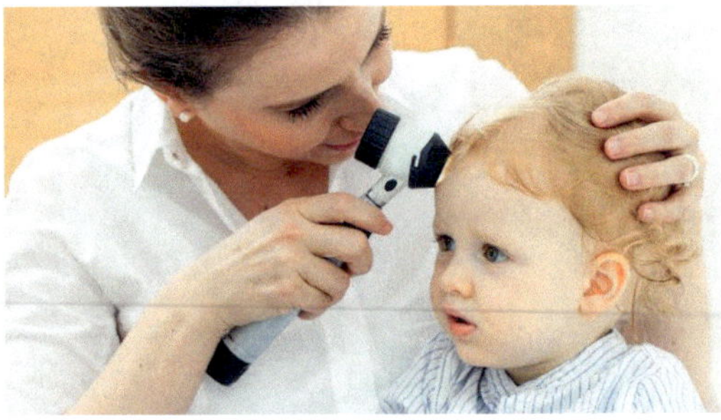

Figure 3.1. The pPediatric dermatology is essential for addressing the unique dermatological needs of infants.

Source: https://medstarhealth-delivery.sitecorecontenthub.cloud/api/public/content/services%2FPediatric-Dermatology?v=608fa78e.

Definition of Pediatric Dermatology

Pediatric dermatology is the expert branch of medicine dedicated to the diagnosis and treatment of skin conditions in infants, children, and adolescents. Pediatric dermatology deals with a wide r conditions, from common problemssuch as, such as eczema and acne to more complex conditions, including congenital cutaneous disorders and skin cancers. It is vital to recogni specific physiological differences among between children's skin and adult skin because these differences would have implications on the presentation, course, and treatment of cutaneous diseases. Secondly, pediatric dermatologists are likely to deal with psychosocial problems related to skin disease because disfigurement as a result of cutaneous lesions would affect a child's self-image and interpersonal relationships. With the increase in demands for specialized treatment, effective communication among pediatric dermatologists and other medical professionals ensures the optimal outcomes of patients (Spelich et al., 2022). Interprofessional collaboration integrated treatment and patients are taken wellwell taken care of in their developmental needs (Lucero et al., 2017).

Importance of Dermatology in Pediatrics

A thorough understanding of the importance of dermatology in pediatrics is essential since dermatological conditions occur differently in children compared to adults. Pediatric patients areble to different dermatological conditions, such as, such as eczema, psoriasis, and infections, that have a profound effect on their general health and quality of lifonally, with the appearance of new diseases, such as, such as multisystem inflammatory syndrome in children (MIS-C) linked with COVID-19, dermatologists must stay updated on new conditions andtations, which can resemble familiar diseases s, such as Kawasaki disease (Esposito & Principiet al., 2021). Effective management of pediatric dermatological issues is important since sn lead to complications and psychosocial complicationsissues. Therefore, pediatric dermatology not only addresses immediate health issues but also provides long-term health, highlighting the necessity for specialist knowledge and research in this field (Jecca et al., 2021). With deliberate intervention, health practitioners can ensure healthier futures for younger patients (Figure 3.2).

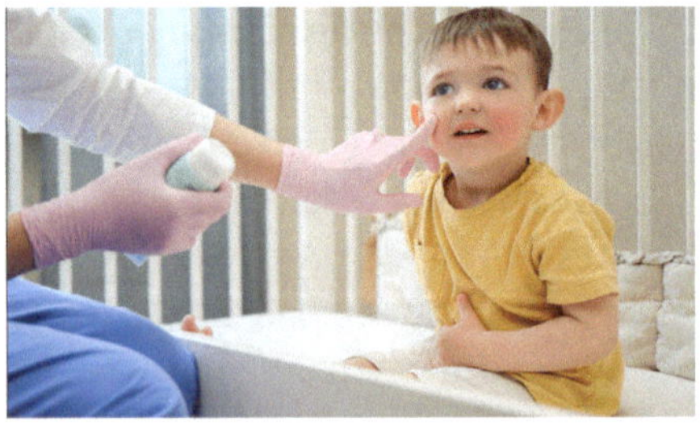

Figure 3.2. Understanding dermatologys significance in pediatrics.

Source: https://southernderm.com/wp-content/uploads/2024/06/Pediatric-dermatology-header--e1720810058857.png.

Overview of Common Skin Conditions in Children

An understanding of the most common skin diseases of children is essential for accurate dia and best therapy in pediatric dermatology. Diseases such as, such as atopic dermatitis, impetigo, and warts are frequently encountered in practice and can have a significant effect on a child's quality of life. Atopic dermatitis, for instance, not only can cause physical distress but can also lead to emotional distress with signs of itching and inflammation. Recent studies have shown that crisaborole, a nonsteroidal phosphodiesterase 4 inhibitor, has led to the improvement of quality of life in such patients, as evidenced by tremendous reductions in the Children's Dermatology Life Quality Index scores (Boguniewicz et al., 2018). Iion, there is a strong correlation between skin diseases such as, such ass, and thus it is crucial for psychiatrists and dermatologists topsychiatrists and dermatologists must collaborate to optimize patient results (Benea et al., 2015). This integrated approach is central to tackling the multifactorial origin of pediatric skin diseases.

Historical Development of Pediatric Dermatology

The historical development of pediatric dermatology reflects a gradual recognition that skin diseases in children are distinct from those in adults. Early practitioners often applied universal dermatologic concepts without considering the unique features of pediatric cases, resulting in inconsistent and sometimes ineffective treatments. Over time, increased awareness of children's specific dermatologic needs prompted reforms in medical education, clinical training, and healthcare policies. Family physicians played a pivotal role during this period, serving as the first line of defense in diagnosing and treating common pediatric skin conditions. Research subsequently revealed that pediatric dermatology was underrepresented in medical curricula, highlighting a critical educational gap. Addressing this deficit has been essential for improving pediatric dermatologic care, fostering integration of child-specific management strategies, and laying the foundation for research and evidence-based education in the field (Bousquet et al., 2016; Khalid et al., 2023).

Role of Pediatric Dermatologists

Pediatric dermatologists have a key role in the care of the unique skin disorders of children, whose expertise is specialized in the diagnosis and management of dermatologic disorders unique to this age group.

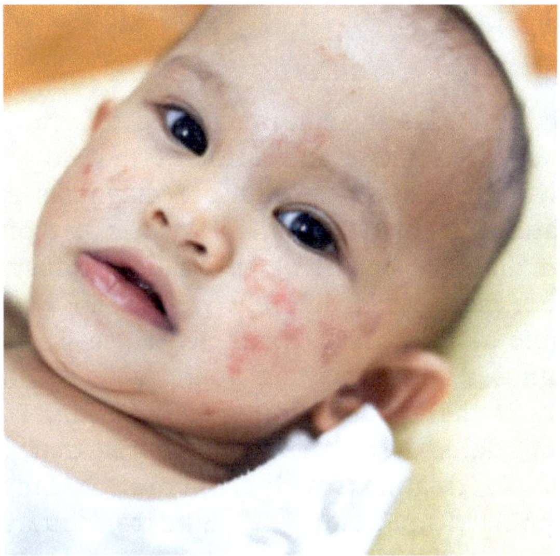

Figure 3.3. Infant with visible facial skin lesions, illustrating a common presentation encountered in pediatric dermatology.

Source: https://cutis.org.in/assets/img/services_dynamic/pediatric-dermatalogy/wat-is-pediatric-dermotology.jpg.

They address an extensive variety of problems ranom common diseases like warts and eczema to complex disorders such as, such as congenital dermatoses or cutaneous manifestations of systemic disease. Pediatric dermatologists play a significant role in assessing the skin problems associated with genetimes, which may extend from finding potential complicainfancy infant development. Together with other professionals, such as, such as pediatricians or geneticists, they ensure comprehensive care tailored to the unique needs of each child. The significance of their work is realized by the ongoing innovation in pediatric dermatology, which seeks to improve therapeutic benefits and the quality of life of the children so affected. Their work is essential, particularly with regard to the psychological impact that suc have during formative years (Lopes et al., 2020; Marilynet al., 2022; Zuberbier et al., 2021) (Figure 3.3).

Differences between Adult and Pediatric Dermatology

It is essential to understand the differences between pediatric and adult dermatology in order to make an appropriate diagnosis and treatment. Pediatric dermatology acts on typical skin diseases occurring in children, most of which manifest in different ways from adults. Atopic dermatitis, for example, which is often diagnosed in infants and young children, has distinct therapeutic strategies quite different from adults. Studies have discovered that, for example, treatment with crisaborole ointment in pediatric patients with mild to moderate atopic dermatitis leads to significant quality-of-life improvement over that in adults, and highlights the importance of individualized therapy (Boguniewicz et al., 2018). Certain autoimmune disorders present in atypical forms in children, e.g., dermatomyositis, and need diligent identification by pediatric dermatologists to prevent misdiagnosis (Cartron et al., 2020). Thus, the specialty of dermatology in adults and children needs differentiated knowledge and practice to address the respective needs of their population efficiently.

Impact of Skin Conditions on Child Development

The impacts of skin illnesses on a child's development extend beyond the physical, also interfering with psychological well-being and sociaopment. For instance, children who have visible dermatological illnesses such as, such as eczema or psoriasis, are stigmatized, hence develop anxiety as well as low self-esteem, influencing social developmen school performance. Healthy management of these conditions is necessary to make ensure healthy emotional growth; as with the concept of a thyroid-skin axis, in which imbalance can influence more than the particular body part, it is necessary to comprehend this in terms of support and interventions. In addition, pediatric neurocutaneous syndromes likewise demonstrate this interaction because dermatologic signs and symptoms of the syndromes may provide early hints at diagnosis while concurrently affecting cognitive and emotional health, necd approach to care (Lopes et al., 2020; Cammisa et al., 2024; Alyamani et al., 2024). It is in managing both skin health and developmental concerns that children are given the coordinated care they need to thrive in every aspect of life.

Goals of Pediatric Dermatology

The goals of pediatric dermatology go beyond mere diagnosis and treatment and include a holistic approach to care with the needs of children with skin disease in mind. A foremost goal is enhancing the quality of life of children through physical and psychosocial management of their dermatological conditions. With proper management measures, pediatric dermatologists attempt to minimize the psychological and emotional burden of seemingly evident skin conditions, which have a profound influence on a child's self-perception and interpersonal relationships. Further, the specialty d to investigating and refining clinical procedures in of many diseases, such as, such as juvenile idiopathic inflammatory myopathies, in order to establish precise classification criteria and treatment plans, especially in the case of children. Ultimately, the long-term objective is to encourage healthy skin development and inform families about good care measures, ong children with skin ailments (Lopes et al., 2020Daniel et al., 2018; Ingrid et al., 2017).

3.1. Common Pediatric Skin Conditions

Learning Outcome

1. Eczema (Atopic Dermatitis)
2. Psoriasis in Children
3. Impetigo and Bacterial Infections
4. Fungal Infections (Tinea)
5. Viral Infections (e.g., Warts, Molluscum)
6. Acne in Adolescents
7. Diaper Dermatitis
8. Birthmarks and Vascular Malformations
9. Allergic Reactions and Rashes

Pediatric dermatology encompasses a wide variety of frequent skin diseases, common in children, that need specialized knowledge and care. The most common conditions encountered are acne, eczema, and infections, which also encompass fungal infections. In a research study conducted at a referral center for specialist pediatric dermatology, the most frequent reasons for consultation were acne and eczema, corroborating thh frequency of presentation within this age group (Boffa et al., 2013). In addition, conditions such as, such as xerosis and lichen simplex chronicus that have the potential to develop from behavior associated with obsessive-compulsive disorder prove the interconnection between dermatological and psychological conditions (Benea et al., 2015). Understanding such common skin ailments and etiology is crucial in management as well as in patient care. As pediatric dermatology evolves, ongoing communication between clinicians of all specialties is ever more critical to the satisfaction of the multifaceted needs of this population of children (Figure 3.4).

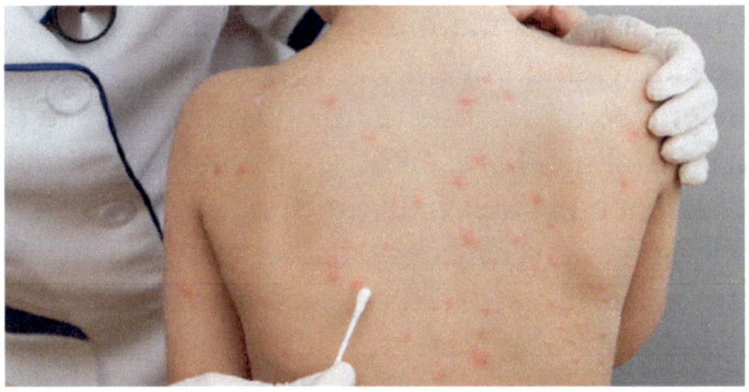

Figure 3.4. Pediatric dermatology encompasses a wide array of common skin conditions that commonly affect children.

Source: https://cutis.org.in/assets/img/blogs/change/4.jpg.

3.1.1. Eczema (Atopic Dermatitis)

Atopic dermatitis (AD) or eczema is a chronic and common cutaneous disease in children that must be well understood in pediatric dermatology. The complexity of the multifactorial cause, which is generated by a broad diversity of interrelated host and environmental determinants, makes its treatment and diagnosis more complex (Abreu et al., 2020). The immunologicromise that accompanies AD is the cause of the chronicity and could also be the cause of comorbidities such as, such as asthma and allergic rhinitis, which exacerbate the patients' condition (Eichenfield et al., 2016). Treatment modalities are multidisciplinary, with topicals like corticosteroids and calcineuribitors, while advances in biologic therapy have been promising in managing moderate-to-severe disease (Abreu Lopes et al., 2020). Notwithstanding the above advancement, inconsistency in immunoglobulin E (IgE) levels is a challenge for treatment direction aniveness (Eichenfield et al., 2016). Hence, ongoing research and clinical evaluation are fundamental to advance advancing therapeutic effectiveness and the quality of life among the suffering children.

3.1.2. Psoriasis in Children

In pediatric dermatology, psoriasis presents a particular challenge, as it is frequently under-recognized and prone to misdiagnosis due to its variable clinical presentation in children. Clinical experience is such that children with psoriasis may present with a myriad of manifestations from well-demarcated erythematous eruptions to less obvious presentations on various body areas, including the vulva. A study noted that most girls who were diagnosed with vulvar psoriasis presented an erythematous vulvar outbreak, occasionally accompanied by perianal involvement, indicating that the conditions had diverse presentations (Wu et al., 2024). Moreover, with advancements in the available treatment, like biologics secukinumab and ustekinumab, pediatric psoriasis has seen a renewed hope to efficiently manage it (Robin et al., 2024). These therapies represent a significant deviation from the traditional practice of treating patients with old technology, offering improved efficacy and safety compared to traditional treatment. The current evolution of psoriasis treatment in children thus underscores the importance of accurate diagnosis and personalized treatment modalities for the child patient.

3.1.3. Impetigo and Bacterial Infections

Impetigo is a freqacterial infection in der It is typically brought about by infection of Staphylococcus aureus*Staphylococcus aureus* or Streptococcus pyogenes*Streptococcus pyogenes*, with honey-colored crusted papules and brings serious pain and potential complications if not treated. Impetigo not only affects the physical well-being of the child but can also inflict significant emotional distress in the form of parental anxiety and perceived stigma in the child (Gashaw et al., 2022). Appropriate treatment is necessary; topical antibiotic therapy in the form of fusidic acid and retapamulin is commonly practiced, with comparablel., 2019). Given the high incidence rate of skin infections in children, it is essential for pediatric practitionerspediatric practitioners need to understand and manage impetigo. This is in itself an indication for an early detection and treatment process aimed at minimizing physical expressions and psychological impacts of the infection (Figure 3.5).

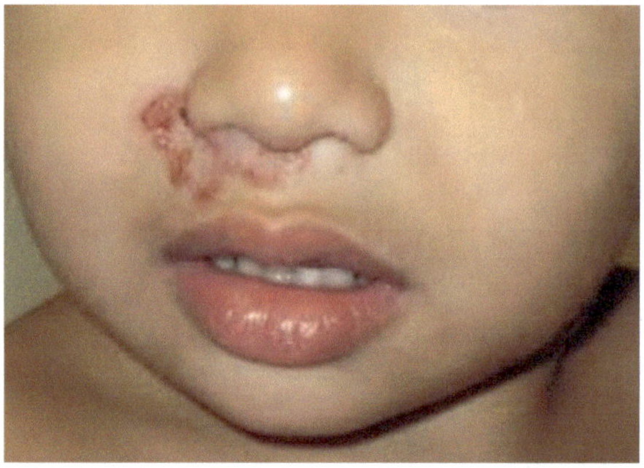

Figure 3.5. Child with perioral crusted lesions, characteristic of impetigo, a common bacterial skin infection in pediatric patients.

Source: https://encrypted-tbn0.gstatic.com/images?q=tbn:ANd9GcStlk8Au3xwuYnc0iLasJGdlb8Ax6cUFfjziA&s.

3.1.4. Fungal Infections (Tinea)

Fungal infections, tinea in particular, represent a significant challenge in pediatric dermatology, especially in prepubopulations. Among the various types of tinea, tinea capitis is surprisingly widespread, caused by dermatophytes such as, such as Trichophyton and Microsporum, of which *T. tonsurans* and *M. canis* are the most common culprits worldwide. As identified in the research, infections account for approximately 26.1% of dermatological diseases that affect children, and 8.1% of this group suffer from tinea capitis (Ayanlowo et al., 2018). Since topically apifungal medications cannot reach through the hair follicle efficaciously, systemic interventions are required in order to be effective. Griseofulvin has been the usual mainstay of treatment; however, more recent treatments like terbinafine are just as effective but shorter in duration, possibly making patient compliance more co(Bennassar et al., 2010). Therefore, pediatricians should be aware of the epidemiology and treatment of tinea in order to provide comprehensive dermcal treatment.

3.1.5. Viral Infections (e.g., Warts, Molluscum)

Among pediatric dermatology, viral infections such as, such as warts and molluscum contagiosum are prevalent and can really impact a child's quality of life. Warts, which are mostly caused by human papillomavirus (HPV), are the most common viral cutaneous infection with high prevalence reported in young children as noted by recent reports suggesting wart prevalence at about 22.1% among children's derlaints (Alam et al., 2024).

Concurrently, molluscum contagiosum in the guise of smooth dome-shaped papules has a tendencytends to occur in immunocomincluding those with HIV, where its prevalence compared to other viral dermatoses is also documented (Diatta et al., 2023Lopes et al., 2020). Clinical management of such infections has a tendency to be patient-dependent in terms of general health and potential underlying immunological status, and hence they form focal areas of expertise in practice in pediatric dermatology. Hence, early detection and awareness are essential to minimize the emotionalysical distress these infections put adolescent patients through (Figure 3.6).

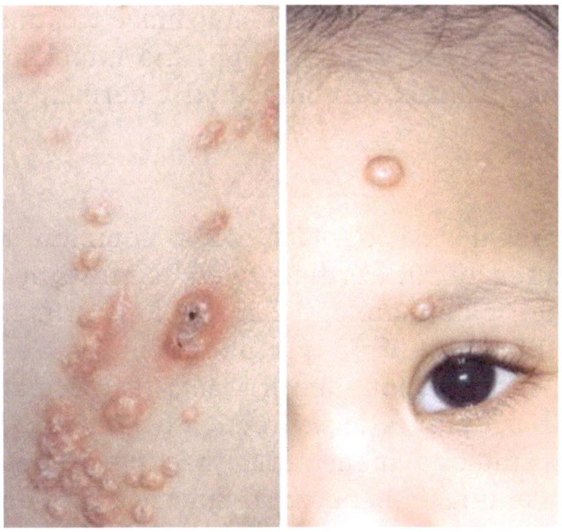

Figure 3.6. The viral infections such as, such as warts and molluscum contagiosum, are prevalent and can significantly impact a child's quality of life.

Source: https://www.mayoclinic.org/content/dam/media/global/images/2023/04/05/molluscum-contagiosum.png.

3.1.6. Acne in Adolescents

Teen acne is a chief problem in pediatric dermatology because of its prevalence and powerful emotional burden. It not only affects the appearance of the skin but also has a profound effect on causing considerable distress, which influences the self-esteem and lifestyle of the individual. Acne vulgaris was found to be more common in this phase of development, and its effective management techniques must be implemented to minimize its effects. Individualized treatment protocols are increasingly becoming essential to address the unique needs of adolescent patients, considering the seof acne and the psychological and social aspects of the disease (Satish et al., 2024). Furthermore, novel treatments such as, such as cold atmospheric plasma (CAP) have proved effective in managing acne with equivalent advantages of being cost-effective (Korotkiy, 2024). By prioritizing both clinical efficacy and psychological wellness in adolescents, dermatologists are able to maximize treatment outcomes and thus highlight the importance of personalized care in pediatric dermatology.

3.1.7. Diaper Dermatitis

Diaper dermatitis (DD) is a common but frequently underdiagnosed condition in pediatric dermatology that develops primarily in infants due to prolonged exposure to moisture, friction, and irritants in the diaper area. DD occurs most frequently in neonates, with studies demonstrating that approximately 34% of infants in neonatal intensive care units develop DD. Risk factors for DD are NICU stay length because longer lengths have a greater incidence of dermatitis, which serves as an indication for effective prevention (Khalid et al., 2023). Resolving the issue is not only necessary for comfort but also for the prevention of secondary infections that may complicate this most common of conditions. Since family doctors are most often the first line of defense in treating and diagnosing pediatric dermatological diseases, increased education and awareness on DD would be to the betterment of the overall healthcare response for these diseases (Khalid et al., 2023). Promoting awareness of this disease will ultimately benefit both healthcare providers and their children.

3.1.8. Birthmarks and Vascular Malformations

Birthmarks and vascular malformations are of significant concern in pediatric dermatology due to their prevalence and influence on patient management. Of these, port-wine birthmarks (PWBs) are capillary vascular malformations in nature, characterized by their classic reddish-purple color and, more frequently than not, appearance on the neck and head. They became darker and thickened over time, necessitating early treatment to optimize outcomes. The gold standard for the management of PWBs is pulsed dye laser (PDL) therapy, which treats the affected vascular structures selectively and successfully with a minimal impact on surrounding tissues. Current standards recommend early use of this laser therapy in the initial weeks of life to achieve the best possible outcome (Lindsay et al., 2023). Moreover, studies have established the potential benefits of combining PDL with sirolimus, namely a macrolide antibiotic, whose mechanism is angiogenesis inhibition, although this combination may involve certain side effects in the form of delayed ulceration and systemic absorption issues (Hobayan et al., 2023). This new scenario indicates the necessity of early referral and customized treatment protocols for such affected children (Figure 3.7).

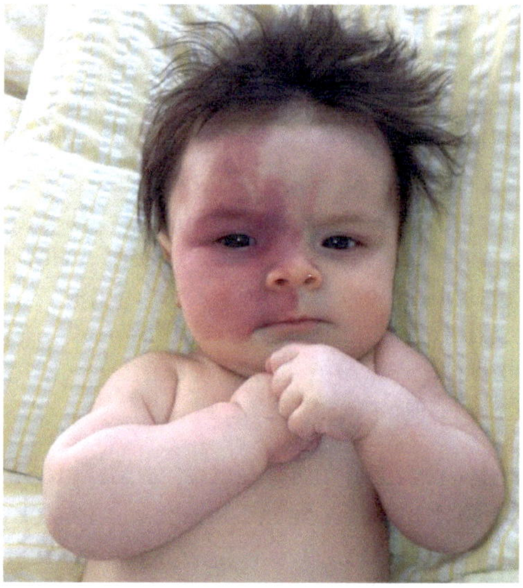

Figure 3.7. Infant with a capillary malformation (port-wine stain) on the face, a congenital vascular anomaly often observed in pediatric dermatology.

Source: https://craniofacialteamtexas.com/wp-content/uploads/2017/01/Capillary-malformations-of-the-face.jpg.

3.1.9. Allergic Reactionsshes

Allergic reactions are prevalent in pediatric populations and will often manifest as several dermatological manifestations such as, such as rashes. Allergic reactions may be of any origin, ranging from environmental allergens to food items and, more recently, vaccines. In the field of vaccination, the development of mRNA-based platforms for COVID-19 vaccines has been associated with an unexpected but alarming incidence of severe allergic reactions and, in a few instances, anaphylaxis. Such events need careful monitoring and emphasize the importance of implementing safe methods for vaccination in children, especially those known to be allergic (Ankermann et al., 2021). Specifically, a study showed that while allergy screening before vaccination is usually not needed for most children, those who have suffered a severe allergic reaction should be assessed (El-Owaidy et al., 2014). Understanding of the dermatologic implications of these allergic phenomena is significant in pediatric dermatology, as early diagnosis and treatment can profoundly affect patient outcome and family distress.

Test Your Knowledge

1. What are the main causes, symptoms, and management strategies for eczema (atopic dermatitis) in children?
2. How do impetigo and other bacterial skin infections typically present and spread among pediatric patients?
3. What are the common types and treatments of fungal infections (tinea) seen in children?

3.2. Diagnosis and Treatment Approaches

Learning Outcome

1. Clinical examination techniques
2. Importance of patient history
3. Diagnostic tests and procedures
4. Topical treatments and medications
5. Systemic treatments for severe conditions
6. Role of phototherapy
7. Importance of multidisciplinary care
8. Patient education and family involvement
9. Emerging therapies and research

In pediatric dermatology, effective diagnosis and treatment modalities require a tender appreciation of the unique skin conditions and the individual characteristics of children. The states of atopic dermatitis and eczema require close examination because their presentations in children can be quite different from those in adults. Recent trends highlight the inclusion of allergen immunotherapy (AIT) as a promising treatment modality in certain allergic dermatologic conditions in children. AIT is a critical intervention in the early stages of respiratory allergic diseases, with long-term health implications. Methodological challenges, however, involve heterogeneity of treatment protocols that complicate clinical trials to compare and hamper standardization across treatment modalities (Arasi et al., 2018). Furthermore, constant endeavor should fill in the evidence gaps around AIT to maximize its utilization in the pediatric population to eventually improve overall management plans for skin diso (AgacheBousquet et al., 2016).

3.2.1. Clinical Examination Techniques

Appropriate clinical examination skills are most crucial in pediatric dermatology because they allow for the appropriate diagnosis and management of dermatological conditions in children. Appropriate history-taking begins with an appreciation of the pediatric patient's anatomical and physiological differences, which can influence presentation and interpretation of dermatological presentations. For instance, utilization of innovative learnls such as, such as virtual reality (VR) and augmented reality (AR) is found more often to advance clinical education and refine examination skills in dermatological clinics but their practical application remains scarce in the literature up to this point (Dellavalle et al., 2020). Moreover, specialists have to be experienced in managing such a disorder as ectodermal dysplasia, for which a well-thought-out strategy of prosthetic care may significantly influence the quality of a child's life, overcoming functional and psychological problems (Angelopoulou et al., 2016). For this reason, knowledge of these examination techniques is required in order to make the best pediatric dermatological treatment (Figure 3.8).

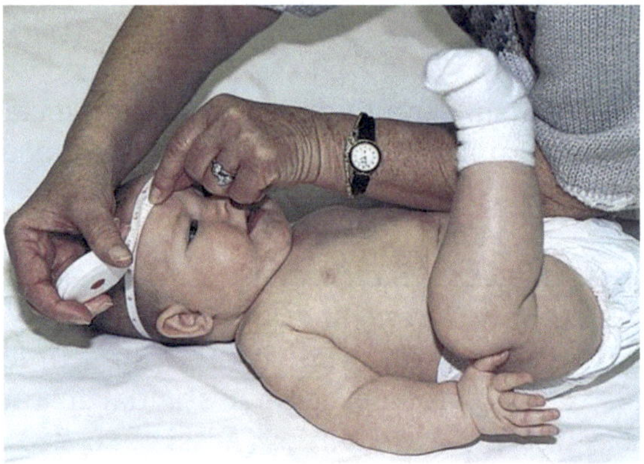

Figure 3.8. The clinical examination techniques are paramount in the realm of pediatric dermatology.

Source: https://nursekey.com/wp-content/uploads/2016/10/F000332f33-02-9781437727753.jpg.

3.2.2. Importance of Patient History

In pediatric dermatology, a thorough patient history is critical to accurate diagnosis and effective treatment. An understanding of a child's medical history, family history, and social history allows practitioners to identify patterns of dermatologic disease that are likely linked with hereditary factors or environmental exposures. For instance, in diseases like atopic dermatitis, improvement in quality of life among the children with the disease has been observed to occur quite significantly with effective interventions, as observed through evaluations of treatments like crisaborole ointment, which has been established to raise quality of life scores for patients and their families (Boguniewicz et al., 2018). Similarly, conditions like diffuse cutaneous mastocytosis illustrate the serious consequences of delayed diagnosis and treatment, highlighting that a comprehensive patient history can avoid life-threatening complications (Akin et al., 2018). Overall, a complete patient history is important for personalized therapeutic approaches in child dermatology.

3.2.3. Diagnostic Tests and Procedures

In pediatric dermatology, the application of diagnostic tests and exams plays a key role in detecting and curing diseases of the skin effectively. The procedures represent a combination of clinical examination and laboratory examinations, unique to what dermatologists experience with pediatric patients. For instanconditions such as, such as Hereditary Angioedema (HAE), with nonspecific symptoms and poorly understood, a concordance of diagnostic criteria helps clinicians to make sound decisions and therefore improve outcomes for patients (Aygören-Pürsün et al., 2012). The relatively infrequent occurrence of certain skin conditions, like localized scleroderma, also emphasizes the necessity for evidence-based practice grounded in clinical experience as well as on current evidence (Hidv et al., 2018). Implementing in-depth diagnostic evaluations not only permits better understanding of skin diseases in children, but also improves collaboration among specialists, ultimately enabling children to receive uniform and effective care.

3.2.4. Topical Treatments and Medications

Topical drugs and agents are among the major cornerstones of pediatric dermatology, managing a variety of skin illnesses prevalent among children and adolescents. As an example, a combination of betamethasone dipropionate and calcipotriene has emerged to be safe and effective in treating extensive scalp psoriasis among adolescents aged between 12 and 17 years, with one study revealing dramatic disease control reduction and an overall acceptable side effect profile henfield et al., 20142019). Similarly, acne vulgaris, the chronic condition of the pediatric age grooften treated that isin a multifaceted. Clindamycin and benzoyl peroxide are the standard, with fixed drug combinations having been encouraging in managing moderate-to-severe cases. The combination regimen best meets efficacy and tolerance, and this underscores the need for careful consideration of treatment regimens unique to young patients (Eichenfield et al., 2015). These cases highlight the importance of topical therapy to control dermatology within pediatric practice (Figure 3.9).

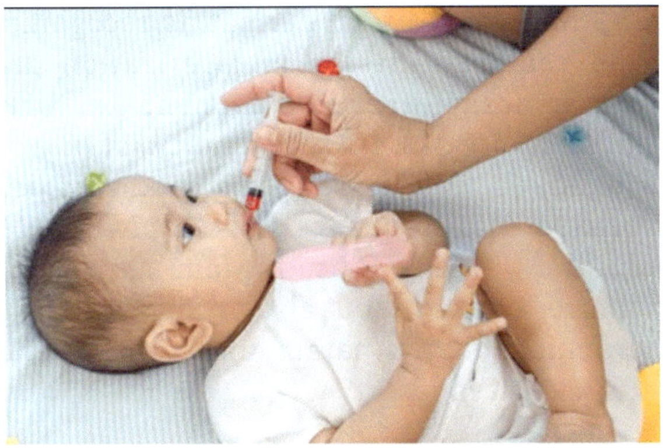

Figure 3.9. Topical treatments and medications serve as foundational components in pediatric dermatology.

Source: https://www.shutterstock.com/image-photo/baby-feeding-liquid-medicine-260nw-437115634.jpg.

3.2.5. Systemic Treatments for Severe Conditions

In pediatric dermatology, effective management of severe disease states is often a matter of systemic therapies that address both cutaneous and underlying systemic derangements. The familial hyperlipidemias are an excellent example because they present in the forcal skin lesions, such as, such as eruptive xanthomas, which, if left untreated, portend severe cardiovascular risk. Early diagnosis is underscored in studies highlighting the necessity of proper dermatological examination for such presentations to be diagnosed early (Morales et al., 2024). Likewise, SCARs like Stevens-Johnson syndrome (SJS) and toxic epidermal necrolysis (TEN) are severe childhood conditions in which early systemic treatment can minimize mortality risk in such instances (Bangxang et al., 2024). Thus, a comprehension of the interconnection between cutaneous presentations and overall health can lead to improved prevention and treatment strategies in pediatric dermatology.

3.2.6. Role of Phototherapy

The use of phototherapy in pediatric dermatology has drawn a lot of attention due to its high rate of success in the management of a variety of skin conditions, particularly in children. A harmless method of treatment, phototherapy employs different wavelengths of light to elicit healing and pain reduction responses. Phototherapy is particularly vital in the management of such skin conditions as psoriasis, atopic dermatitis, and neonatal jaundice, where traditional therapy may be more dangerous or less successful. Experiments have illustrated how modalities like psoralen-UV-A (PUVA) and narrowband UV-B (NBUVB) have achieved dramatic advancements in diseases like early mycosis fungoides, a skin T-cell lymphoma, with good response rates and acceptable side effects (Phan et al., 2019). In addition, the photobiomodulatory effects of laser therapy can stimulate cell proliferation and tissue repair mechanisms, thus enhancing outcomes in children as a whole (Domp et al., 2020). This serves to emphasize the key role played by phototherapy in contemporary pediatric dermatology.

3.2.7. Importance of Multidisciplinary Care

The role played by multidisciplinary management of children's dermatology cannot be overstated because it forms the basis for successful management and compliance by patients. The team approach between dermatologists, general practitioners, and pharmacists helps ensure that homogenized and accurate inon on condition management such as, such as atopic dermatitis,is given to families. This is of especial interest in that the parents are at high risk of anxiety and miscommunication about treatment choices, notably the use steroids (TCS) (Smith et al., 2017Smith, 2017).

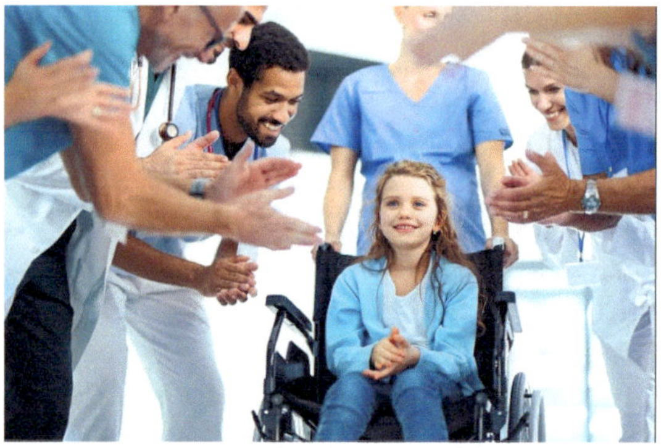

Figure 3.10. The importance of multidisciplinary care in pediatric dermatology cannot be overstated.

Source: https://static.wixstatic.com/media/58e90e_13a72d837e2740b8b264904214356a76~mv2.jpg/v1/fill/w_724,h_482,al_c,q_80,usm_0.66_1.00_0.01,enc_avif,quality_auto/58e90e_13a72d837e2740b8b264904214356a76~mv2.jpg.

The literature indicates that non-concordant recommendations by the care team will further intensify non-adherence to treatment, with a pressing need for alignment of the multidisciplinary team inesive messaging (Smith et al., 2017Smith, 2017). Effective communication in this team not only nhances the care for skin diseases, but also helps families in enhancing trust and adherence to therapy regimens. Last but foremost, placing multidisciplinary care at the forefront is essential to give well-integrated and effective dermatological care to child patients (Figure 3.10).

3.2.8. Patient Education and Family Involvement

Accurate patient education and family involvement are key components in the treatment of children's dermatologic diseases, particularly diaper dermatitis and atopic dermatitis. Education programs equip the caregivers with knowledge related to the prevention and control of skin conditions, which enhances compliance with treatment protocol. For instance, the ABCDE mnemonic, —air, barrie, cleansing, diaper, and education, —is a comprehensive method of curing irritant diaper dermatitis, encouraging education among families about how to defend the skin and prevent recurrence (Helms et al., 2021). Similarly, in atopic dermatitis, recognition of the requirement for moisturization and proper topically directed treatment can make significant strides in the quality of life of the child, as well as reducing medical costs associated with frequent pediatric visits (Eller et al., 2015). Finally, educating families not only maximizes outcomes but also produces a caring environment that is paramount to the overall health of the child.

3.2.9. Emerging Therapies and Research

With ongoing expansion in pediatric dermatology, new studies and evolving treatments are of absolute necessity in further enhancing results in the young patient. New ideas are being explorticularly in treating diseases such as, such as dermatomyositis and acne vulgaris. Diagnosis of dermatomyositis by using myositis-specific antibodies, for example, allows for more specific therapeutic planning and offers hope for improved prognoses through newer treatments like intravenous immune globulin therapy, which has been very effective in severe cases (Cartron et al., 2020). Similarly, the pathogenesis of acne vulgaris is evolving with the advent of combination therapies. The introduction of clindamycin and benzoyl peroxide fixed combinations, specifically more recently the 3.75% gel, is a promising advance aimed at maximizing efficacy and tolerance over the typical limitation of irritation at sger strengths (Eichenfield et al., 20152019). They underscore the dynamic nature of pediatric dermatology and the imperative of ongoing exploration of new treatments (Figure 3.11).

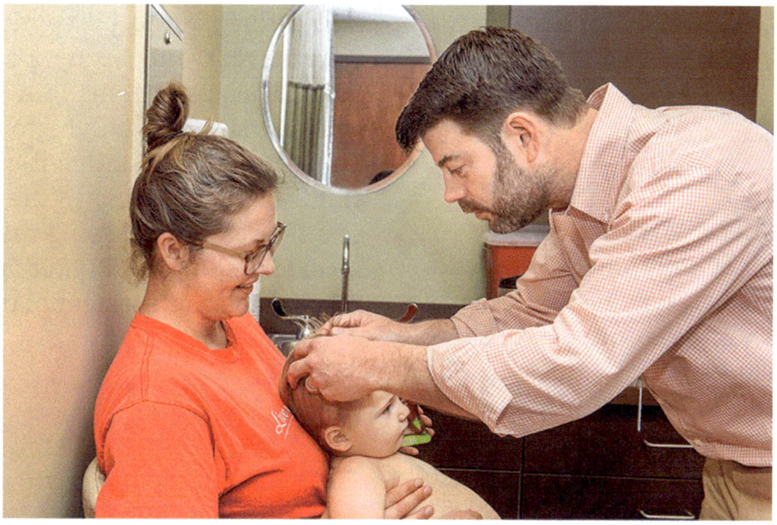

Figure 3.11. Emerging therapies and research.

Source: https://www.muhealth.org/sites/default/files/inline-images/PedsDermatology-760-compressor.png.

Test Your Knowledge

1. What diagnostic tests and procedures are commonly used to identify pediatric skin conditions?
2. How do topical treatments and medications help manage common pediatric skin disorders?
3. What is the role of phototherapy in treating chronic skin conditions in children?

3.3. Psychological and Social Implications

Learning Outcome

1. Impact of skin conditions on self-esteem
2. Social stigmas associated with skin disorders
3. Psychological support for affected children
4. Role of parents and caregivers
5. School environment and peer relationships
6. Coping strategies for children
7. Long-term effects of skin conditions
8. Importance of support groups
9. Advocacy for pediatric dermatology

The psychosocial effect of skin diseases in children is gigantic, not only on the patients themselves but also on their families. Childrenith cutaneous disorders visible to the eye become more depressed, anxious, and withdrawn due to stigmatization from such conditions. This emotional expense is compounded by the stress experienced by family members, who may also have trouble in their daily lives due to the child's illness. According to the research, 92% of the family members surveyed reported emotional impact d by the disease, which reflected the wide wide-reaching ripple effects in the family liBasra et al., 2013). Additionally, the sub sub-treatment of mental health within dermatological clinics exacerbates these problems, with healthcare providers often omitting the psyccal correlates of skin disease (Kraftet al., 2024). As such, it is crucial for pediatric dermatology to have a holistic approach, offering appropriate mental health care alongside physical therapy to enhance overall family quality of life.

3.3.1. Impact of Skin Conditions on Self-Esteem

The psychological impact of skin disorders on the self-esteem of children is a vital concern that should be taken carrehensively. There are many dermatoses, such as, such as congenital melanocytic nevi and atopic dermatitis, that significantly affect a child's body image and psychological health. Kids with abnormal skin diseases normally endure socially, leading to low self-esteem and depression. For instance, (Sanchez et al., 2023) identi atopic dermatitis-suffering children patients are more prone to mental illness compared to their peers and hence the need to screen for mental illness among such groups. In addition, therapy for skin diseases can also influence the perception of a child about themselves; one study proposes comparing surgical excision and lnital melanocytic nevi, with the aim of studyingto study their impact on quality of life and self-esteem by using the children's dermatology life quality index (Lai et al., 2018). Addressing these issues is crucial in establishing resilience and facilitating the psychosocial adjustment of the affected children.

3.3.2. Social Stigmas Associated with Skin Disorders

The social stigmas which are associated with skin diseases have a very strong impon the psychological and emotional health of the individuals afflicted with them, particularly children. Stigmas can cause negative self-concept, social rejection, and even depression in children since they become targets of bullying and discrimination by their peers because they have visible skin diseases. The social perceptions of skin diseases are also complicated by a lack of knowledge, resulting in an atmosphere of prejudice and discrimination. Moreover, the pervasive use of social media amplifies these issues as children are constantly shown unrealistic beauty standards and comparisons that further alienate them. Research indicates that social networking sites may be both remedial and contributory to these stressors, with platforms like TikTok producing upward social comparisons that are harmful to self-esteem (Talbot et al., 2024). Thus, those stigmas must be addressed in the process of creating an empathetic setting for children in pediatric dermatology and eventually improving their qualie and mental health (Bousquet et al., 2016N/A, 2017) (Figure 3.12).

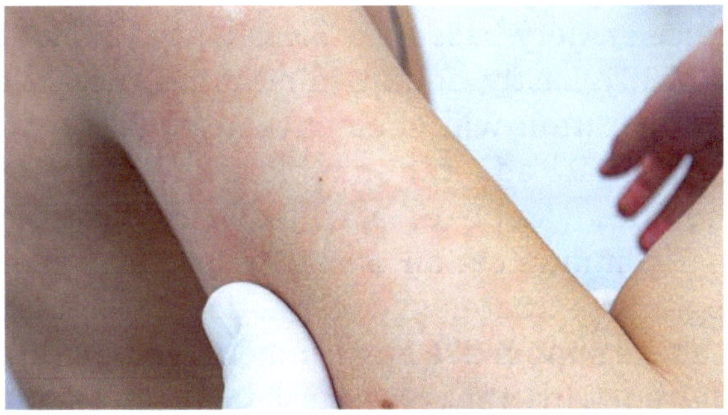

Figure 3.12. Examination of a child's arm showing a widespread erythematous rash, commonly associated with viral exanthems or allergic reactions.

Source: https://cdn.provaeducation.com/cache/93/af/93afef40938e53172d8dc29a169d5802.jpg.

3.3.3. Psychological Support for Affected Children

The psychological impact of skin diseases among children can be extreme, and proper psychological care is required to sustain their well-being. Children with skin diseases tend to develop anxiety, depression, and suicidal thoughts, as established in qualitative research with UK health workers (Hughes et al., 2024). These mental health disorders not only affect the children but also have serious implications for their caregivers, who may experience increased levels of stress and emotional burden. The necessity of specialized supportive interventions is understood, as previous research indicates that early and formal psychological intervention may decrease posttraumatic stress symptoms and enhance resilience in affected families (Yan et al., 2025). However, disparities in the provision of these services between zones can hinder access to these resources. Therefore, integrating psychological support into the daily care routine of pediatric dermatology patients is imperative for promoting holistic patient care and improving overall health outcomes.

3.3.4. Role of Parents and Caregivers

In pediatric dermatology, parents and caregivers are a key force for meeting the unique challenges of various skin disordncluding those associated with genetic diseases such as, such as Down syndrome and tuberous sclerosis complex. Parents are not just the first advocates for their child's health but also crucially important facilitators of medical care, helping to monitor and check up regularly on dermatological symptoms that may arise in these conditions. Their active involvement can contribute substantially to the success of treatment approaches, as early interventions largely rely on diligent observation and reporting of skin changes. Furthermore, parents and caregivers are also important in the compliance with ordered skin care regimens, preventing such complications as xerosis or eczema, thereby improving the quality of the child's life. The interprofessional relationship between the healthcare professionals and families indicates the necessity for intensive support systems in pediatric dermatology, as reflectt et al., 2016Marilyn et al., 2022; Northrup et al., 2021).

3.3.5. School Environment and Peer Relationships

The school environment is a critical place for the formation of relationships between peers and children, and these may significantly influence their dermatological and psychological healtstance, children who have visible skin disorders, such as, such as atopic dermatitis, tend to experience stigma or bullying that may exacerbate their feelings of loneliness and isolation. As evidenced by research, social interactions at school may have a significant impact on a child's self-esteem and stress levels, contributing further to their dermatological conditions. The interrelatedness of the variables underscores the significance of a positive school climate that fosters inclusivity and compassion, as well as the potential for interventions in peer relations. By focusing on healthy social processes, schools can potentially enhance outcomes for health, as healthier peer relationships could be associated with higher levels of treatment adherence or healthier self-care. Thus, offering solutions to the school environment and the impact on peer relationships is important for an integratequet et al., 2016Bernstein et al., 1973; Gallo et al., 2019) (Figure 3.13).

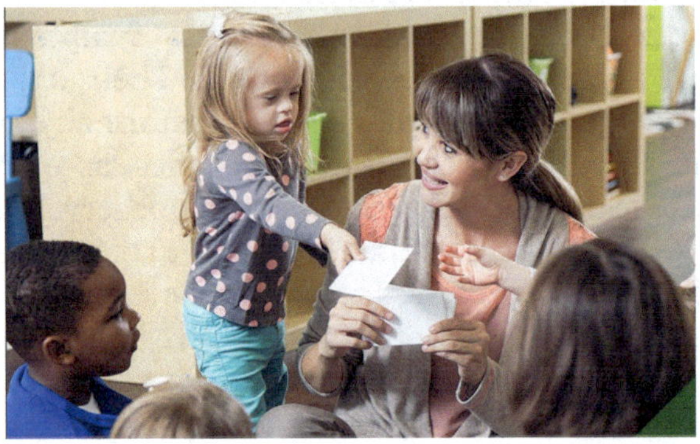

Figure 3.13. The school environment plays a pivotal role in shaping peer relationships among children.

Source: https://www.rasmussen.edu/images/rasmussenlibraries/blogs/what-is-inclusive-education-s.jpg.

3.3.6. Coping Strategies for Children

Children with chronic illnesses, including dermatological disorders such as atopic dermatitis, face unique challenges that require effective coping strategies to manage associated stress and discomfort. These strategies typically combine emotional and functional approaches that promote resilience and adaptive behavior. Psychosocial interventions, such as individual therapy, support groups, and structured counseling, can provide children with opportunities to express themselves, strengthen self-confidence, and develop skills to better manage their condition. In addition, education of the children and their families about the disease, its signs, and therapy will be crucial to reduce anxiety based on uncertainty (Bhatia et al., 2023). Lastly, adding mindfulness activities and relaxation will enhance emotional control and facilitate adaptation to flare and treatment schedules (Jacob et al., 2023). Encouraging open communication among the family about progress on treatment and emotional well-being creates a supportive environment, empowering children with the necessary tools to manage their dermatological experience effectively.

3.3.7. Long-term Effects of Skin Conditions

The chronic consequences of skin conditions, particularly in children, are substantial and long-lasting, with a physical and psychological impact. A common example is atopic dermatitis (AD), even though it is common in children, is chronic, leading to long-term pain and itching that disrupts activities. Psychological distress due to AD can exacerbate its symptoms, creating a negative feedback cycle in which depression and anxiety enhance skin symptoms, hence affecting quality of life.

Treatment is multipl to be tailored to the individual child's presentation, such as, such as topical treatment and systemic therapies like biologics for severe presentations. Although immunotherapy has succeeded in treating diseases like asthma and allergic rhinitis, its efficacy in treating AD remains uncertain due to variable proof of its long-term effveness and its reliability as therapy (Eichenfield et al., 20162019). Finally, treating the dermatologic as well as the psychological aspect n conditions is needed for increasing long-term outcomes (Abreu Lopes et al., 2020).

3.3.8. Importance of Support Groups

Support groups play an important role in the overall management of children's dermatological diseases by providing emotional, educational, and social support to the families and patients. Cophanisms and information about chronic disease management such as, such as acne and atopic dermatitis, are learned by families through collective experiences. For instance, the complex nature of atopic dermatitis, such that it typically co-occurs with other atopic disorders, emphasizes the need for a support group that understands the complexity of the challenge in treatment and management (Eichenfield et al., 2016).

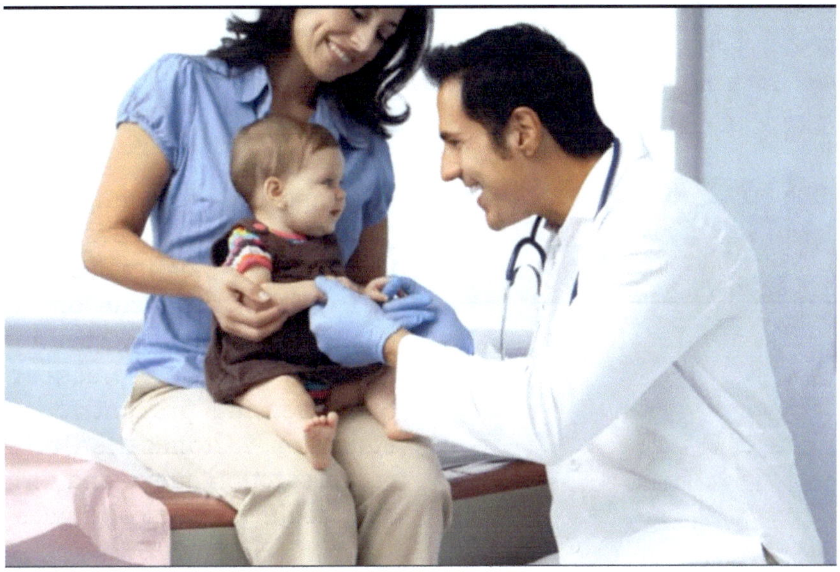

Figure 3.14. Support groups play a vital role in the holistic management of pediatric dermatological conditions by providing emotional.

Source: https://res.cloudinary.com/broadcastmed/image/fetch/q_auto,c_fill,w_1300,h_731,g_faces:center,f_auto/http%3A%2F%2F55933-bcmed.s3.amazonaws.com%2Fbcp%2Fmigrated%2Fimages%2Fvmm%2FimgSource%2FiStock_000022315032_Large.jpg.

Secondly, because children with dermatological issues are socially ostracized or stigmatized, support groups offset such feelings by fostering belongingness and understanding. This common environment not only promotes comprehension but also allows families to more effectively negotiate the health care system, ultimately increasing medication adherence with regimens like tretinoin for acne, ffective in children (Eichenfield et al., 2019Bhatt et al., 2019) (Figure 3.14).

3.3.9. Advocacy for Pediatric Dermatology

It requires advocacy of pediatric dermatology to generate increased awareness and maximize treatment results in children with various skin conditions. Such organizations work tirelessly to inform healthcare workers and the general public about the unique problems related to pediatric patients, particularly those presenting with chronic conditions like atopic dermatitis. Such a promotion is particularly significant since, in addition to raising awareness about good management practice, it also emphasizes addressing the psychological impact these conditions have on the adolescent. Through understanding that adolescence is a pivotal stage whereby self-management is paramount, healthcare professionals must come to appreciate the contribution educational interventions provide to enabling disease management knowrategies in patients (Eichenfield et al., 2019Beaure et al., 2019). Lastly, effective advocacy efforts can lead to improved patient care and a significant boost in the quality of life for impacted children with dermatological conditions (Hwang et al., 2017).

Test Your Knowledge

1. How can chronic skin conditions affect a child's self-esteem and emotional well-being?
2. What social stigmas are commonly associated with visible skin disorders in children?

3.4. Preventive Care and Health Promotion

Learning Outcome

1. Importance of skin care education
2. Sun protection strategies for children
3. Managing allergies and irritants
4. Role of nutrition in skin health
5. Regular dermatological check-ups
6. Awareness of skin changes
7. Community health initiatives
8. Resources for parents and caregivers
9. Future directions in preventive dermatology

Preventive health and health promotion are critical in pediatric dermatology, particularly in the prevention of skin cancer in children. As skin cancer is one of the most prevalent cancers diagnosed in the United States, protection against it is needed, most of which is due to ultraviolet radiation exposure (Bowlds et al., 2020). Research indicates that mothers often prioritize sun protection for their children over themselves, underscoring the need for targeted sun safety campaigns for younger age groups. Equally important is understanding the psychographic profile of adolescents, particularly females, whose behaviors regarding sun exposure are strongly influenced by social perceptions and personal comfort rather than simple negligence (Eichenfield et al., 2019). With the inclusion of these results in health promotion interventions, clinicians can facilitate sun safety practices more effectively by increasing preventive action and health education customization to enhance families' sun protection habits and ultimately long-term skin health outcomes (Figure 3.15).

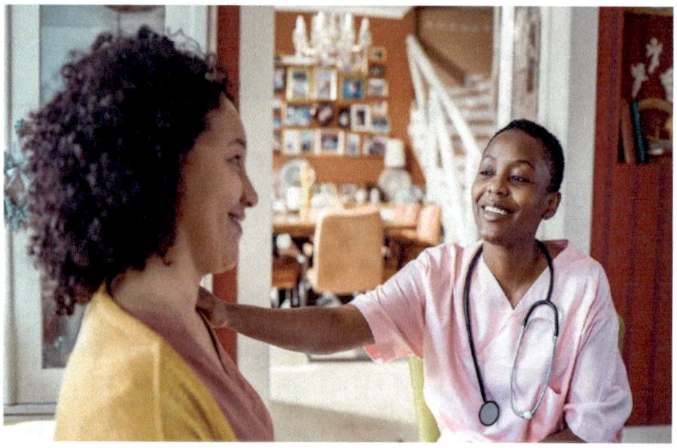

Figure 3.15. Preventive care and health promotion play a critical role in pediatric dermatology.

Source: https://i0.wp.com/post.healthline.com/wp-content/uploads/2023/02/caregiver-taking-care-of-a-senior-woman-header.jpg?w=1155&h=1528.

3.4.1. Importance of kin Care Education

The significance of skin care education should not be over-stressed, particularly as it relates to pediatric dermatology, where conditions of children's skin typically necessitate special management and care. Effective skin care education stimulates parents and health professionals to detect, prevent, and manage dermatological conditions at an early stage. Learning a good foundation of skin care knowledge not only results in healthier consequences but also instills active prevention of skin diseases. Family practitioners, being the first-line treatment experts, are responsible for educating families on common pediatric skin infections and self-care measures. This interactive activity can respond to any shortcomings of medical training when it comes to dermatological disorders, which are usually overlooked, as indicated in the National survey, quoting the significance of increased awareness in the medical training (Alikhan et al., 2014). Health-promoting educational programs can ultimately lead to enhanced detection and treatment of skin diseases in children.

3.4.2. Sun Protection Strategies for Children

Effective sun protection measures in children are a prerequisite to prevent the long-term consequences of sun exposure, which can lead to skin cancer and other dermatoses in adulthood. As children are very vulnerable to the harmful effects of the sun, it is critical to include multi-dimensional protective measures. Key strategies include repeated application of broad-spectrum sunscreen with an S0 or more, utilization of protective wear, and utilization of accessories such as, such as hats and sunglasses. In addition, informing parents and children about avoiding the sun during peak periods can reduce risks significantly. The Brazilian Society of Dermatology identifies education as an intervention due to the fact that the majority of children despise applying sunscreen; hence, the new format of the products and community awareness ientions arey to its effective use. Furthermore, pedicians are highly core committed in to advocating for the health outcomes of the children by practicing and enforcing sun safety measures (Saloni et al., 2024).

3.4.3. Managing Allergies and Irritants

Proper management of irritants and allergens is the backbone of pediatric dermatology, particularly where the condition involves such issues as atopic dermatitis and vernal keratoconjunctivitis. The prevalence of allergic skin diseases among children requires a wide scope of all the potential agents from environmental exposure to food allergens. Prolonged exposure to allergens worsens the conditions through added inflammation and discomfort.

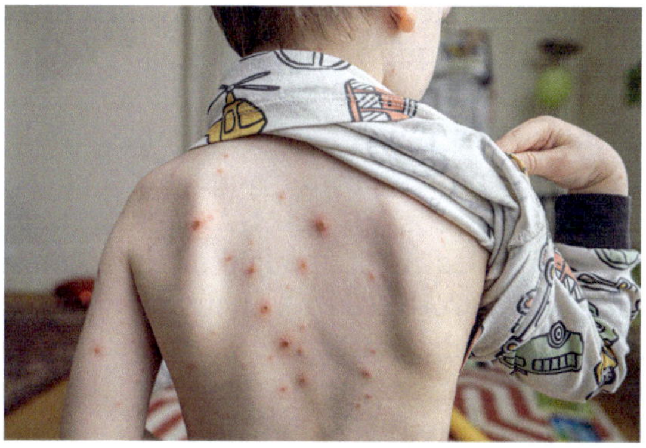

Figure 3.16. Effective management of allergies and irritants is a cornerstone of pediatric dermatology.

Source: https://www.westchestercosmeticdermatology.com//files/2024/09/pediatric-skin-treatment-scaled.jpeg.

Healthcare practitioners should promote individualized management plans, which can include the use of a well-documented eczema action plan (EAP) to guide families on the identification and avoidance of irritants (Heather et al., 2021). Furthermore, focus on the ical aspects of compliance with treatment is necessary; behavioral methods, such as, such as positive reinforcement, can significantly enhance compliance with treatment and results. Meanwhile, a treatment protocol for diseases like VKC is the challenge of achieving balance in care methodologies between different regions due to varying diagnostic and treatment standards, with implications for the need for harmonized protocols (Jodhbir et al., 2022) (Figure 3.16).

3.4.4. Role of Nutrition in Skin Health

Nutrition plays a pivotal role in skin health, particularly in children, as developing skin requires certaients to develop and become resistant. Poor nutrition leads to skin conditions such as, such as atopic dermatitis and psoriasis, which emphasize the need for a nutrient-rich diet with the required vitamins and minerals. For instance, omega-3 fatty acids in fish oil and flaxseeds have been demonstrated to suppress inflammation and enhance skin barrier function, whereas vitamins A, C, and E play significant roles in the repair of the skin and antioxidative protection. Furthermore, the effect of a poor diet may exacerbate a disease like acne, which is typical among adolescents. Nutrition education coupled with pediatric dermatology not only improves healthier skin but also overall wellbeing as children learn to maormed food choices that are able to prevent skin issues in the long run (Keglowichet al., 2014).

3.4.5. Regular Dermatological Check-Ups

Regular dermatological assessment is significant in pediatric practice because it's part of early detection and treatment of skin disease that potentially could impair a chealth and wellbeing. Routine its are not ony a chance to assess common issues such as, such as ecr acne, but it they also makes screening for risk factors for more serious diseases such as, such as skin cancer, feasible. Moreover, studies emphasize the importance of age-specific information and counseling, e.g., for lichen sclerosus vulvar in children, where patients showed the necessity for personalized treatment and counseling on their condition (Burger et al., 2024). Recurrent its stimulate active thinking on dermatological health, enhancing the child's knowledge on of their condition and prophylactic measures. These check-ups are ultimately a part of a broader system of humane care that responds to pediatric patients' evolving needs, and they emphasize their pivotal role in public health.

3.4.6. Awareness of Skin Changes

A critical aspect of pediatric dermatology is heightened surveillance by caregivers and doctors of alterations in the skin since such changeresent signs of disease in children. Early detection of dermatological presentation, such as, such as rashes or color change, is essential for early diagnosis and effective management. For instance, genetic diseases may be apparent through some skin abnormalities; tuberous sclerosis complex (TSC) may be presented with typical skin lesions, demanding careful monitoring and surveillance as outlined in updated diagnostic criteria. Similarly, the presence of skin xanthomas will signal familial hypercholesterolemia, equating dermatological presentations with severe cardiovascular risks, demanding treatmeat an early stage (Harada et al., 2018). Engaging parents and guardians in teaching them on about skin changes makes good healthcare habits, allowing children to get referrals to specialists in time when needed, thereby enhancing the quality of pediatric care and outcomes (Figure 3.17).

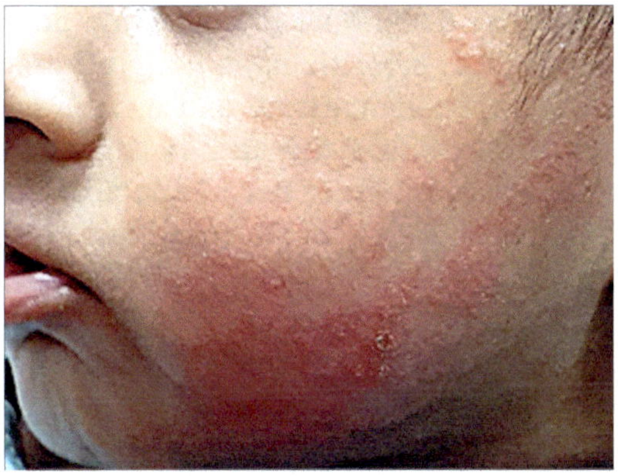

Figure 3.17. Child with inflamed, erythematous, and scaly lesions on the cheek, indicative of pediatric eczema.

Source: https://jsstd.org/content/102/2023/5/1/img/JSSTD-5-028-g003.png.

3.4.7. Community Health Initiatives

In pediatric dermatology, community health programs play an essential role in raising awareness and promoting proactive treatment of skin disease in children. Effective outreach programs make learning about common dermatological disorders and the importance of early intervention easier to deliver enhanced outcomes. Of special interest are programs thaporate evidence-based practice, which has been demonstrated to lower the disease burden such as, such as atopic dermatitis, by quite a margin. For instance, the establishment of core outcome sets in clinical trials is now required to standardize treatment efficacy and improve decision-making in pediatric management. Also, the incorporation of progress in data science, can improve such initiatives by optimizing community health data, keeping pediatric dermatology clinics tethered to actionable research. Combined, these efforts illustrate the potential of community health programs to better bridge gaps in access to healthcare, ultimately increasing families' ability to regulate the skin health of their children.

3.4.8. Resources for Parents and Caregivers

Navigating the difficulties of pe dermatology can be daunting for caregivers and parents alike, particularly with diseases such as, such as atopic dermatitis (AD). As a useful tool, the implementation of a written eczema action plan (EAP) has been extremely encouraging in enhancing caregiver self-efficacy as well as patient outcomes. Studies indicate that caregivers employing an individualized EAP along with educational information from the American Academy of Dermatology and the National Eczema Association enjoy a remarkable improvement in eczema severity, approximately 65%, along with increased ratings of self-efficacy. Added to this, recognition of the vast impact of AD on quality of life highlights the importance of helping caregivers with specialized resources; families suffer from immense psychological and social stresses, especially as the severity of the disease increases. Thus, empowering parents with vast resources is important in helping them cope effectively with their children's skin diseases (Figure 3.18).

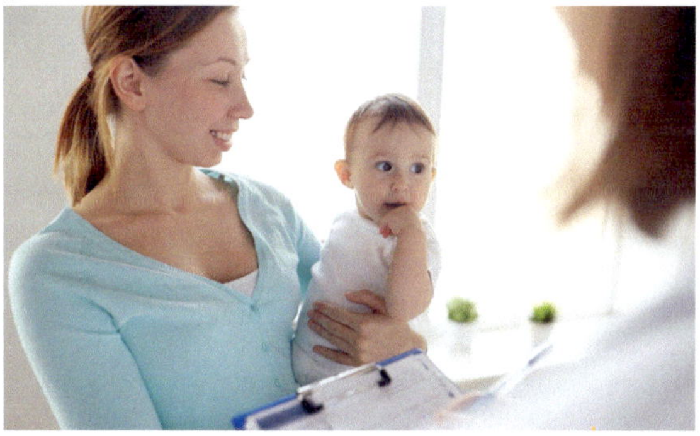

Figure 3.18. Resources for parents and caregivers.

Source: https://www.epiphanydermatology.com/wp-content/uploads/2019/11/pediatric-dermatology.png.

3.4.9. Future Directions in Preventive Dermatology

The future of preventive dermatology awaits fundamental change, particularly among the pediatric community, as medicine continues to expand in line with what has been learned from the COVrience. Among the key changes is increased focus on the application of e-health technologies, and these which are capable of expanding access to dermatology services and improving prevention of skin disease among children. Because normal screening was disrupted during the pandemic, the urgent need for innovative techniques in healthcare delivery was witnessed, prioritizing, among others, the need to adopt telemedicine and mobile health applications towards the end of early ds and ongoing management of dermatological issues. Besides, incorporation of advanced technologies such as, such as IoT and Big Data analytics, would help entification of risk groups and personalization of preventive interventions to suit populations (Helena M da Fonseca et al., 2021). Taking a cue from these advances, future advancements in preventive dermatology not only aim to restore access to care but also enhance patient outcomes on the whole in pediatric dermatology.

Test Your Knowledge

1. What sun protection strategies are most effective for maintaining healthy skin in children?
2. How can managing allergies and avoiding irritants help prevent common pediatric skin conditions?
3. Why are regular dermatological check-ups and preventive care important for children's long-term skin health?

SUMMARY

Pediatric dermatology is both demanding and rewarding, requiring specifically tailored treatment strategies for children. Recent studies on acne treatment, for example, have shown that tretinoin 0.05% lotion produced remarkable improvement in both inflammatory and non-inflammatory lesions among pre-adolescents, establishing its superiority over vehicle treatments (Eichenfield et al., 2019). Similarly, crisaborole ointment for atopic dermatitis significantly improved the quality of life of young patients and their families, highlighting the profound psychosocial effects of cutaneous diseases in children (Boguniewicz et al., 2018). These findings underscore the importance of selecting appropriate, age-adapted therapies that not only address clinical features but also enhance overall well-being. Continued research and clinical innovation remain essential to optimizing pediatric dermatology practice and outcomes. In pediatric dermatology, awareness of the multifactorial nature of atopic dermatitis (AD) is crucial, given its rising prevalence in children, now affecting approximately 13% of this population (Eichenfield et al., 2019). Effective management is often hindered by treatment non-adherence, largely due to misconceptions about the safety of topical corticosteroids (TCS) (Smith, 2017). Parents frequently receive conflicting advice from healthcare providers, relatives, and online sources, fostering a culture of 'TCS phobia' that negatively impacts adherence and treatment outcomes. Educational interventions, such as individualized written Eczema Action Plans, have been shown to enhance caregiver confidence and reduce disease severity (Smith, 2017). A coordinated approach, with consistent messaging from healthcare providers, is therefore essential to improve outcomes and ensure appropriate long-term care for children with AD.

KEY TERMS FROM THIS CHAPTER

- Allergic reactions
- Biologic therapies
- Cold atmospheric plasma (CAP)
- Crisaborole
- Eczema
- Fungal infections
- Human papillomavirus (HPV)
- Infants
- Atopic dermatitis (AD)
- Calcineurin inhibitors
- Complex diseases
- Diaper dermatitis (DD)
- Emotional growth
- Genetic disorders
- Immunoglobulin
- Port-wine birthmarks (PWBs)

CRITICAL THINKING QUESTIONS

1. **What is the most common inflammatory skin condition in children?**
   a. Psoriasis
   b. Seborrheic dermatitis
   c. Atopic dermatitis
   d. Contact dermatitis
2. **A 2-month-old infant presents with greasy, yellowish scales on the scalp. What is the most likely diagnosis?**
   a. Tinea capitis
   b. Cradle cap (seborrheic dermatitis)
   c. Psoriasis
   d. Impetigo
3. **Which skin infection is most commonly caused by Staphylococcus aureus** *Staphylococcus aureus* **in children?**
   a. Molluscum contagiosum
   b. Tinea corporis
   c. Impetigo
   d. Erythema infectiosum
4. **What is the hallmark of diaper dermatitis caused by Candida albicans?**
   a. Dry, scaly patches
   b. Beefy red plaques with satellite lesions
   c. Vesicular eruptions
   d. Lichenification
5. **Which viral infection causes umbilicated papules on the skin in children?**
   a. Herpes simplex
   b. Molluscum contagiosum
   c. Varicella
   d. Hand, foot, and mouth disease

Short Answer Questions

1. Define atopic dermatitis and list its common triggers.
2. Differentiate between irritant and candidal diaper dermatitis.
3. What are the clinical features of impetigo?
4. Describe the presentation and treatment of cradle cap.
5. What is molluscum contagiosum and how is it managed?

Answer to Critical Thinking Questions

1. (c); 2. (b); 3. (c); 4. (b); 5. (b)

REFERENCES

1. Al-Akhras, M. (2024). Editorial: Evaluating generative AI-based models in healthcare. *Jordan Medical Journal.* https://www.semanticscholar.org/paper/3b212070acb5b2d98ccad8e9f566d764e188ee5d (accessed on 16th June 2025).
2. Alikhan, A., Fazel, N., Gorouhi, F., Rezaei, N., et al. (2014). Dermatology residency selection criteria with an emphasis on program characteristics: A national program director survey. https://core.ac.uk/download/323068807.pdf (accessed on 16th June 2025).
3. Arasi, S., Corsello, G., Pajno, G. B., & Villani, A. (2018). The future outlook on allergen immunotherapy in children: 2018 and beyond. https://core.ac.uk/download/286528686.pdf (accessed on 16th June 2025).
4. Aygören-Pürsün, E., Bork, K., Bowen, T., Boysen, H., et al. (2012). WAO guideline for the management of hereditary angioedema. https://core.ac.uk/download/17179867.pdf (accessed on 16th June 2025).
5. Beaure d'Augères, G., Belousova, E., Benedik, M. P., Carter, T., et al. (2019). The TOSCA registry for tuberous sclerosis—Lessons learnt for future registry development in rare and complex diseases. https://core.ac.uk/download/286270878.pdf (accessed on 16th June 2025).
6. Benea, V., Georgescu, S. R., Matei, C., Sarbu, M., et al. (2015). Common dermatoses in patients with obsessive compulsive disorders. https://core.ac.uk/download/144552344.pdf (accessed on 16th June 2025).
7. Eichenfield, L. F., Sugarman, J. L., Guenin, E., Harris, S., & Bhatt, V. (2019). Novel tretinoin 0.05% lotion for the once-daily treatment of moderate-to-sevey treatment of moderate-to-severe acne vulgaris in a preadolescent population. https://core.ac.uk/download/323310744.pdf (accessed on 16th June 2025).
8. Bowlds, J. (2020). The effect of a sun damage simulation photography app on the skin-protective behavior intentions of women with children age 18 or younger. https://core.ac.uk/download/322984951.pdf (accessed on 16th June 2025).
9. Cartron, A. M., Chung, C., Osler, M., Trinidad, J., et al. (2020). Nuclear matrix protein 2 antibody-positive adult dermatomyositis: A case report and review of the literature. https://core.ac.uk/download/322493868.pdf (accessed on 16th June 2025).
10. da Fonseca, M. H., Kovaleski, F., Picinin, C. T., Pedroso, B., & Rubbo, P. (2021). E-health practices and technologies: A systematic review from 2014 to 2019. *Healthcare, 9*, 1192–1192. https://doi.org/10.3390/healthcare9091192 (accessed on 16th June 2025).
11. Dehner, L. P., Gonzalez, I., Rais, R., Saito, Y., et al. (2018). Infantile hemangioma presenting as colocolic intussusception in an infant: Case report with review of pathologic lead points. https://core.ac.uk/download/212868622.pdf (accessed on 16th June 2025).
12. Dellavalle, R. P., Obagi, Z. A., & Rundle, C. W. (2020). Widening the scope of virtual reality and augmented reality in dermatology. https://core.ac.uk/download/287622747.pdf (accessed on 16th June 2025).
13. Diatta, B., Nibirantije, P., Diop, K., Diatta, R., Sarr, M., Mendy, P., Diadie, S., et al. (2023). Dermatological manifestations during HIV infection in children in Dakar, Senegal. *Our Dermatology Online.* https://www.semanticscholar.org/paper/f06d66d3ba46fdb90fddcfa57d8e093bffe4fc5c (accessed on 16th June 2025).

14. Eller, E., Kjær, H. F., Høst, A., Andersen, K. E., & Bindslev-Jensen, C. (2015). Treatment of childhood atopic dermatitis and economic burden of illness in Asia Pacific countries. *Annals of Nutrition and Metabolism, 66*, 18–24. https://doi.org/10.1159/000370221 (accessed on 16th June 2025).

15. Esposito, S., & Principi, N. (2021). Multisystem inflammatory syndrome in children related to SARS-CoV-2. *Pediatric Drugs.* https://doi.org/10.1007/s40272-020-00435-x (accessed on 16th June 2025).

16. Gallo, R. L., Irvine, A. D., Kong, H. H., Luger, T., et al. (2019). The microbiome in patients with atopic dermatitis. https://core.ac.uk/download/323064499.pdf (accessed on 16th June 2025).

17. Helms, L., & Burrows, H. L. (2021). Diaper dermatitis. *Pediatrics in Review, 42*, 48–50. https://doi.org/10.1542/pir.2020-0128 (accessed on 16th June 2025).

18. Hidvégi, B., & Bali, G. (2018). Diagnostic and treatment strategies of dermatologists for treating morphea in Hungary. https://core.ac.uk/download/212467162.pdf (accessed on 16th June 2025).

19. Hwang, B. (2017). Educational interventions targeting adolescents with atopic dermatitis. https://open.bu.edu/bitstream/2144/26735/5/Hwang_bu_0017N_13190.pdf (accessed on 16th June 2025).

20. Keglowich, L. F. (2014). Airway wall remodeling in asthma: Novel mechanisms of human bronchial smooth muscle cells in the induction of angiogenesis. https://core.ac.uk/download/33299347.pdf (accessed on 16th June 2025).

21. Kraft, E. (2024). It's more than skin deep: Evaluating mental health care in dermatology settings. https://core.ac.uk/download/624274604.pdf (accessed on 16th June 2025).

22. Lai, Y. (2018). Comparing congenital melanocytic nevus treatment effect on children's health-related quality of life. https://core.ac.uk/download/475688229.pdf (accessed on 16th June 2025).

23. Lucero, S. (2017). Defining the scope of practice for nurse practitioners in MIAM. https://core.ac.uk/download/147839616.pdf (accessed on 16th June 2025).

24. Mustonen, R. (2018). Social media as a healthcare tool: Case study analysis of factors influencing pediatric clinicians' behavioral intent to adopt social media for patient communication and engagement. https://core.ac.uk/download/236295247.pdf (accessed on 16th June 2025).

25. Sena, T. (2019). Managing childhood atopic dermatitis: Utilizing a written eczema action plan to improve caregiver self-efficacy. https://core.ac.uk/download/214384237.pdf (accessed on 16th June 2025).

26. Shah, S. A., & Jahnke, M. N. (2024). Nevi–when to refer. *Current Opinion in Pediatrics, 36*, 411–417. https://www.semanticscholar.org/paper/c960bc17617d5f25d55966ad4b0cd63c600882e2 (accessed on 16th June 2025).

27. Smith, S. D. (2017). Pediatric atopic dermatitis and treatment adherence: Exploring factors contributing to topical corticosteroid phobia as a contributor to poor treatment adherence. https://core.ac.uk/download/212692517.pdf (accessed on 16th June 2025).

28. Szeto, M. D., Barber, C., Ranpariya, V. K., Anderson, J., Hatch, J., Ward, J., Aguilera, M. L., et al. (2022). Emojis and emoticons in health care and dermatology communication: Narrative review. *JMIR Dermatology, 5*, e33851–e33851. https://doi.org/10.2196/33851 (accessed on 16th June 2025).

PEDIATRIC ENDOCRINE DISORDERS

4

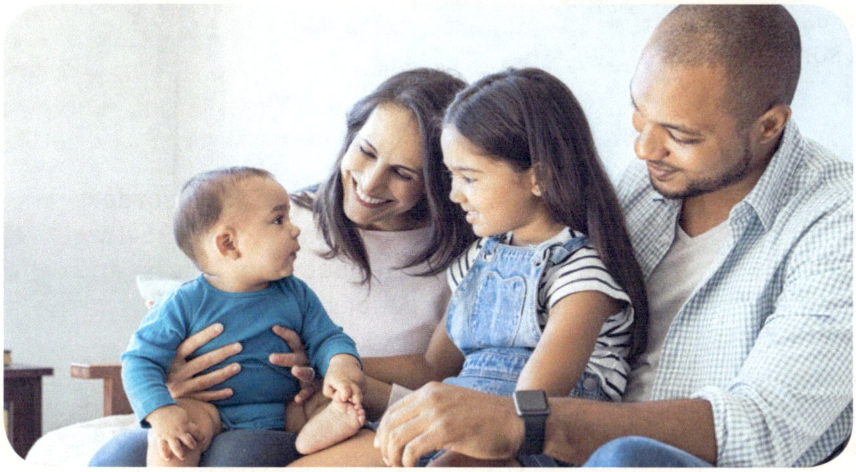

LEARNING OBJECTIVES

After studying this chapter, you will be able to:

1. Explain the categories of pediatric endocrine disorders
2. Discuss etiology and risk factors
3. Focus on emphasize symptoms and diagnosis
4. Learn about treatment options
5. Understand long-term management
6. Know recent advances in research

Introduction

Endocrine disorders of childhood encompass a wide range of conditions in children that are the result of hormonal imbalance and dysfunction of the endocrine system. The conditions may have pivotal impacts on growth, metabolism, and overall health, leading to long-term effects if not diagnosed and treated early. The endocrine system is an intricate network that regulates many of the body's functions through the release of hormones, which play ceoles in functionssuch as, such as growth, development, and maintenance of homeostasis. Notably, detection and control of endocrine diseases at an early level are crucial since they are likely to affect the physical as well as psychological growth of a child, with long-term implications being involved. This introduction sets the background for a complete study of the extent of pediatric endocrine disorders and emphasizes the need for caution while practicing to facilitate early intervention. Among the many forms of pediatric endocrorders, conditions such as, such as diabetes mellitus, thyroid function, and growth hormone deficiency are particularly common. Diabetes, types 1 and 2, in most cases, is increasingly present in the pediatric population, and the significance of effective management of blood glucose to prevent complications cannot be overestimated. The thyroid condition also leads to hypothyroidism and hyperthyroidism, both of which have specific clinical manifestations and effects on growth and development, and mental function, in children. Growth hormone disorders, either due to deficiency or excess, can have a significant effect on a child's somatic pattern of development.

Treatment is based on an understanding of the complicated hormonal mechanisms involved and the potential impact of various therapeutic interventions. Readers may gain an understanding of these diseases, diagnosis methods, and treatment regimens, illustrating the intricacy of pediatric endocrine health. Management of pediatric endocrine disorders is not merely a clinical issue but a challenge to interdisciplinary collaboration among physicians. Involvement of pediatric endocrinologists, dietitians, psychologists, and family physicians is important to provide holistic care that addresses the multifaceted needs of participating children and families. A multidisciplinary team guarantees that therapies take into account not only the biological aspects of the disorders but also the emotional and social aspects of chronic endocrine illnesses. There is also growing awareness of patient-oriented strategies that involve the family in making decisions on treatme As the development of medicine, such as, such as stem cell therapy, comes into consideration as future treatment options, the debate about these disorders becomes more vibrant (Duc et al., 2022). Seconderstanding associated conditions such as, such as cerebral palsy again emphasizes the importance of early intervention and multidisciplinary management (Dilip et al., 2020). This introduction accounts for the necessity of awareness and intervention in pediatric endocrinology and sets the stage for a critical review of all the various conditions and treatment modalities (Figure 4.1).

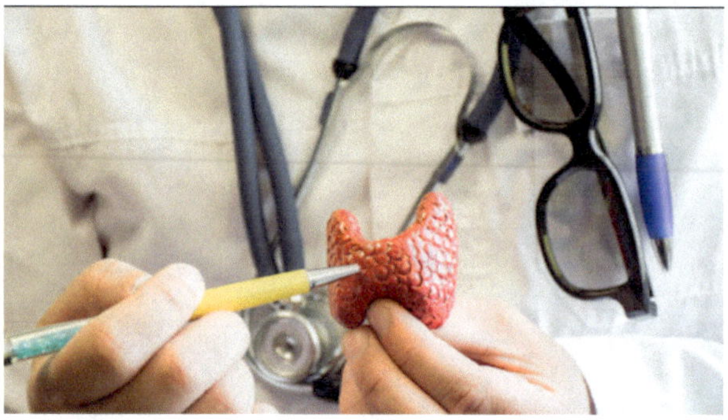

Figure 4.1. Pediatric endocrine disorders encompass a range of conditions affecting children due to hormonal imbalances and dysfunctions of the endocrine system.

Source: https://lh5.googleusercontent.com/proxy/oV6oYbjRHaJ2sGXpAEa4pXXcjLtyTsuvTQhqq6FWZrscpa_XC2ocH97NstBub yCy aDHAdX QWMJBnWQA2PSF3pOwMZQV6hy- u_isHfLzZ91YQ1Zcbhwy_i85-.

Definition of Pediatric Endocrine Disorders

Pediatric endocrine disorders represent a diverse category of illnesses in the endocrtem of children, encompassing glands such as, such as the pituitary, thyroid, and adrenal glands. Pediatric endocrine disorders are characterized by abnormal hormone levels that potentially have a significant impact on growth, metabolism, and development. Hormones are chemical messengers in the body that function to regulate various physiological processes, and any type of disruption in their secretion can lead ed expressions. For instance, conditions such as, such as congenital adrenal hyperplasia and growth hormone deficiency illustrate the potential of aberrations in the levels of hormones to retard normal growth patterns as well as metabolic processes. Timely diagnosis and treatmeediatric endocrine diseases have the capability tocan lead to long-standing problems of health problems if left untreated. Due to the complicated nature of such diseases, a multi-disciplinary approach is mostly required for effective management and treatment. Genetic breakthroughs have unraveled the complex mechanisms of the majority of pediatric endocrine disorders. With advances in research, technologies like long-read next-generation sequencing (NGS) have emerged as instrumental tools in the identification of genetic differences associated with such disorders. A technique of this nature is beneficial to the diagnosis of disorders involving complicated genetic factors, allowing for a better understanding of the etiology of the disorder. For instance, science has determined that long-read NGS can uncover structural changes and repeat expansions that might be overlooked through traditional methods (Cho, 2024). Such advancemize haplotype phasing, improving our ability in tracingto trace the inheritance history of such conditions. Therefore, the use of cutting-edge genetic technology in pediatric endocrinology not only aids in accurate diagnosis but also provides ways of opening the doors to optimized treatment strategies suitable for a patient's individual genetic makeup. Apart from the physiological effect, being aware of the implications of pediatric endocrine disorders involves coping with psychological aal factors as well. For example, endocrine disorders such as, such as polycystic ovary syndrome (PCOS) are not only medical conditions but enormous psychosocial implications. Common symptoms, such as, such as weight gain, acne, and hirsutism, may adversely affect a child's self-esteem and social relationships. Endocrine diildren and adolescents may develop additional issues, such as, ullying or solitude, due to their visible symptoms (N/A, 2024Wang et al., 2019). This highlights the importance of holistic care that includes medical treatment but psychological care as well. By adopting a whole-person approach to treating these patients, health professionals can maximize quality of life and well-being in general, highlighting the importance of an integrated approach in the management of pediatric endocrine disorders.

Importance of Early Diagnosis and Treatment

The importance of early detection and treatment of endocrine disorders in children cannot be overstated. These conditions, which disrupt hormonal balance and growth, often arise during critical stages of development and can profoundly affect overall health and maturation. Early detection of such disorders facilitates early intervention, which reduces potential complicatght about by delayed treatment. Some of these disorders, such as, such as precocious puberty or growth hormone deficiencies, have the potential to dramatically affect the growth and psychosocial development of a child. Early intervention not only aligns development and growth with peers but also avoids long-term complications, like emotional distress or social isolation. Hence, health professionals must prioritize routine endocrine tests as part of routine pediatric examinations so that any deviations can be addressed in time for optimum development. Additionally, in conditions like cryptorchidism, early diagnosis is extremely crucial to prevent future reproductive complications. When either or both testicles do not lie within the scrotum, for example, in cryptorchidism, fertility abnormalities and malignancy threats are significantly increased if they are not treated. The National Endocrinology Comm has underscored that early detection of the condition will have allow for timely surgical intervention, primarily orchiopexy, best performed before the age of 12 ths. Delayed treatment will bear irreparable consequences, such as, such as decreased fertility and cancer risk, which is why awareness and surveillance are crucial. Thus, pediatricians and parents must be vigilant to identify early signs of such disorders in order to implement proper management strategies and provide long-term health results (Viviana et al., 2024). Moreover, early diagnosis and effective management have a relationshipach other for the case of other common endocrine disorders such as, such as PCOS and thyroid abnormalities. The complexities described in treating PCOS emphasize the requirement of immediate and precise diagnosis. Delaying treatment of disorders concerning hormonal imbalances can lead to severe complications like infertility, metabolic syndrome, and increased cardiovascular risks. Early plans of management not only enhance the quality of life of those affected but also equip them for lifestyle adjustment and interventions that can prevent further more severe health issues. It is then so vital to recognize the symptoms and understand the intricacies of such disorders as to validate the role of early intervention in shaping positive health outcomes in children (Azam et al., 2025) (Figure 4.2).

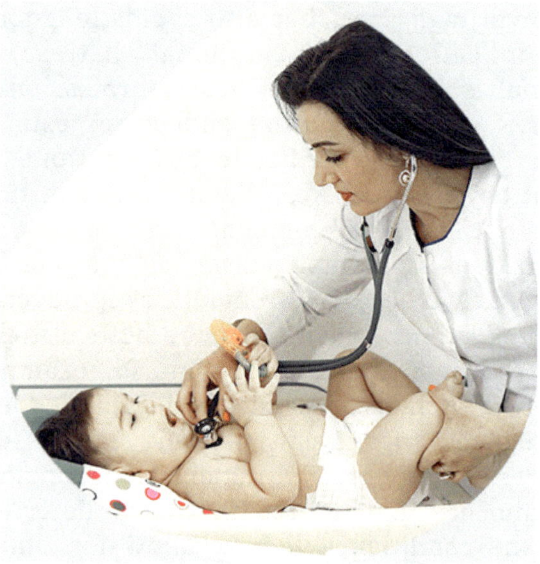

Figure 4.2. Importance of early diagnosis and treatment.

Source: https://gshri.com/wp-content/uploads/2023/11/Pediatric-Onco-surgery.png.

4.1. Types of Pediatric Endocrine Disorders

Learning Outcome

1. Diabetes mellitus
2. Growth hormone deficiency
3. Thyroid disorders

The spectrum of pediatric endocrine disorders encompasses a range of hormonal abnormalities that can significantly impact a child's growth, development, and overall health. The most prevalent endocrine disorder in children is diabetes mellitus in the form of type 1 diabetes. This autoimmune disorder results in the destruction of insulin-producing β-cells in the pancreas, resulting in hyperglycemia. The treatment of diabetes in children requires a comprehensive plan, including insulin therapy, diet control, and constant checking of the blood glucose level. The American Diabetes Association (ADA) recommends that adequate education for the patient and his/her famil crucial for effective management of diabetes (Wang et al., 2019N/A, 2018). Other endocrine diseases apart from diabetes include growth hormone deficiency, which can lead to short stature if untreated. It is important to recognize the implications of these disorders to intervene early and treat them. Thyroid dysfunction is another major category of endocrine disorders in children, either as hypothyroidism or hyperthyroidism. Hypothyroidism due to insufficient thyroid hormone production, in childhood, may initially become evident through developmental delaargy, and failure to grow. Conversely, hyperthyroidism, due to disorders such as, such as Graves' disease, generates signs and symptoms of weight loss, hyperactivity, and tachycardia. Thyroid conditionsrough hormonal replacement therapy or antithyroid drugs with the aim of achievingto achieve hormonal balance. Pediatricians and endocrinologists usually collaborate to diagnose and prescribe treatment plans for such disorders. Follow-ups and monitoring cannot be overemphasized since hormone levels may change over time, necessitating a shift in treatment methodsthe best health benefits are delivered to affecteang et al., 2019N/A, 2017). Also, endocrine disorders of the adrenal gland, such as, such as congenital adrenal hyperplasia (CAH), represent another significant field in pediatric endocrinology. CAH results from enzyme deficiencies that lead to a deficiency in cortisol and impair the body's ability to handle stress. It is most frequently identified in infancy through newborn screening programs, and it is of utmost priority to make such an early diagnosis as not to miss life-threatening adrenal crises. Treatment most often involves hormone replacement, aiming to normalize the hormones and opment. The psychosocial impact of such disorders in children as well as on families is significant, given the chronicity of management and implications for everyday life. Through thorough education and care, medical professionals can make families more comprehensively aware of the complexity that comes with adrenal disorders and thus emphasize the need for a multidisciplinary team when treating children with endocrine disorders (Figure 4.3).

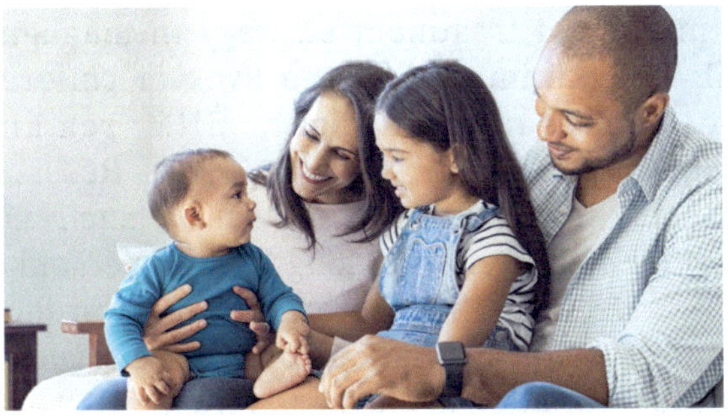

Figure 4.3. Types of pediatric endocrine disorders.

Source: https://ochsner-craft.s3.amazonaws.com/www/services/_960x540_crop_center-center_80_none/692564/GettyImages-696311644.jpg.

4.1.1. Diabetes Mellitus

The rising prevalence of Diabetes Mellitus among children has emerged as a reason for serious concern among pediatric endocrine diseases. Diabetes Mellitus, which is typified by hyperglycemia, is brought about by either a lack of production of insulin or the non-sensitivity of the body towards insulin. Type 1 diabetes tends to be diagnosed in childhood or adolescence and is defined by an autoimmune destruction of pancreatic insulin-secreting beta cells. On the other hand, Type 2 diabetes, increasingly being encountered among children, is linked to obesity, lack of exercise, and genetics. The complex interplay of these problems addsof treating diabetes among younger populations, as interventions need not only to tackleto tackle not only medical issues but also social determinants of health. The effects of diabetes extend beyond glucose control; they encompass numerous biopsychosocial issues that affect the general healwell-being of the child. Children with diabetes are at risk for long-term sequelaesuch as, such as neuropathy, retinopathy, and cardiovascular disease into adulthood. Moreover, psychosocial stressors inherent in chronic illness may also lead to anxiety, depression, and social isolation among affected children. The impact of the COVID-19 pandemic has even amplified such challengeisruptions in routine care and the creation of pathological lifestyle adaptations, such as, such as poor eating habits and decreased physical activity, resulting in worsening diabetes control. Addressing these areas is a must if outcomes are to be optimized and the quality of life for children and families is to be improved. Nutrition is the most vital area in the management of diabetes mellitus. Appropriate dietary interventions significantly influence glycemic control and prevent the complications of the disorder. A balanced diet based on natural foods combined with decreasing refined sugars is a crucial intervention in children with diabetes. Educating the patients about carbohydrate counting, glycemic index information, and healthier foods empowers the children and their families to manage daily challenges effectively. Moreover, vitamin D has been an area of interest in the management of diabetes due to its roles in immune function and insulin sensitivity. Vitamin D insufficiency can lead to other complications; hence, understanding its implications is necessary in the comprehensive control of diabetes in children. Addressing these concerns in a comprehensive manner will encourage a more integrated model of diabetic children's care, considering both medical and lifestyle issues, and ultimately better long-term health outcomes (Figure 4.4).

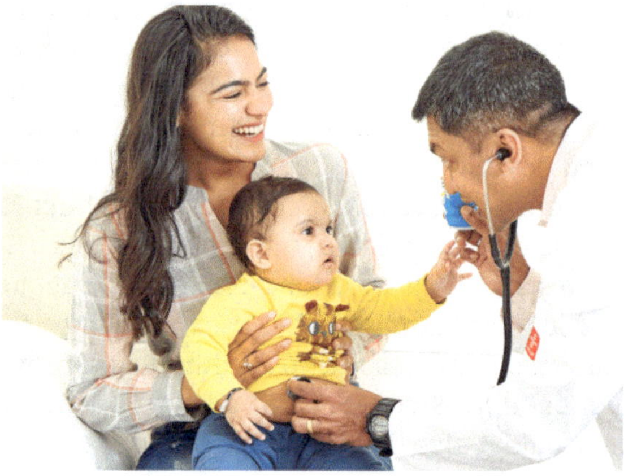

Figure 4.4. Diabetes mellitus.

Source: https://www.manipalhospitals.com/uploads/specialities/Why_MH-Whitefield_570x420_10.png.

4.1.2. Growth Hormone Deficiency (GHD)

GHD is the most frequent endocrine cause of short stature in children and adolescents, with very significant physical, emotional, and social implications. Since pediatric endocrinologists encounter issues with growth quite frequently, it becomes imperative to distinguish GHD from other causes of short stature. The etiology of GHD onset is due to genetic mutations, hypothalamus or pituitary trauma, or idiopathic etiology, affecting various aspects of development in young patients. The psychological impacts are particularly concerning; GHD children have difficulty with lower self-esteem and social withdrawal, compromising their health-related quality of life (HRQoL) at critical adolescent years (Guerra et al., 2025). Identification of GHD and treatment early on are therefore essential, not only for the development of stature but also in the development of emotional strength as they navigate significant phases of life. The management of GHD in children is typically growth hormone replacement, which has been reported to have a good capability for inducing growth and enhancing overall well-being. The therapy does, however, require close monitoring og to its mixed effect on metabolic parameters and overall health. Pediatric endocrinologists do find use in a multi-disciplinary approach that incorporates regular psychological assessments alongside physical therapy. Such an integrative process recognizes the relationship between psychological development and emotional development, where psychological screening can be a useful tool in establishing the underlying issues that may be exacerbated if left untreated (Guerra et al., 2025). Incorporating these assessments in practice not only aids in individualizing treatments to meet specific needs but also emphasizes the importance of an integrated treatment strategy in managing GHD and its impact on the lives of children. Dee improvementeatment, GHD remains underdiagnosed and underreported. Research indicates how that factors such as, such as a shortage of awareness among medical personnel, ineffective screening protocols, and differences in referral policies play a role in the issue. In addition, variation in diagnostic cra may produce variation in reported rates of prevalence, making it challenging to understand GHDs its actual contribution. New research suggests that enhanced knowledge and education regarding GHD can significantly enable early detection and initiate timely interventions that enhance the quality of life in affected adolescents. This is particularly critical, as untreated GHD has the potential to lead to long-term psychosocial morbidity and reduce overall health statufore, breaking through the impediments to successful treatment and diagnosis is essential towards for enhanced management of pediatric endocrine disorders, and Growth Hormone Deficiency is a case in point.

4.1.3. Thyroid Disorders

Disorders of the thyroid in children form a very significant group of endocrine pathology, with the occurrence of hypo- and hyperthyroidism prevailing. Hypothyroidism, either due to autoimmune conditions like Hashimoto's or congenital failure of the glands, can result in a variety of developmental complications ranging from growth retardation to impaired intellect. Hyperthyroidism, caused mostly by Graves' disease, can manifest itself in the form of weight loss, tachycardia, and enhanced nervousness. These disorders not only disrupt the usual physiological processes but can further complicate the treatment of underlying health issues, hence warranting early diagnosis and therapeutic management. Moreover, long-term results of thyroid disease left untreated in formative years justify the necessity of universal pediatric screening programs encompassing thyroid function testing, not merely on an individual basis but also on a broad public health basis to prevent exposure to potential developmental sequelae of such conditions. The intricate interplay between thyroid illness and other disease conditions is particularly noteworthy among children with autism spectrum disorder (ASD). Early evidence suggests that the prevalence of thyroid dysfunction in pediatric populations with ASD could be more than 50%, highlighting the need for judicious screening practices among the population. Patients with ASD are likely to have multiple gastrointestinal, nutritional, and metabolic disorders complicating their health profile. Diagnosis and management of thyroid disorders in such individuals can greatly improve the quality of life and control of symptoms. To this end, pediatric practire advised to adopt a holistic response that entails comprehensive assessment of associated conditions, such as, such as extensive thyroid evaluation, in their treatment of children with ASD, balancing medical therapy with the interrelated needs of this patient population (Nicolás et al., 2020). Technological improvements in the medical knowledge of rare endocrine diseases have unraveled the complexities of the management of thyroid diwithin a spectrum of rare endocrine diseases. Thyroid disease belongs to a group of rare endocrine diseases, which although rare per se, collectively affect a significant number of children globally. The European Society for Endocrinology has identified that over 440 discrete rare endocrine disorders can impact pediatric populations, making the need for robust systems to enable timely diagnosis and emerging therapies even more important. Pediatric endocrinologists are tasked with addressing these issues, striving to provide quality care amid often multifactorial rare endocrine disease.

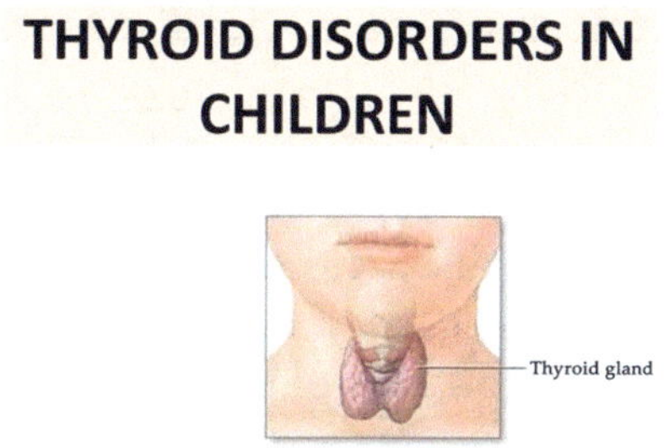

Figure 4.5. Thyroid disorders in pediatric populations represent a significant category of endocrine dysfunction.

Source: https://cdn.slidesharecdn.com/ss_thumbnails/thyroiddisordersinchildren-200619210229-thumbnail.jpg?width=640&height=640&fit=bounds.

Coordination to better enable European Reference Network development can drive diagnostic accuracy and treatment efficacy further for pediatric thyroid disease, ultimately contributing to improved health outcomes (Reincke et al., 2021) (Figure 4.5).

Test Your Knowledge

1. What are the common causes, symptoms, and management strategies for diabetes mellitus in children?
2. How does growth hormone deficiency affect a child's physical development and overall health?
3. What are the typical presentations and treatments of thyroid disorders in pediatric patients?

4.2. Causes and Risk Factors

Learning Outcome

1. Genetic predispositions
2. Environmental influences
3. Autoimmune conditions

The etiology of pediatric endocrine disorders is heavily burdened with several causes and risk factors that markedly impact children's health. Genetic predisposition is one dominant contributing factor among these, since most endocrine disorders, like obesity and diabetes, are genetic. Children whose immediate families have histories of the same disorders are at increased risk, and this suggests thagene-environment interactions may trigger the development of these disorders. Furthermore, some endocrine diseases such as, such as thyroid disease, may be caused by genetic mutations that affect the control of hormones. It is crucial to learn how genetics and endocrine function correlate to identify high-risk populations and implement early intervention strategies that can avoid chronic health consequences. Besides genes, environmental and behavioral factors significantly contribuhildhood endocrine disorders common among all of them is childhood obesity, which is now a global epidemic within among millions of ch Sedentary A sedentary lifestyle accompanied by unhealthy eating habits makes this issue acute and leads to diseases such as, such as type 2 diabetes and metabolic syndrome. Most notably, scientific studies have pinpointed social media and screen time as influencers of children's consumption patterns and activity levels, and these have been linked to an uptick in unhealthy weight trends (Czeczotka et al., 2024). Addressing these determinants in the environment requires an all-inclusive approach of attention that focuses on education on healthy lifestyle choices alongside the provision of physical activity.

These interventions are essential for the prevention of endocrine disorders caused by lifestyle factors. Also, the psychosocial setting can be a causative factor in the development of endocrorders in children. Family stressors, peer issues, and societal stressors tend to lead to unhealthy coping strategies such as, such as bad dietary habits and lack of physical activity. The empirically established connection between psychological well-being and the onset of eating disorders makes it imperative that mental well-being is made a primary focus of prevention (Voroncova et al., 2024). The establishment of a support network and making available resources specifically geared toward overcoming these psychosocial factors can help healthcare providers aid in preventing the possibility of endocrine problems. This holistic approach becomes pivotal not just for the management of existing health issues but also for the prevention of disease in adulthood, eventually fostering the well-being of vulnerable children in the long run.

4.2.1. Genetic Predispositions

Understanding genetic predispositions is essential in the study of pediatric endocrine disorders because these genetic predispositions significantly affect the development and progression of many diseases. Genetic predispositions are the increased risks of disease formation based on one's genes. In children, the predispositions may be caused by inherited mutations within genetics that affect hormones, growth patterns, or metabolism. For instance, identification of diseaseg mutations in genes involved in immune deficiency disorders can enlighten the pathogenetic mechanism of complex diseases such as, such as Evans syndrome. Research has identified that a significant number of children with pediatric patients harbor these genetic variants, which complicate their clinical presentation and courses of treatment (Crickx et al., 2023). By grasping the role of genetic predispositions, medical professionals can tailor interventions most effectively in respo the unique needs of children at risk for certain endocrine illnesses. Further, recent research acknowledges the interaction among between environmental factors and genetic predispositions in shaping the health outcomes of children. The mother's state of health and behavior during pregnancy and the consequent genetic expression form a critical part of this interaction. For example, maternal overnutrition and obesity have been shown to have an impact on the metabolic profiles of the offspring, thus making them more susceptible to obesity and the related endocrine abnormalities in adulthood. This epigenetic inheritance is an estimate of the extent to which environmental factors might interact with genetic susceptibility to alter health pathways in populations of children (Panera et al., 2022). This clarificf these dynamics not only sheds light on the complexity of the endocrine disorders but also underscores preventive interventions such as, such as maternal well-being, nutrition, and lifestyle modifications during pregnancy to lower risk in future generations. Lastly, the significance of genetic predispositions for childhood endocrine disorders calls for the institution of aggressive genetic counseling and testing programs. Hereditary factors decide the likelihood of inherited endocrine issues, and hence, the significance of proactive evaluations. At times, the low rate of genetic diagnoses among adults compared to children with conditions like Evans syndrome shows that early genetic testing among pediatric populations is most likely to provide significant insight into clinical care (Crickx et al., 2023).

Secondarily, by elucidating the underlying genetic mechanisms, clinicians can facilitate informed decision and specific health care modalities. Ultimately, the adoption of a holistic awareness of genetic predispositions will strengthen the fields capacity for effectively managing pediatric endocrine disorders, leading the way to better patient outcomes and individualized therapeutic interventions (Figure 4.6).

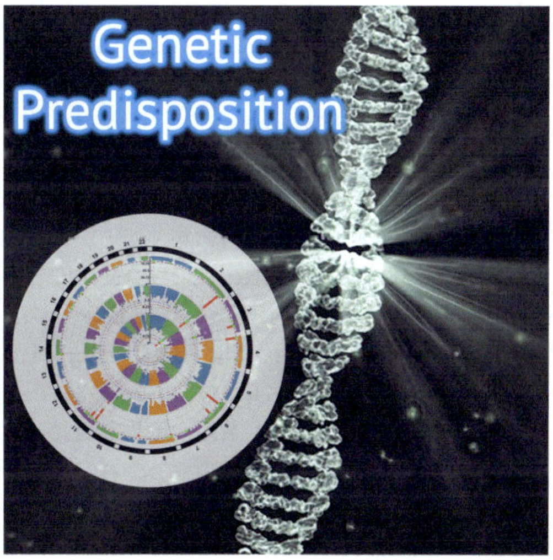

Figure 4.6. Genetic predispositions.

Source: https://diskinlab.org/wp-content/uploads/2019/08/Research-headings_Predis_v3.png.

4.2.2. Environmental Influences

The environmental determinants of pediatric endocrine disease are vast and pervasive, encompassing influences that shape physical and psychosocial health at critical junctures of development. Diet is just one of these determinants that sets the stage for normal endocrine function, with evidence indicating that a compromised diet in early life lays the ground for obesity and metabolic disease in adult life. Particularly, malnutrition at these early stages has been linked to long-term deficits of growth trajectory and hormonal control. Indeed, children with nutritional deficiencies have a higher likelihood of exhibiting retarded growth and impaired metabolic response, which underscores the importance of sustained exposure to sufficient, well-planned diets (Soliman et al., 2025). Parental stress is yet another important environmental factor influencing the endocrine function of children. Increased cortisol levels resulting from excessive stress have the ability to suppress growth hormone release, which is fundamental for optimal physical growth. Epidemiologic research has revealed that children who are brought up under stressful conditions tend to exhibit lower height-for-age and weight-for-age measurements than their counterparts exposed to more stable environments. In addition, the implications of stress are not merely temporary growth effects; they can indeed influence overall metabolic health and lines of development, calling for the need for sound systems of parental support to mitigate these stressors. Parental stress reduction interventions would thus fortify children's growth and predestined outcomes of health simultaneously (Soliman et al., 2025). Furthermore, exposure to excessive screen time has become more problematic, particularly with its association with disordered sleep patterns and endocrine imbalance. Chronic use of digeen correlated with reduced melatonin levels, a hormone with a close association with sleep regulation and growth hormone posed childrenChildren exposed to high screen exposure over four hours per day can be at increased risk of stunting growth and obesity. Following rResearch also indicates that children's circadian rhythms can be drastically affected, leading to additional complexity in their metabolic functions. Adjusting screen use and promoting healthy media usage behaviors, therefore, could have a crucial role to play in making endocrine protection for future generations.

4.2.3. Autoimmune Conditions

Autoimmune illnesses prevail in pediatric endocrine disease due to the complex interaction they have with the hormonal pathways. Of these, Type 1 diabetes mellitus is a classic example, wherein autoimmune cell-mediated destruction of pancreatic β-cells leads to insulin deficiency. It is one of the most prevalent chronic endocrine diseases in childhood and has an amazing predisposition to develop and advance rapidly. In fact, children with Type 1 diabetes are more likely to develop additional autoimmune diseases, which suggests the polyvalency of autoimmune pathologies in children. Identification of unique clinical and laboratory findings in these children is significant for the creation of effective treatment protocols and enhancing their quality of life, as evident from the awareness of the comorbidities and complications involved in this condition (Vikhrova et al., 2025). Autoimmune disorders' relationship with the pediatric endocrine system is also made complex by the co-occurrence of other diseases, autoimmune thyroiditis. This condition is relatively prevalent in pediatric patients with Type 1 diabetes, which addresses the sheer need for appropriate screening and evaluation. Patients of autoimmune thyroiditis often present with growth and metabolic disturbances, which can have cascading effects on their overall health and well-being. A more increased risk of thyroid dysfunctions developing, therefore, necessitates integrated care with endocrinologists and healthcare workers handling cases of autoimmune diseases. Furthermore, understanding the prevalence and importance of thyroid disease in children presenting with non-diabetic endocrine disorders not only helps with the management of diabetes but also with broader treatment strategies that consider the child's complete health status (Vikhrova et al., 2025). More significantly, the emerging field of study of avoidant restrictive food intake disorder (ARFID) introduces another source of pediatric endocrine and autoimmune disease complexity. Studies have indicated that children with ARFID may have varied neurodevelopmental and endocrine problems, which may make their already existing health profiles more complex. Although autoimmune disorders are described less frequently in this group, the associated conditions, like pituitary conditions, indicate a unique overlap among metabolic, nutritional, and psychological aspects of health. The significant psychological wellbeing implications associated with ARFID have been connected to an increased hospital stay and higher specialist treatment demand. This crossroads explains the necessity of comprehensive healthcare models addressing the polyvalent needs of children with both endocrine and autoimmune diseases and thus enhances long-term outcomes for this susceptible population (Figure 4.7).

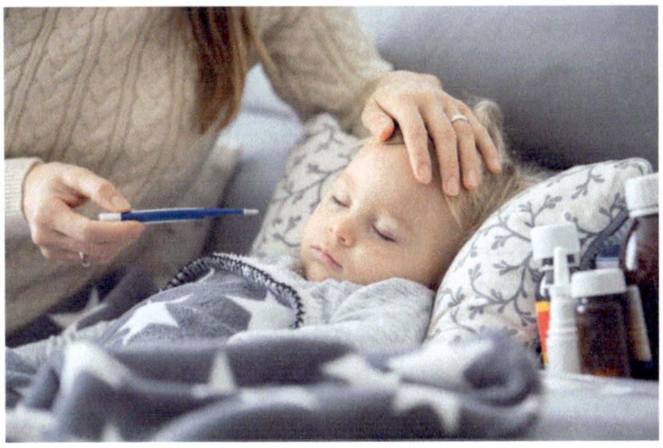

Figure 4.7. Autoimmune conditions.

Source: https://www.ankurahospitals.com/wp-content/uploads/2024/10/autoimmune-disorder-in-children.jpg.

Test Your Knowledge

1. How do genetic predispositions contribute to the development of pediatric endocrine disorders?
2. What environmental factors can influence hormonal balance and endocrine function in children?

4.3. Symptoms and Diagnosis

Learning Outcome

1. Common symptoms in children
2. Diagnostic tests anedures
3. Importance of differential diagnosis

Clinical manifestation of endocrine disorders of childhood can be quite distinctive, typically dependent on the onset age and type of consequent hormonal derangements. Unusual symptoms may develop as disturbances in growth, sexual maturation, or metabolism. Precocious puberty, for instance, in which children are noted to exhibit signs of sexual development before the typical age, is one of the notable signs of endocrine dysfunction. This condition may be precipitated by other etiologies, including tumors or hormone therapy, as is observed in research showing presentation of precocious puberty in children who have been placed on mitotane therapy for adrenocortical carcinoma. Accordingly, pediatric patients manifesting symptoms must undergo extensive evaluations to determine the source of hormonal imbalances and to apply appropriate interventions and therapies specifically designed for their requirements (Elżbieta et al., 2024). The diagnosis of pediatric endocrine disorders necessitidisciplinary practice involving clinical assessment, laboratory tests, and imaging studies. A careful physical and history taking will reveal subtle clues, such as, such as delayed growth or atypical secondary sexual development, that will prompt further investigation. Hormonal assays play an important diagnostic role through the measurement of certals of specific hormones in the blood and thereby the identification of deficiencies or excesses associated with most endocrine disorders. Imaging modalities such as, such as ultrasound or MRI may be employed to assess anatomical abnormalities, like tumors or structural endocrine gland pathologies. PANDAS, for example, depicts specialized symptoms that are inextricably linked to hormonal malfunction and necessitate a sensitive, integrative diagnostic strategy that incorporates the polyfacetic character of these childhood endocrine diseases (Eissa, 2024). The complexity of pediatric endocrine disorder diagnosis further underscores the significance of an interdisciplinary team-based approach among pediatric endocrinologists, radiologists, and mental health professionals. Some disorders have comorbidities that complicate the diagnostic process and ultimately lead to misdiagnosis and late treatment. With treatment for mitotane, children may present a range of symptoms from neurological disturbances to hormonal imbalance, where they need close observation during treatment. It is critical that healthcare providers are sensitive to the spectrum of endocrine disorders and their effects on development and health. Early detection not only alleviates short-term suffering but also results in better long-term prognosis, demonstrating the importance of prompt recognition and response to the subtle presentation that may be present in children with endocrine disorders (Elżbieta et al., 2024).

4.3.1. Common Symptoms in Children

For pediatririne diseases, the expected symptoms are very heterogeneous and typically constitute a management and diagnostic issue. Symptoms in children with conditions such as, such as congenital adrenal hyperplasia (CAH) pose a spectrum of symptoms directly related to endocrine disturbances. CAH can lead to ambiguous genitalia in infant females or premature virilization in males with psychosocial and social implications. These are manifestations due to deficiencies of enzymes that disrupt cortisol and aldosterone synthesis, causing presentation requiring emergency intervention. Moreover, heterogeneity of clinical presentations of CAH, ranging from salt-wasting to non-classical presentation, mirrors the requirement of high clinical suspicion and patient-by-patient evaluation. Early intervention is crucial because untreated severe cases lead to life-threatening complications, proving that screening for such symptoms is part of pediatric medicine and endocrine disease care (Dudnyk et al., 2025). Another endocrine disease fhildren is type 1 diabetes mellitus (T1D), which is characterized by its chronic nature and intense physiological and psychological effects. Symptoms of T1D, such as, such as polyuria, polydipsia, and unexplained weight loss, usually develop insidiously, and therefore early diagnosis is critical for maximum treatment. Moreover, children with T1D may also develop psychosocial complications, as the insulin regimen and dietary restrictions can be demoralizing. Research has indicated that adolescents with T1D also have a higher level of anxiety and depression, which makes it difficult to manage their disease and negatively influences metabolic control. This brings to the forefront the necessity of recognizing mental as well as bodily symptoms of children who have T1D so that they can be provided with comprehensive care, promoting a balanced treatment and care strategy (Silina et al., 2025). As endocrine disorders in children can manifest differently and thus present a diverse range of symptoms, it is extremely necessary for medical practitioners to adopt a cautious strategy. The common presentations of these conditions are often manifestations of intrinsic hormonal disturbances that have the potential to influence a child's growth and overall development. Symptoms like retardation of growth, fatigue, and sexual developmental abnormalities require extensive clinical investigations. Diseases like thyroid disease, for instance, can potentially result in growth retardation in children and thus must be diagnosed and treated early. By fostering an awareness of such common symptoms, health care providers are better positioned to contribute to early diagnosis and treatment. Not only does this enhance the possibility of positive health outcomes, but it also improves the quality of life for children who have endocrine disorders, further underscoring the significance of holistic and proactive health care (Figure 4.8).

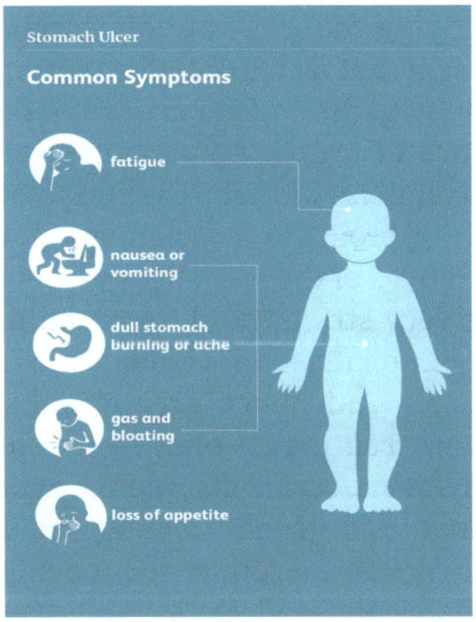

Figure 4.8. Common symptoms in children.

Source: https://www.verywellhealth.com/thmb/9QBpq0eV1Ln-NVhO0XaeNPkCDtA=/1500x0/filters:no_upscale():max_bytes(150000):strip_icc()/peptic-ulcers-in-children-1742814-5c454b38c9e77c0001b24888.png.

4.3.2. Diagnostic Tests and Procedures

Diagnosis of endocrine disorders in children may necessitate a sequence of diagnostic tests and procedures that yield critical information on individualized treatment plans. Genetic testing has proven to be a valuable asset, with data supporting its superior diagnostic yield over regular imaging or metabolic workups. For instance, a prospective study of inexplicable global developmental delay revealed that genetic diagnosis was established in nearly half the cases and that metabolic screening and magnetic resonance imaging (MRI) had limited utility for diagnosis (Veronese et al., 2024). These findings suggest that genetic testing must be accorded priority in clinical practice, especially when primary assessment cannot account for the clinical presentation. Therefore, pediatric practitioners are increasingly taking advantage of the promise of advanced genetic testing technology in their clinics to better establish underlying causes of endocrine conditions among affected children, thereby speeding up targeted management interventions. Apart from genetic testing, biochemical tests are also an integral part of the diagnostic process for pediatric endocrine disorders. Such tests tend to measure hormone and metabolite levels, providing useful information regarding the functioning of individual endocrine glands. For example, abnormalities in thyroid hormone levels might indicate hyroidism or hyperthyroidism, both of which are prevalent in the pediatric age group. Furthermore, regular testing for growth hormone and adrenal function is useful since they it can diagnose such intricate disorders as Growth Hormone Deficiency or Cushing's Disease. Biochemical investigations of this kind are generally supplemented by imaging tests if necessary. However, while these tests are very helpful, they also need to be used cautiously in the context of the complete clinical situation to avoid misdiagnosis or unwarranted intervention. Imaging tests like MRI and ultrasound are also important for diagnostic evaluation of endocrine disorders in children, particularly for visualization of anatomical defects. For instance, in the case of diseases like congenital adrenal hyperplasia or pituitary or adrenal gland tumors, advanced imagilogies can delineate the physical anatomy and guide therapeutic interventions. But this reliance on imaging needs to be weighed against the recognition of its limitations, such as, such as in certain research, wherein MRI yielded diagnostic information minimal percentage of cases of unexplained developmental delay (Veronese et al., 2024). Pediatric patients may also pose special problems when being imaged diagnostically, such as, such as anxiety or sedation. Hence, the clinicians have to use a discerning policy, choosing the most suitable diagnostic investigations while keeping the child as comfortable and happy as possible during this process (Figure 4.9).

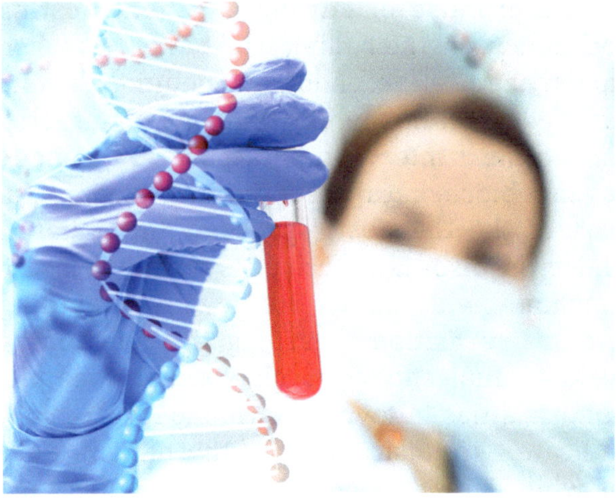

Figure 4.9. Diagnostic tests and procedures.

Source: https://www.nchealthinfo.org/wp-contends/2019/08/LabTestsAndDiagnostic.jpg.

4.3.3. Importance of Differential Diagnosis

In pediatric endocrine disease, differential diagnosis cannot be overemphasized. Symptoms such as, such as these could suggest any of a number of hormonal disturbances, and the ability of the clinician to accurately differentiate disease is essential for optimal therapy. For instance, diseases like congenital adrenal hyperplasia or growth hormone deficiency can present alike but demand entirely disparate therapeutic protocols. An obvious differential diagnosis allows health care practitioners to target conditions that would lead to severe morbidity if left untreated, facilitating timely intervention and best results. Therefore, regular meticulous examinations that encompass clinical evaluation, laboratory investigations, and diligent patient history are pivotal to the minimization of the vast array of potential endocrine diseases in a child. Besides, there is a crucial knowledge deficit in pediatric tremor disorders that can misguide clinical practice unless differential diagnosis is used with strictness. Pediatric tremors can result from a vast variety of causes ranging fronign physiological tremors to less auspicious neurological or systemic illnesses (Ghadery et al., 2025). Accurate identification of the underlying cause is not only crucial for the management, but also to comfort parents about their child's condition. The majority of the time, the absence of proper epidemiological data in children compels clinicians to extrapolate adult-normative approaches, which might not be true representatives of the pediatric presentation. By adhering very strictly to differential diagnosis models, clinicians can reduce the risks of misdiagnosis and hence greatly enhance the quality of treatment offered to pediatric patients with endocrine disorders. Furthermore, advancements in genetic testing, for example, long-read next-generation sequencing (NGS), have further enhanced differential diagnosis of pediatric endocrine disorders by making complex genetic mechanisms more understandable. By enabling the idenn of structural variants and variants of unknown significance, such advanced methods facilitate improved diagnosis of otherwise indeterminate conditions (de Vries et al., 2023Cho, 2024). Not only does the application of NGS technologies assist in distinguishing between hereditary and acquired endocrine disorders, but it also interprets the inheritance mode, particularly in autosomal recessive diseases. Therefore, the integration of such varied diagnostic tools in clinical practice reflects the evolving scenario of pediatric endocrinology and emphasizes the utmost importance of differential diagnosis in offering maximum patient-centered care.

Test Your Knowledge

1. What are the common symptoms that may indicate an endocrine disorder in children?
2. Which diagnostic tests and procedures are commonly used to evaluate pediatric endocrine function?
3. Why is differential diagnosis important in identifying specific pediatric endocrine disorders?

4.4. Treatment Options

Learning Outcome

1. Hormone replacement therapy
2. Lifestyle modifications
3. Surgical intons

Pediatric endocrine disease management is often multifaceted, including wide-ranging treaat considers both medical and technological interventiomore conditions such as, such as diabetes mellitus in children, are on the rise, the healthcare system more and more invests investing in ways to enhance disease control. Advances such as, such as insulin pumps and continuous glucose monitoring systems are pivotal in maximizing glycemic control and preventing complications. There is evidence that diabetes technology adoption plays a large role in rising treatment costs through augmented monitoring and treatment options. However, lower hospitalization rates associated with it have implications for potential long-term health benefits that could make such expenditure worthwhile (de Vries et al., 2023). Maximizing utilization of resources and creating treatment modalities are, therefore, imperative in addressing the pediatric endocrine disorder burden. Pharmacotherapy is another essential feature in treating endocrine disorders among children. Chifflicted with growth hormone deficiency or other hormonal imbalances can, for example, make significant improvements from hormone replacement therapy. The initiation of treatments such as, such as synthetic growth hormone early can lead to dramatic changes in physical growth and overall health. Also essential is the aspect of psychological support since the majority of children have a hard time dealing with the long-term effects of endocrine disorders. Resilience may be imparted through counseling in a supportive environment that fosters obedience to treatment regimes. Therefore, the inclusion of pharmacotherapy combined with psychological support is an integral approach to treatment that guarantees pediatric patients receive care that considers physical and emotional elements of heaurgical interventions are also indicated in some pediatric endocrine disorders, particularly when the treatment with drugs is unresponsive. For instance, interventions for diseases such as, such as congenital adrenal hyperplasia or tumors of specific types may necessitate the surgical repair or removal of the affected structures. For these, there must be a coordinated approach by the pediatric endocrinologists, surgeons, and other care providers to organize a comprehensive treatment. The need for early surgery is a testament to the importance of a tailored approach that meets the specific condition and growth needs of the child. Early detection and treatment can lead to favorable outcomes, reducing the risks of complications resulting from undiagnosed endocrine disorders. Such integration of surgery in the overall treatment model, thus, serves as proof of the importance of a tailored treatment in the treatment of pediatric endocrine disorders (Eliaçık et al., 2023) (Figure 4.10).

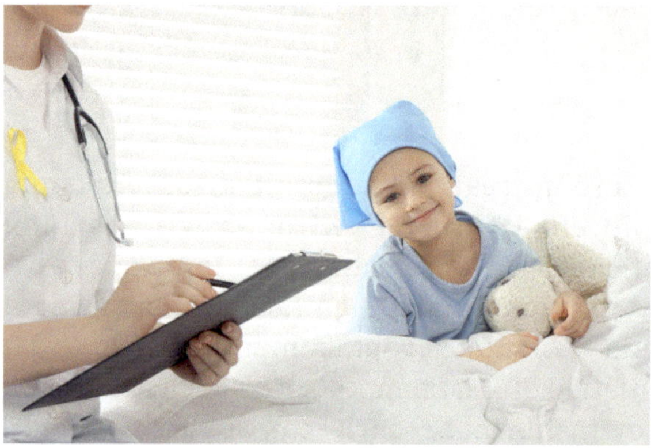

Figure 4.10. The treatment options for pediatric endocrine disorders are often multifaceted.

Source: https://healthyturkiye.com/storage/media/4299/pediatric-oncology-treatment-option.jpg.

4.4.1. Hormone Replacement Therapy

In the context of pediatric endocrine disorders, hormone replacement therapy (HRT) emerged as an important treatment measure for children's growth deficits. Growth hormone therapy (GHT), the most commonly practiced form of HRT, is very effective in children suffering from Growth Hormone Deficiency (GHD), Turner syndrome, and chronic renal insufficiency. Studies have also shown that early intervention with GHT can lead to significant gains in height, body composition change, and overall psychosocial adaptation in such children. With the treatment setting for children evolving, not only is the focus on the physical growth, but also on the long-term quality of life improvement, highlighting the diversified benefits of HRT in pediatric endocrinology, which calls for careful assessment and follow-up during treatment (Penna et al., 2024). Physiological reasoning behind hormone replacement therapy is complex and calls for an advanced approach by the medical professionals. Growth hormone therapy, for example, triggers the release of insulin-like growth factor 1 (IGF-1) by the liver, which is crucial in triggering growth. Longitudinal studies confirm that a majority of GHRT patients exhibit normal IGF-1 levels, affirming the success of the intervention in restoring hormone balance and triggering growth (Carmichael). More critical, however, is that such therapies must be tailored to individual patients, taking into account patient-specific issues, underlying illness, and potential side effects. In so far asIf there are positive results involving HRT, health care providers must still monitor patients closely for side effects or complications, emphasizing the importance of a team effort in properly treating pediatricndocrine conditions. Additionally, psychological sequelae of hormone replacement therapy in children warrant careful examination. Growth hormone-deficient children typically manifest with intensive emotional and social disturbances, like poor body image and self-esteem. Some of these conditions can be corrected by HRT, particularly GHT, through enabling actual growth outcomes, which have a positive influence on psychosocial development (Penna et al., 2024). Second, the availability of treatment for their condition can enhance confidence among children and families, causing them to feel that they are not different after all. As evidenced by recent systematic reviews, the benefits of HRT extend beyond body size, influencing the child's overall mental health and relationships. This intersection between body development and mental health reiterates the significant role played by health practitioners in identifying and acting on both in the care of children with pediatric endocrine disorders (Figure 4.11).

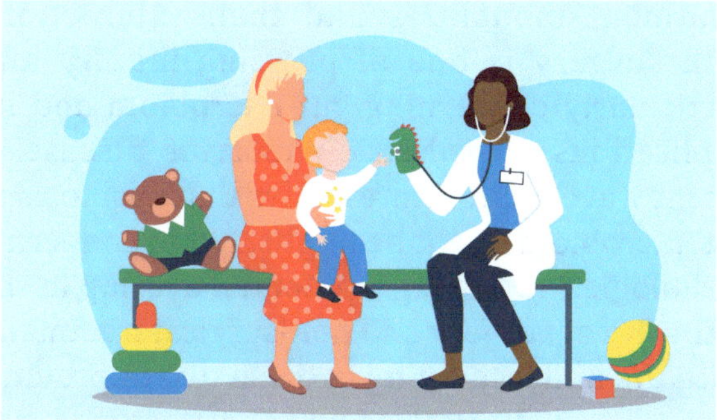

Figure 4.11. Hormone replacement therapy (HRT) has emerged as a pivotal intervention for managing growth-related deficiencies in children.

Source: https://assets.clevelandclinic.org/transform/15052375-063d-4af9-98c5-211020f98f19/growth-appointment-child-1341126662.

4.4.2. Lifestyle Modifications

Lifestyle modifications are the cornerstone of the management of endocrine disease in children, particularly obesity and its consequent disorders such as, such as polycystic ovary syndrome (PCOS). The adoption of healthier lifestyle paterns in the form of improved diet and increased physical activity has the potential to greatly enhance the health prognosis in the involved children anents. Evidence suggests that the life-style modification interventions are vital in sustaining metabolic health since they not only aid in weight maintenance but also regulate comorbidities, such as, such as insulin resistance and emotional status. Additionally, the emphasis on education in lifestyle decisions is essential itaining long-term behavioral change. By enabling children and their families to make educated choices, healthcare professionals are able to develop an active model that reduces the risk factors with of pediatric endocrine disorders (Teede et al., 2018). When examining lifestyle adjustments, their multidimensional effect on patient outcomes must be weighed. Actions like personalized exercise routines and nutritional education have proven effective in not only improving physical well-being, but also mental health. Given the complex interrelationship of endocrine disorders and obesity, follow-up should be regular and patient-centered. This is through the inclusion of feedback from patients and families in coming up with responsive health plans that shift with the changing needs of the child. While medical systems ever so well understand the importance of lifestyle interventions, putting evidence-based practice into actreover, the necessity of researching how lifestyle changes are successfully sustained in the long term is vital because most patients have constraints hindering sustainable change(Dennis et al., 2017). Lastly, the effective management of pediatric endocrine disorders requires an extensive knowledge of lifestyle changes as an integral aspect of care. Health care providers must not only advocate for diet and exercise modification but also create supportive environments that help to reverse the social and economic determinants that mold these behaviors. Through the use of an integrated model that addresses the individual patient context, health care providers can enhance adherence to lifestyle recommendations as well as overall treatment effectiveness. Furthermore, ongoing collaboration between pediatric endocrinologists, dietitians, and mental health professionals can facilitate the establishment of robust support structures for children and families. With ongoing expansion in pediatric endocrine illnesses, prioritizing lifestyle modifications in clinical practice will prove vital in promoting the health outcomes and quality of life of individuals (Teede et al., 2018).

4.4.3. Surgical Interventions

Surgical intervention in childhood neoadjuvant disease typically becomes necessary when conservative therapy is not productive or if complications arise that require instantaneous intervention. Of the most common endocrine diseases requiring a surgical approach, thyroid pathology is most significant, particularly where neoplasia or large formations of goiter are involved. The indication for surgery is further evidenced by findings in a 10-year review study that showed 63.2% of children who had thyroid surgery were diagnosed with thyroid neoplasia, among which a significant number had papillary thyroid carcinoma (Asya et al., 2025). The statistics highlight the urgent necessity for proper diagnosis and early surgical intervention to prevent risks to the developing endocrine system. Surgical management is complex and often includes multidisciplinary therapy, balancing the requirement for urgent management against possible long-term effects on the child's endocrine function. The technical complexity of surgical management of pediatric thyroid disease implies that special attention must be paid to this age group. Children possess a developing anatomy that will complicate surgery more than in adults. Surgical complications like vocal cord paralysis or hypoparathyroidism are serious factors that demand the surgeon's great skill and expertise (Asya et al., 2025). In the retrospective review, instances of complications like transient vocal cord paralysis and transient hypocalcemia highlight the underlying complications. Not only do they affect the early stage of recovery, but complications can also cause lasting effects on a child's development and quality of life. Thus, a careful weighing of all risks of surgery against the possible benefits is crucial in the pediatric situation. Moreover, the place of developing treatment modalities and their interactions with surgery is one of pressing inquiry and particularly concerning gut microbiota and its implications in pediatric endocrine disease. A recent wave of literature shows that dysbiosis of gut microbiota might be implicated in endocrine pathologies, including a potential overlap in the pathways of surgery and non-surgical treatment. With the understanding of these two improving, it may alter surgical choice and postoperative care. The use of probiotics in conjunction with other therapies may offer additional avenues for lowering the risks associated with endocrine surgery as well as enhancing patient outcomes in general. Therefore, a comprehensive treatment process involving both surgery and adjunct therapies may well be the most effective modality available for treating children's endocrine diseases (Figure 4.12).

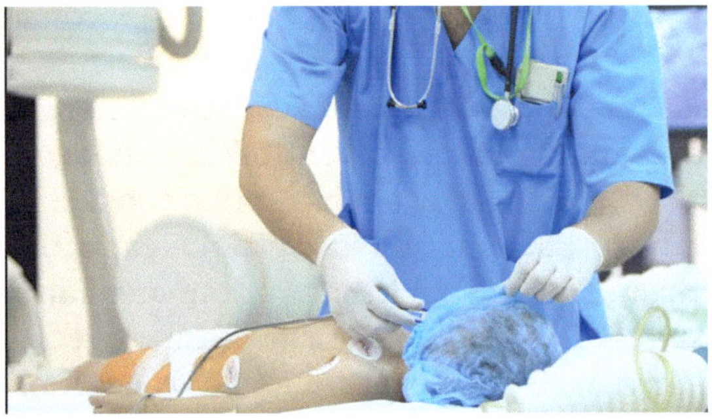

Figure 4.12. Surgical interventions in pediatric endocrine disorders.

Source: https://res.cloudinary.com/drdawan/image/upload/pediatric-surgery-1550055448.jpg.

Test Your Knowledge

1. How does hormone replacement therapy help manage pediatric endocrine disorders?
2. What lifestyle modifications can support treatment and improve outcomes in children with endocrine conditions?
3. When are surgical interventions considered necessary in the management of pediatric endocrine disorders?

4.5. Long-term Management

Learning Outcome

1. Monitoring and follow-up care
2. Psychological support for affected children
3. Education for families and caregivers

Endocrine disorder management in children over the long term calls for interdisciplinary care that addresses the unique needs of chthrough development. Effective management techniques are not only significant insofar as they operate to manage short-term symptoms, but also insofar as they can forestall long-term disease complications such as, such as obesity, polycystic ovary syndrome (PCOS), and adrenal insufficiency. An integrated management plan must include rout monitoring, lifestyle alteration, and drug therapy according to the age of the child and the specific condition. For instance, in pediatric obesity, new strategies like the use of nutraceuticals can be added on to traditional treatment modalities, treating related conditions like hypertension and psychopathology. Therefore, the intricate nature of these disorders must be tac a bid to ensure optimal health outcomes, an aspect that speaks volumes regarding the essence of individualized care in pediatrics. Beyond an interdisciplinary framework, long-term management of disorders such as, such as adrenal insufficiency also includes being certain that the patient is continually educated and reassured. Children with this endocrine condition require close observation to maintain their growth and development in line while reducing the likelihood of adrenal crises. Routine follow-up and modifications of glucocorticoid replacement therapies based on the child's constantly changing needs can significantly improve their quality of lrthermore, education of families regarding manifestations of adrenal insufficiency and the importance of drug adherence is an important consideration in the prevention of medical complications. Facilities such as, such as learning materials and support groups can empower families so that they can be a part of their child's management and remain active towards health. The psychosocial aspect of long-term management in pediatric endocrine disorders cannot be overlooked. Research has shown that children with chronic conditions are prone to experiencing psychological distress, which in turn goes on to complicate their disease further and makes treatment compliance even more difficult. The illnesses, like obesi, are linked not only with physical diseases but also with mental illnesses like depression and anxiety, thus the requirement for complete care. Endocrinologists, psychologists, and dieticians can collaborate inteams to develop integrated management plans tsical and emotional requirements of the child. As attested in the testimony concerning the long-term management of child obesity (Street et al., 2025) and adrenal insufficiency (Teede et al., 2018Itzel et al., 2025), an all-encompassing, multidisciplinary treatment plan is not only vital for upholding health but also for developing resiliency and improving the overall quality of life of children with such complex endocrine conditions.

4.5.1. Monitoring and Follow-Up Care

Monitoring and post-treatment care in pediatric endocrine disorders are crucial aspects that ensureent treatment of the underlying complicated conditions. Ongoing evaluation allows medical professionals to track patterns of growth, metabolic changes, and overall growth of children with endocrine disorders such as, such as adrenal insufficiency or diabetes. By implementing systematic follow-up regimens, clinicians can detect potential complications at an early stage, adjust treatment plans accordingly, and inform families in an appropriate manner about the handling of the disease. Not only is this useful for maintaining maximal health status, but also for establishing a facilitative milieu in which families can actively participate in their child's care. Such interaction is critical, as it has the potential to greatly enhance treatment regimen compliance and improve the quality of life in the child. In addition, the application of longitudinal follow-up cannot be overemphasized in endocrine r children. With children's growth and changes in their physiological demands, the monitoring process needs to adjust in order to provide age-targeted intFor instance, thmanagement of conditions such as, such as precocious puberty or growth hormone deficiency involves periodic evaluation to reassess therapeutic impact and to alter dosing. Such follow-up adjustively matters because a mismanagement may have psychosocial impacts or initiate sexual development delay. After the incorporation of the findings from ongoing assessment with best practices, clinicians can enhance the optimisation of treatment modalities. Furthermore, systematic follow-up care facilitates the transfer of these patients into adult health care settings, with continuity of care through several stages of life. Aside from clinical evaluation, the importance of psychosocial monitoring for cildhood endocrine disorders is clearer today. Adolescents and children with chronic diseases often have chronic psychological issues, including anxiety and depression, which complicate follow-up and adherence to cinfluence the quality utcomes. Therefore, integrating mental health assessments in the follow-up treatment is essential. Health care teams must collaborate to treat the emotional stability of the patients, such as, such as integrating the mental health practitioners into the treatment plan. Support services for families also play an important role in providing coping tools and adaptation strategies for handling the intricacies of their child's sickness. Through the management not only of the endocrine aspect but also the understanding of the broader psychosocial environment, health professionals will be able to enhance monitoring and follow-up care, eventually leading to more effective outcomes for the treatment of pediatric endocrine disorders (Figure 4.13).

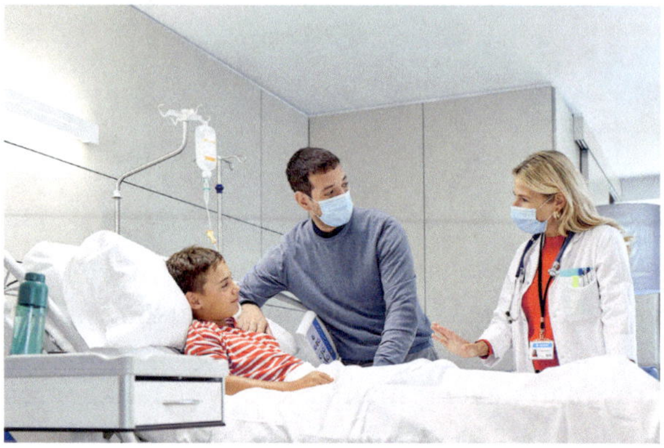

Figure 4.13. The monitoring and follow-up care are critical components that ensure the effective management of these complex conditions.

Source: https://assets-us-01.kc-usercontent/6239a81e-8f0f-0040-a1df-b4932a10f6ae/8767a311-71bf-43-416e96bdf5be/3404009.jpg?q=75&w=1920&auto=format&fm=webp&lossless=true.

4.5.2. Psychological Support for Affected Children

Psychological counseling for the children suffering from pediatric enisorders such as, such as Type 1 diabetes, plays a vital role in cultivating mental and physical health. Adolescents undergoing this challenging period are likely to face an entire range of psychological issues, such as, such as depression and anxiety, and these can greatly interfere with their ability to properly care for themselves. Studies reveal that approximately 30% of adolescents with Type 1 diabetes exhibit severe anxiety symptoms, and they have a troubling convergence with diabetes distress. These psychiatric issues may resent themselves in the form of behaviors that dsrupt proper diabetes care, leading to less-than-optimal glycemic control and increasing health complications. Therefore, generating a psychological climate of support, —via therapy, peer relations, and family support, —becomes paramount for assisting these children in managing their condisensitivity toward the psychological effects of diabetes is essential for medical practitioners to construct successful treatment regimens for the multifaceted needs of these children (Teede et al., 2018John et al., 2022). Incorporating mental health intervention into the treatment regimen of pediatric endocrirders can facilitate enhanced diabetes control results. Multidisciplinary diabetes management addresses the disease not only as a physical condition but also as one linked with psychological health. Interventions such as, such as cognitive-behavioral therapy (CBT) have been identified as useful modalities in the management of anxiety and depression symptoms among children. Family functioning also plays a critical role in influencing health outcomes; positive and authoritative parenting correlates with better glycemic control among adolescents. Family therapy to educate positive communication and emotional support can minimize diabetes-related distress and enhance coping abilities in children. Successful diabetes control is thus a natural function of optimal psychological treatment, with evidence of theen mental health and chronic disease outcomes in such vulnerable children (John et al., 2022). Given the fundamental medical impacts, weight stigma that includes obesity and other endocrine conditions has the capacity tocan exacerbate the psychological distress felt by such kids. Studies determine that individuals who are obese often encounter discrimtization, particularly in healthcare settings, which acts as a constraint for them to access necessary medical treatments. This social stigma not only disrupts their ability to manage their health needs in an effective waeffectively but also contributes to the production of further mental stress, which creates a cycle of negative health states. Public health initiatives must be focused on educating not just healthcare professionals but the public at large regarding the ill effects of weight stigma, developing a discourse that is incion and advocacy interventions for proactively addressing these social challenges, we can develop an atmosphere conducive to the development of children with endocrine disorders to develop in a positive and healthy mannerpositively and healthily, ultimately enhancing their quality of life.

4.5.3. Education for Families and Caregivers

Effective education of caregivers and parents of children with pediatric endocrine diseases is most critical in ensuring the best management and outcomes. The educational programs should therefore entail not only the biomedical characteristics of the conditions but also the psychosocial components, which are an essential determinant of the quality of life in children with such conditions. For instance, families of children with conditions such as type 1 diabetes must recognize that caregiving extends beyond routine blood glucose monitoring to include ongoing emotional and psychological support.. Research shows that teenagers have worsening glycemic control at develonal phases due to a number of reasons, including physiological change and increasing independence, so it is essential that family engagement continues to attain better health outcomes (Teede et al., 2018John et al., 2022). Arming caregivers with communication and support strategies is building a good climate, favoring treatment adherence and emotional resilience in the child. Furthermore, family education needs to be interactive in form, addressing the individualized needs of each family and being culturally sensitive when attempting to untangle medical complexities. Pediatric endocrinology also often overlh several different medical specialties, so family caregivers must be well-educated, well-informed advocates for their children. Developmental stages pose unique challenges, particularly during the formative years such as, such as adolescence, where the psychological aspects of chronic disease care become increasingly difficult. Effective educational interventions must include trainingskills, identification of potential complications, and psychosocial monitoring methods to detect early warning signs of anxiety or eating disorders prevalent with endocrine disorders (Teede et al., 2018Northrupet al., 2021). By making this information available to families, caregivers are encouraged to take part in their child's health care, facilitating ongoing communication with healthcare providers and ensuring their child receives complete care. Lastly, community and peer support within education cannot be underscored. Familaregivers can potentially reap fantastic rewards from shared experiences and knowledge from other caregivers who have to work with the same pediatric endocrine disorders. Establishing platforms for shared learning, such as, such as support groups or online forums, serves as a critical avenue for emotional support and practical advice. These interactions can demystify the complexities of managing endocrine disorders and provide valuable perspectives on coping strategies, encouraging resilience through shared narratives. Integration of such community resources into curriculum components can assist in strengthening fay of patient care, and contribute to the improvement of health outcomes in children who are confronted with the challenges involved in pediatric endocrine disorders (Teede et al., 2018John et al., 2022; Northrupet al., 2021) (Figure 4.14).

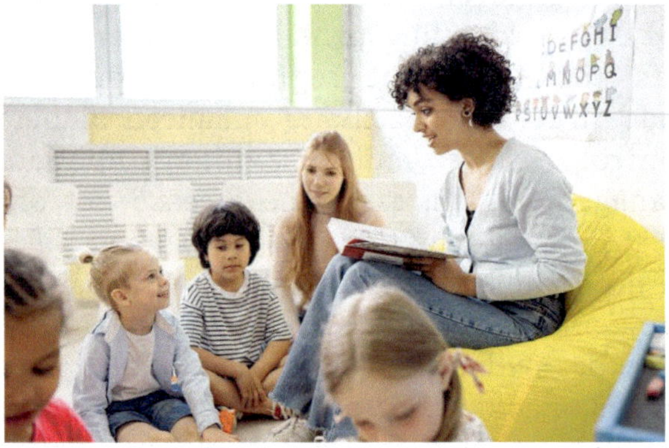

Figure 4.14. The education for families and caregivers of children with pediatric endocrine disorders is paramount for optimal management and outcomes.

Source: https://www.canr.msu.edu/contentAsset/image/46dfc557-92ab-4500-bb76-29970ef0bed4/fileAsset/filter/Resize,Jpeg/resize_w/750/jpeg_q/80.

Test Your Knowledge

1. What are the main goals and types of hormone replacement therapy used in children with endocrine disorders?
2. How can lifestyle modifications, such as diet and physical activity, support endocrine health in pediatric patients?
3. Under what circumstances are surgical interventions required in the treatment of pediatric endocrine diseases?

4.6. Recent Advances in Research

Learning Outcome

1. New treatment modalities
2. Genetic research and implications
3. Innovations in diagnostic techniques

Recent pediatric endocrine disorder research has shed light on new treatment strategies, most notably regarding congenital adrenal hyperplasia (CAH), a common disorder in this age group. Published guidelines by the Endocrine Society have mental role in guiding clinical practice. These updated best practices managed care that incorporates published information in conn with recommendations from experts, addressing key concerns such as, such as cost, quality of life, and patient safety (Teede et al., 2018Speiser et al., 2018). Individualized care assures that patient characteristics such as, such as psychosocial concerns and genetic background, guide treatment choices. This multifaceted treatment plan is not merely meant to improve clinical outcomes, but it also aims to ensure overall quality of life for both affected children and their families. Therefore, recent advances reflect an investment in not merely curıng the disorder, but also in considering the overall welfare of patients. Ongoing research into the etiology of pediatric endocrine disorders has highlighted the merit of personalized medicine, employing genetic and phenotypic variation to customize treatment. Advances in genomic technology now enable researchers to analyze particular mutations responsible for such conditions as CAH and other endocrine disturbances. For example, identification of specific genetic markers provides for early detection and treatment, which ca extremely valuable for long-term prognosis. In addition, this precision medicine approach enables clinicians to more closely monitor therapy responses, leading to interventions that prevent probable complications. In diseases such as, such as adrenal crisis, immediate responses can prevent fatal health outcomes, supporting the imperative for research-based innovation in managing complex pediatric endocrine . Through implementing these innovations, health care providers are better positioned to address the unique requirements of a growing patient population. The use of immunotherapy in the treatment of childhood endocrine disease also isis also a very promising advancement in current research. This new arena follows on from developments under consideration for cancer therapy, particularly in brain tumors of children, where standard treatments have often proved to be woefully inadequate. Recent evidence indicates that chimeric antigen receptor T (CAR-T) cell therapy holds not only potential in hematologic malignancies but also in the treatment of refractory disease, conceivably even tumor-associated endocrine dysregulation (Wang et al., 2019). Despite ongoing concerns regarding safety and efficacy in children, the adaptability of such therapies forms the basis for new treatment strategies. Growing research underscores the value of multi-specialty collaboration and highlights the potential of an agnostic approach to endocrine diseases. In this context, immunotherapy is emerging as a promising avenue with the capacity to redefine treatment paradigms for complex pediatric endocrine disorders

4.6.1. New Treatment Modalities

Pediatric endocrine disease is evolving, and this is primarily being fueled by the introduction of new therapeutic modalities that are making developments in medical technology and pharmacology. These new approaches are aimed at maximizing efficacy with reduced side effects, an important factor in children since longtatus is of top priority. New therapies such as, such as biologics and gene therapy are becoming more prominent, and these ected at specific endocrine dysfunction at the molecular level. By individualizing treatment in relation toconcerning genetic and metabolic profiles, clinicians are better equipped to effectively manage the complexity of diseases such as, such as growth hormone deficiencies and thyroid dysfunctions. These advances not only promise enhanced outcomes, but also set a precedent for treatment protocols that provide individualized patient management, with a goal directed towards an improved quality of life in children suffering from these diseases. Moreover, coordination between multidisciplinary treatment teams has been found to be essential in delivering these new modalities of treatment effectively. Pediatric endocrinologists, nutritionists, psychologists, and other experts collaborate to create combined care plans that are specifically tailored to each patient's individualized needs. This integrative approach is particularly important in the sense that endocrine disease often intersects with other diseases like obesity and metabolic syndrome. Recent research underscores the importance of such a collaborative strategy, with improved clinical outcomes increasingly being linked to coordinated care interventions. For instance, children with ongoing monitoring and synchronized support experience greater rates of treatment compliance and exhibit better emotional well-being, thus underscoring the worth of total management in pediatric endocrine therapy. Lastly, no account of recent improvement of treatment modalities would be complete witt a consideration of the worth of technology. Telemedicine and online health platforms are transforming pediatric endocrine disease monitoring and management. These technologies allow real-time tracking of hormone levels and symptoms, and to offer timely interventions and adjustment of the treatment regimen. Further, the accessibility facilitated by these technologies promotes ongoing patient-cr interaction, providing an enabling environment for family support in managing complex regimens. Studies have found that these electronic interventions not only increase levels of adherence but also empower patients nd families, who becomeare able to take an active role in managing endocrine disorders. As the technologies improve further, they can reshape the treatment landscape for pediatric endocrine disorders so that children can gain from effective, and also comprehensive, care (Figure 4.15).

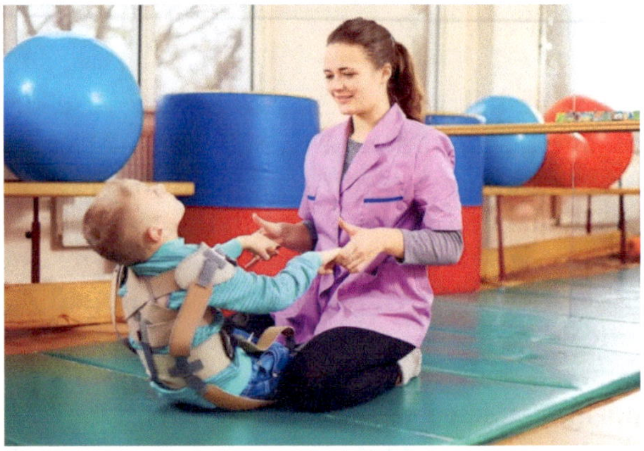

Figure 4.15. Pediatric physical therapist working with a child with cerebral palsy, emphasizing the rolebilitation in improving motor function.

Source: https://pebblestherapycentre.in/wp-content/uploads/2024/01/Cerebral-Palsy-Pediatric-Physical-Therapy-1024x676.webp.

4.6.2. Genetic Research and Implications

The role of genetic research towards in unraveling endocrine diseases in children cannot be overestimated. The breakthroughs in the area of genomics have revealed e of genetic factors in thyroid dysgenesis, congenital adrenal hyperplasia, and diabetes mellitus. The presence of specific mutations in genes has provided insights into the pathophysiology of these conditions. For example, in illnesuch as congenital adrenal hyperplasia, often caused by 21-hydroxylase deficiency, genetic testing can make a diagnosis and guide treatment protocols. This increased knowledge of genetic involvement aids the healthcare professional to personalizein personalizing treatment strategies, thereby improving patient care. Moreover, with advancing genetic research, the expectation of gene therapy and other advanced treatments that can prevent or even reverse genetic abnormalities makes more effective management of such endocrine disorders in children an eventual reality. Besides the identification of genetic factors, the function of environmental factors acting on such genetic susceptibiliis also significant. Factors like chemical exposures have been identified to play a part in exacerbating genetic susceptibilities, affecting endocrine regulation and overall well-being. Pesticides and heavy metals, which pervade most environments, have pose risks with the ability to impact the severity and development of endocrine disease. For instance, endocrine-disrupting chemical exposure has the capability of combining synergistically with existing genetic suslity. It is therefore crucial to comprehend these interactions in developing more comprehensive treatment and prevention strategies. A model that incorporates both environmental and genetic issues can result in more useful interventions and health policy policies to protect vulnerable pediatric populations. This multidisciplinary model underscores the complexity of pediatri endocrine disorders and the need for multifaceted research efforts. Emerging areas of investigation, notably gut microbiota research, add another level of complexity to the dynamics of ding pediatric endocrine disorders. Recent data substantiates that a healthy gut microbiome is crucial for metabolic and immune functions, both of which can affect endocrine function. Gut microbiota development is influenced by a variety of factors, such as, such as genetics, diet, and exposure to antibiotics. Dysbiosis will be the result of an imbalance in gut microbiota, and, as research affirms, it has been associated with a range of disorders beyond the gastrointestinal tract, potentially including endocrine dysfunctions. Therefore, the addition of gut microbiome health to the research on genetic predispositions for pediatric endocrine disease could potentially create new knowledge anctions has the potential to bring new strategies for maintaining or restoring balance in the body and, through that, more effectively managing endocrine disease and the child's quality of life (Teede et al., 2018Alengebawy et al., 2021; Rinninella et al., 2019).

4.6.3. Innovations in Diagnostic Techniques

The most recent advances in pediatric endocrine disease diagnostic techniques have significantly improved previous detection and intervention outcomes. e significant advances includes the application of deep enteroscopy techniques, like push enteroscopy and balloon-assisted enteroscopy. These technologies have revolutionary potential for the diagnosis and treatment of gastrointesract disorders, such as, such as obscure gastrointestinal bleeding and pediatric Crohn's disease. Balloon-assisted enteroscopy offers greater access to the small bowel, enabling not only improved diagnostic capability but also therapeutic interventions such as, such as stricture dilation and polypectomy. The availability of these new techniques permits much better insight into the intricate pathologies responsible for pediatric endocrine illness, ultimately paving the way for more personalized and effective treatments (Brett, 2025). Apart from endoscopic innovation, the development of machine learning approaches has now started to impact the diagnostic landscape of pediatric endocrine disorders, particularly short stature. Traditional methods of diagnosis are not very sensitive and specific, given the multifactorial aetiology of growth disorders. To address this void, machine learning techniques have been employed in recent studies to prxplainable prediction models, improving diagnostic accuracy for normal-variant short stature. For example, following an analysis of 33 medical features and conditional logistic regression, researchers were able to identify influential protective factors such as, such as parental height and children's weight. This new approach provides not only a more robust diagnostic model but also underscores the key rol played by environmental and family influences in development, thereby enriching clinical understanding and guiding preventive interventions (Liu et al., 2025). Moreover, developments in diagnostic techniques have raised debate regarding their use in pediatrics endocrinology. The integration of artificial intelligence into standard diagnostic procedures is likely to optimize both effectiveness and accuracy in the diagnosis of endocrine disease. As testified to by current studies, the interface of machine learning and traditional clinical assessment is able to significantly advance the detection of high-risk persons and enable earlier intervention. However, even with the promise that accompanies these developments, there are still barriers in regards to educating healthcare practitioners as well as codifying standard procedures for these advanced methods. Through overcoming these challenges, the specialty can optimize diagnostic methods and offer efficient management of pediatric endocrine diseases, ultimately leading to improved patient outcomes and quality care (Brett, 2025; Liu et al., 2025) (Figure 4.16).

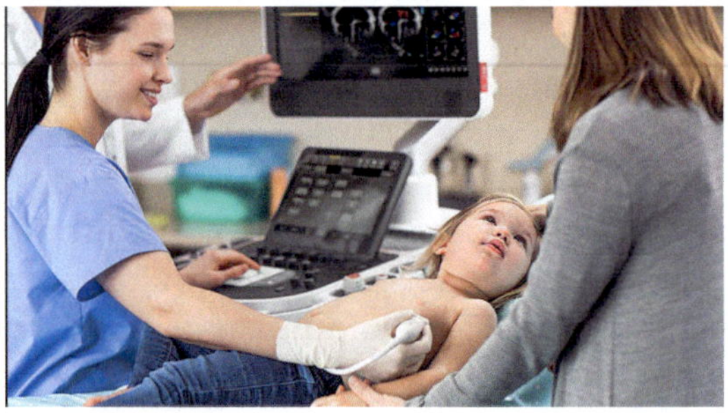

Figure 4.16. Pediatric ultrasound exam showing non-invasive imaging in child healthcare.

Source: https://www.philips.com/c-dam/corporate/innovation-and-you/global/jun-2021/teaser-child-being-scanned.jpg.

Test Your Knowledge

1. What new treatment modalities are emerging for managing pediatric endocrine disorders?
2. How is genetic research improving understanding and treatment of endocrine diseases in children?
3. What innovations in diagnostic techniques have enhanced early detection of pediatric endocrine disorders?

SUMMARY

The pediatric endocrine disorders represent a daunting and complex issue in the realm of pediatric health. These disorders, representing a wide range of complications affecting hormonal regulation and metabolic function, result in significant impacts on the health, development, and growth of affected children. As more is learned about such diseases, it has increasingly become clear that successful management requires a program that includes not only pharmacological interventions but diet. The addition of nutritional elements to the therapeutic program can play an important role in patient outcomes by allowing hormonal homeostasis and metabolic health, consistent with findings demonstrating that the contribution of nutrition cannot be ignored in treating endocrine disorders (Ullah et al., 2025). In addition, research into personalized medicine for the management of pediatric endocrine disorders has great promise for achieving new therapeutic advances in the future. By tailoring dietary counsel and medical interventions based on individual metabolic and genetic features, clinicians can more effectively tdren who have these disorders. Precision health strategies along these lines are particularly relevant in light of the heterogeneity of etiologies for pediatric endocrine disorders and their varied clinical presentations among individuals. With increasing research enhancingenhancements, the incorporation of evidence and development of comprehensive clinical guidelines will play a crucial role in the successful implementation of these focused strategies (Ullah et al., 2025). Finally, the urgent need for further research and method standardization within both the clinical and dietary approaches cannot be overstated. A focus on rigorously planned randomized controlled trials would enhance the role of nutrition in the management of pediatric endocrine disorders, filling existing gaps in evidence-based practice guidelines. Long-term trials could also elucidate causal relationships between dietary interventions and clinical endpoints, opening the gate for less toxic and more effective forms of management. Pediatric endocrinology and nutritional science is a key area of intersection for future clinical application and investigation that has the potential for improved health in affected children.

Pediatric endocrine disorders is a collection of diseases that affect the growth, development, and metabolism of children. Diabetes, congenital adrenal hyperplasia, and hypothyroidism are the disorders that directly affect the health as well as the quality of life of a child. Early diagnosis and treatment is an extremely important factor concerning the knowledge of these disorders. Early detection is likely to achieve better outcomes as most of these conditions are easily manageable with an optimal treatment protocol. Diabetic children, for instance, require intensive monitoring and insulin treatment to prevent the consequences of suboptimal glycemic control. The role of health professionals in detecting the signs and referring patients for appropriate diagnostic tests is important to effectively manage such endocrine conditions. But another essential argument in pediatric endocrine disorders is the necessity for interdisciplinary treatment. Cooperation between pediatricians, endocrinologists, dietitians, and psychiatric staff ensures comprehensive treatment. Coordination is particularly significant in the treatment of chronic diseases like polycystic ovary syndrome (PCOS), where hormonal management as well as lifestyle modifications are both critical to patient health. The most recent worldwide consensus regarding PCOS emphasizes an interdisciplinary care model, with involvement of various specialists to provide individualized care (Teede et al., 2018). It not only addresses the medical management of the condition but also the psychological and emotional aspects, and thus delivers a better overall experience for families and patients. Such holistic care models are necessary to provide for the demand of children with endocrine disorders, which are complex in nature. Apart from that, ongoing research and shifting clinical practice recommendations are paramount to pediatric endocrine disease treatment. As technology advances and more is understood about such diseases, clinicians can more effectively offer evidence-based care that guarantees enhanced patient outcomes. The recommendation of ongoing education and improvement in management protocols emphasizes the need for healthcare systems to adapt to new information (Rychik et al., 2019). This adaptation is crucial in managing the subtleties of disorders that could pose significant long-term health threats. Therefore, while pediatric endocrine disorders are a serious challenge, developing research and dynamic clinical practices promise better clinical outcomes and quality of life for the children.

KEY TERMS FROM THIS CHAPTER

- Autism spectrum disorder (ASD)
- Congenital adrenal hyperplasia (CAH)
- Glucose
- Growth hormone
- Hormone deficiency
- Hypothyroidism
- Paramount
- Pediatric patients
- Complex network
- Diabetes mellitus
- Glycemic control
- Growth Hormone Deficiency (GHD)
- Hyperglycemia
- Next-generation sequencing (NGS)
- Pediatric endocrine
- Polycystic Ovary Syndrome (PCOS)

CRITICAL THINKING QUESTIONS

1. **What is the most common endocrine disorder in children?**
   a. Hypothyroidism
   b. Type 1 Diabetes Mellitus
   c. Growth hormone deficiency
   d. Addison's disease
2. **Which hormone is deficient in Type 1 Diabetes Mellitus?**
   a. Glucagon
   b. Cortisol
   c. Insulin
   d. Adrenaline
3. **A child presents with polyuria, polydipsia, and weight loss. What is the most likely diagnosis?**
   a. Nephrotic syndrome
   b. Hyperthyroidism
   c. Type 1 Diabetes Mellitus
   d. Diabetes insipidus
4. **The most common cause of congenital hypothyroidism is:**
   a. Iodine deficiency
   b. Thyroid agenesis
   c. Pituitary adenoma
   d. Thyroid cancer
5. **Which test is used to screen for congenital hypothyroidism in newborns?**
   a. TSH and T4 levels
   b. HbA1c
   c. ACTH stimulation test
   d. Glucose tolerance test

Short Answer Questions

1. Describe the etiology, clinical features, diagnosis, and management of congenital hypothyroidism in neonates.
2. Discuss the types of diabetes mellitus in children, with emphasis on pathophysiology, diagnostic criteria, acute complications, and long-term management strategies.
3. Explain the pathophysiology and clinical presentation of congenital adrenal hyperplasia (CAH), and outline the steps in its diagnosis and treatment.
4. Describe the causes, clinical evaluation, and treatment options for short stature in children, including the role of growth hormone therapy.
5. Compare and contrast central (true) and peripheral (pseudo) precocious puberty, including causes, diagnostic approach, and management.

Answer to Critical Thinking Questions

1. (b); 2. (c); 3. (c); 4. (b); 5. (a)

REFERENCES

1. Alengebawy, A., Abdelkhalek, S. T., Qureshi, S. R., & Wang, M.-Q. (2021). Heavy metals and pesticides toxicity in agricultural soil and plants: Ecological risks and human health implications. *Toxics, 9*, 42–42. https://doi.org/10.3390/toxics9030042 (accessed on 16th June 2025).
2. Browne, N. T., Snethen, J., Greenberg, C. S., Frenn, M., Kilanowski, J. F., Gance-Cleveland, B., Burke, P. J., et al. (2020). When pandemics collide: The impact of COVID-19 on childhood obesity. *Journal of Pediatric Nursing, 56*, 90–98. https://doi.org/10.1016/j.pedn.2020.11.004 (accessed on 16th June 2025).
3. Chang, S.-W., & Lee, H.-C. (2019). Vitamin D and health–The missing vitamin in humans. *Pediatrics & Neonatology, 60*, 237–244. https://doi.org/10.1016/j.pedneo.2019.04.007 (accessed on 16th June 2025).
4. Etienne Crickx, Jehane Fadlallah, Morgane Cheminant, Jeremie Rosain, Jeremie Dion, Marion Malphettes, David Boutboul, Clement Gourguechon, Mikael Ebbo, Anne Marie Ronchetti, Thomas Moulinet, Delphine Gobert, Jerome Hadjadj, Julie Graveleau, Marie-Claude Stolzenberg, Bertrand Godeau, Lionel Galicier, Jean-Francois Viallard, Sy3-174512Crickx, E., Fadlallah, J., Cheminant, M., Rosain, J., Dion, J., Malphettes, M., Boutboul, D., et al. (2023). Whole exome sequencing of patients with adult-onset Evans syndrome: A cohort of 80 patients. *Blood.*https://www.semanticscholar.org/paper/91d92e2245cc9cf66a20ce7c06270f1c993eaa35 (accessed on 16th June 2025).
5. de Vries, S. A. G., Bak, J. C. G., Verheugt, C. L., Stangenberger, V. A., Mul, D., Wouters, M., Nieuwdorp, M., et al. (2023). Healthcare expenditure and technology use in pediatric diabetes care. *BMC Endocrine Disorders, 23.* https://www.semanticscholar.org/paper/3a67fdf0f19f2969e15755a6b2cc2cc8260339a0 (accessed on 16th June 2025).
6. Ghadery, C. M., Gorodetsky, C., & Lang, A. E. (2025). Tremor in pediatric populations: Clinical characteristics, differential diagnosis, and management challenges. *Movement Disorders Clinical Practice.* https://www.semanticscholar.org/paper/ee51b00f529d1168364f3a6d0bbb747c145b45ef (accessed on 16th June 2025).
7. Hoang, D. M., Pham, P. T., Bach, T. Q., Ngo, A. T., Nguyen, Q. T., Phan, T. K. T., Giang, N. H., et al. (2022). Stem cell-based therapy for human diseases. *Signal Transduction and Targeted Therapy, 7.* https://doi.org/10.1038/s41392-022-01134-4 (accessed on 16th June 2025).
8. Hoskins, B. J. (2025). Deep enterostomy in children: Techniques, applications, and future directions. *Frontiers in Pediatrics, 13.* https://www.semanticscholar.org/paper/7870dd6eaae7ad8e039e309647e7e69b6ae2b1ad (accessed on 16th June 2025).
9. Koshizaka, M., Eguchi, A., Takaguchi, K., Yamamoto, M., Takatani, R., Hisada, A., Kawanami, A., et al. (2024). Second phase Chiba study of mother and child health (C-MACH): Japanese birth cohort study with multimers analyses. *BMJ Open, 14.* https://www.semanticscholar.org/paper/81ee6853e9a18e47e4a9eacb0e71851457bb1d28 (accessed on 16th June 2025).
10. Patel, D. R., Neelakantan, M., Pandher, K., & Merrick, J. (2020). Cerebral palsy in children: A clinical overview. *Translational Pediatrics, 9*, S125–S135. https://doi.org/10.21037/tp.2020.01.01 (accessed on 16th June 2025).

11. Pipman, V. R., Arcari, A., Alonso, G. F., Bengolea, S. V., Boulgourdjian, E., D'Amato, S. P., Keselman, A., et al. (2024). [Cryptorchidism: An update of advances in its diagnosis and treatment]. *Archives Argentinos de Pediatric.* https://www.semanticscholar.org/paper/6ab3062832589f003bb3407fa3491f6f96246afb (accessed on 16th June 2025).

12. Rosenberg, A. G. W., Mochèl, K., Hähner, L. M., Ruules, L., Davidse, K., Bos-Roubos, A., van Dijk, S. A., et al. (2024). Endocrine and non-endocrine causes of fatigue in adults with neurofibromatosis type 1. *Frontiers in Endocrinology, 14.* https://www.semanticscholar.org/paper/0d6b6452736b1e82f56e1a58fc3678b97223566a (accessed on 16th June 2025).

13. Rubino, F., Puhl, R. M., Cummings, D. E., Eckel, R. H., Ryan, D. H., Mechanick, J. I., Nadglowski, J., et al. (2020). Joint international consensus statement for ending stigma of obesity. *Nature Medicine, 26*, 485–497. https://doi.org/10.1038/s41591-020-0803-x (accessed on 16th June 2025).

14. Rychik, J., Atz, A. M., Celermajer, D. S., Deal, B. J., Gatzoulis, M. A., Gewillig, M., Hsia, T.-Y., et al. (2019). Evaluation and management of the child and adult with Fontan circulation: A scientific statement from the American Heart Association. *Circulation, 140.* https://doi.org/10.1161/cir.0000000000000696 (accessed on 16th June 2025).

15. Teede, H., Misso, M., Costello, M., Dokras, A., Laven, J. S. E., Moran, L., Piltonen, T., et al. (2018). Recommendations from the international evidence-based guideline for the assessment and management of polycystic ovary syndrome. *Clinical Endocrinology, 89*, 251–268. https://doi.org/10.1111/cen.13795 (accessed on 16th June 2025).

16. Thakur, Y., Meshram, R., & Taksande, A. (2024). Navigating pediatric cor pulmonale: A comprehensive review of diagnosis and management. *Cureus, 16.* https://www.semanticscholar.org/paper/0c55d708784169569baf14219459599de5d6815e (accessed on 16th June 2025).

17. Wang, S. S., Bandopadhayay, P., & Jenkins, M. R. (2019). Towards immunotherapy for pediatric brain tumors. *Trends in Immunology, 40*, 748–761. https://doi.org/10.1016/j.it.2019.05.009 (accessed on 16th June 2025).

ASSESSMENT AND MONITORING IN PEDIATRICS

5

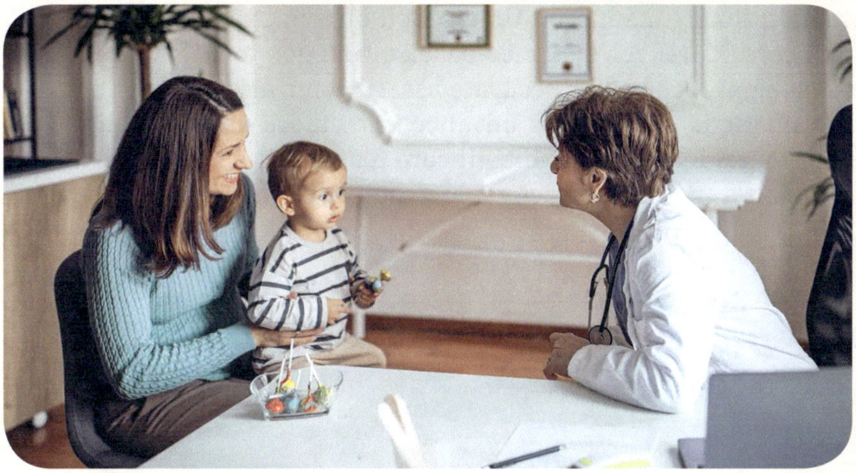

LEARNING OBJECTIVES

After studying this chapter, you will be able to:

1. Describe developmental milestones
2. Emphasize growth assessment
3. Explain the assessment of health history
4. Identify physical examination techniques
5. Understand diagnostic tests and instruments
6. Describe monitoring chronic disease

Introduction

Pediatric patient monitoring and assessment are key elements of medical care aimed at enhancing maximal growth and development through targeted interventions. Pediatric assessment is a multi-dimensional process that encompasses not only physical examination but also developmental screening, psychosocial evaluation, and more. It is essential to be aware of the distinctive aspects of pediatric care because children present different heals from adults because ofdue to their growth physiologically and emotionally. Thus, the healthcare providers need to use child-centered methods that establish a calm environment, allowing for open communication with the children and even their parents. Such a simple awareness is supportive of effective monitoring practices and allows clinicians to identify indicators of potential health issues early on, thereby optimizing health benefits. Moreover, the significance of surveillance in pediatrics cannot be overemphasized, as it represents an ongoing monitoring of a child's progress through the stages of development. Surveillance entails a whole host of activities, including regular check-ups, screenings, and assessment of signs of health like weight, height, and intellectual milestones. Effective monitoring not only tracks a child's physical health but also provides critical information regarding behavioral and emotional development, which is of the highest priority for integrative care. Deliberate tracking of these indices can help support recognition of trends that indicate developmental delay or illness complications. Incorporation of systematic monitoring protocols into pediatric practice, then, is paramount in directing treatment planning in ensuring interventions to bare timely and appropriate. Lastly, the application of evaluation and monitoring strategies in pediatrics is also supported by advances in technology and evidence-based practice. Electronic health records, telemedicine, and mobile health apps have revolutionized the provision of pediatric care through enhanced data gathering and availability. All these advances provide real-time data analysis, enabling healt inform decisions in a timely manneron time based on evidence, as well as empowering families through participatory care. Moreover, evidence-based evaluation tools have also been developed to standardize the monitoring procedure for accurate assessments among children of diverse demographics. As pediatric evaluations continue to advance with these advances, the over-riding significance of multidisciplinary interaction among healthcare teams becomes a reality, leading to improved healthcare delivery tailored to address each child's unique needs (Figure 5.1).

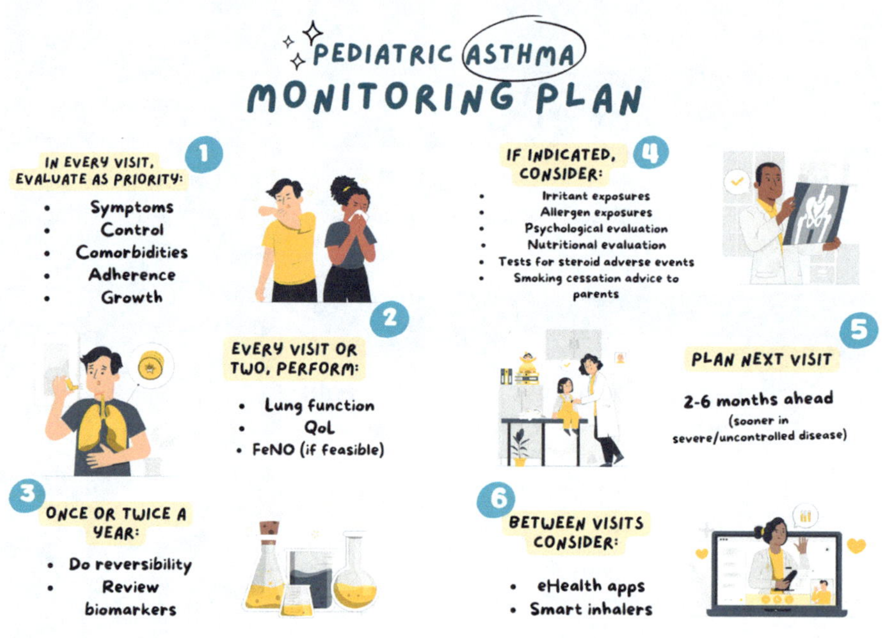

Figure 5.1. The assessment and monitoring of pediatric patients.

Source: https://onlinelibrary.wiley.com/cms/asset/2166a914-2a2a-43fd-b3bb-8e587c996589/pai14129-fig-0001-m.jpg.

Definition of Pediatric Assessment

The word pediatric assessment covers an inclusive evaluation process that is vital in the pediatric care of children from infancy to adolescence. Unlike adult exams, pediatric exams need a grasp of the physiological, psychological, and developmental differences that come with children. This prcomplex, covering multiple aspects, such as, such as physical wellness, developmental milestones, and psychosocial aspects. Clinicians use a variety of tools and techniques to gather information, tailor interventions, and monitor progress over time. A successful pediatric evaluation not only evaluates the child's health status at the moment but also considers family and environmental determinants that affect the child's health, highlighting the need for an integrative approach to health care. With accurate and broad-ranging assessments, health professionals can identify early signs of developmental problems and put timely interventions in place, thereby enhancing pediatric patient outcomes. Incorporation of evidence-informed interventions in pediatric assessment enhances coordination of care among educators, families, and healthcare providers. The utilization of a variety of assessment methods gives a multi-dimensional understanding of a child's developmental trajectory and health. instance, standardized tools may be applied for to various areas of assessment, e.g., functional or behavioral assessments. The model of the childhood health assessment is supportive of interdisciplinary collaboration, as evidenced by the support for an integrated system in order to link care fo and family support (Antonelli Jeanne W McAllister et al., 2009). This is a strategy that encourages ongoing care, allowing health providers to share critical information that may affect treatment decisions and outcomes. By this, pediatric evaluations become an integral part of successful monitoring plans that ensure holistic care. In addition to that, knowledge of the importance of different methodologies in pediatric evaluation is crucial in the provision of quality care. Subsequent studies have focused on diverse measuremategies, particularly for chronic conditions such as, such as diabetes, that reveal the intricacies of the interaction between adherence and outcomes. As an illustration, research has pointed out that elf-report measures can vely align adherences with clinical measures such as, such as Hemoglobin A1c levels in adolescents with Type I Diabetes Mellitus (Alemzadeh et al., 2011). This necessitates the application of multiple assessment methods to maximize the reliability of results and determine the most powerful variables for application in health status monitoring. The evaluation process not only offers evidence for timely clinical decision-making but also improves the depth of comprehension of a child's health dynamics over time, reinforcing the necessity for continuous and varied assessment in children's healthcare centers (Figure 5.2).

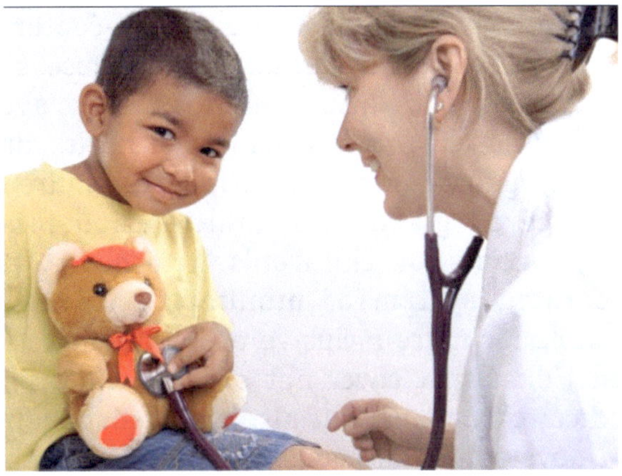

Figure 5.2. Pediatrician engaging a child with a stethoscope and toy, promoting a comforting clinical environment.

Source: https://media.licdn.com/dms/image/v2/C4D12AQGiX_m1ssagvw/article-cover_image-shrink_600_2000/article-cover_image-shrink_600_2000/0/1545411786875?e=2147483647&v=beta&t=ddiyjJwTAakEvfVQ2V2Hv1Bt-1grp2Hbo82-etMecdc.

Importance of Monitoring in Pediatric Care

Pediatric monitoring is necessary in order to establish the optimum health outcome for infants at various phases of development. With the continuous physical and mental development during this stage, continuous observation allows medical professionals to identify any potential issues with health at an early stage. Monitoring is necessitated not only for more than the immediate needs of health but also for continuous assessment of developmental milestones and behavioral wellbeing. Specifically, the existence of a system to measure patient and family experience can significantly enhance the process of care. For instance, through utilizing the Child Hospital Consumer Assessment of Healthcare Providers and Systems Survey, hospitals can make nationwide pediatric experience comparisons. These findings are significant because they provide something to be worked on as well as create an environment where patient-centered care is a reality (Hays et al., 2020). Successful monitoring can also result in improved coordination between providers of healthcare, something that is especially critical in children's healthcare, given the multi-dimensional requirements of children's healthcare. An integrated system of monitoring makes it possible for more inclusive observations to be made, ones that cover not only the children's medical care needs but also their educational and developmental needs. In addition, routine monitoring of data has the potential to create trends that might necessitate changes in health practice or policy. For example, when a trend is highlighted by monitoring that there is a chronic underavailability of developmental services, it can prompt reassessment of national preventive care standards and training for health professionals. Such interventions, aside from improving the care of individual patients, also bring system-level changes that the quality of pediatric care in general (Halfon Stevens et al., 2005). Furthermore, the importance of monitoring in pediatrics can be magnified by creating best practices that promote quality improvement (QIties. Evidence indicates that effective QI projects, such as, such as the application of evidence-based practices and operational communication systems reporting back to employees on patient satisfaction, are most critical. These strategies allow for ongoing feedback and fine-tuning of care practices, ultimately resulting in patient and family sat. Healthcare facilities can maximize their services in order to create a more responsive healthcare environment by implementing the optimal times and means of gathering feedback. This model is evidence of an ongoing improvement culture from traditional pediatric models and develops an overarching framework that focuses on the worldwide health and well-being of children (Hays et al., 2020).

5.1. Developmental Milestones

Learning Outcome

1. Key milestones in infancy
2. Milestones during early childhood
3. Importance of tracking developmental progress

Developmental milestones refer to major points of measurement by which pediatricians monitor a child's growth and development. They are a combination of many skills that encompass motor skills, language skills, social behavior, and mental processes. Monitoring these milestones helps in identifying any delay or unexplained patterns of development that may reflect the need for follow-up examination or intervention. For instance, tools like the Parents Evaluation of Developmental Status (PEDS) are created to evaluate children's developmental status through parental report. Despite their perceived value, heterogeneity in their utility has recently been demonstrated, particularly in the capacity to diagnose communication delay in infants aged 6–12 months. This inconsistency is an indicator of the requirement for pediatricians to utilize various methods of assessment and avoid exclusive dependence on formal tools in an attempt to ensure roervision andvision of care for children's development (Glascoe Dix et al., 20162015). The developmental monitoring context is particularly highlighted in those regions with limited resources, where the prevalence of communication delays is increasing. The picture is bleak in low- and middle-income nations, where more than 200 million children suffer developmental delay and disability. In South Africa, the Road to Health Booklet (RTHB) has been used as the mainstream developmental screen throughout the health system.

This checklist has been shown to miss more than half of at-risk infants and frequently does not identify correctly those in need of further assessment in studies. This inefficacy reflects a widespread disconnect within early identification processes that have lasting effects on the well-being and health of a child. Without accurate detection mechanisms, children stand to lose valuable early interventions teer their path of development (Dix et al., 2015Glascoe et al., 2015). With these limitations in mind, it is critical that healthcare providers not merely refine existing screening measures but also advocate for the implementation of validated and effective instruments with the potential to address the specific needs of at-risk children with developmental delay. High sensitivity of screening measures, as seen in studies comparing the PEDS measures, is important for optimizing outcomes for at-risk populations. Moreover, adaptability of screening behaviors to settings could enhance their relevance and validity. Therefore, ongoing research and commitment to enhancing developmental testing techniques are needed to facilitate better identification and support systems for children, eventually making the overall pediatric healthcare system robust. Incorporation of advocacy and community involvement can also play an important role in fostering awareness and guarapropriate resources by families (Dix et al., 2015Glascoe et al., 2016) (Figure 5.3).

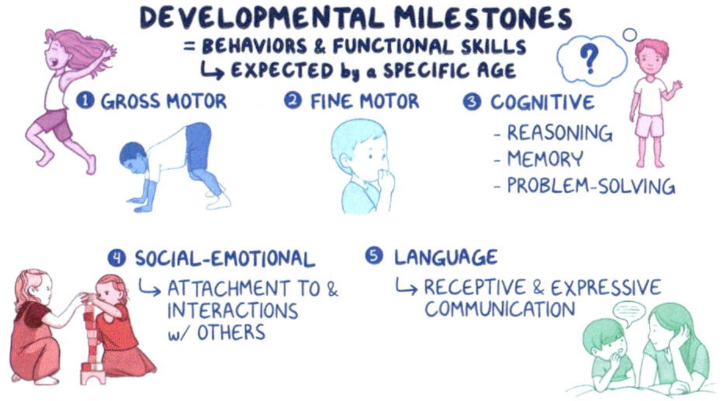

Figure 5.3. Developmental milestones serve as essential benchmarks through which pediatricians gauge a child's growth and development.

Source: https://www.osmosis.org/_next/image?url=https%3A%2F%2Fd16qt3wv6xm098.cloudfront.net%2FJSv2Qr7gTg_vDffkHrmG3XTwT6a20jpg%2F_.jpg&w=3840&q=75.

5.1.1. Key Milestones in Infancy

Infancy is a vulnerable stage of development with rapid growth in the physical, intellectual, and social spheres. The important milestones during this stage can provide valuable clues regarding the overall health and development of an infant. All aspects of development, including gross and fine motor skills, language, and social-emotional development, are addressed by these milestones. Identification of these milestones accurately becomes necessary to identify potential developmental delays and treat them accordingly. The measurement of motor skills, for instance, is commonly done dized testing tools, which assist medical health care providers to determinein determining the course of an infant's development over time. The tests not only gauge the course of movement but also permit early intervention whenever there has been a determination of delays, so that the child may be assisted to excel. The applicability of standard tests becomes apparent, particularly when considering the diverse factors that are likely to influence infant development. Research comparing latent structure in motor milestone assessment established that there was a distinct separation between gross and fine motor skills assessment, and tests should consider nuanced metrics for each (Bardid et al., 2022). This differentiation is critical, as infants can mature at varying speeds within these domains, thus reinforcing the necessity for tailor-made evaluations that take individual differences into account.

	6 TO 12 MONTHS	12 TO 24 MONTHS
MOTOR DEVELOPMENT	• Holds head steady. • Sits in lap without support; grasps book, puts in mouth drops, throws book.	• Hols and walks with books. • No longer puts books in mouth right away. • Turns board pages.
COMMUNICATION AND COGNITION	• Smiles, babbles, coos likes, and wants your voice. • Likes pictures of baby faces. • Begins to say 'ma', 'ba', 'da'. • Responds to own name • Pats picture to show interest.	• Says simple words, then 2 to 4-word phrases. • Gives book to adult to read. • Points at pictures. • Turns book right-side up. • Names pictures, follows simple stories.
ANTICIPATORY GUIDANCE	• Talk back and forth with your baby; make eye contact. • Cuddle, talk, sing, read, and play. • Point at and name things; nose, ball, baby, dog... • Follow baby's cues for 'more' or 'stop'. • Play games such as 'peek-a-boo' or 'pat-a-cake'.	• Smile and answer when your child speaks or points. • Let your child help turn the pages; keep naming things. • Use books in family routines; naptime, playtime, bedtime; on the potty; in the car, bus. • Use books to calm or distract your child while walking.

Figure 5.4. Infant developmental milestones chart.

Source: https://images.template.net/103276/infant-developmental-milestones-chart-swlre.jpeg.

The research also lends further evidence to the validity of gross and fine motor scores regardless of infant traits like sex, birth weight, and gestational age. By altering assessments to take into consideration these variables, pediatric clinicians can create more reliable monitoring of developmental milestones, which is central to early and effective intervention. Despite the availability of tools for monitoring significant milestones during infancy, primary care providers underdetect developmental delay. This gap in developmental monitoring underscores the importance of systematic screening practices going beyond casual observation (Sices, 2007). Having effective monitoring systems in place can significantly increase the early detection of developmental delays, allowing early intervention that is crucial to long-term developmental outcomes. Improving communication and collaboration between parents, educators, and healthcare workers can enhance monitoring practices and raise awareness of developmental pathways. Finally, fixing the shortages of current practices of measurement will not only advance improved health in infancy but also make the importance given to vigilance in monitoring milestones across populations even more solid (Figure 5.4).

5.1.2. Milestones During Early Childhood

Early childhood is a critical period for achieving developmental milestones that serve as predictors of healthy growth and overall well-being. These milestones encompass physical, cognitive, social, and emotional domains. Pediatric practitioners must conduct regular evaluations and monitoring during this period to detect potential developmental delays. For example, infants typically progress from cooing at two months to producing meaningful words by one year of age. Such benchmarks allow parents and clinicians to assess whether a child is developing within expected time frames. Early detection through vigilant monitoring enables timely intervention, ultimately improving outcomes for children with atypical developmental patterns. However, despite the availability of developmental screening tools, some early communication delays remain undetected. The Parents' Evaluation of Developmental Status (PEDS), for instance, has shown limited validity in addressingn groups, such as infants aged 6 to 12 months (Dix et al., 2015Glascoe et al., 2016). This finding underscores the importance of using validated tools to monitor milestones consistently. For instance, the sensitivity scores in relation to expressive and receptive language development were seen to be quite low, reflecting a high need for further research into effective methods of screening communication delay. Not only is the difficulty in finding such issues, but also taking up action for effective monitoring that can aid early intervention. Further, underdetection of developmental delays must include how primary care providers collectively work to strengthen their monitoring practices. Most children endure delays that are not addressed during crucial development stages, according to literature (Sices, 2007). More effectively preparing providers to spot these delays earlier would be a tremendous step toward improving the future health of children. Strategies may include intensified training for health practitioners and the application of a standardized model for developmental evaluation. By establishing an environment that emphasizes regular and thorough assessments, pediatric services can become more centered on meeting the needs of every child so that critical milestones are achieved and received appropriately throughout early childhood.

5.1.3. Importance of Tracking Developmental Progress

Pediatric populations need to have their developmental progress monitored in order to identify and address potential health challenges at an early stage. Developmental milestones provide the most important indicators that help healthcare providers know what the course of growth for a child should be. With more regular monitoring, healthcare providers can easily detect abnormal patterns that may reflect health, behavior, or development problems. Creating policies that increase participation in Medicaid and the Children's Health Insurance Program can greatly increase the number of Well-Child Visits and screenings and the quality thereof, allowing for timely intervention (Genevieve et al., 2010). Not only does this preventative measure allow for early detection, but allows for the implementation of targeted measures that can greatly impth outcomes as children grow. In addition, developments in screening methods, such as, such as accelerometry, can potentially revolutionize the monitoring of pediatric developmental progress.

Monitoring children's motor behavior using wearable technology to gather real-life data can potentially provide rich information regarding their developmental health. For instance, accelerometry measures bilateral motor activity, enabling clinicians to differentiate between typically developing children and motor-impaired children. These quantitative assessments are also crucial when assessing motor milestones, which serve as markers of greater trends within development. (Dosenbach et al., 2019) When using a referent group of typically developing children, health care providers can identify a baseline that can be utilized for comparative assessmehat deviations from normal development are identified and addressed in a timely mannerpromptly. Finally, continuous education and training of health professionals on the significance of developmental monitoring is also required. By fostering a culture that enhances developmental monitoring, pediatricians and other health workers can enhance their ability for early detection of red flags in childhood. This commitment has to be evident both in the practice and policy-making roles so that new screening tools and intensive training programs can be implemented. The long-term goal is to give all children the support they need to reach their full developmental potential, and thus reduce long-term disparities in health and well-being. Taken together, the worth of tracking developmental achievement cannot be exaggerated; it is not merely a clinical necessity but a critical component of improving children's overall health and attainment (Figure 5.5).

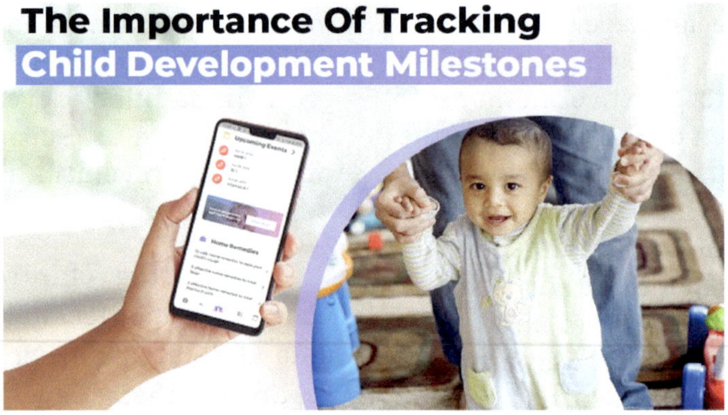

Figure 5.5. Importance of tracking developmental progress.

Source: https://kidscur.com/blog/wp-content/uploads/2022/07/Child-development-milestone-1.png.

Test Your Knowledge

1. What are the key physical, cognitive, and social milestones that occur during infancy?
2. Which major developmental milestones are typically achieved during early childhood?
3. Why is it important to track and monitor a child's developmental progress over time?

5.2. Growth Assessment

Learning Outcome

1. Measuring height and weight
2. Understanding growth charts
3. Identifying growth disorders

Growth assessment in pediatrics is a significant part of monitoring the overall health and development of a child. There are various measures used to evaluate growth by pediatricians, including height or length, weight, and head circumference, with the use of body mass index (BMI) when appropriate. The figures must be interpreted against the background of growth charts, which provide normative data to search for evidence of growth disorders or nutritional deficiencies. One has to stick to acceptable norms because variations from expected percentiles will be indicative of underlying health problems. Researchers have examined pediatric nursing-sensitive outcomes (PNSOs) that help in early identification of growth issues in lower and medium-complexity care units. The future direction not only aids in early diagnosis but also allows for more effective management practices for healthy growth in children, which leads to improved long-term health results (Batino et al., 2024). The worth of growth measurement extends beyond figures; it encompasses the psychosocial variables of significance to the health of a child. Obd stunted children are socially stigmatized and psychosocially stressed, a condition which that may reflect in poor overall mental health and low self-esteem. Frequent and accurate monitoring of growth can enable early intervention, an intervention critical during the vulnerable formative years of childhood and adolescence. Moreover, practices focused on family-based care play a significant role, as the engagement of families in the assessment process supports improved habits at home. Educating parents regarding a balanced diet and exercise may have substantial effects on a child's physical and emotional growth. Based on a thorough assessment that is geared towards these areas, healthcare practitioners are then able to offer care towards children's development (Batino et al., 2024). Population-specific issues, such as, such as those related to chronic health conditions or developmental delay, also increase the intricacy of growth evaluation in children. Children with a human immunodeficiency virus (HIV) diagnosis, for instance, have unique growth challenges concurrent with their specific requirements and therapy for their illness. Infected infants and children occasionally require specialized follow-up to consider the impact of antiretroviral treatment on growth and the nuance of perinatal acquisition of infection. In addition, age-associated changes in immunologic assessments, including CD4+ T cell counts, affect health and growth trajectories. This identification calls for individualized growth evaluation in proportion to the specific condition of each child to facilitate healthcare providers in thoroughly addressing the compounded issues embodied in complex pediatric cases (Figure 5.6).

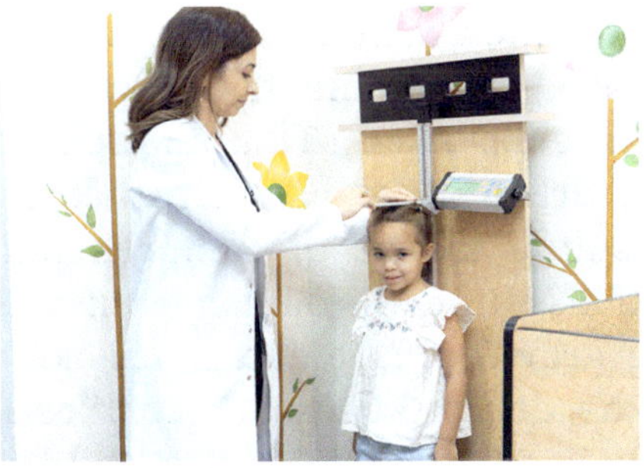

Figure 5.6. Pediatrician measuring a child's height during a routine health check-up.

Source: https://mypediaclinic.com/wp-content/uploads/2022/12/Hearing-Screening-1.png.

5.2.1. Measuring Height and Weight

Measurement of height and weight is an integral part of pediatric surveillance and assessment, capturing important markers of the growth and development of a child. Correct measurement not only provue about the general health condition of the child but also shows potential risks to health, such as, such as obesity or malnutrition. It is crucial in routine check-ups, enabling workers in the health sector to track growth patterns. Further, continuous measurement of weights and heights provides for prompt action in case of deviations from anticipated growth. As an example, identifying a child who has drastically altered percentile rank may warrant inquiry into diet, activity, or medical status so that problems can be addressed early. The accuracy of measurement methods cannot be emphasized enough, as they can result in incorrect diagnosisunsuitable health advice. Standardized apparatus, including calibrated scales and stadiometers, are is needed to acquire accurate measurements. Proper training of healthcare personnel also improves the accuracy of data obtained. In addition, the environment where measurements are being made plays a role because, for example, clothing and time of day can have an effect on readings. By putting the focus on systematic approachesmeasure height and weight, pediatric health professionals can determine that the data collected are is accurate in quantifying a child's state of growth. This focus is important, particularly while comparing data between populations or in doing epidemiology, as addressed in Bement et al. (2019). In contemporary pediatric practicement of height and weight is also useful in assessing the risk of developing chronic disease, such as, such as hypertension and metabolic syndrome. Weight status, particularly for overweight and obesity in a has in some studies been shown to be linked to highly significant metabolic health risks in spite ofdespite superior physical fitness levels. As depicted in Bement et al. (2019), obese and overweight teens manifested metabolic syndrome characteristics that highlight the need for frequent measurements. Furthermore, increasing numbers of hypertension cases among children require an all-encompassing approach toward height and weight monitoring as a component of comprehensive cardiovascular assessments, as noted in. This justifies the fact that routine anthropometric screening can lead to early identification of possible health issues, thus resulting in improved long-term outcomes for children and adolescents (Figure 5.7).

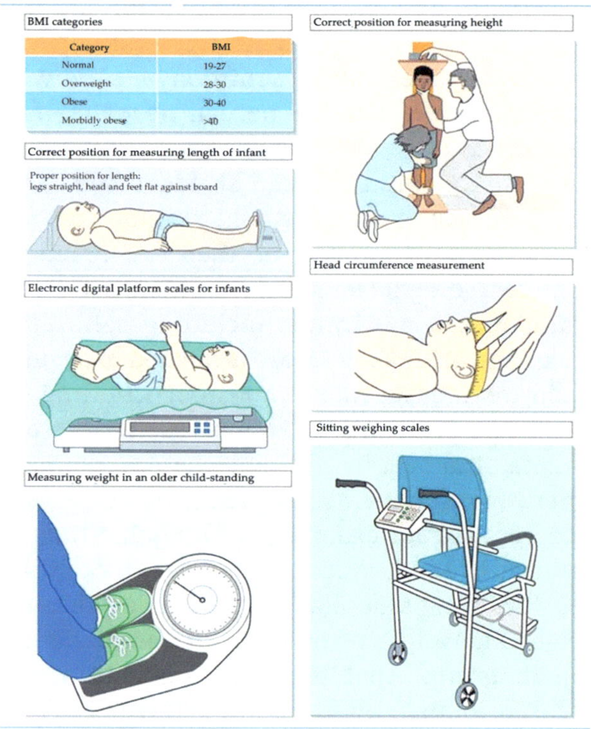

Figure 5.7. Weight, BMI, height/length and head circumference.

Source: https://i0.wp.com/nursekey.com/wp-content/uploads/2018/10/c17f001.jpg?w=960.

5.2.2. Understanding Growth Charts

Growth charts are an essential component of pediatric health monitoring and assessment, having the capacity to graphically represent a child's growth pattern against population norms. The plotting over time of such parameters as head circumference, height, and weight on charts makes it possible for clinicians to detect early potential growth abnormalities. For instance, deviations from predetermined percentiles can indicate underlying disease or nutritional deficiencies. The importance of head circumference is especially significant, as it strongly correlates with neurological development. Deviations in head circumference measurements can indicate developmental abnormalities, mandating further investigation and intervention (Corsello et al., 2019). As such, growth charts not only allow for regular health assessments but also provide the ability to monitor targeted developmental surveillance, rendering them essential tools in pediatrics. The establishment of growth charts is founded on comprehensive data from populations, usually representing varying demographics and age ranges. Such data provide percentile ranges that categorize growth patterns into normal, at risk, or abnormal. This numerical approach makes it possible for practitioners to compare sensibly based on an individual child's own background, e.g., socioeconomic status and ethnicity. Additionally, growth charts can be adapted longitudinally to reflect evolving growth patterns of children, synchronizing with changing health trends and environmental realities. Through the deployment of such contextual intelligth professionals will be in a better position to customize their assessment and intervention activity activities to meet the personalized requirements of various groups (McCarthy et al., 2004). Thus, the application of growth charts is more than mere measurement; it is a subtle means of comprehending the implications of health outcomes in pediatrics. Reading growth chart data does not merely involve the identification of percentiles. Instead, it is a holistic evaluation of a child's health and developmental status. For example, while a child may be within the normal range for height and weight, simultaneous measurement of head circumference can determine critical information regarding neurodevelopmental well-being (Corsello et al., 2019). Such multidimensional evaluation underscores the merit in the utilization of a composite of multiple growth parameters in the quest for an overall picture of child health. Pediatricians are required to consider various determinants, including genetics, eating habits, and environmental factors, in interpreting growth charts. Besides, continuous monitoring via ongoing appraisal allows for tracking of changes in the course of time, with valuable information present that is capable of informing health care management and interventions. Comprehension of growth charts thus constitutes an introductory aspect within the broader framework of pediatric monitoring and evaluation.

5.2.3. Identifying Growth Disorders

Growth disorder detection in children is a critical component of health assessment because it allows clinicians to diagnose and treat conditions that have detrimental effects on long-term physical and psychological well-being. Growth disorders, like growth hormone deficiency, nutritional insufficiency, and growth retardation associated with chronic illness, are usually determined by deviations in growth parameters. The assessment typically involves tracking a child over time, with growth charts used to track height, weight, and body mass index (BMI) plotted against standardized age and sex distribution. Regular monitoring enables the early identification of significant deviations that can indicate underlying disorders, so that intervention steps are implemented at an early period, critical in promoting good development. With the changing conceptualization of weight and illness correlations, even in disorders like anorexia nervosa and atypical anorexia nervosa, advanced techniques for tsessment of growth are needed. Recent research suggests that attention to the child's current weight only alone might not optimally represent a child's health status, esy when previous weight data are considered. For instance, research indicates that severity markers such as, such as serum phosphorus and heart rate may provide additional information on nutrition-related issues regardless of admission weight, thus supporting the multifactorial etiology of growth disorders (Accurso et al., 2019). This wide-ranging assessment is important since it allows practitioners to detect patterns that may suggest nutritional deficits or more subtle endocrine disorders, thu more effective treatment approaches.

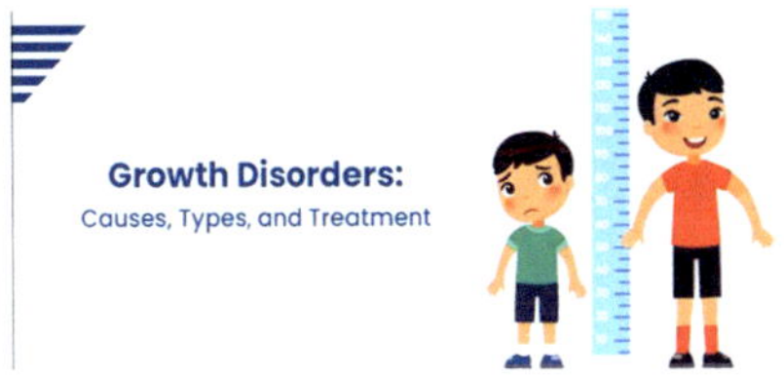

Figure 5.8. Identifying growth disorders in pediatric populations.

Source: https://www.sprintdiagnostics.in/blog/images/growth-disorder-causes-types-treatment.webp.

Furthermore, overlap among specific developmental conditions, such as, such as autism spectrum disorder (ASD), and growth monitoring is an added confounding factor in identifyh disorders. Individuals with ASD may have unique challenges that can affect their growth patterns, such as, such as behavioral issues that affect diet and activity level. A recent intervention study indicated that the implementation of a parent-based weight-loss intervention in children with ASD was effective, reporting improvement in weight as well as dietary behavior (Boutelle et al., 2019). This brings into prominence the importance of addressing growth assessments from a comprehensive viewpoint with respect to behavioral, environmental, and biological aspects. Healthcare providers must be vigilant in their assessments, employing a variety of strategies in an effort to accurately identify growth disorders while modifying interventions to accommodate the diversity of pediatric patients (Figure 5.8).

Test Your Knowledge

1.How are height and weight accurately measured to assess a child's growth?
2. What information do growth charts provide about a child's physical development?
3. What signs or patterns may indicate the presence of a growth disorder in children?

5.3. Health History Evaluation

Learning Outcome

1. Importance of Comprehensive Health History
2. Family Medical History Considerations
3. Assessing social and environmental factors

A comprehensive health history evaluation is a cornerstone of sound pediatric assessment and follow-up. It not only gives a baseline against which to compare the health status of a child, but also discloses risk factors and potential health issues. Putting clinical information, including family history, previous illnesses, and developmental milestones together, health care providers are able to produce a general idea of the health status of the child that will guide future practice. Also, by taking the time to thoroughly evaluate, it becomes possible to identify patterns that indicate genetic risk or environmental impact on health, an especially important consideration within the pediatric context, where the early identification of issues can revolutionize outcomes. Therefore, the dedication to meticulous health history evaluation allows practitioners to better tailor care to the unique needs of each child. The importance of proper documentation of health history cannot be overstressed, particularly in pediatrics, where growth and development are dynamic and rapid in nature. A child's health history is a valuable roadmap to monitoring progress through the various areas elopment, i.e., physical, mental, and emotional development. It also offers a means of detecting trends which that can initiate the demand for additional screening or intervention. For instance, a history of recurrent urract infections (UTIs) highlights the requirement for further assessment to prevent future complications such as, such as renal scarring. Such a preventive strategy is crucial, as evident from the findings of the study, which show a lack of consistency with routine imaging among these patients, suggesting a targeted plan to be a necessity (Biggi et al., 2005). Thus, assessment of health history is at the forefront of enhancing pediatric health care management. In addition to the clinical function of health history assessment, most critical is family communication. Communicating with parents or guardians not only enhances the quality of information obtained but also maintains an open method of management of health. This collaborative communication serves to guarantee that significant health problems are addressed in the right manner and that families are notified of necessary preventive measures. Additionally, leveraging educational potential within health history taking can aid families in taking an active part when it comes to the health of their child. For instance, training immunization managers within various areas has been recognized as an effective intervention for building local capacities and sustaining health programs (Rinderle et al., 2012). These efforts have a direct impact on the health outcomes of communities, illustrating the extensive reach of comprehensive health history assessments in pediatrics.

5.3.1. Importance of Comprehensive Health History

In the area of pediatric monitoring and evaluation, the importance of the complete health history cannot be overstated. Having a written health history is an invaluable element to understand the status of a child's current health and can contribute significantly toward clinical decision-making and treatment planning. Having detailed information on a child's past medical history, family history, and psychosocial setting helps health proals identify potential health risks and adjust interventions accordingly. By incorporating holistic aspects such as, such as diet, physical development, and behavior, clinicians are provided with information that goes beyond mere symptomatology. This holistic approach to practice supports optimal pediatric practice and allows for a greater understanding of those forces shaping the health of children, with improved outcomes. Second, incorporating the adverse childhood experiences (ACEs) and social determinants of health (SDOH) into the pediatric health history is required for early identification of risk factors that may influence long-term health. Research has demonstrated robust correlations between ACEs and child health in generalh negative experiences have major effets on both physical and mental health throughout life. Having kowledge aboutKnowing a child's social environment, —family relationships, economic status, and community resources, —is how healthcare workers can bring in interventions that not only address the chidiate health concerns but also address the grander scheme of a child's life. Current practices in most areas, such as, such as work-family-neighborhood policies in New Hampshire community-based providers, recognize the emerging recognition of these influences within the context of pediatric primary care, further supporting the role of a thorough health history in guiding interventions (Corvini et al., 2018). Practice The practice of comprehensive health history taking further involves not only the clinical information but also points to the role of interactive communication with families. Involving caregivers within the process facilitates the release of sensitive information that might not emerge via routine questioning, enabling a better appreciation of a child's health. Useful dialogue can reveal information regarding environmental stresses, habits, and even cultural impacts on health behaviors, thus adding value to the assessment data. As noted in successful immunization capacity-building initiatives, a critical needs assessment that puts local contexts first leads to more effective health interventions tailored to the specific needs of the community (Rinderle et al., 2012). The value of comprehensive health histories, thus, extends beyond mere data gathering; it is an important factor in establishing a strong and resilient healthcare system in pediatrics (Figure 5.9).

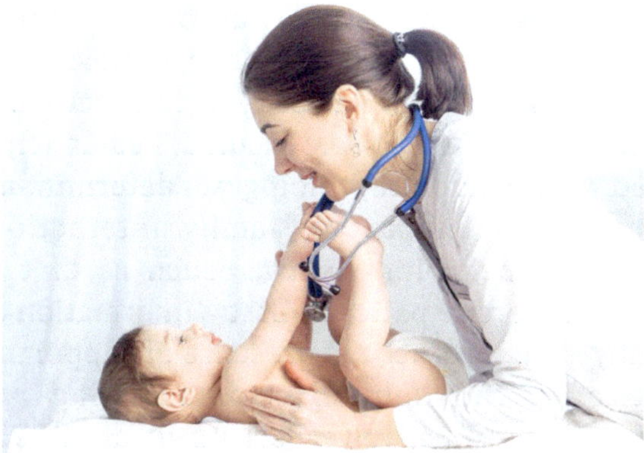

Figure 5.9. Pediatrician interacting playfully with an infant during a check-up, fostering trust and comfort.

Source: https://images.squarespace-cdn.com/content/v1/6487334be849e87dffd73f5c/1713250029772-T7ZT6MEZNNMTG2VJFA1A/3736.jpg.

5.3.2. Family Medical History Considerations

Family medical history knowledge is essential in pediatrics because it is a clue to the assessment of risk for various genetic and chronic conditions in children. A full family medical history is exceedingly useful in the recognition of inherited diseases, psychiatric illnesses, and disease susceptibility that may develop in adults. By compiling comprehensive information about the disease and health behavior among a child's family members, medical professionals can better assess potential hazards to health. An example would be a history of ADHD among family members, which would raiseelated risk fhe child and require intense follow-up and specialized assessment plans in pediatric settings (Gavin Neto et al., 20172018). This future position enables the establishment of preventive care and interventions earlier that can significantly change patient outcomes in the long run. Moreover, the significance of family medical history goes beyond the identification of inherited diseases. It is vital to the psychosocial aspect of pediatrics, giving insight into the child's environment and way of life. Family structure, stress, and behavior patterns can affect a child's health directly or indirectly and hence, need to be closely studied. Pediatricinly need to consider the biological determinants but also the impact of family interactions on health behavior, such as, such as diet or physical exercise patterns. Lastly, information on family structure, i.e., the presence of supporting networks, can help in communicating and intervening effectively (Perkins et al., 2005). Developing such connections can encourage improved treatment compliance, ultimately leading to optimal health for children. It is also important to realize the limitations of relying solely on family medical history in the absence of integrating it with a model of comprehensive assessment. While family history provides a preliminary awareness of potential health hazards, it should be supplemented by clinical assessment, lifestyle evaluation, avidual health screenings. For example, while a family history of diabetes is of concern, personal living habits such as, such as diet and exercise must be evaluated in an effort to develop an optimal management plan. Finally, there is also a risk in inaccurately reporting family histories, and therefore, clinicians must critically utilize this information. This combined strategy assists pediatricians in customizing preventive measures and therapeutic interventions that address both g predispositind environmental influences, thereby maximizing the overall child health surveillance strategy (Gavin Neto et al., 20172018).

5.3.3. Assessing Social and Environmental Factors

Understanding the social and environmental determinants of health is crucial to the effective appraisal and monitoring of children's populations. Children are extremely vulnerable to adverse conditions engendered by the environmtating far-reaching measures that consider socio-economic status, family dynamics, and regional resources. Interaction The interaction between variables has a tremendous influence on health status and lines of development. For instance, it has been found through research that adolescents who live in rural areas are faced with certain challenges, like limited access to healthcare and social services, which may enhance physical as well as mental health issues. This refinement attests to the fact that healthcare practitioners need to approach the assessment of chi's needs holistically, not only observing clinical symptoms but also the broader social environment affecting their life lives and prospects for recovery. Furthermore, the importance of including environmental factors in children's evaluations cannot be exaggerated enough, particularly for neurodevelopmental health. The central nervous system of humans is highly susceenvironmental poisons, which can disrupt development and negatively impact cognitive and behavioral functioningnegatively. Many children are exposed to various toxic chemicals in the environment, which can lead to conditions like attention deficit disorder or autism spectrum disorder. Applying strict measures of assessment that prove exposure to neurotoxicants along with corresponding social influences, researchers are able to define a more nuanced perspective towards child development. Incorporating these aspects in evaluation makes it possible to identify vulnerable populations so that early intervention and focused intervention can decrease the detrimental effect on long-term children's health outg., studies on principles of pediatric neurotoxicology (AACN et al., 2005). Finally, with new assessment methods, such as, such as tele-assessment batteries, monitoring and support for children with different nimproved, especially among disadvantaged groups. It is adaptive in data gathering and can reach families who otherwise arare otherwise hampered in seeking care in traditional health centers. Current evidence provides evidence of the acceptability and feasibility of distance assessment in the measurement of social functioning among adolescents with TBI. Through analyzing quantitative and qualitative data, researchers can come up with valuable information about the lived experiences of the impacted families and the determinants of social functioning. Such a deep understanding can prove to be highly influential in the creation of interventions for promoting the use of environmental resources and overcoming challenges for overcoming hurdlest children afed by TBI and other environmental adversity are able to develop resiliently and grow positively (Rennie Neto et al., 20152018) (Figure 5.10).

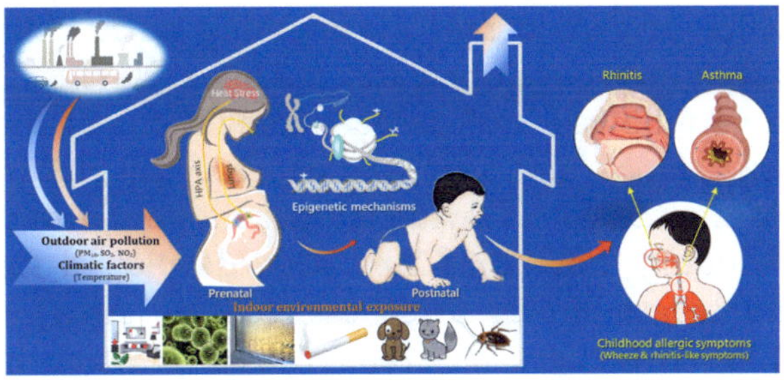

Figure 5.10. Assessing social and environmental factors.

Source: https://ars.els-cdn.com/content/image/1-s2.0-S0360132322009702-ga1_lrg.jpg.

Test Your Knowledge

1. Why is obtaining a comprehensive health history essential in evaluating a child's overall health?
2. How can family medical history help identify potential hereditary health risks in children?
3. Why is it important to assess social and environmental factors during a pediatric health evaluation?

5.4. Physical Examination Techniques

Learning Outcome

1. Standard Procedures in Pediatric Exams
2. Age-specific examination techniques
3. Importance of a thorough physical assessment

Proper physical examination skills are central to pediatric evaluations, as they are key sources of information about a child's overall health and developmental status. The pediatric physical examination is frequently in need of special adjustments since children are generally more apprehensive or less capable of describing their symptoms. Clinicians will need to incorporate elements that support trust and cooperation, including the use of child-friendly terminology, provision of a comfortable setting, and inclusion of caregivers in the assessment process. Furthermore, age-related differences in mportant; for example, examination of infants may often be performed with the infant on the caregiver's lap in an effort to reassure. Having a longer examination protocol not only enhances diagnostic precision but also establishes a good rapport between the medical caregiver and pediatric patient, paving the way for ongoing health monitoring and intervention as necessary. A complete physical examination involves meticulous observation, palpation, auscultation, and percussion to assess severasystems. The practitioners are recommended to begin with the general appearance of the child, noticing parameters such as, such as height and weight, which are important in assessing nutritional status and developmental milestones. This is to be followed by focused examinations of the heart, lungs, abdomen, and neurological status. plementation of evidence-based guidelines, including those that have been developed for the treatment of diseases such as, such as MPS VI, focuses on standardized practice in assessment across various healthcare settings. Practitioners are guided by these guidelines in monitoring needs in normal practice and the potential of medical treatments. The consistency created byparadigms allows it to be feasible for healthcare providers not only to monitor pediatric patients efficiently but to alsalso to identify deviations from typical results that may necessitate further examination or referral for professional treatment (Akyol et al., 2019). Tracking growth throughout the process by using physical examination techniques is essential in regard to early intervention and treatment of disabilities within pediatric care. Related services, as established under special education legislation, focus on the requirement of integrated assessments that include health assessments at all stages of a child's growth. Assessment of physical health, which includes developmental screens, and utilization of interagency resources, are all channels utilized to benefit children with disabilities, deriving useful information to be incorporated in Individualized Education Programs (IEPs). Through the use of physical examination techniques in conjunction with a multidisciplinary framewoitioners can deliver improved results for children with special education needs. By making heterogeneity of input, such as, such as the caregivers, a priority, the quality of the assessment is enhanced, besides adhering to policies for the improvement of adaptive educational and health services for disabled students (Dennis et al., 1999) (Figure 5.11).

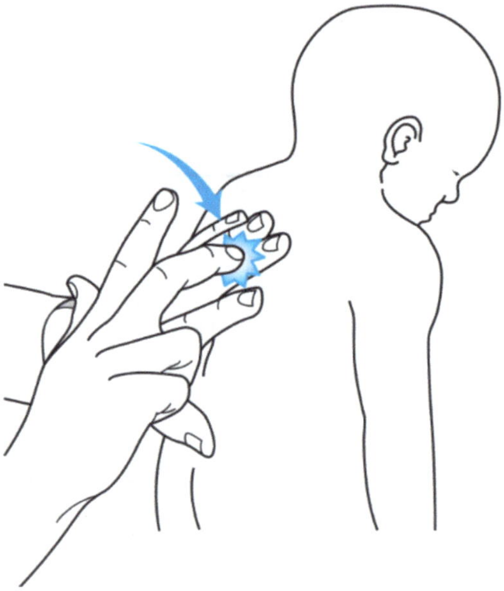

Figure 5.11. Physical assessment.

Source: https://connect.springerpub.com/binary/sgrworks/0b6a59722a2097a2/5236fe374b8e2b742480bd98f373456dbadf353576e034b2f75c5678da79cbdb/9780826174512_fig1_2.png.

5.4.1. Standard Procedures in Pediatric Exams

In child check-ups, standard practices are crucial in ensuring effective check-ups and follow-up of children's health. The practices are aimed at providing healthcare professionals with a comprehensive guideline to evaluate developmental milestones, physical health, and psychosocial health. Generally, such check-ups entail a sequential appginning with the history taking of the child's medical history, followed by physical examination of growth markers, such as, such as height and weight. This disciplined procedure for evaluation not only allows for the determination at an early point of those problems which may become health issues, but also serves to secure a trusting doctor-patient relationship between healthcare providers and pediatric patients. Secondly, compliance with these standard practices ensures uniformity within various healthcare settings, ultimately having a beneficial effect on health outcomes. Integration and coordination of preventive care are also fundamental to standard procedures in pediatric exams. Specifically, quality improvement programs under the Medicaid framework have emerged to offer proper developmental services to young children. External quality review organizations are reported to haveal role in this regard through reviewing the quality of preventive and developmental services for enrolled children (MarkusKrissik et al., 2008). By putting a lot of stress on routine monitoring, such organizations encourage an orderly process of healsessment capable of identifying areas of gaps in services and outcomes. With good protocols, healthcare providers are well well-positioned to offer comprehensive care that not only treats immediate health concerns but also long-term development needs, which are reflective of the complex nature of pediatrics. Aside from traditional testing methods, the integration of new technologies wd the parameters of standard practices in pediatric examination. Clinical ultrasound (CUS) is one of the methods that have has become invaluable in several medical specialties, indicating that the practice is shifting toward advanced diagnostic tools. Researchers have advocated for the creation of guidelines that cover all aspects of CUS use in hospitals and healthcare organizations with a focus on leadership, competency, and quality assurance (Abo et al., 2018). Standardization of these new methodologies in enforcing uniformity and effectiveness in the evaluation process allows for accurate tracking of pediatric patients. As such, incorporation of new technologies supports conventional evaluations, increases diagnostic potential, and ultimately fosters a more complete approach to pediatric health surveillance and treatment (Figure 5.12).

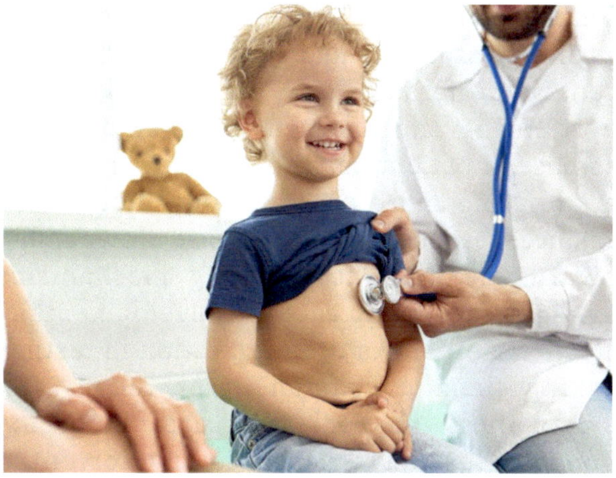

Figure 5.12. Standard procedures in pediatric exams.

Source: https://images.squarespace-cdn.com/content/v1/6487334be849e87dffd73f5c/06540c11-6fa7-4867-8662-7d2286da9f99/pediatricians+in+oklahoma+city.

5.4.2. Age-specific Examination Techniques

Pediatric practice assessment involves the utilization of appropriate examination techniques compatible with the child's developmental stages. Newborns, for example, must be touched softly to provide room for their bodily fragility and intellectual naivety. Observation-based techniques are used in assessment, for example, assessing a newborn's reflexes or monitoring their development through standardized growth charts. As children progreddlerhood and beyond, health professionals adapt these approaches to incorporate play so that the examination is continuingcontinues to be stimulating and less intimidating for the child. This adaptive development is critical to rapport building and allowing for more accurate results, ultimately making the experience less stressful for the child and caregivers. In working with older children, their level of understanding and communication shifts, necessitating adjustments in examination technique. In preschoolers, for instance, the explanation is tempered to utilize comprehensibogies so that the examination becomes less frightening. In children and teens, medical professionals try to use self-report reprt-encing and participatory methods. The increase in patient participation not only helps in gathering more accurate data, but it also enhances responsibility and a sense of ownership towards health. These coping mechanisms highlight the importance of developmentally effective methods of communication in testing, making them a component of the overall effectiveness in pediatric care. Emerging technologies havprogressed age-oriented methods of testing, particularly in surveillance and diagnostic tests. The creation of systems such as, such as the NEOREG system, which is designed to monitor and analyze neonatal data effectively, is one of the innovative approaches of age-appropriate testing. This technology supports an unproblematic combination of information, allowing systematic observation and improved clinical results in neonates with conditions like congenital cytomegalovirus (cCMV) infection that require close monitoring (Backere et al., 2013). Utilization of contrast-enhanced ultrasound (CEUS) also has a potential avenue for pediatric condition evaluation with minimal radiation exposure, thereby meeting the particular demands of younger patients (Cantisani et al., 2016). The ongoing development of these approaches serves to reinforce the dynamic process of pediatric assessment and the necessity for continuous evolution in response to shifting best practices.

5.4.3. Importance of a Thorough Physical Assessment

A thorough physical examination is a critical component of pediatric practice because it serves as the foundation for accurate diagnosis and management planning. The examination allows clinicians to detect early signs of potential health issues, parti in neonates and infants who can have subtle presentations due to their physiological immaturity. For instance, disorders such as,s hyperbilirubinemia are extremely prevalent among newborns and may lead to extreme morbidity unless diagnosed and treated at oncepromptly. A deliberate physical examination ensures that clinicians are able to monitor vital signs, evaluate growth parameters, and conduct a focused examination necessary to diagnose abnormalities. Thus, this proactive measure is paramount to mitigating the risk of complications arising froions, thus highlighting the significance of frequent and comprehensive examinations within the pediatric setting (Boo et al., 2015Olusanya et al., 2015). Furthermore, physical examination is also essential to the process of monitoring, allowing for the monitoring of developmental milestones as well as overall health milestones. The physical check-up not only assesses the curth of a child but also educates one about their pattern of growth. Detection of departures from patterns of growth, such as, such as reduced fetal movements during pregnancy, may be suggestive of underlying conditions such as, such as developmental dysplasia or other pathologies that have to be asd and addressed. Through the repeated assessment of these parameters, one can formulate a proactive model of healthcare that lays places strong importance on preventive interventions. This ongoing process facilitates timely referrals and the necessary adjustments in intervention strategies so that each child receives optimum care according to his or her unique needs (Nowlan et al., 2015). In addition to facilitating early identification and intervention, complete physical exams also facilitate proper communication between healthcare providers and families. This interaction is essential, as caregivers possess first-hand, intimate knowledge of their child's behavior and nuances, and can greatly inform the assessment pxplaining physical examination results to families creates a sense of partnership and collaboration, allowing them to be activist active stakeholders in their child's care. Since parents are becoming more knowledgeable regarding potential health issues and why they are being tested, they are more likely to become advocates for their child's needs. Thus, the benefit of a thorough physical examination extends beyond clinical considerations, both highlighting its benefit as an educational and empowering tool, ultimately enhancing pediatric health outcomes as families become their child's allies in assessment and monitoring (Figure 5.13).

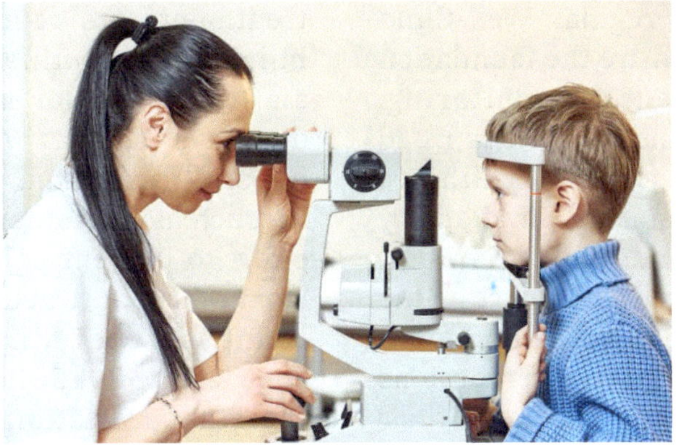

Figure 5.13. Pediatric eye exam using a slit lamp for vision screening.

Source: https://cchclinic.com/wp-content/uploads/2020/07/THE-IMPORTANCE-OF-PHYSICAL-EXAMINATION-IN-PEDIATRICS.jpg.

Test Your Knowledge

1. What are the standard procedures followed during a routine pediatric physical examination?
2. How do examination techniques vary according to the child's age and developmental stage?
3. Why is performing a thorough physical assessment crucial for accurate pediatric diagnosis and care?

5.5. Diagnostic Tools and Tests

Learning Outcome

1. Common Laboratory Tests in pediatrics
2. Imaging Techniques Used in Pediatric Assessment
3. Role of screening tools in early detection

In children's assessment, diagnostic instruments and tests are crucial in early diagnosis of opmental disorders to facilitate interventions in time. A good case in point is the Autism Detection in Early Childhood (ADEC) that which serves as a Level 2 screening tool targeted at toddlers. A retrospective study on toddlers referred to an Australian child development service evidently refers to the clinical usefulness of ADEC. The results showed an outstanding sensitivity of 87.5% and a moderate specificity of 62%. Such accuracy makes ADEC a valuable tool for clinicians diagnosing autism spectrum disorders (ASDs). By making proper discrimination among children with ASDs and other communication disorders, ADEC not only helps in precise diagnosis but also helps in making appropriate developmental intervention reach children at optimal formative ages (Ahmad et al., 2015). In addition, application of screening tools like ADEC is required, but is faced with several barriers that can hinder on-time pediatric health issue identification. Research emphasizes that better access to diagnostic screenings ought to be offered through policies designed to increase membership in Medicaid and the Children's Health Insurance Program. These efforts can enable regular Well-Child Visits and screenings, which are the foundation of pediatric developmental monitoring. Highlighting the importance of widespread use of data can further facilitate healthcare policies, ultimately increasing the availability and quality of developmental screenings. Overcoming all these challenges is part of the ongoing effort to improve early detection tools, so that at-risk children are given interventions as soon as possible and thus maximize their developmental attainment (Genevieve et al., 2010). Moreover, the integration of diagnostic equipment into a comprehensive model of child care is essential for effective assessment and monitoring. Early diagnosis success does not lie in the tools alone, but also in training and facilities accorded to medical professionals. For instance, clinicians must learn how to conduct these screening tests and interpret them properly. Continuing professional development and provision of best evidence-based practices can do a tremendous amount to enhance the effectiveness of diagnostic assessment. Apart from this, stimulating collaboration among health providers, teachers, and families facilitates a supportive environment for early identification of developmental problems. Lastly, utilizing well-validated diagnostic measures through a structured pediatric health system will extend timely and individualized care to children and yield improved longer-term health benefits (Ahmad et al., 2015).

5.5.1. Common Laboratory Tests in Pediatrics

A critical element of pediatric evaluation is laboratory testing, which plays a critical role in diagnosing and treating a range of conditions in children. Routine tests include complete blood counts (CBC), which aid in diagnosing anemia, infections, and other hematologic conditions. What the clinician evaluates through a CBC allows them to make vital decisions on whether or not additional investigations or treatments are required. In addition, serum bilirubin is routinely tested in neonates in an attemcreen for jaundice, a common issue durinays of life. With every detection of hyperbilirubinemia, immediate therapy such as, such as phototherapy can be initiated in an effort to prevent pgic consequences stemming from bilirubin toxicity, especially in developing countries with varied treatment protocols (Boo et al., 2015Olusanya et al., 2015). With the standardization of laboratory testing in pediatrics, the quality of care and appropriate assessment can be enhanced by healthcare providers. Urinalysis and urine culture are also crucial in the diagnosis of urinary tract infection (UTI) among children, which if not treated, can have serious complications. The process among the young population typically involves checking for the presence of nitrites, leukocyte esterase, and cultureermine infection. Of note, the benefit of many follow-up imaging tests following UTI is controversial, with evaluations such as, such as ultrasounds and renal scintigraphy, found to have limited predictive abilities for outcome events such as, such as renal scarring (Biggi et al., 2005). In view of these findings, clinicians are encouraged to utilize alternative modalities, including conthanced ultrasound imaging modalities, that minimize radiation exposure while still providing effective evaluation of conditions such as, such as vesico-ureteral reflux. The economic value of targeted studies is an expression of the impact that laboratory research has on pediatric UTI treatment. Finally, metabolic and genetic diagnoses in children are especially valuable for the identification of underlying disorders not evident on clinical presentation. Newborn screening panels, for instance, enable the early detection of disorders like phenylketonuria (PKU) and congenital hypothyroidism, both of which, untreated, lead to catastrophic long-term consequences. The adoption of standard protocol in such screenings enables health practitioners to intervene early, with the resultant better prognoses among the affected children. Besides, complete metabolic panels can reveal electrolyte imbalance or hepatic failure, thus informing future treatment interventions. By integrating the latest laboratory practices into pediatric practice, health workers not only enhance the precision of diagnosis but also enhance outcomes considerably to a point where every child receives the finest possible follow-up and assessment as it matures (Figure 5.14).

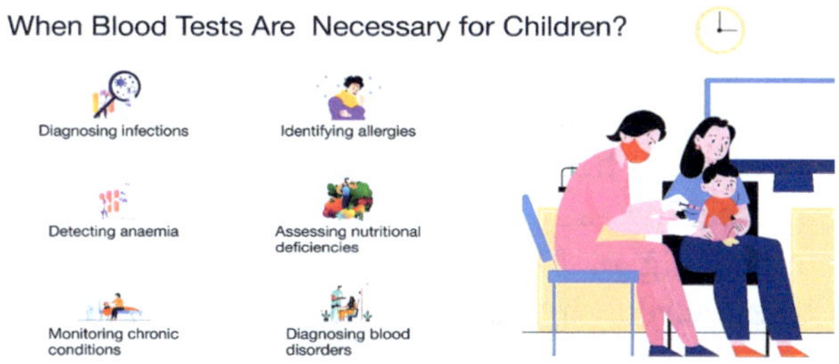

Figure 5.14. Blood test for kids.

Source: https://www.manihospitals.com/uploads/image_gallery/blood-test-for-kids.jpg.

5.5.2. Imaging Techniques Used in Pediatric Assessment

In the diagnosis in of a child, selecpropriate imaging methods lies at the heart of effective diagnosis and monitoring of a large variety of ailments. Imaging devices such as, such as ultrasound, magnetic resonance imaging (MRI), and computed tomography (CT) are commonly utilized due to their capacity to provide valuable information concerning a child's anatomy without necessitating invasive methods. Ultrasound, in particular, is the preferred modality because of its safety profile since it does not expose children to ionizing radiation, which is extremely beneficial when assessing abnormalities like urinary tract anomalies. MRI is also beneficial in imaging soft tissue and neurological conditions, but its higher cost r duration can be disadvantages. It is important for clinicians to know the benefits and constraints of such imaging modalities in order to deliver appropriate diagnosis with limited risks througextra exposure or distress to children. One of the pediatric imaging areas, that of urinary tract infection (UTI), has also been given a thought where imaging modalities play a remarkable role in assessing complications. A systematic review indicated that routine imaging in children with established UTIs might be ineffective in preventing recurrent infection or renal scarring, and hence indicative of a requirement for particular approaches in imaging protocols. Even though ultrasound remains a non-invasive technique, evidence indicates it may not be an appropriate screening imaging for upper urinary tract infection as compared to renal scin Emerging evidence points towards contrast-enhanced ultrasound techniques as a promising alternative to more traditional methods, such as, such as micturating cystourethrography, for detecting vesico-ureteric reflux (VUR). It is non-radiative, but clinically informative, influencing clinical decision-making in pediatric UTI management (Biggi et al., 2005). Evidence-based practice should be incorporated into pediatric imaging pathways to enhance diagnostic accuracy and patient outcomes. With the radiology and pediatric settings evolving, ongoingnto the efficacy of different imaginies are essential. Studies into imaging methods that can be refined can yield data enhancing that enhances everyday practice and reducing reduces unnecessary intervention. For instance, an awareness of the limits of technology-intensive imaging devices like ultrasound, when set against their diagnostic potential, may facilitate better usage of these devices. Furthermore, efforts to evaluate existing methodologies within a clinical setting remain imperative to ensure children are afforded the best possible, effective and safe evaluations. Ultimately, adopting an informed applicimaging modalities will greatly accelerate the end goal of improved health outcomes in pediatric populations (Krissik et al., 2008N/A, 2010) (Figure 5.15).

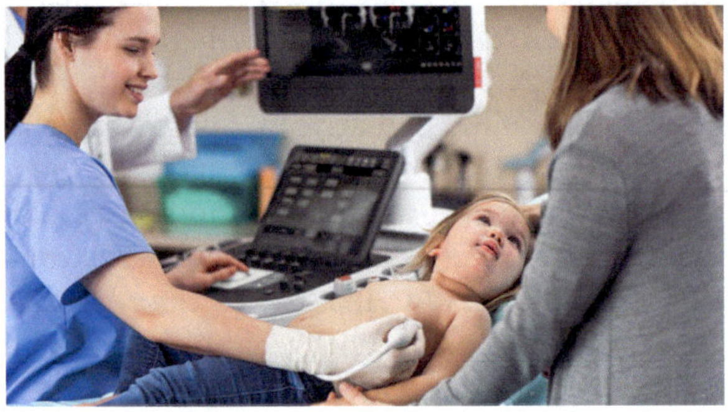

Figure 5.15. Child undergoing ultrasound scan for diagnostic imaging.

Source: https://www.usa.philips.com/c-dam/corporate/innovation-and-you/global/jun-2021/hero-child-being-scanned.jpg.

5.5.3. Role of Screening Tools in Early Detection

Application of screening tools incs is necessary in early identification of developmental delays and other conditions. The tools identify potential concerns before becoming they become significant problems that can slow down the development and quality of a child's life. Developmental delays are underappreciated by most primary care clinicians, and hence, the a necessity for a solid developmental monitoring and screening framework. As noted by Sices (2007), excessive rates of inappropriate detection in early childhood emphasize the need for systematic efforts to improve monitoring and timely intervention. Using standardized screening instruments, medical providers can effectively prioritize high-risk children for timely access to resources and interventions. In addition to developmental screening, screening instruments are important in detecting other conditions that affect newborn health, e.g., hyperbilirubinemia. It is a condition known commonly as jaundind has dangerous implications, particularly in low- and middle-income countries where medical facilities are few. According to Olusanya Boo et al. (2015), appropriate and timely use of screening guidelines must be done to avoid potentially fatal complications of untreated hyperbilirubinemia. Protocols facilitating early recognition and control of hyperbilirubinemia can significantly reduce rates of morbidity and mortality by allowing for optimal care to be given to infants in their initial weeks of life. Thus, the integration of reliable screening instruments into pediatric practice not only aids in the identification of acute health problems but is also vital in aiding overall long-term health outcomes. Furthermore, the applicability of the integration of screening tools extends beyond immediate health assessments; it signifies an assertive approach to the evaluation and monitoring of pediatric health. When doctors utilize screening tools in an efficient manner, they are engaged in an integrated evaluation of a child's development and maturation. This approach facilitates a broadening perspective of a child's course of health, which in turn contributes to more informed clinical decisions. Early identification using screening enables the implementation of indialized interventions that can address a child's particular needs.In the face of recommendations like those in Sices (2007) and Olusanya Boo et al. (2015), with strong calls for the creation of contextually-relevant guidelines, there is further buttressing of the utility of screening instruments. These suggestions can assist healthcare professionals in maximizing practices to achieve better health outcomes for children, affirming the radical potential of early diagnosis in pediatric assessment.

Test Your Knowledge

1. What common laboratory tests are used to evaluate health conditions in pediatric patients?
2. Which imaging techniques are most commonly applied in pediatric assessment and diagnosis?
3. How do screening tools aid in the early detection of developmental or medical issues in children?

5.6. Monitoring Chronic Conditions

Learning Outcome

1. Importance of regular follow-ups
2. Strategies for managing chronic illnesses
3. Family involvement in chronic condition management

The tracking of chronic disease among the pediatric population needs continuous multifaceted evaluation due to the variability of children's health needs. Children are different from adults since they grow and develop constantly, and as a result, healthcare providers need to constantly assess not only their medical status but also the psychosocial environment. Regular assessments allow for timely intervention and adjustment of treatment planning so that therapeutic modalities remain compatible with the child's fluctuating health status. In addition, a comprehensive strategy combining medical intervention with education and family support mechanisms is needed. This concurs with research evidence that proposes a model for pediatric care coordination which links health care, education, early child care, and family support with emphasis on the necessity of an integrated infrastructure in being able to track chronic s effectively (Jeanne et al., 2009). Furthermore, technology in tracking chronic conditions grows stronger. Digital health technologies, such as, such as wearable monitors and mobile health applications, facilitate real-time capture and analysis of data, which engage families in the management of their child's care. In addition to facilitating enhanced communication between medical professionals and families, these technologies are also a platform for managing medication schedules, monitoring symptoms, and general health parameters. Telehealth services, where clinicians remotely consult with families, are an exemplar of improved pediatric healthcare access. In the case of specialist treatments, including oxygen therapy at home in children with respiratory disorders, there have been guidelines that have been developed to inform clinicians and care providers on how to effectively provide care. This is important for the purposes of ensuring the maximum monitoring measures in chronic diseases (Balfour-Lynn et al., 2005). Lastly, the evolving nature of chronic disease in children necessitates ongoing education and training of care providers. Clinicians need to be well-informed regarding contemporary evidence-based care and emerging technologies to ensure high-quality care. This is about knowing how to implement individualized care plans as well as the latest clinical guidelinerious conditions. Training programs focused on care coordination, treatment strategy modification, and family involvement are critical to improve improving outcomes. Through investment in educational resources and development of an environment of collaboration between healthcare, education, and family systems, healthcare providers are better positioned to address the diversified needs of children suffering from chronic diseases, ultimately enhancing their quality of life (Figure 5.16).

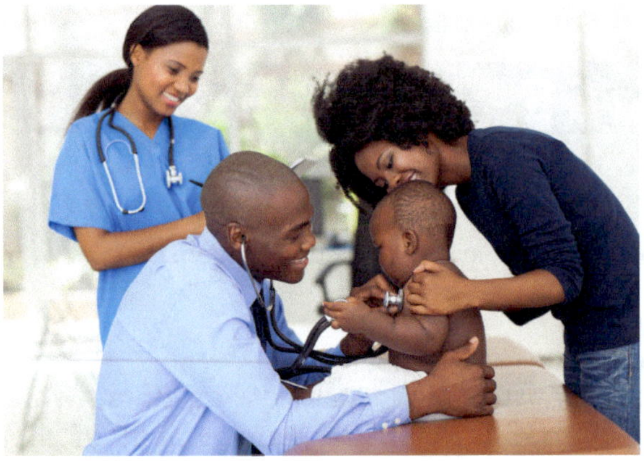

Figure 5.16. Monitoring chronic conditions in pediatric populations requires a multifaceted approach due to the complexities inherent in children's health needs.

Source: https://staticnew-prod.topdoctors.co.uk/files/Image/large/8c13b2ea42f7da8b5f1b66d55025e7e8.jpg.

5.6.1. Importance of Regular Follow-Ups

Follow-ups are critical pillars of good pediatric care, particularly in the management of chronic diseases such as, such as diabetes. Initial diagnosis weighs enormously psychologically and physically on pediatric patients and their familiesty of frequent checks and assessments. By implementing systematic follow-ups, healthcare workers can detect possible complications in a timely manneron time, including diabetic nephropathy, which is among the commonest causes of end-stage renal disease in diabetic children (Nfors et al., 2014). Follow-ups enable interventions to be done in a timely fashion and can significantly change the course of the disease, eventually contributing to enhanced not only clinical outcomes but also patients' and caregivers' quality of life. Besides, routine follow-ups serve to strengthen the doctor-patient and family-doctor alliances, creating the right environment for further disease management. Effective communication during follow-ups offers the ground for the exchange of essential information regarding disease progression and control. For instance, the application of education on domains of self-management skills and psychosocial support can play a critical role in assisting families in managing difficulties of diabetes (Nfors et al., 2014). Health care providers, through frequent interaction, can individualize treatment plans to suit a patient's personal situation. Thus, treatment adherence and improved health outcomes are enhanced. Additionally, follow-up visits are not only useful in terms of mere clinical monitoring but also as empowering and educational occasions. Programs like the International Diabetes Federation Life for a Child (IDF-LFAC) integrate clinical care with education in a way that families receive overall care, ranging from education to technical training and required medical infrastructure. The system emphasizes open communication at every point in time, encouraging active involvement of families in the child's healthcare process. By creating competence and skills in caring for diabetes, health professionals can enable children to enjoy healthier lives with reduced rates of complications and enhanced long-term health maintainability.

5.6.2. Strategies for Managing Chronic Illnesses

Effective management of chronic diseases in pediatric populations involves a robust strategy consisting of firm assessment and monitoring mechanisms. The Pediatric Self-Management Model is employed as the underlying paradigm, emphasizing thcance of behavioral determinants and self-management activities in the shaping of health outcomes. For instance, children with chronic illnesses, such as, such as type 1 diabetes, can be greatly assisted using targeted interventions that focus on enhancing adherence to treatment strategies. Research indicates that self-management swhen supplemented with specially designed educational materials for adolescents, can improve metabolic control as well as overall health outcomes (KaugarsKichler et al., 2012). Therefore, it is crucial to develop settings that encourage active participation by the patients and families to achieve effective management of chronic diseases in children. In addition to patient empowerment, elimination of systemic barriers is essential for effective management of chronic illness. The fragmentation of care, particularly within public insurance programs, is very difficult in referring and accessing treatment for children. The low payment rates and complex billing requirements have a tendency to discourage clinicians from offering routine care, which in turn impacts treatment continuity as well as efficacy (Genevieve et al., 2010). The creation of connected policy reforms that improve communication among primary care and specialist treatment practitioners can enable early intervention and improved health results. Providing pediatric patients with proper resources ensures that healthcare systems can successfully close gaps in the treatment of chronic diseases. Lastly, continuous monitoring of assessment is required to determine that management strategies are modified to include the evolving needs of pediatric patients with chronic diseases. Co monitoring allows care teams to identify changes in health status acy of treatment plans, particularly for dynamic management conditions such as, such as asthma and diabetes. Further, integration with technology, such as, such as telehealth and mobile health apps, allows real-time monitoring and data collection, so healthcare professionals can adjust treatment protocols in a timely fashion. Highlighting the significance of tailored care strategies based on regular assessments can result in better health outcomes and enhance the quality of life for children with chronic conditions. A combination of self-management, systemic support, and ongoing monitoring therefore, forms an overarching approach to chronic illness management in pediatrics (Figure 5.17).

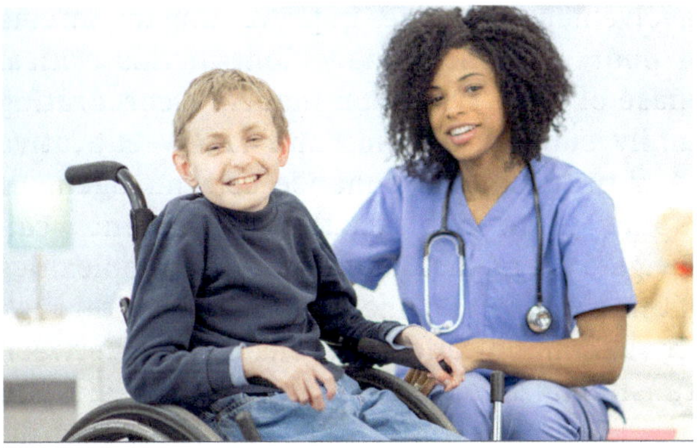

Figure 5.17. Healthcare provider supporting a smiling child in a wheelchair.

Source: https://www.thrivespc.com/wp-content/uploads/2025/04/10.png.

5.6.3. Family Involvement in Chronic Condition Management

Family participation is essential in the management of chronic diseases in children, and their participation determines the outcomes of children's health significantly. When families are actively involved in the care process, they not only help the child but also enhance compliance with medical regimens and self-management behaviors. Family and provider communication is generally typical of this participation, which enhances understanding and compliance with treatments. Furthermore, as has been explained in the Pediatric Self-Mat Model, family interaction is affected by contextual variables directly implicating behaviors associated with the management of chronic conditions such as, such as diabetes. The model stresses the importance of engagement to be integrated into care rategies because it plays a major role in enhanced health outcomes among children with chronic conditions (KaugarsKichler et al., 2012). Transition from a pediatric to adult health care is special, particularly for adolescents with chronic illnesses like Type 1 diabetes. Proper transition during this time is not just the duty of the health care system but also of involved families. Research has identified the involvement of families in preventing the threats of poor glycemic management in this critical phase of care. Transition models incorporating family support systems and family educative been promising to enhance self-management capacities in adolescents. Adolescents can navigate the medical and emotional complexities of this phase with of life more effectively through active communication and collaboration between transitional care teams, healthcare workers, and families (Bagnall et al., 2013). Subsequently, promoting family roles in transitional programs has the potential to promote long-term health and adherence. In conclusion, the value of family engagement in chronic disease management cannot be overstressed. Families are focal support systems, which help pediatric patients become more engaged in their treatment through education and collaborative decision-making. Incorporating family dynamics into healthcare frameworks allows comprehensive assessments to meet the unique needs of children with chronic conditions. Furthermore, as research continues to highlight the benefits of family engagement, healthcare providers must prioritize the creation of measures that actively involve families in the treatment. Aside from empowering adolescents with chronic diseases, this for the establishment of a robust support network that contributes to enhanced management of general health and leads to better long-term outcomes (KaugarsKichler et al., 2012).

Test Your Knowledge

1. Why are regular follow-up visits important for children with chronic health conditions?
2. What strategies can help effectively manage chronic illnesses in pediatric patients?
3. How does family involvement contribute to better management and outcomes in children with chronic cos?

SUMMARY

It is evident that effective interventions are critical to mitigating health disparities and maximizing outcomes for children. Initiativessuch as, such as early recognition and appropriate referral for substance abuse or behavioral health problems can really make a difference in the trajectory of a child's life. The study of brief interventions in various health settings has emphasized the importance of taking into account not just the immediate health needs of children but their general social context. Through channels like primary care to implement such kinds of interventions, medical professionals can establish a platform of support systems that encourage healthy behavior in addition to minimizing risks associated with substance abuse and other unhealthy practices, as underscored through the evidence around the value of continued follow-up support (Aisha et al., 2017). In addition to that, attgiven to multi-disciplinary practices in pediatric health assessment cannot be overemphasized. Interdisciplinary collaboration between healthcare workers such as, such as nurses, doctors, and support staff, facilitates better effectiveness of interventions by pooling knowledge and resources. Insights from stakeholders in various healthcare environments confirm the importance of incorporating feedback loops in assessment protocols, thus enabling continuous monitoring and adjustment of strategies to address the specific needs of pediatric populations. Integration of such feedback loops encourages a comprehensive appreciation of a child's health, which is essential for timely interventions. As proposed in many studies, overcoming challenges like organizational support and resource deployment is key to the implementation and sustained use of evidence-based practices (Stout et al., 2015). In summary, the integration of evidence across pediatric health assessment and monitoring brings into focus proactiand multidisciplinary practices as imperative for providing optimal outcomes of development. Future initiatives need to be focused on enhancing intervention quality by through continuous training and support to the professionals, along with more investment in community resources. The commitment to continuous enhancement of pediatric assessment techniques will not only enhance individual care practice but also facilitate broader public health initiatives directed toward strengthening resilience in children. Finally, with increasing understanding of the complexities involved in children's health, being child-focused is still key to successful monitoring and intervention programs, on the way forward towards enhanced futures for all children.

Within pediatric monitoring and evaluation, there is a single most important key point that focuses on the creation of a strong framework for ongoing evaluation. These frameworks must be grounded in rigorous needs assessments that identify the local priorities and problems in health care. By focusing on the special needs of pediatric populations, healthcare professionals can align their strategies toward dealing with children's specific needs. Further, constant M&E are imperative to enable timely program adjustment so that they remain responsive and impactful. Institutions can learn from experiences like those of The Merck Vaccine Network in Africa, pointing out that there is a necessity for monitoring projects to attract more partners as well as finances and eventually enhance health outcomes among childrentions (Rinderle et al., 2012). Another essential element includes the integration of family and patient experience in pediatric care assessments. Focused surveys, such as, such as the Child Hospital Consumer Assessment of Healthcare Providers and Systems Survey, are essential in gaining insightful feedback. Based on knowledge of patient and family experiences, health care providers can identify areas needing improvement and achieve successful quality improvement (QI) interventions. Data collected through these methods may allow for the comparison of performance in healthcare institutions at a country level, promoting an environment of responsibility and excellence. Emphasized in the literature is the emphasis on the application of evidence-based approaches in conjunction with qualitative evidence, leading to better patient outcomes, representing evidence of excellent child-centered care (Hays et al., 2020). Lastly, pediatric health program sustainability is based upon a well-planned strategy that extend the initial stages of funding. Effective programs must be made part of the local health systems and leverage existing infrastructure and resources to maximize the maximum impact in the long run. Setting a plan for sustainability at the onset of the program ensures that return on investment in pediatric evaluation and monitoring is sustained in the long run. This approach not only enhances the effectiveness of programs but also ensures that training and initiative-acquired knowledge is not wasted but is applied and utilized in the comEffective case studies demonstrate how frequent communication and supportive supervision can trigger continuous learning and enhancement in pediatric care, ensuring in turn a system-wide commitment to enhancing children's health outcomes (Rinderle et al., 2012).

KEY TERMS FROM THIS CHAPTER

- Adolescents
- Growth hormone deficiency
- Health complications
- Healthcare professionals
- Infancy
- Parents Evaluation of Developmental Status
- Pediatric care
- Pediatric nursing-sensitive outcomes (PNSOs)
- Body mass index (BMI)
- Health assessment
- Health policy
- Human immunodeficiency virus (HIV)
- Language acquisition
- Pediatric assessment
- Pediatric healthcare framework
- Psychosocial assessments

CRITICAL THINKING QUESTIONS

1. **Which of the following is the most reliable indicator of acute illness severity in a child?**
   a. Respiratory rate
   b. Heart rate
   c. Capillary refill time
   d. Blood pressure
2. **At what age should head circumference measurement typically be discontinued in routine pediatric check-ups?**
   a. 6 months
   b. 1 year
   c. 2 years
   d. 3 years
3. **Which growth chart should be used to assess children under 2 years of age?**
   a. WHO growth charts
   b. CDC growth charts
   c. Local school health records
   d. BMI percentile charts
4. **A 4-month-old infant should be expected to:**
   a. Sit without support
   b. Crawl
   c. Hold head steady when upright
   d. Speak two words
5. **Which of the following is NOT a component of the Pediatric Early Warning Score (PEWS)?**
   a. Behavior
   b. Cardiovascular status
   c. Temperature
   d. Respiratory effort

Short Answer Questions

1. Discuss the comprehensive approach to pediatric history-taking and physical examination across different age groups.
2. Explain the principles and components of growth monitoring in children.
3. How are growth charts used, and what are the clinical implications of identifying failure to thrive or growth acceleration?
4. Describe the assessment of developmental milestones in pediatrics. What tools and techniques are used to evaluate motor, cognitive, language, and social development, and how should delays be investigated?
5. What are the guidelines for vital sign monitoring in different pediatric age groups?
6. Discuss the interpretation of abnormal vital signs and their implications in detecting early signs of clinical deterioration.

Answer to Critical Thinking Questions

1. (c); 2. (c); 3. (a); 4. (c); 5. (c)

REFERENCES

1. Accurso, E. C., Adams, S. H., Buckelew, S. M., Cheng, J., et al. (2019). Weight loss and illness severity in adolescents with atypical anorexia nervosa. https://core.ac.uk/download/323083194.pdf (accessed on 16th June 2025).
2. Lurbe, E., Agabiti-Rosei, E., Cruickshank, J. K., Dominiczak, A., Erdine, S., Hirth, A., Invitti, C., Litwin, M., Mancia, G., Pall, D., Rascher, W., Redon, J., Schaefer, F., Seeman, T., Sinha, M., Stabouli, S., Webb, N. J., Wühl, E., & Zanchetti, A. (2016). 2016 European Society of Hypertenst al. (2016). 2016 European Society of Hypertension guidelines for the management of high blood pressure in children and adolescents. https://core.ac.uk/download/46165193.pdf (accessed on 16th June 2025).
3. Dix, L., Fallows, R., & Murphy, G. (2015). Effectiveness of the ADEC as a Level 2 screening test for young children witctiveness of the ADEC as a level 2 screening test for young children with suspected autism spectrum disorders in a clinical setting. https://core.ac.uk/download/30707627.pdf (accessed on 16th June 2025).
4. Akyol, M. U., Alden, T. D., Amartino, H., Ashworth, J., et al. (2019). Recommendations for the management of MPS VI: Systematic evidence- and consensus-based guidance. https://core.ac.uk/download/323074857.pdf (accessed on 16th June 2025).
5. Bagnall, A., Day, R., & Kime, N. H. (2013). Systematic review of transition models for young people with long-term conditions: A report for NHS Diabetes. https://core.ac.uk/download/29018738.pdf (accessed on 16th June 2025).
6. Balfour-Lynn, I. M., Primhak, R. A., & Shaw, B. N. J. (2005). Home oxygen for children: Who, how and when? https://core.ac.uk/download/58952.pdf (accessed on 16th June 2025).
7. Bardid, F., Cogo-Moreira, H., de Almeida Maia, D., Eid, M., et al. (2022). Is motor milestone assessment in infancy valid and scaled equally across sex, birth weight, and gestational age? Findings from the Millennium Cohort Study. https://core.ac.uk/download/511306047.pdf (accessed on 16th June 2025).
8. Batino, M., Fiorini, J., Frigerio, S., Moraca, A., et al. (2024). Pediatric nursing-sensitive outcomes in lower and medium complexity care units: A Delphi study. https://core.ac.uk/download/621339894.pdf (accessed on 16th June 2025).
9. Olusanya, B. O., Ogunlesi, T. A., Kumar, P., Boo, N. Y., Iskander, I. F., de Almeida, M. F., Vaucher, Y. E., & Slusher, T. M. (2., Kumar, P., et al. (2015). Management of late-preterm and term infants with hyperbilirubinaemia in resource-constrained settings. https://core.ac.uk/download/323066114.pdf (accessed on 16th June 2025).
10. Boutelle, K. N., Drahota, A., & Matheson, B. E. (2019). A pilot study investigating the feasibility and acceptability of a parent-only behavioral weight-loss treatment for children with autism spectrum disorder. https://core.ac.uk/download/323308512.pdf (accessed on 16th June 2025).
11. Corsello, G., Mancuso, G., Martorana, C., Montante, C., Notarbartolo, V., Piro, E., Schierz, I. A. M., et al. (2019). Microcephaly and macrocephaly: A study on anthropometric and clinical data from 308 subjects. https://core.ac.uk/download/287859205.pdf (accessed on 16th June 2025).
12. Corvini, Marguerite; Cox, Katherine; O'Neil, Molly; Ryer, Jeanne EdD; and Tutko, Holly Deblois, "Addressing Childhood Adversity aet al. (2018). Addressing childhood adversity and social

determinants in pediatric primary care: Recommendations for New Hampshire. https://core.ac.uk/download/215540986.pdf (accessed on 16th June 2025).

13. Dennis, R. E., Edelman, S. W., & Giangreco, M. F., et al. (1999). Related services for Vermont's students with disabilities. https://core.ac.uk/download/51067326.pdf (accessed on 16th June 2025).

14. Dosenbach, N. U. F., Everett, E. A., Hoyt, C. R., Koller, J., et al. (2019). Detection of pediatric upper extremity motor activity and deficits with accelerometry. https://core.ac.uk/download/287888133.pdf (accessed on 16th June 2025).

15. Honorio Neto, F., Tatlow-Golden, M., Mulligan, A., Gavin, B., & McNicholas, F. (2018). Attitudes and reported practice of paediatricians aAttitudes and reported practice of paediatricians and child psychiatrists regard Ireland. https://core.ac.uk/download/159108018.pdf (accessed on 16th June 2025).

16. Jessica C Kichler, Ashley Moss, Astrida S Kaugars

17. Kaugars, A. S., Kichler, J. C., & ncing health outcomes in youth with type 1 diabetes. US Endocrinology, 2012;8(2):77-83 DOI: http://doi.org/10.17925/USE.2012.08.02.77https://core.ac.uk/download/213084246.pdf (accessed on 16th June 2025).

18. Kenney, G. M., & Pelletier, J. E. (2010). Improving the lives of young children: The role of developmental screenings in Medicaid and CHIP. https://core.ac.uk/download/71347983.pdf (accessed on 16th June 2025).

19. Krissik, T., Ireys, H. T., Markus, A., & Rosenbaum, S. (2008). *Monitoring and assessing the use of exteessing the Use of External Quality Review Organizations to Improve Services for Young Children: A Toolkit for State Medicaid Agencies.*https://core.ac.uk/download/71353308.pdf (accessed on 16th June 2025).

20. R. C. Antonell, & Antonelli, R. (2009). Making care coordination a critical component of the pediatric health system: A multidisciplinary framework. https://core.ac.uk/download/71352885.pdf (accessed on 16th June 2025).

21. McCarthy, D., & Leatherman, S. (2004). *Quality of Health Care for Children and Adolescents: A Chartbook.* https://core.ac.uk/download/71354153.pdf (accessed on 16th June 2025).

22. Perkins, J., & Youdelman, M. (2005). Providing language services in small health care provider settings: Examples from the field. https://core.ac.uk/download/71354088.pdf (accessed on 16th June 2025).

23. Rennie, B. J. (2015). Social impact of traumatic brain injury in adolescents: A mixed methods study with a focus on rural adolescents. https://core.ac.uk/download/267582993.pdf (accessed on 16th June 2025).

24. Quality of Preventive Health Care for Young ChildrenG., Abrams, M. K., Inkelas, M., & Halfon, N. (2005). Quality of preventive health care for young children: Strategies for improvement. https://core.ac.uk/download/71354158.pdf (accessed on 16th June 2025).

25. Stout, J., Patel, S., Larson, E., Goel, M., Burges, D., Rosenfeld, M., Melbye, H., et al. (2015). Abstracts selected for the PCRJ. https://www.semanticscholar.org/paper/69d94b49bfdcf9803e2c3016b2af2a10c9fc0589 (accessed on 16th June 2025).

PEDIATRIC EMERGENCIES AND CRITICAL CARE

6

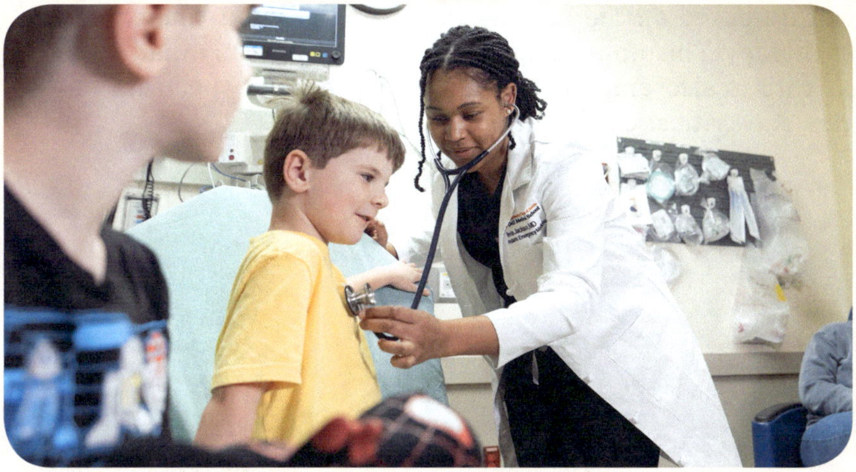

LEARNING OBJECTIVES

After studying this chapter, you will be able to:

1. Enumerate common pediatric emergencies
2. Define assessment and diagnosis
3. Explain the resuscitation techniques
4. Comprehend the management of each condition
5. Define the role of pediatric intensive care units (PICUs)
6. Highlight the ethical aspects of pediatric critical care

INTRODUCTION

The subspecialty of pediatric critical and emergency care is a unique combination of sophisticated medical knowledge and emergency care methods designed to address the unique physiological and developmental needs of children. Children present with a variety of concerns that require specialized approaches, worlds apart from those used in adult emergency care, due to their varying sizes, levels of communication, and stages of development. Understanding the differences between children and adults is imperative to healthcare providers since children may respond differently to disease, injury, and treatment. The requirements for rapidity of pediatric emergencies will serve to compound these problems as conditions grow rapidly and prompt immediate and often definitive action by healthcare providers. Timely response is key in pediatric emergencies, with immediate decision-making having a critical role in determining outcomes. Health care workers not only have to be familiar with specific pediatric diseases, but also possess the requisite skills to perform rapid evaluations and interventions. Such a multi-dimensional strategy includes learning resuscitation skills, familiarity with age-specific medication dosages, and skill at communicating effectively between children and their parents. The subtleties of such emergencies highlight the need for ongoing education and training, emphasizing the importance of technical skill as well as interpersonal communication in providing maximal care to children in extremis. Beyond this, however, the psychological effect of pediatric emergencies extends from the clinical setting to reach families who necessarily find themselves in crisis-like and unaccustomed circumstances. Effective emergency treatment is not merely about meeting a child's initial physical needs, but also providing aid to families during emergency situations. An awareness of the psychological and emotional impacts on caregivers as well as children can help provide an environment for healing and recovery. Therefore, family-centered care practices need to be integrated in pediatric emergency care based on the fact that activation of family members plays a significant role in the process of therapy. This holistic approach ensures not only that care in a medical sense is effective, but that care is also empathetic, addressing the full spectrum of needs that arise in pediatric emergencies and critical care situations (Figure 6.1).

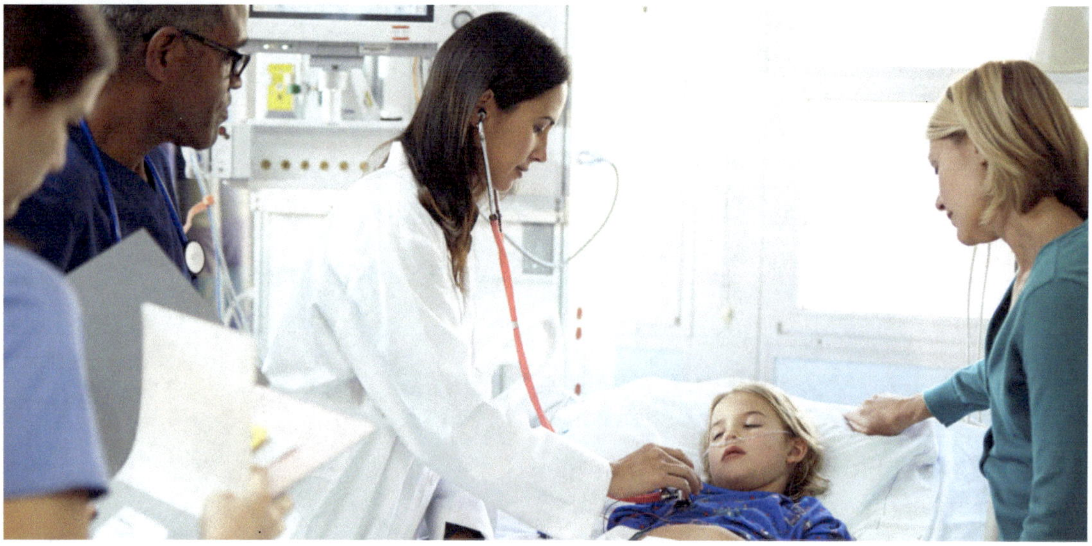

Figure 6.1. Pediatric emergencies and critical care.

Source: https://external-content.duckduckgo.com/iu/?u=https%3A%2F%2Fwww.arnoldpalmerhospital.com%2F-%2Fmedia%2Fimages%2Farnold-palmer-hospital%2Fservices-and-specialties%2Fcritical-care%2Fcriticalcare_465073227.jpg&f=1&nofb=1&ipt=abca01e3f73b9240d0d89b69312da34836e91a661c04ba27f4ce54b7a8a86916&ipo=images.

Definition of Pediatric Emergencies

Pediatric emergencies represent a wide variety of acute medical illnesses that can affect children and adolescents and necessitate immediate intervention and specialist care. Some of these emergencies include respiratory distress, severe infection, trauma, and allergic reaction to life-threatening conditions, to name but a few. The physiological and developmental uniqueness of the pediatric population obliges clinicians to recognize that children's responses to illness will often differ dramatically from those of adults. Therefore, delayed treatment or misdiagnosis can lead to exacerbation. The necessity for urgent classification and treatment of pediatric emergencies is underscored by the need for urgent examination and intervention, since the impact is more severe when children are involved. Consequently, physicians must be adept at identifying and treating such emergencies in order to gain maximum outcomes for children's patients, an integral component of the continuity of pediatric care. In defining pediatric emergencies, one must consider addressing the evolving healthcare environment of challenges that disproportionately impact this group. A key aspect of this definition is the increasing prevalence of specific disorders of health, including among children, hypertension. Current research highlights how the management of long-term conditions can intersect with acute conditions in such a manner as to introduce further complexity into emergency care. For instance, adolescent-like isolated systolic hypertension can result in emergent conditions if not treated immediately, highlighting the necessity for prevention. With the incorporation of scientific breakthroughs and clinical understanding, contemporary guidelines attempt to increase the quality of care for pediatric populations encountered with emergencies by emphasizing the intersection of short-term response procedures with long-term health concerns. The incorporation of such data is imperative to healthcare providers navigating the intricate landscape of pediatric emergency response. Further, the child emergency critical care system requires a comprehensive intervention that covers not only the clinical aspect of care but also systemic factors that can influence the delivery of healthcare. Recent national and state readiness assessments indicate the need for more investment, training, and infrastructure to effectively manage public health emergencies. These are important, as they establish the capacity of health systems to respond quickly in case of emergencies like the H1N1 flu pandemic, which struck disproportionately vulnerable youth populations. An advanced understanding of pediatric emergencies should prompt healthcare policy making to aim for evidence-based interventions for improving care access and response readiness. In so doing, the discussion on pediatric emergencies becomes a situation not only clinical but encompasses broader public health implications, emphasizing the critical intersection of acute cstemic health policy intervention (N/A, 2009; Agabiti-RoseiLurbe et al., 2016).

Imprtance of Critical Care in Pediatrics

The role of pediatrics critical care is of paramount significance, particularions involving emercies that require immediate interferenceintervention. Children patients are distinct from adults due to their physiological composition, developmental phases, and healthcare requirements. Such a group is particularly vulnerable in cases involving health crises; hence, there is a need for critical care units to deal with complex conditions. The ability to be immediately and professionally managed can be of immense value in the resolution of pediatric emergencies. Apart from that, the technological advances in the critical care of children have also promoted improved survival rates of previously incurable conditions, confirming the necessity for specialized centers and trained professionals to manage such emergencies. Preparedness is also achieved in critical care through health practitioners' training and the creation of communication networks. There is evidence to support that systemic education and resource access significantove the preparedness of medical providers to react to cases such as, sac arrest. or instance, Lurbe et al. (2016) (Dahlen et al., 2014) demonstrates that school nurses, who play the focal role in the case of an emergency, testify to varying degrees of preparedness, highlighting the value of standardized training and access to critical resources like AEDs. Besides, open communication and coordination among various health stakeholders may result in an improved response during emergencies. Ongoing education, training, and evaluation of emergency procedures are thus essential in order to ensure that critical care teams are well-equipped and skilled enough to deliver high-quality care. As much as initial response actions are important, the long-term impact of interventi within c careot be overlooked. Pdiatrintensive care is not only saving saves life lives at the moment, but it also entails proper follow-up care that controls the potential long-term effects of disease and therapy. Quality critical care should not only be medical management, but also psychosocial care for the child and the family, focused on the well-being of the child. Also, as indicated through evaluations of pogress in terms of sfederal readiness for public health emergencies, (Lurbe et al., 2016N/A, 2009), there is an ongoing need for improvements in the area of funding and accountability to improve pediatric critical care infrastructures. These include considerations that highlight the worth of critical care in pediatrics as extending to more than short-term medical emergencies, but finding its place in the child's long-term health trajectory to ensure that they receive continued care for optimal recovery (Figure 6.2).

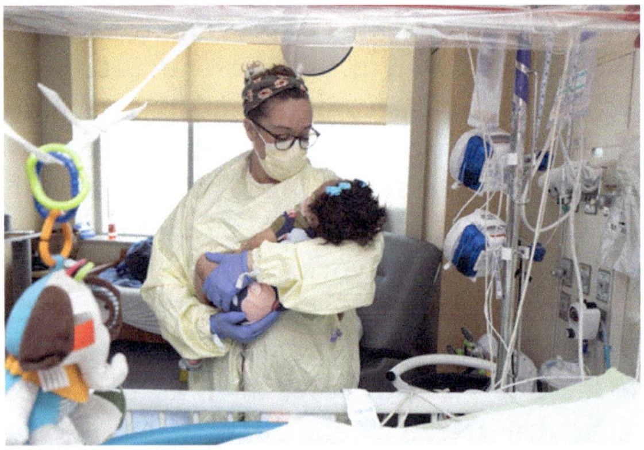

Figure 6.2. The role of critical care in pediatrics.

Source: https://health.ucdavis.edu/media-resources/contenthub/health-library/health-topics/pediatric-critical-care-marquee.jpg.

6.1. Common Pediatric Emergencies

Learning Outcome

1. Respiratory distress and failure
2. Anaphylaxis and allergic reactions
3. Trauma and injury management

Pediatric emergency encompasses a wide variety of health-related emergencies that require immediate medical intervention. Respiratory distress is the most common pediatric emergency, frequently arising in conditions such as asthma attacks and pneumonia. Owing to the unique anatomical and physiological differences between children and adults, respiratory emergencies in children carry a heightened risk of rapid deterioration and require prompt recognition and intervention. For instance, a routine viral illness in a child can suddenly develop into life-threatening respiratory failure. Prompt recognition and treatment of such emergencies are important to prevent long-term morbidity or death. Moreover, the deployment of medical emergency teams (METs) is effective in a dramatic way in such situations because the stabilizes patients and permits critical care intervention when warranted (Alampi et al., 2016Kosoko et al., 2024). Another common pediatric emergency is traumatic injury, often due to a fall, motor vehicle accident, or collision during sports. Children's age of development and high-energy lifestyle make the risk of injury multifaceted. Fractures, concussions, and lacerations are all frequent, and each has its own set of challenges in diagnosis and m. Prompt evaluation by emergency department providers must detect potential complications, such as, such as internal bleeding and neurologic impairment. The psychological impact of trauma on children must also be addressed, as trauma is likely to induce anxiety and long-term emotional issues. Effective communication with pediatric patients and families regarding treatment plans and outcomes is crucial to building a supportive process for these difficult times. Lastly, allergic reactions and anaphylaxis constitute an essential category of pediatric emergencies that need to be addressed immediately. With the increasing prevalence of food allergy among children, knowledge and education about potential causative agents have been more essential than ever. Unexpected anaphylaxis can occur with potentially fatal manifestations of airway obstruction and cardiovascular instability. Immediate epinephrine is still the preferred therapy in such a scenario, and it emphasizes preparation in educators and caregivers. Moreover, the incorporation of emergency protocols in schools and public buildings has the added benefit of enhancing the experience for allergic children, particularly in cases of an emergency. Collaboration between medical practitioners and public forums is important during the planning of environments that concentrate on the welfare and safety of these vulnerable individuals (Garrett et al., 2009).

6.1.1. Respiratory Distress and Failure

Respiratory failure and distress are ominous presentations that are very common in pediatric emergencies and need to be managed promptly and adequately can be a very wide range of etiology for respiratory distress inen, from infectious processes such as, such as pneumonia and bronchiolitis to non-infectious processes such as, such as asthma attack or foreign body aspiration. All of these can lead to impaired airways and impaired gas exchange, eventually leading to respiratory failure. The acuity may manifest as increased work of breathing, alteration in consciousness, or cyanosis, necessitating immediate assessment to determine the urgency and quality of medical intervention to be initiated. An understanding of the pathophysiology is essential for clinicians as it directs the management alternatives and can go a long way toward determining patiet outcomes in emergencies. The treatment of respiratory distress and failure in the pediatric patient is a multi-faceted approach to the individual patient's requirements. First and foremost, airway managemains the primary concern where airway patency should be ensured by providers, typically through maneuvers such as, such as suctioning or intubation. Supplemental oxygen may also be necessary to maintain e levels of oxygen saturation, with more severe presentations potentially necessitating more active therapysuch as, such as mechanical ventilation. Where drug management is called for, bronchodilators or corticosteroids are often of primary significance, particularly in the management of asthma or anaphylaxis. Ongoing monitoring of the patient is necessary at this time to quickly identify any deterioration in the child's condition and to alter therapy accordingly. Thus, optimal coordination among healthcare workers is necessary in order to ensure proper and timely treatment. Furthermore, the education of healthcare professionals in the identification and care for respiratory distress in child patients cannot be emphasized enough. As corroborated in most studies, including those that feature simulation-based training in advanced emergency scenarios, accurate training goes a great distance in providing augmented readiness by clinical staff. Simulation-based practice allows clinicians to hone their practice in the management of acute respiratory presentations while learning teamwork and communication skills in emergency units. This is particularly important in pediatric groups wherein treatment may differ considerably from adult presentations. With the use of low-cost simulation modalities reproducing real events, healthcare personnel can become more competent and assertive, ultimately improving outcomes in high-stakes situations wherein rapid intervention is necessary (Alinier et al., 2018). Also, having a well-trained team with the skills and knecessary to support life-sustaining functions can go a long way in the overall management of pediatric emergencies, such as, such as those due to respiratory distress and failure (Ciomaga et al., 2019) (Figure 6.3).

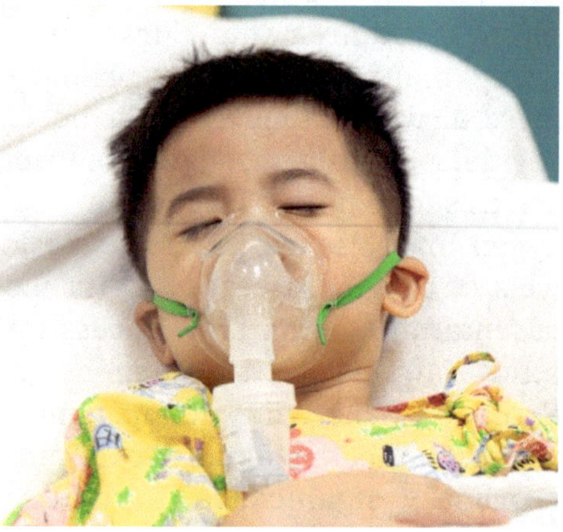

Figure 6.3. Pediatric respiratory distress and failure.

Source: https://external-content.duckduckgo.com/iu/?u=https%3A%2F%2Fson.symphonypreview.com%2Fwp-content%2Fuploads%2F2021%2F12%2Frespiratory-distress-vs-failure.jpg&f=1&nofb=1&ipt=fe093ba46004a5ede2e8f5a06b94f67da08e28b5a3c617b50342fbe5cecdcf08&ipo=images.

6.1.2. Anaphylaxis and Allergic Reactions

Anaphylaxis is a severe, life-threatening allergic reaction that arises soon after the introduction of an recognized allergen. Foods, insect stings, medications, and latex are common causes in children. The presentation of anaphylaxis can be respiratory distress, gastrointestinal upset, cardiovascular collapse, and cutaneous with hives and edema. Rapid recognition and treatment are critical because children may rapidly develop. Epinephrine is the first-choice drug, and its timely administration can be life-saving. Besides this, children who are prone to anaphylaxis also need an epinephrine auto-injector with them and need an action plan, ng importance to awareness among parents and caregivers while adopting preventive measures and prompt intervention on developing the an allergic reaction. Food allergy is a significant issue in the pediatric emergency setting because it can lead to acute presentation of anaphylaxis. The increasing rate of food allergy among children in Western nations, particularly the United States, necessitates proper education and agement of the condition. Consistent with research, food allergies are also predictoccur in 5.6% of mothers and have fluctuated by in prevalence in children, placing increased burdens on healthcare resources (Seitaet al., 2013). The allergies usually manifest psychologically through fear and isolation as children transfer between environments like schools, ere are prevalent food allergens. Health professionals need to collaborate with schools and families to ensure children with food allergy allergies are safe and supported in their activities, taking into account the emotional and social consequences of having an illness with potentially life-threatening consequences. Successful prevention and management of anaphylaxis due to food allergy needs a multidisciplinary team approach. The addition of other allied healthcare professionals contributes to the knowledge and application of measures in preventing accidental exposures. Allergists,pediatricians, nutritionists, and mental health clinicians are some of the stakeholders in this group, each with their respective expertises in characterizing and managing food allergies (Maziarz et al., 2018). Educational interventions for both children and caregivers can empower families with the knowledge to avoid certain allergens and recognize early signs of anaphylaxis. Second, adherence to federal guidelines intended to prevent allergic young people from being accidentally exposed to allergens imposes the system support necessary to ensure successful control. Lastly, a multicomponent model that combines education, clinical management, and psychosocial support can come a great distance toward improving health outcomes in children at risk for anaphylaxis (Figure 6.4).

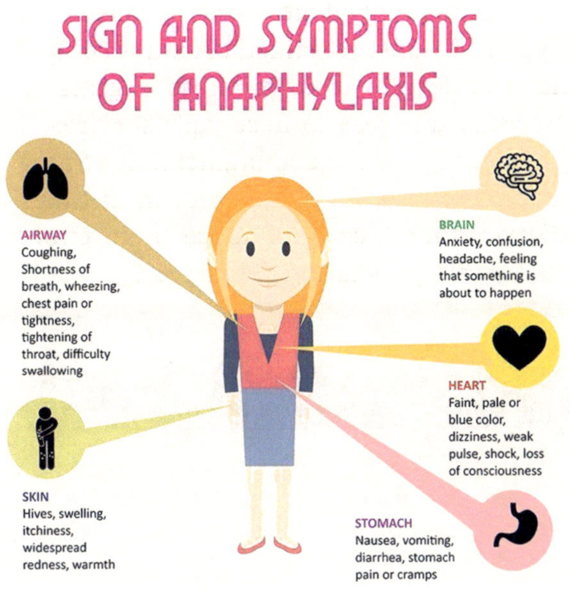

Figure 6.4. Anaphylaxis.

Source: https://external-content.duckduckgo.com/iu/?u=https%3A%2F%2Fcdn.medizzy.com%2FRiMwf_FD8FUB_lV3qTLyY9UCNGM%3D%2F800x800%2Fimg%2Fposts%2F5fbe4fca-1417-4216-be4f-ca1417121614&f=1&nofb=1&ipt=21dc1d2182800419e515de2b445b62f5c67067bb91eceb0d181cddb363d8968c&ipo=images.

6.1.3. Trauma and Injury Management

Effective trauma and injury management in children's emergencies is particularly important due to the unique physiological and anatomical characteristics of children. Children, as opposed to adults, respond uniquely to trauma and require unique assessment and intervention strategies. Emergency medical services need to be responsive to recognizing potentially life-threatening injuries that may be typical froup of children. For example, data from a Danish study reported that approximately one-third of child patients presented severe emergencies which that required instant medical treatment (Bender et al., 2022). This does much to highlight the importance of not only rapid transportation to appropriate medical facilities but also bringing highly advanced out-of-hospital treatments, which play a crucial role in determining the outcomes of younger patients. The spectrum of injury in children is broad, ranging from blunt trauma to severe cases of multi-system injury. For an examination of HEMS missions, 32.2% of hospital diagnoses were attributed to injury, an indication that there is a need for proper triage and effective management of child trauma (Bender et al., 2022). Furthermore, the psychosocial status of trauma must not be ignored; child patients are likely to suffer tremendousonal trauma when under emergency circumstances. Therefore, emergency response teams and medical professionals should have provisions in place which that cater to the bodily and mental needs of young patients in order to facilitate all-around healing.

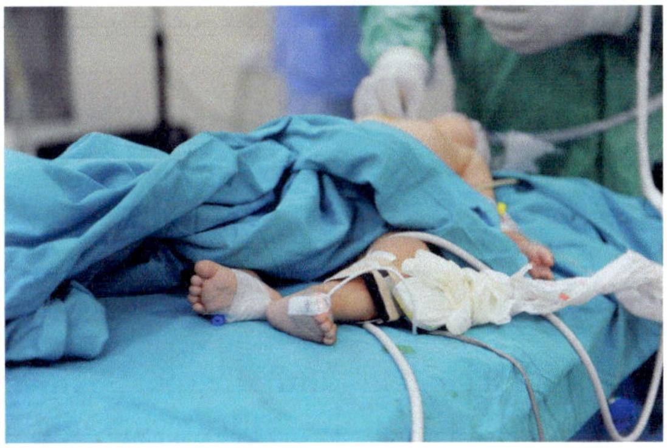

Figure 6.5. Infant undergoing surgery with monitoring and supportive care.

*Source:*https://externalcontent.duckduckgo.com/iu/?u=https%3A%2F%2Fwww.nurse.com%2Fmedia%2Fcatalog%2Fproduct%2Fr%2Fe%2Frel-acu-0-mptp2_coverimage.jpg&f=1&nofb=1&ipt=ce565cd01c919dd3803e73b59a26b1d3d0ca5d974545c746bcaf510a41d176e1&ipo=images.

This all-round approach guaraner outcomes and may even avert eng trauma effects. One of the emerging challenges in trauma management is the impact of external stimuli, such as, such as the COVID-19 pandemic, that which has changed patient behavior and healthcare routines. Research indicates that while dental trauma consultations reduced during the pandemic period, the volume and type of trauma remained constant compared to pre-pandemic periods. Such an observation means that despite disruptions to routine care, pediatric trauma care must transform to ensure uninterrupted access to necessary services. The pandemic has also highlighted the importance of implementing robust communication strategies between the family and healthcare providere timely access to care for children even in times of crisis. It is essential to comprehend the levels of pediatric trauma care influence in an effort to improve management protocols and results for this vulnerable population (Figure 6.5).

Test Your Knowledge

1. What are the main causes and signs of respiratory distress and failure in children?
2. How should anaphylaxis and severe allergic reactions be recognized and managed in pediatric patients?
3. What are the key steps in assessing and managing trauma and injuries in children during emergencies?

6.2. Assessment and Diagnosis

Learning Outcome

1. Pediatric assessment triangle
2. Importance of history taking
3. Diagnostic tools and techniques

Effective assessment and diagnosis in the pediatric emergency are critical components of delivering positive outcomes in the acute care setting. Children can present with a multitude of symptoms that are distinctly different from those of adults, so there are specialized approaches needed for the evaluation. The initial evaluation is typically preceded by a detailed process of history-taking, including information about the child's history of prior medical problems, presenting complaint, and pertinent environmental factors. Clinicians need to possess the ability to recognize distress cues that may portend serious underlying disease. As examples, acute respiratory shortness of breath or dehydration findings can be harbingers of respiratory or gastrointestinal emergencies, respectively. One's role cannot be overemphasized for Point-of-Care Ultrasonography (POCUS) in optimizing diagnostic precision, as this modality allows timely decision-making that can have a huge influence on management and outcome of the patient (Tamimi et al., 2023). Furthermore, the integration of evidence-based clinical algorithms for the early recognition of pediatric emergencies is crucial. This entails the education of health professionals to employ formalized assessment tools and clinical pathh current best practice. In low-resource settings, generalist clinicians are often the first response in pediatric health, and thus it is important that theythey must possess the skills and knowledge required to stabilize critically ill children. A curriculum to develop the skill sets of such generalist practitioners focuses on the detection and treatment of multiple conditions. An emphasis on gastrointestinal emergencie bowel obstruction and gastroenteritis reflects the importance of integraed learning in develoing diagnostic competencies and practice preparedness (GeniscaKosoko et al., 2024). Such learning can improve not only knowledge recall, but also hard skills, and thus make the healthcare workforce more competent. Lastly, the process of pediatric emergency diagnosis and assessment is an illustration of synergy among educational interventions, clinical acumen, and technological advancement. Use of POCUS has proven to be highly effective in many emergency environments to allow clinicians to make confident, timely decisions that alter patient outcomes for the better. As technology advances, continuous education of health care professionals via current diagnostic methods and instrumentation is at the forefront. With an emphasis on training that integrates POCUS into practical pediatric emergency practice comes the ability to drive the transition toward better patient outcomes. Complemented by structured educational curricula, this process serves to prepare clinicians for the demands of pediatric emergencies, justifying the necessity for continued learning and accommodation is sensitive field (Tamimi et al., 2023).

6.2.1. Pediatric Assessment Triangle (PAT)

The PAT is an important tool in the clinicians' hands in pediatric emergencyemergencies. The structured approach enables the clinicians to efficiently observe and assess the clinical status of children during an emergency quickly. The PAT encompasses three key areas: appearance, work of breathing, and circulation to the skin. They offer indispensable insight into the child's health status. By evaluating such factors, medical personnel are able to quickly detect potentially life-threatening disorders and administer appropriate interventions. As documented in recent assessments conducted in various clinical settings, improved understanding of the PAT not only supports identification of risky illnesses but also leads to improved utilization of resources and patient care procedures in emergency rooms (Houten et al., 2018). Full appreciation for the Pediatric Assessment Triangle also highlights the necessity for continuous training within the clinical setting. Since many hospitals have expressed a requirement for increased preparedness to recognize clinical deterioration, focused training can contribute to clinical decision-making in a considerable manner. For instance, simulation training on the PAT equips health practitioners with the knowledge of how to properly interpret signs and respond appropriately in pediatric emergencies. Studies show that when emergency dent staff are trained on the aspects of the PAT, patient outcomes tend to be better, suggesting that training programs of this kind are essential (Clancy-Burgesset al., 2024). As a result, adding simulation-based education on the PAT can not only increase confidence among nurses but ultimately serve pediatric patients by enabling theive timely and effective care.

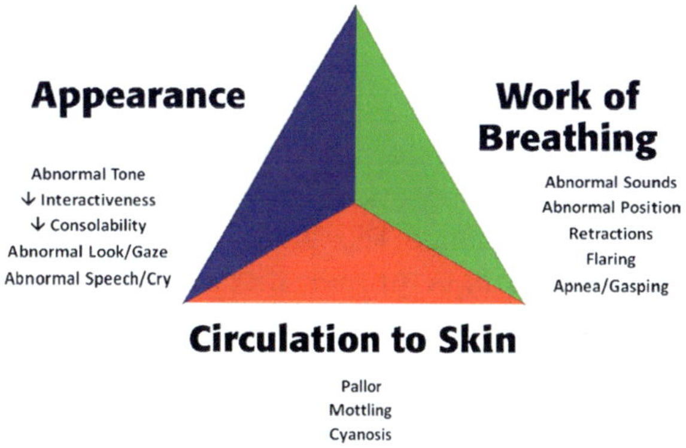

Figure 6.6. Pediatric assessment triangle (PAT).

Source: https://external-content.duckduckgo.com/iu/?u=https%3A%2F%2Fels-jbs-prod-cdn.jbs.elsevierhealth.com%2Fcms%2Fattachment%2F8599c63f-1ce1-4636-90f7-814e6f01932a%2Fgr1_lrg.jpg&f=1&nofb=1&ipt=65f97d9c3e4e895cb4c98d08724ad586f040cd2c8494ff96a9f2cef3a8b70947&ipo=images.

Moreover, the ability to rapidly implement the Pediatric Assessment Triangle can revolutionize the care of symptomatic children, such as, such as respiratory distress or shock. For instance, assessing work of breathing, by observing respiratory effort and breathing patterns, allows clinicians to detect mild and severe respiratory distress. Such a triage role is crucial, particularly in acute settings where timeliness is essential. By combining the results from the PAT, the clinicians can provide appropriate interventions at the right time, achieving optimal resource utilization and patient health outcomes. Training courses focusing on how to use the PAT are therefore essential and e backbone of pediatric emergency training and eventually enhance the quality of critical care provided to vulnerable children (Houten et al., 2018; Clancy-Burgesset al., 2024) (Figure 6.6).

6.2.2. Importance of History Taking

Good history taking is a cornerstone in pediatric emergencies and critical care, and it enhances the diagnostic process and facilitates the selection of appropriate treatment strategies.. A comprehensive medical history taken allows practitioners to ascertain underlying illnesses, previous illnesses, and family medical history that can influence the status of the child's current health. A proper history can enable clinicians to recognize possible patterns of emergencies, which is crucial, particularly with the higher speed of pediatric illnesses. For instance, awareness of a child's history of asthma or allergic reaction can decide emergency procedures and management. Furthermore, parents or guardians often provide important information that might nily be seen or understood by clinicians, enhancing patient care generally in such emergencies. The necessity for taking history is shown in life-threatening conditions such as, such as sudden cardiac arrest (SCA) in children, in which time is of the essence. School nurses are revealed to be important in this scenario by being prepared to manage SCA-emergency scenarios immediately. Literature review shows that despite some limitations concerning budget and equipment, school nurses feel some level of preparedness to manage SCA events. This preparedness is commonly facilitated by the ability to elicit a child's past medical history, especially through history taking, which can inform the urgency and type of intervention required. Proper communication and proper history taking not only facilitate an organized response plan but also enable risk factors to be established which necessitate untervention. Further, history taking is important not only for emergency care but also for post-emergency preparedness and public health interventions. In times of crisis such as, such as the H1N1 flu outbreak, state and hospital indicators of readiness that have a direct impact on effective history taking are directly linked. n previous medical cases can be reviewed by healthcare professionals to better plan public health interventions and allocate resources accordingly. Continuing enhancemestory history-taking practices can lead to more accountability and funding in health systems, and therefore may contribute to the foundation of emergency care. Overall, good history history-taking practices facilitate both immediate response and longer-term public health preparedness, making it a cri element in pediatric emergencies and critical care.

6.2.3. Diagnostic Tools and Techniques

In pediatric critical care and emergency, effective diagnostic agents and methods are most essential in ordave early and accurate evaluations. Pediatric patients tend to have unique challenges e to their ge, and stage of life that need unique approaches. New imaging technologies such as, such as ultrasound and computed tomography (CT), play essential roles in evaluating a conditions such as, such as appendicitis or trauma. These devices allow for quick imaging of the inner structures, shortening therapy delays. Moreover, their use of point-of-care testing, including quick blood tests, makes clinicians even faster at obtaining essential information, allowing instant decision and intervention. These diagnostic technologies simplify the process of care in emergency situations, ultimately leading to improved patient outcomes because life-threatening problems are addressed more efficiently than would otherwise occur. With the rapid development of healthcare, telemedicine use in pediatric emergencies is transforming the way diagnostics are handled, particularly in remote or disadvantaged areas. Telemedicine allows physicians to check patients with digital tools, enabling real-time consultation for emergencies without physical visits. This is especially crpediatrics, where timely assessment can make a huge difference in health outcomes. Through the implementation of telehealth models, providers can leverage multiple diagnostic techniques, such as, such as virtual consultations and examinations, to determine the urgency of cases and guide local treatment practices. Additionally, the incorporation of technology within these procedures helps to cover gaps in care so that continuous monitoring and prompt interventions that are essential in emergent cases become feasible. By the inclusion of a multi-disciplinary team, including pediatricians and emergency specialists, the diagnostic process is maximized, and thorough care is assured. In the field of pediatrics, incorporating psychological assessments as part of diagnostic procedures canverlooked, particularly when it comes to dental anxiety (DA) and its impact on emergency cases. As cited in studies, knowledge about a child's psychological profile plays a critical role towards in appropriate manage critical care areas. Treatment of DA entails a holistic approach with the necessity to assess the underlying conditions, provision of effective communication, and utilization of techniques such as, such as iatrosedation and hypnosis, along with drug therapy. Placed within pediatric emergency, such psychological assessments have a double role: they improve immediate care by mitigating anxiety and finally contribute to long-term management of patients by promoting trust among healthcare staff. Thus, an integrated outlook with both physical and psychological diagnostic tools is needed in order to enhance the quality of children's emergency care as a whole, leading to enhanced short-term and long-term health outcomes (Figure 6.7).

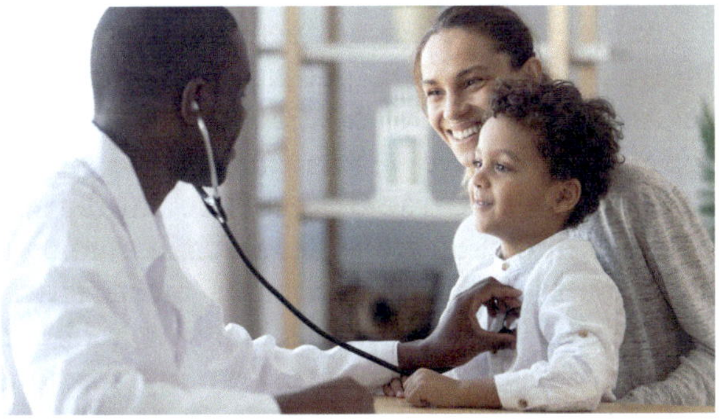

Figure 6.7. Diagnostic tools and techniques.

Source: https://www.toplinemd.com/ana-hpmd/wp-content/uploads/sites/7/2020/10/What-Kind-of-Equipment-Do-Pediatricians-Use.jpg.

Test Your Knowledge

1. What components make up the Pediatric Assessment Triangle, and how is it used in emergency evaluation?
2. Why is thorough history taking important in diagnosing pediatric emergency conditions?
3. Which diagnostic tools and techniques are commonly used to assess critically ill or injured children?

6.3. Resuscitation Techniques

Learning Outcome

1. Basic life support (BLS) for children
2. Advanced cardiac life support (ACLS) protocols
3. Pediatric-specific considerations in resuscitation

Successful resuscitation techniques in pediatric emergencies are the determinants of improving outcomes for critically ill children. The ever-changing nature of pediatric emergencies necessitates comprehensive knowledge of various resuscitative techniques modified according to the unique physiological needs of infants and children. Key areas in pediatric resuscitation include recognition of cardiopulmonary arrest signs, appropriate algorithms of advanced life support, and rapid sequence intubation as and when indicated. Research has shown that simulation-based training is most critical in preparing health professionals to respond adequately to the situation. Training sessions that include careful practice on resuscitation procedures have been shown to unveil profound enhancements in the readiness of medical practitioners, hence a direct relation to better patient care outcomes in emergencies (Brancati et al., 2003). The application of formal curricula in training has worked to advance the comfort and competency of the health professionals when it comes to pediatric resuscitation. For example, a recy evaluated the impact of an intense six-hour pediatric resuscitation curriculum and reported spectacula in confidence levels among resident physicians for different resuscitation skill domains. Prior toBefore training, the majority of residents reported difficulty with performing life-critical activities such as, such as cardioversion and drug administration for intubation. After training, more than 80% reported comfort level with self-assessment, demonstrating the role of targeted pedagogic interventions. Such training not only equips medical personnel with the requisite skills but also inculcates a culture of preparedness, making them better able to deal with pediatric emergencies (Brancati et al., 2003).er, the setting for resuscitation techniques is regularly evolving in accordance with advances in simulation technology. The development of sophisticated simulations, particularly in high-risk situations such as, such as ECMO, further enhances the learning process for clinicians. By mimicking real-world situations in some degree of realism, these simulations habituate healthcare professionals to the complexity they are likely to be confronted with in the context of critical care situations. Emerging new technologies include ECMO simulators that mimic circuit variation and potential complications with high fidelity, offering an even more realistic learning environment. These developments ensure that clinicians not only acquire theoretical education but are also subjected to practical, first-hand experience, ultimately bridging the gap between simulated environments and real patient care (Figure 6.8).

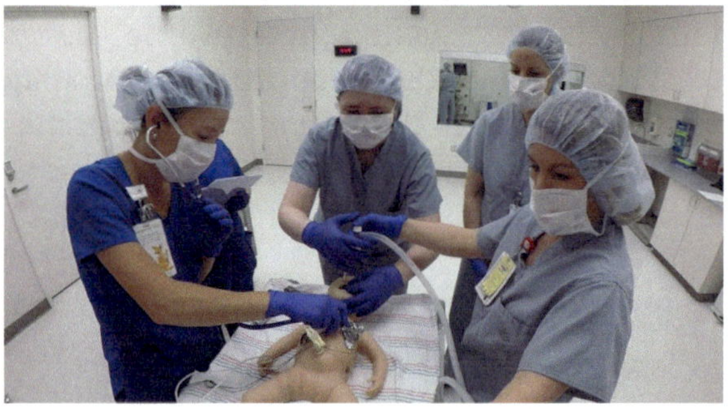

Figure 6.8. Pediatric resuscitation techniques.

Source: https://external-content.duckduckgo.com/iu/?u=https%3A%2F%2Fi.ytimg.com%2Fvi%2FC1yh-1N3A3Q%2Fmaxresdefault.jpg&f=1&nofb=1&ipt=ed895f59f0bdf2a7c69e40baec5fbb406be2f993f764387e7ff465460b50b804&ipo=images.

6.3.1. Basic Life Support (BLS) for Children

BLS for children is an important intervention in pediatric emergencies that fills the time between the triggering of a medical em and definitive medical intervention. The skill that is needed to perform an effective BLS involves identification of cardiac and respiratory arrest and administration of early and appropriate interventions such as, such as chest compressions and rescue breathing. Interestingly, anatomy and physiology in children are unlike that of adults and demand age-related procedures and modifications in resuscitation efforts. For instance, depth and rate of compressions in children are adjusted so that they become useful without causing harm. BLS training equips the caregivers, healthcare providers, and bystanders with the knowledge and confidence required to respond suitably in cases of emergencies, which ultimately increases the survival rate among child patients. Such education has an emphasis on the necessity of continuous education, particularly for medical professionals, to generate preparedness and competency. The use of formal BLS training curricula is necessary to enhance the competence of health professionals in pediatric critical care settings. A pediatric resuscitation curriculum study showed that resident physicians comfort levels with pediatric resuscitation activities significantly improved following program completion (Brancati et al., 2003). This course brings out the significance of not just clinical information but also of procedural skills, which are crucial in real-life emergency settings. Effective BLS in pediatric patients entails accurate technique, including the use of the appropriate compression-to-ventilation ratio and the administration of airway adjuncts if required. Additionally, skills like intraosseous access for the administration of drugs are brought out, indicating that one must be proficient in pediatric-specific interventions. Developing a strong BLS foundation not only enhances the confidence of individual providers but also supports a readiness culture within healthcare settings. Additionally, preparedness for pediatric emergencies extends beyond individual proficiency to encompass systemic frameworks and equipment within healthcare settings. Emergencdness progress is measured through assessment of different components, including state and federal public health program funding and population-level hospital preparedness to respond to emergencies effectively (N/A, 2009Lurbe et al., 2016). With the evolving nature of health threats, whether pandemics or natural catastrophes, integrating BLS into broader emergency response planning is essential. This integrated approach not only equips healthcare professionals with BLS techniques but also empowers them to work within interprofessional teams during emergency conditions. By fostering a cooperative environment founded upon pediatric practice, healthcare organizations are well-positioned to cope with the complexities of pediatric emergencies so that short- and long-term outcomes become optimized for critically ill children who come into contact with life-threatening events (Figure 6.9).

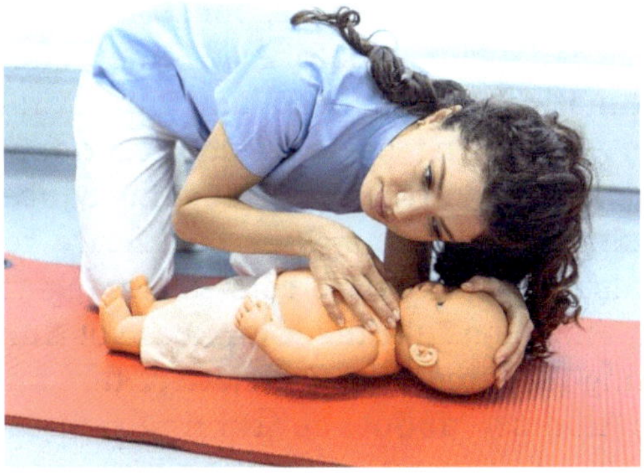

Figure 6.9. Basic life support (BLS) for children serves as a critical intervention in pediatric emergencies.

Source: https://cprcenterofhouston.com/wp-content/uploads/2024/05/Pediatric-Basic-Life-Support-BLS-Certification-feature-image.jpg.

6.3.2. Advanced Cardiac Life Support (ACLS) Protocols

ACLS guidelines play a critical role in the management of pediatric emergencies where timely intervention can significantly alter outcomes. The employment of ACLS in pediatric patients is more than just implementing adult guidelines; it involves recognizing the unique physiological responses and child-related features. Pediatric patients are much different from adults in terms of anatomy, physiology, and common pathologies presented as cardiac arrest. Accordingly, ACLS guidelines are modified to accommodate these differences through age-related drug dosing and resuscitation method guidelines. This difference underscores the need to train medical practitioners in ACLS pediatric-specific practices so they can administer effective emergency intervention during critical situations. Proper application of ACLS guidelines is not only a matter of technical skills but also of effective teamwork and communication among medical practitioners. The dynamic pediatric emergency process often involves miplinary teams like doctors, nurses, and paramedics. Each of the members has an important role to ensure protocols are put into action quickly and effectively. Clearly established roles and responsibilities must be defined prior tobefore an emergency so coordination is enhanced and opportunities for errors during pressurized situations can be minimized. Furthermore, ongoing education and simulation training for healthcare teams can also play a crucial role in honing these skillrganizations like the Iowa Board of Nursing creating resources like newsletters that inform practitioners about continuing education courses, board meetin emerging best practices in pediatric care (Lurbe et al., 2016N/A, 2015). Implementation of advanced technologies in ACLS protocols is also vital, particularly while responding to pediatric emergencies. Advanced technologies such as, such as automated external defibrillators (AEDs), are also being developed in child sizes so that they can safely be applied during emergencies with pediatric patients. Moreover, implementation of telemetry and real-time monitoring of data allows clinicians to assess the effectiveness of interventions almost instantaneously. Such technology does not only enhance the effectiveness of resuscitation procedures but also overall outcomes under emergency interventions. Since pedi being continually developed, practitioners need to stay up to date with developments in ACLS guidelines through ongoing professional development initiatives and resources provided by nursing organizations (Lurbe et al., 2016N/A, 2017) (Figure 6.10).

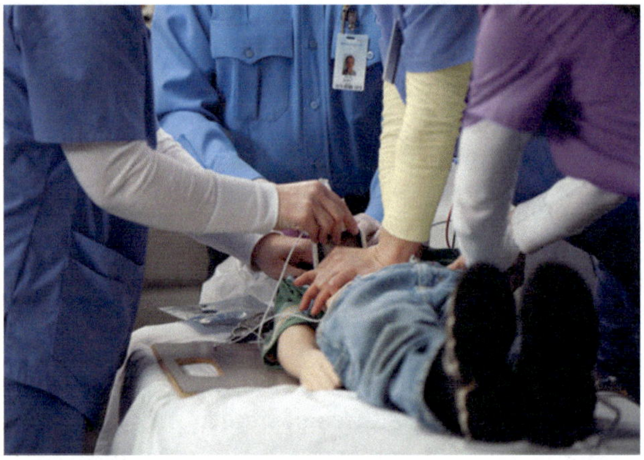

Figure 6.10. Medical team performing emergency care on a pediatric patient.

Source: https://external-content.duckduckgo.com/iu/?u=https%3A%2F%2Fcpr.heart.org%2F-%2Fmedia%2FCPR-Images%2FCourses-and-Kits%2FHeartsaver%2Fteam_triage_child.jpg&f=1&nofb=1&ipt=35bcd2cf61d08a2146e6a845f9f4d4c9da4424e5fa287a022243f89c769a0449&ipo=images.

6.3.3. Pediatric-specific Considerations in Resuscitation

Identification of the specific anatomical and physiological differences between children and adults is critical in pediatric resuscitation since they necessitate special modalities under life-threatening conditions. Pediatric patients, for instance, have different cardiovascular responses whereby they depend on heart rate as opposed to blood pressure in maintaining circulation. Additionally, the pediatric airway is more compliant and is at higher risk of being obstructed by size and anatomical factors. These areas emphasize the importance of higher-level training of healthcare professionals working with child emergencies. The inclusion of rigorous pediatric resuscitation educational programs, as demonstrated by a study assessing the enhancement of resident physicians' comfort levels, can be very effective in enhancing the proficiency of medical professionals in handling such life-threatening situations (Brancati et al., 2003). This curriculum focused on key skills like conducting drug dosing and cardioversion, which are pivotal in successful pediatric emergency care. Medical Emergency Teams (METs) changed the face of acute pediatric care wir quick and specialized interventions in pediatric crises. Involvement of METs not only improves the early management of pediatric crises but also addresses the ethical concerns generally encountered in critical situations. Issues such as, such as end-of-life care choice and patient transfer to intensive care units are more acute among pediatric patients, in whom physicians must reconcile parental pressure with what is medicallld. Surveys among intensivists illustrate the seriousness of the ethical challenges that arise among children in urgent situations, compelling the need for an overt paradigm reconciling medical necessity and compassion (Alampiet al., 2016Kosoko et al., 2024). This dual emphasis on clinical efficacy and ethical concern results in the ultimate goals of pediatric resuscitation as a whole: stabilizing young patients with regard to their unique family dynamics and personal situations. Moreover, ongoing education and competency testing of health professionals on pediatric-specific resuscitative techniques are essential. The rise in levels of confidence among residents identified following systematized training indicates that effectively planned learning approaches can bridge the knowledge gap in pediatric resuscitation cases (Brancati et al., 2003). Standardization of training programs facilitates the implementation of a standardized approach to managing pediatric emergencies, hhancing the quality of care offered to this vulnerable population. Because pediatric emergencies are often complicated conditions in which accuracy and speed are paramount, investment in continuous professional development not only excels equips healthcare professionals with the pertinent expertise but also promotes teamwork as part of a multidisciplinary team ethos. In conclusion, resolution of the special clinical challenges and ethical dilemmas in pediatric resuscitation calls for a balanced solution that is centered on education, team working, and patient-centered care respect.

Test Your Knowledge

1. What are the key steps involved in performing Basic Life Support (BLS) for children?
2. How do Advanced Cardiac Life Support (ACLS) protocols guide the management of pediatric cardiac emergencies?

6.4. Management of Specific Conditions

Learning Outcome

1. Asthma exacerbations
2. Sepsis in children
3. Diabetic emergencies

Among childhood emergencies, the treatment of some medical conditions needs to be holistic and well-informed. An essential part is the detection of preventable or non-emergency conditions that typically prompt families to look for emergency services. According to recent research, most children appear within emergency departments for issues that can actually be treated satisfactorily at primary care facilities, thus creating concerns about the efficiency and allocation of healthcare. The implications of these patterns of use are widespread, including clogging up emergency rooms and placing financial strain on hospital resources. These processes need to be understood so effective measures can be set up that promote priority in correct care pathways, eliminating unnecessary use in the emergency room and ensuring that vital resources are still available for acute needs (DeLia et al., 2009). Pediatric emergency readiness also rests upon systemic preparedness to respond to health emergencies. An example is measuring state and federal readiness to address public health emergencies, for instance, the H1N1 flu pandemic. Reviewing 10 main indicators of readiness indicates increases in funding and accountability but also notable areas where gaps exist. These are important to the quality of care in emergencies, including the treatment of some pediatric conditions. Accordingly, it is vital to meet these deficits in order to establish a sound healthcare system that can respond effectively to pediatric emergencies and ultimately improve patient outcomes (N/A, 2009). Lastly, pediatric emergency management is effective when it is based on a specific approach that can address the specific physiological and developmental demands of children. This practice involves the use of evidence-based protocols that inform clinicians on how to manage individual conditions, from acute asthma attacks to full-blown allergic reactions. Given that children are more likely to report differently than adults, their healthcare providers must be educated to recognize these differences and institute age-appropriate interventions early. Herein, interprofessional communication between pediatricians, nurses, and emergency medical personnel is essential in order to create a continuity of care. Through fostering cooperation and interchange between disciplines, healthcaretems can manage specific pediatric disorders in such a way as to maximize timely and effective emergency intervention while reducing inappropriate use of resources within the pediatric emergency treatment environment (Figure 6.11).

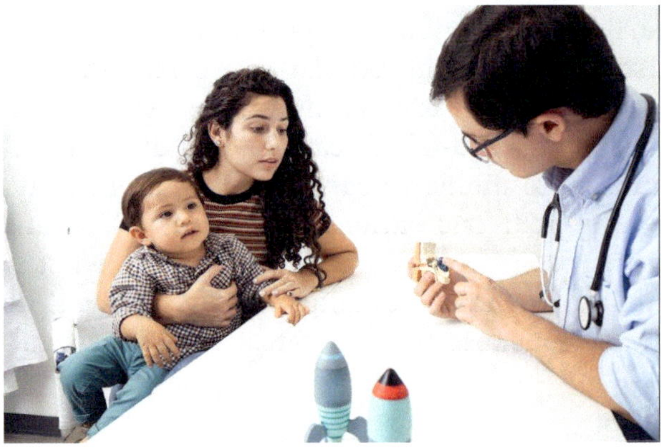

Figure 6.11. ThemManaging specific medical conditions necessitates a comprehensive and nuanced approach.

Source: https://max-website20-images.s3.ap-south-1.amazonaws.com/Pediatric_Diseases_412272b958.jpg.

6.4.1. Asthma Exacerbations

Asthma exacerbations represent a major pediatric emergency, as they can rapidly progress to life-threatening respiratory distress and frequently necessitate hospitalization. Common triggers include allergens, respiratory infections, and abrupt weather changes. During an exacerbation, airway inflammation, edema, and obstruction significantly impair ventilation in children. The high prevalence of pediatric asthma underscores the importance of early diagnosis and timely initiation of treatment. Evidence demonstrates that caregiver education and proper inhalation technique substantially improve long-term disease control, reducing both the frequency and severity of exacerbations.. A study indicates that before educational intervention, 39.4% of children were inappropriately using inhalation techniques, which greatly increased to 62.1% after intervention, supporting the key role of health education in managing this chronic illness (Alijarde-Lorente et al., 2022). In an emergency department setting, asthma exacerbation needs a systematized process to ensure patient safety and effective treatment. A recent series of studies has shown the need for specialized training among health workers in treating pediatric respiratory emergencies, including asthma. Introduction of a new curriculum on pediatric asthma management at Karl Heusner Memorial Hospital Authority, Belize, achieved noticeable clinical benefits, which were defined by improved response time terol administration among trained physicians. The study pinpoints the importance of ongoing education and structured interventions in the emergency room since early treatment with efficient medication is crucial in the prevention of exacerbation severity (GeniscaKosoko et al., 2022). This training impacts not only the case of the individual but also hospital admission as a whole, thereby expressing the significance of best practices in emergency care. Finally, the management of asthma exacerbations in children must be an integrated process that includes both short-term medical care and longer-term management. Integrating both patient and provider education programs can encourage improved health outcomes and maybe reduce the overall burden of asthma-related emergencies. Caregivers must be sensitive to the warning signs of an impending exacerbation and do everything in their power to avoid triggers, establishing a healthy environment in which children will thrive. Formal protocols and guidelines also provide for standardized care within various health care settings and that medical penel have the skills needed to manage acute asthma attacks effectively. Continuing education, training, and clinical excellence will be a part of enhancing the care provided to children with asthma exacerbations (Alijarde-Lorente et al., 2022; GeniscaKosoko et al., 20222024) (Figure 6.12).

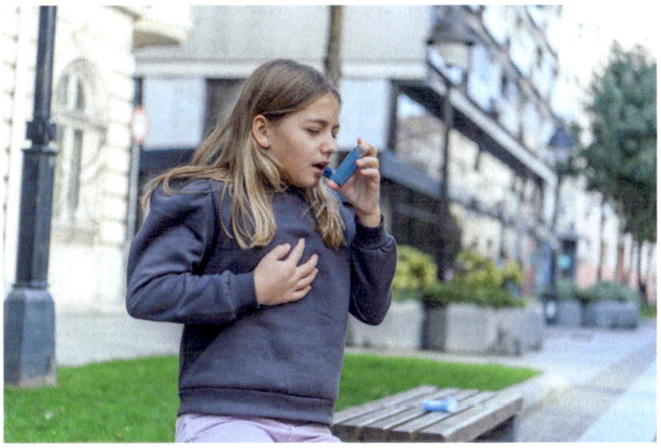

Figure 6.12. Child using an inhaler during an asthma episode outdoors.

Source: https://external-content.duckduckgo.com/iu/?u=https%3A%2F%2Fwww.pulmonologyadvisor.com%2Fwp-content%2Fuploads%2Fsites%2F21%2F2022%2F09%2FChild.Asthma_G_1310226975.jpg&f=1&nofb=1&ipt=0de8bba20db6c9f65b4aaf74e35835ce4473f8b2dd37446fb7c65a78912f8202&ipo=images.

6.4.2. Sepsis in Children

Sepsis in children is a critical public health problem, particularly in resource-poor countries where preventable death among children is still prevalent. Sepsis is characterized by inflammation of the whole body as a result of infection with possible accelerated progression into multi-organ failure and therefore early diagnosis and treatment are very important. Sepsis was identified in Nigeria as the leading cause of mortality among children in hospital-based research with a case fatality rate of 12.6%. Spookily enough, most of the deaths occurred in children under five years of age, which indicates the vulnerability of children in this age bracket to severe infectious diseases. The study highlights that delayed presentation in health facilities exacerbates consequences, and mortality increases as patients present later in their illness course. This requires heightened vigilance and educational practice among communities towards the provision of early medical care for child diseases, particularly for sepsis indicators (Carrol et al., 2014). The use of Pediatric Early Warning systems (PEWs) in clinical practice has been promising towards improved outcome among children who are at risk of sepsis. PEWs have been developed to aid early detection of deteriorating patients, thereby enhancing clinical responses prior to the development of complications. Evidence from a tertiary pediatric hospital revealed that utilization of PEWs resulted in decreased morbidity, as evidenced by decreased pediatric index of mortality (PIM2) scores after implementation. Specific improvement noted included fewer children requiring invasive ventilation and fewer days spent in the pediatric intensive care unit (PICU). These results suggest that early intervention and systematic observation reduce the severity of sepsis and minimize the risk of mortality in vulnerable pediatric populations, once more emphasizing the need for systematic approaches within pediatric emergency and intensive care settings (Carrol et al., 2014). Moreover, the treatment of sepsis in children also demands an integrated approach that includes not only therapeutic actions but also sweeping public health initiatives. Evidence indicates that early detection and treatment are reliant upon robust health systems capable of rapid response as well as effective allocation of resources. Through the reinforcement of sepsis signs and symptoms education at the community level, healthcare providers can encourage timely medical care, which makes a significant difference in death rates. Ongoing tracking of emergency department admissions and outcomes also provides critical information that can inform clinical best practice and allocation of resources. Considering the profound prevalence of sepsis and its accompanying complications, concerted action in both hospital care systems and community outreach is required for improving pediatric health outcomes, especially in resource-poor settings (Ndukwu et al., 2015) (Figure 6.13).

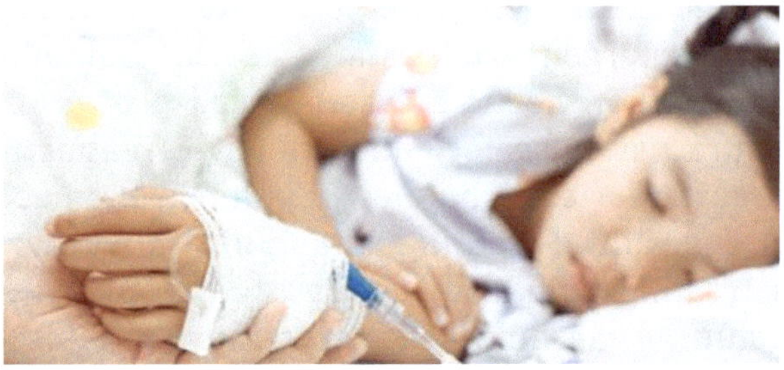

Figure 6.13. Child receiving intravenous treatment while resting in a hospital bed.

Source: https://external-content.duckduckgo.com/iu/?u=https%3A%2F%2Ftse4.mm.bing.net%2Fth%3Fid%3DOIP.iHqCsq-gX3KDAYP6A77WTgHaDd%26pid%3DApi&f=1&ipt=65ba6f096b07febbec896a5ef623f7f3c1840c8f5ac3f2251338041eec717d38&ipo=images.

6.4.3. Diabetic Emergencies

Diabetic emergencies present some challenging conditions in pediatric practice that must be handled immediately and correctly. DKA and severe hypoglycemia are two of the most dangerous emergencies among diabetic emergencies that may lead to severe morbidity. DKA results from a deficiency of insulin, producing ketones and thus a metabolic acidosis. Nausea and vomiting, abdominal discomfort, and altered mental state are some of the conditions that may be presented by children. The consequences of untreated acute DKA are devastating, with risk of cerebral edema, multi-organ failure, and death. Hence, prompt identification followed by immediate medical intervention is paramount in order to prevent the acute life-threatening condition from worsening and highlights the need for ongoing family and medical practitioner educatearly identification of DKA. In addition, hypoglycemicondition that has to be handled immediately by children with diabetes, especially T1DM. These include factors of an excess of insulin, skipping meals, or too much exercise. The symptoms range from mild signs such as, such as shakiness and irritability to severe signs such as, such as seizure and loss of consciousness. One recent study has shown that 75.4% of school staff possess adequate general knowledge about diabetes, but there are none who can manage hypoglycemic incidents adequately in schools (Duraywish et al., 2017). This indicates a need for comprehensive diabetes education programs for parents and school with hypoglycemia and enhance overall management of diabetic children's care during school hours. Because of the prevalence of childhood diabetes, particularly in schools, there is a need to establish supportive infrastructures that manage such emergencies in a systematic waysystematically manage such emergencies. Schools are pivotal in diabetes care among children, and the lack of professionals can lead to dangerous outcomes if there are medical emergencies. Only 16% of educators reported that their schools have employed staff trained to deal with diabetes emergencies, a problem that raises serious concern for the health and well-being of T1DM students (Duraywish et al., 2017). Implementation of teacher training, creation of a robust system of health support made up of school nurses, and institution of cooperation between healthcare workers and schools are highly effective steps towards ensuring health protection for diabetic students. These actions can lead to improved outcomes and reduced levels of emergencies, allowing these youngsters to pass their coursework while properly managing their condition.

Test Your Knowledge

1. What are the key steps in managing acute asthma exacerbations in children?
2. How is sepsis identified and treated in pediatric patients to prevent severe complications?
3. What are the main types and management approaches for diabetic emergencies in children?

6.5. Role of Pediatric Intensive Care Units (PICUs)

Learning Outcome

1. Structure and function of PICUs
2. Multidisciplinary team approach
3. Family-centered care in PICUs

The PICU plays a crucial role in the care of very sick children requiring advanced medical therapy and crvation. The units are designed to handle a wide array of severe medical conditions ranging from respiratory distress to traumatic injuries. The significance of PICUs is underlined by their ability to provide advanced therapies not available on general pediatrics wards, such as, such as invasive monitoring and mechanical ventilation. Significantly, well-functioning PICUs strive to feed into completely integrated pediatric emergency and critical care systems that serve a crucial role in improving health outcomes upon the occurrence of an emergency. They facilitate rapid assessment and intervention, which are the key under circumstances of pediatric mass casualty events, thus the need for regionalized systems that can manage such incidents proficiently (N/A). Alongside, collaborative strategy applied in PICUs is a multidisciplinary team working together to meet the optimal patient outcomes. It can consist of pediatric intensivists, nurses, respiratory therapists, and pharmacists, among others. Shrehensive medical knowledge of the professionals allows individualized treatment protocols taking into account the children's particular physiological requirements and response patterns. For instance, more recent research has shown various ways to deliver respiratory support, such as, such as the use of vibration therapy, which, while it did not reduce ventilation time, has been effective in shortening the course of continuous positive airway pressure (CPAP) in preterm infants (Goudoever et al., 2008). This is a demonstration of the creative mechanisms with which PICUs improve conservative care and ventilation in high-risk patient populations. Outside of direct clinical care, PICUs are also a vital part of pediatric education and research. PICUs are a site for clinical trials that provide insight into critical care interventions and, ultimately, treatment protocols and outcomes. Information generated in PICUs can be used to inform subsequent pediatric emergency guidelines, especially in the setting of large-scale disasters where surge capacity remains an issue. In ordto bridge gaps in emergency preparedness, it is essential that local health systems engage in meticulous planning for pediatric mass critical care, on the needs basis of legislation and operational standards supportive of the unique needs of critically ill children (Lurbe et al., 2016N/A). Owing to their complex functions, PICUs not only save lives but also create avenues for future innovations in pediatric medicine (Figure 6.14).

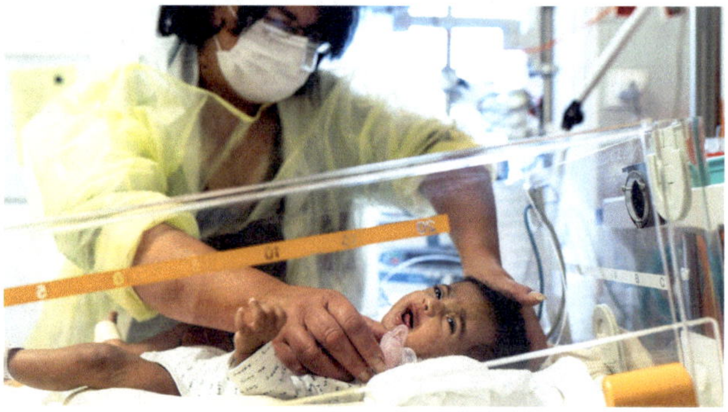

Figure 6.14. Role of pediatric intensive care units (PICUs).

Source: https://external-content.duckduckgo.com/iu/?u=https%3A%2F%2Fassets.medpagetoday.net%2Fmedia%2Fimages%2F110xxx%2F110151.jpg&f=1&nofb=1&ipt=d6edbb9652f91fcea3ce5b0c8b12119f9bb5d45c8640b982126e52a494a0c416&ipo=images.

6.5.1. Structure and Function of PICUs

PICUs design and organization are critical in the care of the complex illnesses of critically ill children. PICUs,compared to general pediatric wards, are equipped with state-of-the-art technologies and staffed by skilled caregivers trained in pediatric critical care. The units offer a multidisciplinary framework that includes pediatricians, surgeons, nurses, respiratory therapists, and social workers, to offer comprehensive treatment for patients with serious health complications. The configuration of a standard PICU prioritizes access and surveillance, complete with sophisticated bedside machinery that provides constant monitoring of vital signs, oxygen saturation, and hemodynamic status. This kind of setup is pivotal in the detection of quick changes in patient status so that timely interventions may be provided, which are inevitable in emergencies among children. In the study of patients in the PICU, the definition and impact of long-stay patients (LSPs) have become a major area of concern. Research in a South African PICU setting has characterized LSPs and described a model of identifying the patients in terms of length of stay and complexity of care level (Nupen et al., 2015). The study investigates the profiles and impacts of LSPs, revealing their extreme rate of resource utilization, which tends to outweigh the short-stay patients. The findings strongly indicate that not only do LSPs consume longer medical care, but they also raise significant questions about resource utilization and PICU care efficiency. By acquiring the demographics and clinical nuances of LSPs, healthcare administrators and clinicians can further optimize staffing, resource utilization, and ultimately, patient care in such specialized settings. Besides this, the operational efficiency of PICUs relies on the extent to which they can match fluctuating patient needs while maintaining optimal standards of care. Ongoing quality improvement programs in these units strive to achieve optima patients and minimize turnaround times during pediatric emergency surges for admissions. Anoperations review is often followed by guidelines on how to manage patients effectively, in a way that the most severely ill children are given prompt and appropriate care (Lurbe et al., 2016N/A, 2007). Implementing evidence-based practice and integrating technological advancements into every-day work is necessary for enhanced patient safety and results of care. Thus, the intricate interplay between structure, function, and continuous betterment in PICUs is important to address the unique PICU challenges in pediatric emergencies and critical care, highlighting the need for continued research and innovation in this vital healthcare field (Figure 6.15).

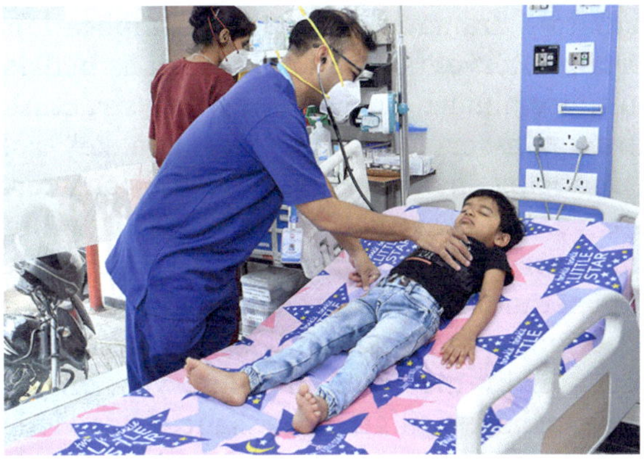

Figure 6.15. The structure and function of pediatric intensive care units (PICUs).

Source: https://cradlehospital.com/wp-content/uploads/2023/05/picu.jpg.

6.5.2. Multidisciplinary Team Approach

The multidisciplinary team philosophy is at the core of managingc emergencies and critical care. The team approach shuns the traditional discipline-based boundaries of medical treatmenn favor of overall patient care. In situations of crisis, for instance, when ECMO is warranted, the treatment type demands a diverse category of health professionals, such as, such as physicians, nurses, respiratory therapists, and pharmacists. Each member contributes high-level expertise, thus the an environment where high-level individual and team performance is feasible. The mixture of ideas allows for early detection of looming complications and swift intervention, thereby greatly enhancing patient outcomes. For instance, simulation education, highlighted in ECMO cases, stresses the importance of teamwork and forcing the idea that effective communication and teamwork are essential in high-pressure situations (al., 2018). Also, applying a multidisciplinary team approach can lead to major improvement in the management of tracheostomy patients with airway emergencies. A study indicates that strict adherence to team-based protocols leads to a dramatic decrease in complications. Certain interventions, such as, such as bedside multidisciplinary team rounds and structured nursing in-services, have played a key role in reducing incidence rates at the long-term care ventilator unit (LTCVU). Such a unified effort, on the basis of cooperative objectives and methods, allows for effective monitoring of complication rates and active prevention measures by the team. Impointerventions are shown to have significantly enhanced knowledge from a mean pre-education score of 49% to 98% after education. Such enhancement highlights how concentrated training in a team environment can lead to increased readiness and responsiveness in intensive care units (Anderson et al., 2019Anderson & Samuels, 2019). Furthermore, the multidisciplinary model optimizes the learning environment and ensures lifelong professional growth. When healthcare professionals collaborate, they learn from one another's expertise, particularly in pediatric emergencies where quick decision-making is important. Regular interdisciplinary meetings to discuss case studies, review complications, and share best practices not only enhance clinical skills but also promote a safety and responsibility culture. This blended approach in pediatric critical care settings ultimately leads to enhanced patient care and outcomes, driving incy from real-time feedback and collaborative problem-solving. Therefore, with the establishment of the specialty of pediatric emergency and critical care, the focus on a multidisciplinary model remains a pillar for achieving excellence in healthcare provision (Hssain et al., 2018; Anderson et al., 2019Anderson & Samuels, 2019).

6.5.3. Family-Centered Care in PICUs

In the context of PICUs, family-centered care is the reason why patient outcomes are shaped and why families are provided with a more improved overall experience during times of critical health crisis. It establishes the family as part of the child's healing environment and encourages an approach in which family members are empowered by family-centered care through collaborative care throughout their child's hospitalization. Contemporary research illustrates that through active involvement of families in decision-making and care, there is a clear improvement in the psychological health of children and caregivers. The shift towards family care also aligns with overall healthcare trends, emphasizing the importance of treating not only physical but also emotional and social aspects of pediatric care, as well, redefining normative care in contemporary healthcare contexts. Family-based care in PICUs demands a significant revision of the medical practices to accommodate the unique needs of families with children suffering from serious health problems. The revisions could entail generous visiting policies, involvement of the family members during rounds, and providing extensive support services for coping with emotional and practical problems. For children with complex chronic conditions, an recent reports, the coordination of care is all that distinguishes their management from effective management. Since families tend to bear heavy emotional and financial responsibilities, offering them resources like care coordinators or avenues to psychosocial services can golong way toward relaying relieving stress and enhancing the overall health care experience, thus establishing the imperative role of a family-centered philosophy in the PICU environment (Hamilton et al., 2012). Moreover, family-oriented care principles extend beyond involvement and attendance to entailingistic support systems that recognize the contribution of the family to the recovery process of the childhis fosters the participation of medical professionals to have open channels of communication with famil fostering trust and ensuring decisions about care are made in collaboration. In the light of increasing recognition of the mental health issues of children in the emergency setting, it is as important that family-focused care be supplemented with the integration of mental health care. Not only addresses does this address the urgent health concerns ofthe child, but this also allows for the accessibility of services to families after discharge within the community, thus improving continuity of care and assistance provided to them (Cooper et al., 2007). Generally, the emphasis on family-focused care in PICUs is a revolutionary approach towards pediatrics care that puts the wellness of both patients and their families above everything else during times of turmoil (Figure 6.16).

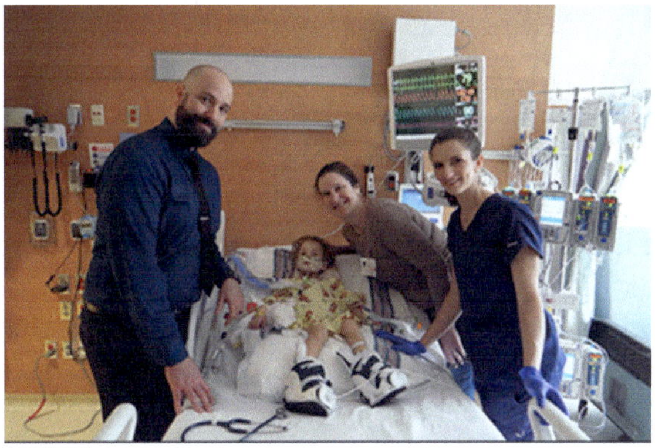

Figure 6.16. The family-centered care plays a pivotal role in shaping patient outcomes and enhancing the overall experience for families navigating critical health crises.

Source: https://www.urmc.rochester.edu/MediaLibraries/URMCMedia/childrens-hospital/critical-care/images/2020PICU-child-mom-team-org.JPG.

Test Your Knowledge

1. What is the structure and primary function of Pediatric Intensive Care Units (PICUs)?
2. How does a multidisciplinary team approach improve patient outcomes in the PICU?
3. Why is family-centered care important in the management of critically ill children in the PICU?

6.6. Ethical Considerations in Pediatric Critical Care

Learning Outcome

1. Informed consent and assent
2. End-of-life decisions
3. Resource allocation and equity

Pediatric critical care is plagued with ethical challenges that significantly influence decision-making within the clinic. The most significant challenge for healthcare providers includes crossing the fine line between aggressive treatment interventions and pediatric quality of life. This is the dilemma that will more frequently necessitate end-of-life conversations, particularly when intervention will prolong suffering without great hope for recovery. The function of the medical emergency teams (METs) is invaluable in such situations since t amounts of medical expertise to the bedside. Their multi-disciplinary strategy is central to evaluating not just the child's medical needs but also their psychological and emotional welfare, highlighting the need for a sensitive multi-dimensional ethical strategy in pediatric emergencies (Alampi et al., 2016Kosoko et al., 2024). In addition to end-of-life care, the ethical consequences of invasive interventions and procedures need to be examined. Children, frequently not able to state their preferences or fully understand the connotations of their medical treatment, present special challenges to informed consent. Medical providers should enter such circumstances with increased sensitivity, taking care that parents or guardians are adequately informed. Additionally, best-interest factors for the child need tding careful examination of possible advantages against risks in the context of intervention. This is compounded when handling tracheostomy complications, which present varied emergency case rates across healthcare facilities and reinforce sticking to the conducted protocols to prevent ris et al., 2019Anderson & Samuels, 2019). Besides, the ethical scenario in pediatric critical care involves equal resource allocation, which is often a contentious matter, particularly in crisis situations. Pediatric patients may require immediate access to intensive care services, particularly in emergency situationies where time is critical. Unequal distribution of healthcare resources may dissuade access on an equal basis, and hence ethical issues arise about fairness and justice. This is best understood when analyzing the assessment of how health systems might assist in ensuring quality care. Merging effective interventions andhe solution to bridging these gaps, allowing for a more equal response that prioritizes vulnerable groups. Hence, constant discourse regarding ethical practice within pediatric critical care is essential in order to advance clinical practicll as ethical standards within healthcare delivery (Alampi et al., 2016Kosoko et al., 2024).

6.6.1. Informed Consent and Assent

Under the context of pediatric critical care and emergencies, informed consent and assent also present its own limitations, particularly in addressing the needs of vulnerable patients such as, such as adolescents and children. Informed consent is a process in which approval is obtained from the parent or guardian prior to the administration of a treatment. However, obtainnsent also must consider the child's comprehension of what their treatment involves. Minors, especially in emergency scenarios, may not be mentally equipped to fully comprehend their medical treatment options. Hence, health care workers must strike a balance between ethical obligations ande reality of offerings so as to ensure that informed consent captures the wishes of guardians as well as increasing adolescent patient autonomy, while placing importance on giving an accurate explanation of treatment options and potential risks to both parties. Assent, as distinct from informed consent, is also equally as important in the pediatric setting, as it acknowledges the increasing autonomy of the child. Informed assent involves incorporating the child into discussions regarding their treatment to the extent that they can comprehend them. This is achieved in a manner that fosters a cooperative environment, allowing young patients to have their wishes and attitudes towards the treatment heard. For instance, in emergency cases involving children, where decisions sometimes have to be taken in haste, healthcare workers need to try to include the child in such decision-making whenever it becomes feasible. The ethical requirement of staying attuned to a child's changing perception is a patient-oriented care virtue that is particularly important within the acute care setting, where pressure and anxiety may interfere with communication. Considering cultural and individual differences is core in the process of acquiring assent, making children heard and respected during their health experiences. Applying standards of ethics in pediatric intervention and research is also pivotal to safeguarding vulnerable populations. According tinical practice (GCP) guidelines, conducting trials or interventions on minors calls for careful observance of ethical standards, which accentuate patient safety and welfare. Difficult problems with informed consent and assent become ever more complex when conducting research with populations of higher vulnerability, such as, such as those with mental health issues. Latina adolescents with depressive symptoms, for instance, can have distinct barriers to research involvement that need individualized strategies recognizing their particular needs and context (McCord et al., 2017). Following ethical practices to ensure compliance minimizes risks and guarantees interventions provided to these clients are properly planned and responsibly designed, with the final result of a more inclusive environment for pediatric health care (Mohammadi et al., 2017) (Figure 6.17).

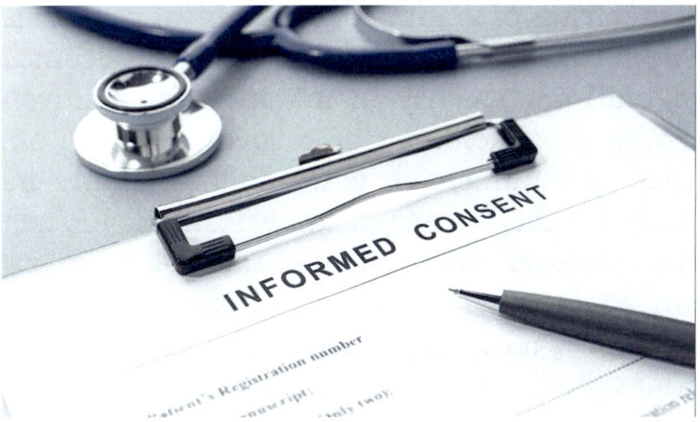

Figure 6.17. The informed consent and assent present unique challenges, particularly when addressing the needs of vulnerable populations.

Source: https://irp.cdn-website.com/f84ff235/dms3rep/multi/Informed+Consent.jpeg.

6.6.2. End-of-life Decisions

In pediatric intensive care and emergency departments, end-of-life decision-making poses an especially challenging ethical dilemma. Doctors typically are trapped in the conflict of maintaining or terminating life-sustaining measures, especially where a child has a poor prognosis. Ethical considerations demand thorough consideration of the child's best interests, which is difficult in an emotionally charged environment. This is compounded by the involvement of a number of stakeholders, including parents, guardians, and the medical team, each differing perceptions regarding what constitutes proper care in such extreme circumstances. Additionally, the role played by Medical ETeams (METs) in such circumstances is essential, as they tend to be cal making timely decisions on end-of-life care and potential ICU admissions (ALAMPI et al., 2016Kosoko et al., 2024). Such considerations highlight the necessity for standardi processes that guide these difficult decisions and ensuring ensure that the voices of families are heard through the process. When making the decisiondeciding to transition from curative approaches to palliative care, the medical team must navigate a spectrum of emotional and ethical concerns. The meaning of comfort care is thus becomes pivotal, particularly in instances of children where the likelihood of recovery i doing so, open communication with families should be sought to facilitate their understanding of such changes' consequences. Good end-of-life choices indeed depend on good communication, which minimizes misinterpretation and encourages an atmosphere of cooperation. Util communications strategies, such as, such as joint decision models, can also improve the quality of the talks significantly. Moreover, palliative care option education for families of sick children is fundamental because they may not be aware of what centers they can utilize during this challenging time (Anderson et al., 2019Anderson & Samuels, 2019).

Through educating the families and healthcare professionals, the caring spirit is sustained even in the face of loss. Lastly, the practice of end-of-life decision-making in pediatric crisis is not just a medical necessity but a most ethical practice. This will typically involve consideration of the quality of a child's life, values, and beliefs as understood and imagined by the family and treatment team. Parents and guardians are integral to the discussion, given that they possess intimate knowledge of the child's likes and dislikes. When medical professionals are engaged in such critical debates, a constant display of emotional support towards the families is imperative to enable them to manage their own fears and grief. The pediatrics' ethics of end-of-life care challenge medical professioalancing technical mpassion and empathy. Hence, training and policy must also adjust to reflect the intricate processes of these discussions, drawing upon ethical underpinnings, medical information, and the rich emotional landscape navigated by families in these painful circumstances (Alampi et al., 2016Kosoko et al., 2024; Anderson et al., 2019Anderson & Samuels, 2019).

6.6.3. Resource Allocation and Equity

In the case of pediatric critical care and emergency, the principles of rationing and equity are of prime importance in ensuring all children have access to timely and effective medical treatments. The resource allocation process often grapples with balancing clinical need and available technology, skilled staff, and fiscal constraints. For instance, in emergency settings, healthcare professionals need to be prepared to act promptly and efficiently; therefore, interactive education of healthcare professionals is essential. However, evidence exists that is uncertain regarding the impact of such training on clinical outcomes, as evidenced by low-certainty evidence of improved patient survival and practice adherence (Barnard et al., 2019). This gives rise to significant questions about the deployment of educational resources and how such initiatives could be made available on an equitable basis to all healthcare providers involved in pediatric emergencies. Aside from training, the availability of medical materials and advanced healthcare technologies also plays a valuable role in the equity of pediatric care. Inequitable deployment of resources may lead to disproportionate exchange of information, treatment capacity, and f health outcomes between groups. For instance, the COVID-19 vaccine rollout shows how inequality can be amplified where access is not equally managed (Afolabi et al., 2020). Policymakers must examine the distribution systems that various settings adopt to ensure that minority groups are not left behind but rather prioritized above over being excluded based on logistics or socioeconomic status. This calls for a deep understanding of local demand, so that resource distribution in an equitable manner is not just a moral necessity but a strategic requirement for the success of healthcare. Equitable resource distribution also raises ethical considerations in triage in emergencies, particularly in pediatric emergencies. Emergency care most commonly encounters scenarios where medical resources are limited, and health workers are compelled to make rapid decisions that determine survival rates. Developing clear-cut guidelines that place priority on the needs of the most vulnerable, such as, such as critically ill children, is important in facilitating fair healthcare delivery. Programs should be aimed at developing guidelines to guarantee transparency and equity in resource distribution, considering the heterogeneity of pediatric patients' needs. Further, relying on existing mechanisms of continuous evaluation to apply to resource allocation systems will ensure they remain responsive to emerging healthcare issues, which ultimately will provide an environment where equity can be achieved for pediatric emergencies and critical care settings.

Test Your Knowledge

1. What are the key principles of informed consent and assent in pediatric critical care settings?
2. How are ethical challenges addressed when making end-of-life decisions for critically ill children?
3. Why are resource allocation and equity important ethical concerns in pediatric intensive care?

SUMMARY

The intrinsic complexities in pediatric emergencies demand robust groundwork in cognition and managing critical care needs. As reiterated through the discussion, the high level of variability in emergency presentation among children underscores the necessity for specialized interventions and the necessity for healthcare professionals to have sufficient knowledge in terms of pediatric-specific protocols. This is corroborated by findings that formal pediatric resuscitation curriculum not only enhances residents' comfort levels but also ensures they acquire requisite competencies for effective management of critically ill children (Brancati et al., 2003). These learning programs are the backbone in filling knowledge gaps and cultivating a preparednessatric departments. Moreover, quality improvement initiatives can make a profound impact on outcomes in the critical care setting. Outcomes from recent campaignsg-term care ventilator units, show that systematic programs, including multidisciplinary team-based approaches and continuous training, can reduce significantlysignificantly reduce the incidence of airway complications in tracheostomy patients. Despite the initial increase in rates of complications post-implementation (Anderson et al., 2019Anderson & Samuels, 2019), ongoing monitoring and improvement are likely to bring about improvement over time, showcasing the dynamic nature of quality assurance in healthcare environments. All these findings establish that ongoing observation and tweaking of care practices are essential in maintaining high standards in pediatric critical care. Therefore, the future of pediatric critical care and emergency lies with an all-around approach that encompasses education, quality improvement,. The emphasis on simulation-based education and strategic implementation of evidence-based principles is critical in establishing the skill base for health professionals. As shown by the positive outcomes of resuscitation training courses (Brancati et al., 2003) and targeted intervention studies with high-risk populations (Anderson et al., 2019Anderson & Samuels, 2019), the creation of large-scale training modules and quality care programs has the potential to contribute strongly to pediatric emergency preparedness. Continuous research and collaboration between disciplines will be critical as we work towards a higher level of care and outcomes for the smallest and most at-risk patients.

In pediatric emergencies and critical care, the most vital element in this instance involves the recognition of the subtleties surrounding airway management in tracheostomy patients. Tracheostomy patients are at great risk of severe complications upon interference with their airway, demonstrating the seriousness of effective intervention. From epidemiological data, the range of complications is from a mere 3.2% to 30% in tracheostomy patients, a rate that demonstrates the seriousness of stringent clinical protocols. In a long-term care ventilator unit, compld in about 40% of the cases, prompting urgent quality improvement. By applying evidence-based practices from the Johns Hopkins Nursing Evidence-Based Practice model, healthcare professionals aim to enhance the level of care with a focus on the severity of airway management in children at risk of respiratory failure and distress (Anderson et al., 2019Anderson & Samuels, 2019). Collaboration and continued education become paramount factors in maximizing outcomes in pediatric critical care units. A quality improvement project demonstrated the efficacy of multidisciplinary rounds and in-services for nurses to enhance the quality of care provided to patients. Pre-education testing resulted in an alarming 49% average score among nurses, which signifies knowledge deficiencies in managing airway care. The use of systematic education interventions contributed to a striking post-education average of 98%. This stark difference underscores the crucial role that traininfer contribute in enabling healthcare professionals to learn skills that can enable timely and effective response to emergencies as a result of tracheostomy care. Continuous professional development therefore, gains significance in reducing complications as well as enhancing a safety culture in pediatric critical care environments (Anderson et al., 2019Anderson & Samuels, 2019). Public health crises like pandemics H1N1, make pediatric emergencies and critical care practices even more cohe readiness of the healthcare system includes analysis of different indicators at both the federal and state levels to ensure adequate funding, accountability, and infrastructure are in place. Although improvements have bed in certain emergency response capacities, issues remain about the capacity of hospitals to handle efficiently patient surgespatient surges efficiently amidst crises. The consideration of these evaluations indicates that, while preparedness is better, challenges are still present and require ongoing review and sharpening of emergency procedures. Effective An effective and strategically funded response is important in the care of pediatric patients, particularly those in intensive care, to ensure that they receive effective and timely intervention in the midst of growing healthcare needs.

KEY TERMS FROM THIS CHAPTER

- Anaphylaxis
- Cyanosis
- Diabetic ketoacidosis (DKA)
- Hypoglycemia
- Injury management
- Respiratory distress
- Social ramifications
- Vulnerable populations
- Cardiac Arrest
- Dehydration
- Emergency medical services (EMS)
- Infectious causes
- Medical emergency teams (METs)
- Social isolation
- Trauma

CRITICAL THINKING QUESTIONS

1. **What is the first step in assessing an unresponsive child in an emergency?**
   a. Check for breathing and pulse
   b. Call emergency services
   c. Start chest compressions immediately
   d. Place the child in a recovery position
2. **Which of the following is a common sign of respiratory distress in children?**
   a. Slow breathing
   b. Nasal flaring and retractions
   c. Normal skin color
   d. Quiet, effortless breathing
3. **What is the most common cause of cardiac arrest in children?**
   a. Heart attack
   b. Respiratory failure
   c. Stroke
   d. High blood pressure
4. **Which condition is a medical emergency in children and requires immediate intervention?**
   a. Mild fever
   b. Croup
   c. Anaphylaxis
   d. Common cold
5. **What is the recommended depth of chest compressions for a child during CPR?**
   a. About 1 inch
   b. At least 2 inches
   c. About 1.5 inches or one-third of the chest depth
   d. No compressions, only rescue breaths

Short Answer Questions

1. What are the components of the pediatric assessment triangle (PAT)?
2. How do you differentiate between mild, moderate, and severe respiratory distress in children?
3. What are the causes of pediatric cardiac arrest?
4. What are the first steps in managing a child with an altered level of consciousness?
5. What is the ABCDE approach in pediatric trauma resuscitation?

Answer to Critical Thinking Questions

1. (a); 2. (b); 3. (b); 4. (c); 5. (c)

REFERENCES

1. Abrahamsson, T., Abramiuk, M., Aitken, M., Ajram, J., Akers, K., Aldhouse-Green, S., Andrews-Hanna, J., et al. (2017). The odyssallocation and prioritization of COVID-19 vaccination. https://core.ac.uk/download/337890488.pdf (accessed on 16th June 2025).

2. Agabiti-Rosei, E., Cruickshank, J. K., Dominiczak, A., Erdine, S., et al. (2016). 2016 European Society of Hypertension guidelines for the management of high blood pressure in children and adolescents. https://core.ac.uk/download/46165193.pdf Lurbe, E., Agabiti-Rosei, E., Cruickshank, J. K., Dominiczak, A., Erdine, S., Hirth, A., Invitti, C., Litwin, M., Mancia, G., Pall, D., Rascher, W., Redon, J., Schaefer, F., Seeman, T., Sinha, M., Stabouli, S., Webb, N. J., Wühl, E., & Zanchetti, A. (2016). 2016 European Society of Hypertension guidelines for the management of high blood pressure in children and adolescents. *Journal of hypertension*, *34*(10), 1887–1920. https://doi.org/10.1097/HJH.0000000000001039 (accessed on 16th June 2025).

3. Ait Hssain, A., Al Disi, M., Alhomsi, Y., Alinier, G., et al. (2018). Addressing the challenges of ECMO simulation. https://core.ac.uk/download/287580894.pdf (accessed on 16th June 2025).

4. Al Duraywish, A. A., & Nail, A. M. (2017). Assessment of the primary and intermediate school staffs' knowledge, attitude and practice on care of children with type 1 diabetes at school, Al-Jouf, Saudi Arabia. https://core.ac.uk/download/478395375.pdf (accessed on 16th June 2025).

5. Al Tamimi, A. A. A., Alruwaili, A. M. S., Alruwaili, E. M., Alenazi, F. M., Almoammar, N. A., Alwayli, N. S., & Alfayer, T. A. (2023). The utility of point-of-care ultrasound (POCUS) in the emergency department: A systematic review. https://core.ac.uk/download/603897418.pdf (accessed on 16th June 2025).

6. Alcala-Van Houten, L. (2018). A pediatric respiratory care curriculum for emergency department nurses. https://core.ac.uk/download/159400973.pdf (accessed on 16th June 2025).

7. Alijarde-Lorente, R., Benito-Ruiz, E., de Vicente, C.k/download/535115879.pdf (accessed on 16th June 2025).

8. Alinier, G. (2018). Cost-effective extracorporeal membrane oxygenation simulation. https://core.ac.uk/download/288394195.pdf (accessed on 16th June 2025).

9. Anderson, B., & Samuels, J. (2019). Quality improvement on the long-term care ventilator unit: Interventions to increase patient safety and prevent patient harm. Anderson, Billie and Samuels, Joanne, "Quality Improvement on the Long-term Care Ventilator Unit: Interventions to Increase Patient Safety and Prevent Patient Harm" (2019). DNP Scholarly Projects. 19. https://scholars.unh.edu/scholarly_projects/19 (accessed on 16th June 2025).

10. Barnard, K., Burden, C., Caldwell, D. M., Draycott, T., et al. (2019). The effects of interactive training of healthcare providers on the management of life-threatening emergencies in hospital. https://core.ac.uk/download/323195508.pdf (accessed on 16th June 2025).

11. Bender, L., Bruun, N. H., Christensen, E. F., Kløjgård, T., et al. (2022). Pediatric emergencies in helicopter emergency medical services: A national population-based cohort study from Denmark. https://core.ac.uk/download/534429600.pdf (accessed on 16th June 2025).

12. Brancati, D. O., David, S., Dobson, J. V., Nagel, T., et al. (2003). Pediatric resuscitation: Evaluation of a clinical curriculum. https://core.ac.uk/download/pdf/85708.pdf (accessed on 16th June 2025).

13. Carrol, E. D., Lane, S., Lisboa, P. J. G., McGrath, J., et al. (2014). What impact did a pediatric early warning system have on emergency admissions to the pediatric intensive care unit? An observational cohort study. https://core.ac.uk/download/42136646.pdf (accessed on 16th June 2025).

14. Ciomaga, I. M., Frăsinariu, O., Nistor, N., Rugină, A., et al. (2019). Poisoning in the pediatric intensive care unit. https://core.ac.uk/download/322441124.pdf (accessed on 16th June 2025).

15. Clancy-Burgess, S. C. (2024). Implementing change: Training for adult emergency assessment, recognition, and stabilization for novice and non-critical care nurses. https://core.ac.uine curriculum on asthma outcomes in Belize. https://core.ac.uk/download/619409594.pdf (accessed on 16th June 2025).

16. Genisca, A. E., Kosoko, A. A., Adekunbi, M., Mackey, J., et al. (2024). A simulation and small-group pediatric emergency medicine course for generalist healthcare providers: Gastrointestinal and nutrition emergencies. https://core.ac.uk/download/622191535.pdf Kosoko, A. A., Genisca, A. E., Peoples, N. A., Tompkins, C., Sorensen, R., & Mackey, J. (2024). A Simulation and Small-Group Pediatric Emergency Medicine Course for Generalist Healthcare Providers: Gastrointestinal and Nutrition Emergencies. *Journal of education & teaching in emergency medicine*, *9*(4), C1–C120. https://doi.org/10.21980/J8WH2K (accessed on 16th June 2025).

17. Hamilton, L. J., Kelly, R. B., Klitzner, T. S., Lerner, J. M., et al. (2012). Medical transport of children with complex chronic conditions. https://core.ac.uk/download/484113461.pdf (accessed on 16th June 2025).

18. Maziarz, L., McCartney, M., Raker, C., Welch, A., et al. (2018). Food allergy in youth: A primer for allied health professionals. https://core.ac.uk/download/215366035.pdf (accessed on 16th June 2025).

19. McCord, A. L. (2017). Ethical considerations for involving Latina adolescents in mental health research. https://core.ac.uk/download/161627594.pdf (accessed on 16th June 2025).

20. Mohammadi, M. R., & Mostafavi, S. A. (2017). Good clinical practice in children and adolescents. https://core.ac.uk/download/322432390.pdf (accessed on 16th June 2025).

21. Ndukwu, C. I., & Onah, S. K. (2015). Pattern and outcome of post neonatal pediatric emergencies in Nnamdi Azikiwe University Teaching Hospital, Nnewi, South East Nigeria. https://core.ac.uk/download/478302384.pdf (accessed on 16th June 2025).

22. Nupen, T. L. (2015). Characteristics and outcome of long-stay patients in a pediatric intensive care unit in Cape Town, South Africa. https://core.ac.uk/download/185459829.pdf (accessed on 16th June 2025).

23. Seita, H. M. (2013). Food allergies in pregnant women: A study of prevalence in expecting mothers and association with neonatal outcomes. https://open.bu.edu/bitstream/2144/12219/6/Seita_Helene_2013.pdf (accessed on 16th June 2025).

24. van Goudoever, J. B., Helder, K. O., & Hop, W. C. J. (2008). Vibration therapy reduces CPAP need in a prospective randomized controlled trial. https://core.ac.uk/download/18523604.pdf (accessed on 16th June 2025).

COMMON PEDIATRIC PSYCHIATRIC DISORDERS

7

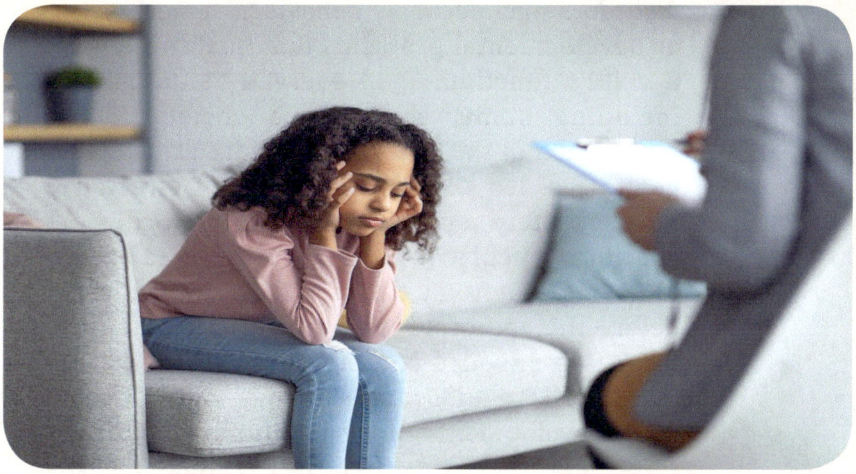

LEARNING OBJECTIVES

After studying this chapter, you will be able to:

1. Discuss the attention-deficit/hyperactivity disorder (ADHD)
2. Emphasize anxiety disorders
3. Explain the depression in children
4. Learn about autism spectrum disorder (ASD)
5. Emphasize oppositional defiant disorder (ODD)
6. Understand eating disorders

Introduction

It is important to know the landscape of child psychiatric disorders for both treatment and diagnosis. The disorders encompass many kinds of conditions that significantly impact children's, adolescents', and families' well-being and mental health. In the past few years, the prevalence of such disorders has increased, and these have been of interest to healthcare workers and researchers. Above all, conditio as, such as attention-deficit/hyperactivity disorder (ADHD), anxiety disorders, and eating disorders have emerged as key concerns in the field of pediatric psychiatry. The rising recognition of these conditions requires massive study in order to address a multitude of determinants, including etiology, symptoms, and effects on development, thus opening avenues for effective interventions. The convergence of cultural, social, and economic factors complicates the diagnosis and treatment of pediatric psychiatric illness. Historical stereotypes of limited populations for these disorders have been dispelled as they can appear in individuals of multi-ethnic and multi-racial descent. This shift in perspective identifies the need to examine differentials in diagnosis and access to care. For instance, while eating disorders have comparable prevalence rates for differing demographic groups, studies reveal enormous clinical gaps for under-treated patient groups. As is evident from new studies, specific examinations of minority ethnic groups' experiences and challenges reveal the necessity for culturally modified methodologies for treatment (Tuomainen et al., 2024). The influence of these disorders is not only personal but also reaches family and society. For example, pediatric ADHD patients not only struggle with impulse control but are at higher risks for coms, such as, such as unnecessary hospital readmission following physical injury (Halevi et al., 2024).

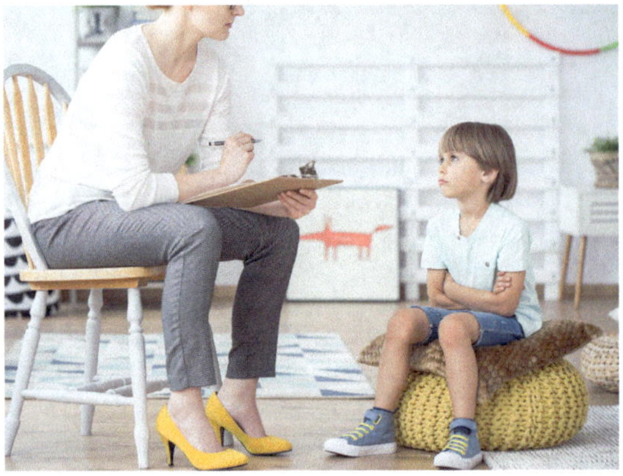

Figure 7.1. The landscape of pediatric psychiatric disorders.

Source: https://blog.boardvitals.com/wp-content/uploads/2019/10/psychiatric-disorders-in-children.jpg.

Such interdependence highlights the fact that pediatric psychiatric disorders require whole-person management strategies that incorporate family engagement and community intervention. i-dimensional multi-dimensional approach, health workers can better respond to the unique needs of mentally ill children, ultimately enhance outcomes and facilitate resilience. Building awareness through accelerated research and effective communication among stakeholders remains key in combating pediatric psychiatric disorder stigma so that all children receive their rightful treatment (Figure 7.1).

Definition of Pediatric Psychiatric Disorders

Child psychiatric disorders represent a cluster of mental illnesses that deeply influence children and young people. Pediatric psychiatric disorders may occur as behavioral, emotional, or developmental problems that interfere with a child's functioning in everyday situations, including home, school, and society. The recognition of the salience of children's mental health has led to more focus being directed at accurately specifying these disorders. Specifically, pediatric psychiatric disorders refer to having symptoms that are likely to manifest before the age of 18 and can include anxiety disorders, mood disorders, attention-deficit/hyperactivity disorder (ADHD), and other neurodevelopmental disorders. Understanding these definitions is necessary since early detection and treatment can reduce the long-term impacts of the disorders. The nuances encompassed in pediatric psychiatric disorders require a stristic process. Current models, such as, such as the Diagnostic and Statistical Manual of Mental Disorders (DSM-5), specify criteria for categorization of these disorders. The criteria consider the developmental stage of the child because symptoms also vary significantly in younger versus older children. A diagnosis of ADHD, for instance, may be dissimilar in a toddler versus an adolescent based on changing behavior and expectations in society. This developmental process allows clinicians to be able to effectively investigate the children's symptom presentation and ultimately lead to improved treatment methods. Multidisciplinary collaboration between pediatricians, psycholod other medical professionals should beis necessary in order to offer complete care. With society seeing the rise of pediatric psychiatric disorders, genes, environment, and social pressure need to be considered in establishing and understanding these. Studies confirm that chronic stressors like domestic instabilityues, and even bullying have the ability tocan trigger or worsen psychiatric disorders in susceptible children. Moreover, the increasing prevalence of technology and its impact on social interactions is also an essential area of concern. The symptoms expressed in disorders like anxiety or depression are often intertwined with extraneous factors, rendering it a complex process to diagnose. Given these nuances, further research and concurrence by experts, including the establishment of extensive diagnostic criteria, are required to characterize and adequately treat pediatric psychiatric disorders in practice, with children being provided with appropriate education and emotional care that is tailored to their particular requirements (Fadl et al., 2023; Dharmaraj et al., 2023).

Importance of Early Diagnosis and Treatment

Early diagnosis and treatment of children's psychiatric disorders cannot be overstated since timely action noticeably tips the scales in favor of improcomes. Early diagnosis of conditions such as, such as anxiety disorders, ADHD, and depression allows families and professionals to initiate appropriate interventions before the symptoms accumulate to the point of becoming difficult to manage. Research shows that undiagnosed and untreated psychiatric illnesses in children most frequently lead to long-term problems, including low academic achievement, social difficulties, and a higher risk for developing comorbid rders in adulthood. Treating and diagnosing the illnesses during the formative stages of development prevents irreversible impairments and supports healthier developmental trajectories. Early intervention promotes resilience and coping skills, allowing children to successfully transcend adversity and ultimately enhance their own quality of life. Besides, tment of pediatric psychiatric disorders in its their early stages can significantly alleviate the emotional suffering of children and their families. The impact of psychiatric illness also reaches beyond the sick individual, imposing on the family and causing parental stress. Treatment is not only successful if it eliminates the symptoms of the child, but also because it enhances interamilial relations, leading to a healthy home eent conducive to recovery. Interventions such as, such as cognitive-behavioral therapy can supply children with everyday skills for regulating emotions and behaviors, as well as support parents in utilizing tools to meet their child's mental health requirements. Regular screening and involvement in school settings are prevention measures that assist in the early identification of children at risk, so problems do not intensify. Thus, the combined benefits of early diagnosis and treatment emphasize the value of employing systematic methods to approach mental well-being in pediatric populations. Second, the evolving character of psychiatric research serves to emphasize the value of continuing education and awareness among healthcare workers in the broad array of symptoms and presentations of pediatric mental health disease. As hinted at by differences in treatment response and symptom change by diagnosis, as highlighted in recent studies, clinicians in mental health must exercise care in discriminating between normal variations of development and clinically significant disorders. Multidisciplinary integration is essential because a number of various forms of treatments may be appropriate for the unique needs of a ghild. Moreover, consideration of thos factors which that affect treatment effectivenss, —social, psychological, and biological factors, —can help ensure individualized care. Family participation in treatment fosters collaborative decision-making, and hence, care is appropriately contextual and adheres to the special needs of the child. Overall, the need for early diagnosis and treatment is well established in the knowledge that early and context-specific interventions have a huge impact on the mental health outcomes of children afflicted with psychiatric disorders (Figure 7.2).

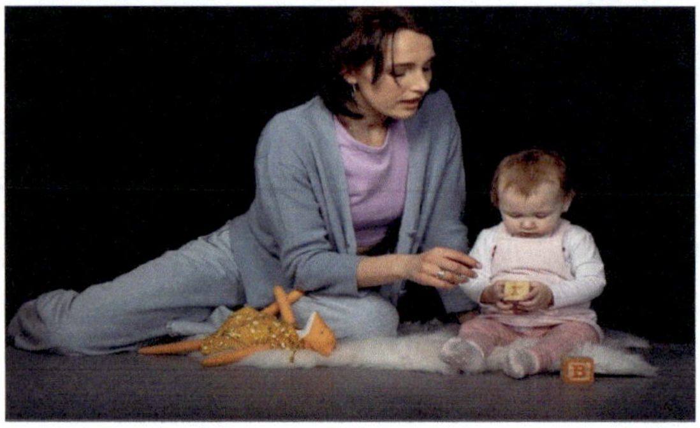

Figure 7.2. Therapist supporting a toddler in developmental play therapy.

Source: https://littlebones.org/wp-content/uploads/2024/10/Child-Developmental-Disorders-Treatment-In-Indore-1024x536.jpg.

Overview of Common Disorders to be Discussed

Pediatric psychiatric disorder onset is variable, and every disorder has specific challenges and symptoms that impact children differently. Some of the most frequently treated disorders include attention deficit hyperactivity disorder (ADHD), anxiety disorders, and depressive disorders. Diagnosis of ADHD is characterized by chronic histories of inattention and/or hyperactive-impulsive behavior, which have the potential to significantly compromise a child's functioning academically and socially. Prevalence rates of ADHD indicate that it is linked with approximately 5–10% of children worldwide, suggesting the importance of effective identification vention strategies. Considering anxiety disorders, such as, such as generalized anxiety disorder and separation anxiety disorder, it is evident that these disove significant effects on developmental milestones through by impairing a child's participation in daily tasks, including school attendance and interaction with peers. The far-reaching implications of these disorders require widespread comprehension and sensitivity among caregivers, educators, and medical professionals. As children grow through the myriad stages of development, depressive disorders represent a second major concern. Depression in children may present itself as irritability, withdrawal, and alterations of appetite or sleep, which can complicate diagnosis. The National Institute of Mental Health says that 3–5% of children are apt to experience depressive disorders at some point, and half of all mental illness begins before the age of fourteen. Understanding childhood depression is based on an awareness of environmental, biological, and psychosocial forces acting together to affect a child's mental well-being. The recognition of depression early warning signs can lead to early intervention and appropriate therapeutic modalities, such that the suffering children are afforded the assistance they need to thrive emotionally and academically. The complexities of depression among children thus highlight the importance of meticulous monitoring and holistic treatment modalities. Apart from ADHD, anxiety, aessive disorders, there are also behavioral disorders such as, such as oppositional defiant disorder (ODD) and conduct disorder (CD), which should be mentioned in pediatric psychiatric disorders. With its angry, irritable mood pattern, argumentative behavior, and vindictiveness, ODD typically occurs early in childhood and often co-exists with ADHD. On the other hand, Conduct Disorder, which involves a more serious violation of social norms and infringement on others' rights, typically occurs in later childhood or adolescence. The difference between the two conditions is critical to developing successful treatment programs and requires precise clinical evaluation and targeted interventions to address unique child needs. The impact of behavioral disorders extends beyond the child to affect family relationships and interpersonal relations. Undersding such disorders thus becomes essential in the enabling of conducive environments for affected children and f comprehensive care and intervention (Zuberbier et al., 2021; Steven et al., 2020; Zuberbier et al., 2021).

7.1. Attention-Deficit/ Hyperactivity Disorder (ADHD)

Learning Outcome

1. Symptoms and diagnostic criteria
2. Prevalence and demographic factors
3. Treatment options and interventions

ADHD is one of the most prevalent childhood psychiatric conditions, which is characterized by persistent behaviors of inattention, hyperactivity, and impulsivity. Symptoms of ADHD can lead to significant impairment in school function and social interactions in a child. Epidemiologic research has shown that ADHD affects approximately 5% of children and often continues into the teen and adult years. The diagnosis of ADHD is based primarily on behavioral assessment rather than on laboratory tests in terms of quantity, raising controversy among clinicians regarding its authenticity and treatment approaches. Stereotypes and misinformation generate misconceptions regarding ADHD that typically stigmatize the afflicted, rendering them less acceptable in society and postponing medical attention (Stephen et al., 2021). It requires accurate evaluation in thclto exclude ADHD from other imitative behavior disorders, ; thus the children would receive appropriate support and apply intervention methods that suit their respective difficulties. The effects of ADHD extend beyond the apparent behavioral symptoms, across a broad educational and phological spectrum of influence, from academic difficulty to be even underachievers with low self-esteem. Included is the fact that der is often co-morbid with other psychiatric disorders, such as, such as depression and anxiety, and these contribute to the challenges faced by affected children. Etiological theories regarding ADHD suggest a matrix of genetic, neurological, and environmental factors as responsible for its development. Important in the ongoing controversy around ADHD is the reminder of the need to recognize the heterogeneity of symptom presentation in individuals and the utility of tailoring treatment protocols to consider co-morbid conditions.

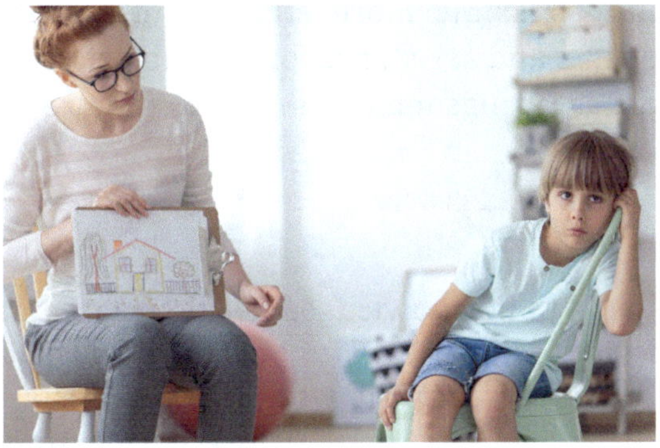

Figure 7.3. Attention deficit hyperactivity disorder (ADHD).

Source: https://external-content.duckduckgo.com/iu/?u=https%3A%2F%2Ftnvoices.org%2Fwp-content%2Fuploads%2F2020%2F08%2FAttention-Deficit-Hyperactivity-Disorder-ADHD-The-Basics-tn-voices-nashville.jpg&f=1&nofb=1&ipt=8d2283d8de2a751e83be376e510202a7818e2128d7f07f6c5a5a0b222bff6330&ipo=images.

Management of ADHD is optimally gained through multidisciplinary collaboration, with education, behavioral, and, if necessary, pharmacological interventions. Early diagnosis and individualized management for children with ADHD are stressed by recent research because the delay in treatment will lead to higher symptoms and impairment. Parent training and classroom accommodation are the primary elements of management as part of behavioral interventions. Pharmacological treatment with stimulant medications has also been effective in treating core symptoms, but is no panacea and often requires close management to control side effects. While clinicians strive to optimize treatment success, they must also be vigilant for comorbidities, including learning disabilities and conduct disorders, which may need oher treatments. Ideally, knowledge of the complex nature of ADHDs is essential for clinicians, educators, and families. Greater awareness and debunking of myths about ADHD are important, making possible more efficient intervention measures and assistance for the subjects of this disorder (Pringsheim et al., 2021) (Figure 7.3).

7.1.1. Symptoms and Diagnostic Criteria

It is vital to be knowledgeable about symptoms and diagnostic criteria of pediatric psychiatric disorders so that they can be appropriately identified and treated. ADHD is one of the most prominent disorders observed among children, which is characterized by chronic types of inattention, hyperactivity, and impulsivity that disrupt functioning or development. Diagnostic criteria for ADHD, as outlined in the DIAGNOSTIC and statistical manual of mental disorders (DSM-5), require symptoms to last at least six months, be developmentally inappropriate for the child, and impair social, academic, or occupational functioning. Patterns of symptoms may be highly varied across children, so it is critical to have a comprehensive evaluation process involving consideration of behavioral, emotional, and cognitive factors. Efficient diagnosis permits clinicians to tailor interventions that can significantly enhance the child's functioning in multiple settings. Obsessive-compulsive disorder (OCD), with the occurrence of obsessions, compulsions, or both, is another significant pediatric psychiatric disorder. Obsessions are intrusive and unwanted thoughts that induce anxiety, while compulsions are repetitive behaviors performed to alleviate this anxiety. Diagnostic criteria for OCD include the awareness that the obsessions or compulsions occupy more than one hour a day and consume time and are excessive. It is critical to differentiate between normal childhood functioning and clinically significant symptoms, as children may exhibit repetitive behavior or magical thinking without meeting full diagnostic criteria for OCD. Additionally, as many as 41% of those with eating disorders also endorse symptoms of OCD, highlighting the comorbidity and complexity of symptomatology among pediatric groups (Gorbis et al., 2024).

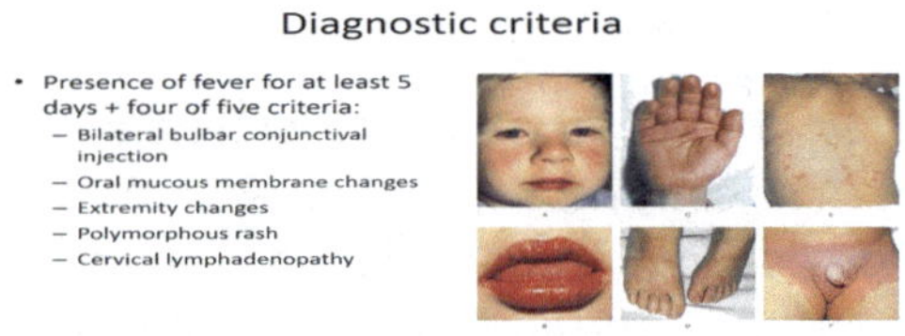

Figure 7.4. The symptoms and diagnostic criteria associated with pediatric psychiatric disorders.

Source: https://i.ytimg.com/vi/o3_n2clyyjA/maxresdefault.jpg.

This overlap makes diagnosis more challenging, requiring clinicians to be cautious. Similar to other psychiatric conditions, clinicians should be aware that the presentation of symptoms ry from one diagnostic group to another. For instance, disorders such as, such as generalizety disorder and major depressive disorder share common symptoms such as, such as irritability, fatigue, and concentration problems in children. Recent studies have shown significant improvements in the symptom severity in most psychiatric disorders in placebo conditions and suggested that diagnostic evaluations need to consider placebo effects seriously while evaluating the response to treatment. In particular, it has been shown through a meta-analysis that pre-post placebo effect sizes overall differed significantly between diagnoses, thus implying that subjective experience of symptoms and responsiveness to treatment in children can be quite heterogeneous. Such findings have therapeutic implications and highlight the necessity for full assessment and monitoring in estimating the efficacy of treatments of pediatric psychiatric disorders (Bschor et al., 2024) (Figure 7.4).

7.1.2. Prevalence and Demographic Factors

Child psychiatric disorder prevalence is very diverse among different demographic groups and is influenced by the roles of ar, and socio-economic status. Recent studies depict some disorders, such as, such as depression and anxiety, as having higher incidence rates among adolescent populations. Females have been disproportionately affected compared to males, as research has ed that females are more likely to develop mental health illnesses, such as, such as depressive disorders and self-harm (DSH). Specifically, a research on DSH in children admitted to hospital in China reported 16.90% of patients with self-injurious acts, and 71.55% of them were female (Jiang et al., 2024). These results indicate the necessity to take into account individualized characteristics of various population groups while determining the prevalence of psychiatric disorders in children and adolescents. Besides gender disparities, socio-economic determinants play a decisive role in pediatric psychiatric disorder prevalence. Younger children who belong to lower socio-economic statuses often face more than one stressor, like a lack of adequate access to mental health care, which can exacerbate existing psychiatric disorders. The above study highlights the relationship between DSH and parental marital status, implying that children raised in distressed or dysfunctional family environments are at higher risk of engaging in self-injury behavior (Jiang et al., 2024). These findings point to a crucial crossroads between family lives and the onset of psychiatric disease, not only calling for family-involvement interventions but also overcoming socio-economic barriers. Identification of these demographic measures supports more effective resource targeting and application of prevention strategies that are targeted to high-risk populations. Correlations between the intensity of psychiatric diseases and demographic variables are also of significant importance in treating disorders like anorexia nervosa (AN). One study recently demonstrated that 57.7% of children with AN exhibited cardiac abnormalities, illustrating the dire medical ramifications of untreated psychiatric illnesses. Remarkably, the study did not discover a significant relationship betwec complications and AN severity, and that implies demographic factors, such as, such as gender and age, can be an essential part of assessing patient risk. Consequently, it is important to establish individualized care plans that not only address the severity of the disorder but also demographic variables, enabling comprehensive care to better address the multidimensional needs of child psychiatric patients. Therefore, increased understanding of both prevalence rates and demographic variables provides gains in treatment approaches for common pediatric psychiatric disorders.

7.1.3. Treatment Options and Interventions

Most pediatric psychiatric disorders have treatment and intervention that is multifactorial, with both pharmacoland non-pharmacological interventions. Psychotherapeutic interventions such as, such as cognitive-behavioral therapy (CBT) are often allocated a first-line treatment for most of the conditions, including depression and anxiety. CBT helps children develop coping skills and modify unhelpful modes of thinking, eventually enhancing emotional regulation. The effectiveness of these treatments is based on sound clinical evidence, validating their use in creating the mental well-being of children.

Adding family therapy can also enhance treatment outcomes, as this incorporates the parents and siblings of the child into the treatment, thereby cultivating a more nurturing environment for the child. Inclusion of such therapy emphasizes the role of holistic management in pediatric psychiatric disorders where child as well as family dynamics have a pivotal role to play in recovery. Pharmacological interventions are also integral to the treatment of pediatric psychiatric disorders. In the face of continued controversy over the use of drugs by the younger population, antidepressants are widely used, particularly for depression and anxiety disorders. According to research, fluoxetine is generally the first choice among SSRIs, which have been proven to be effective and well-tolerated in children and adolescents with depression. However, it has been seen that approximately 31% to 48% of adolescent patients can be non-responsive to them, thereby necessitating close mnitoring and individualized treatment. Second,the potential for side effects, —estimated to happen in up to 25% of patients, —reminds clinicians that they have to weigh benefit and risk when they are thinking about pharmacologic treatment in th The better-growing evidence regarding the effectiveness of other SSRIs, such as, such as sertraline and escitalopram, is also accessible alternatives to use and investigate in the clinic, indicating the evolving face of pediatric psychiatric treatment. Moreover, the contribution of large-scale screening for psychiatric comorbidities cannot be devalued, particularly in adolescents who come with disorders like scoliosis. Results from studies indicate that nearly 58% of these adolescents presenting show anxiety, depression, or body-image disturbance, typically diagnosed after significant delays in distress regarding their underlying disorder. This correlation emphasizes the grave necessity of healthcare providers to implement regular mental health screening among at-risk populations. Treatment of such comorbid conditions not only enhances the overall course of treatment but also optimizes psychosocial benefits for the affected youths. By recognizing the intricate relationship between physical and mental health, practitioners can better tailor interventions to meet individual needs, with the potential to address both the physical and emotional dimensions of the child. This multi-dimensional treatment strategy demonstrates a commitment to building overall wellness in pediatric populations, ultimately enhancing their development and mental wellness throughout the course of their developing years (Figure 7.5).

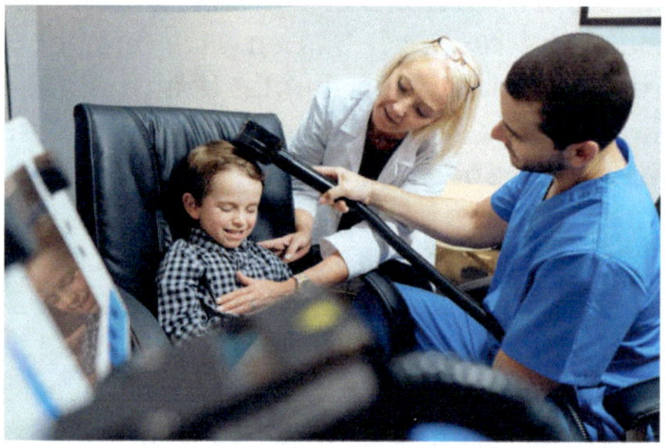

Figure 7.5. The treatment options and interventions for common pediatric psychiatric disorders.

Source: https://dramitvatkar.com/assets/images/services/best-child-neurologist-in-mumbai.jpg.

Test Your Knowledge

1. What are the key symptoms and diagnostic criteria used to identify ADHD in children?
2. How do prevalence rates and demographic factors influence the occurrence of ADHD?
3. What treatment options and interventions are most effective in managing ADHD symptoms?

7.2. Anxiety Disorders

Learning Outcome

1. Types of anxiety disorders in children
2. Signs and symptoms to recognize
3. Therapeutic approaches and coping strategies

Anxiety disorders are a significant area of concern in pediatric psychiatry and affect a high proportion of children and adolescents. They present in the form of excessive worry or fear, which has the potential to disrupt functioning, social interactions, and academic achievement. The increasing prevalence and impact of anxiety disorders among children and adolescents have become significant, particularly in view of the rising trends of these disorders that have been noted in more recent studies. For instance, children with hypermobile Ehlers-Danlos Syndrome (hEDS) provide evidence of a staggering prevalence of anxiety, with research indicating that approximately 80% of them possess at least one or more anxiety diagnoses. It is in this fact that the relationship between body chronic illnesses and psychiatric illnesses is reflected, and it is advised that care givers carefully follow the mental status of children, particularly those who are chronically ill (Amanda et al., 2025). The effect of anxiety disorders extends beyond personal symptomatology, significantly affecting health-relity of life (HRQoL) in children. In examination of various pediatric populations, such as, such as patients with systemic lupus erythematosus (cSLE), clinically significant anxiety has been demonstrated to correlate with lower quality of life scores. In fact, nearly half of the patients in a recent study had significant symptoms of anxiety, indicating the degree to which such disorders may impact overall quality of life. The comorbidities that accompany them generally involve poor academic performance at school, impaired interpersonal relationships, and amplified physical symptoms, thus complicating the impact on both the child and the family as a whole. Treating these issues comprehensively, both medicinally and psychologically, is vital for improving HRQoL outcomes (Duangmala et al., 2025). Effective treatment of pediatric anxiety disorders needs to be multifaceted and multidisciplinary in addressing the unique needs of the child.

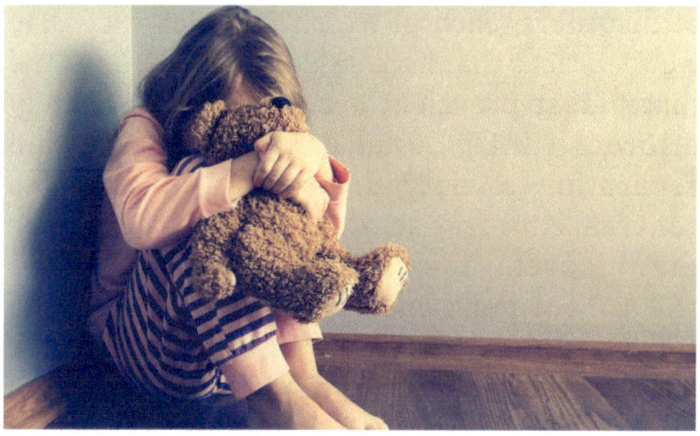

Figure 7.6. Anxiety disorders.

*Source:*https://external content.duckduckgo.com/iu/?u=https%3A%2F%2Fwww.thelist.com%2Fimg%2Fgallery%2Fwhat-it-really-means-when-you-have-separation-anxiety-disorder%2Fsymptoms-of-separation-anxiety-disorder-1658881946.jpg&f=1&nofb=1&ipt=cfafe5f9d53bec116512e708335967d1edee0f755aea04ef3b5c78bc29650dff&ipo=images.

This can involve cognitive-behavioral therapy (CBT), which has proven effective in alleviating symptoms of anxiety, and pharmacotherapy when appropriate. Interdisciplinary close collaboration between mental health professionals, family physicians, and families is essential in developing individualized treatment plans that address not only the psychological issues but also physical health issues related to anxiety disorders in children. This collaborative practice enhances resilience as well as equips children with coping strategies effective for the management of their condition, thus enabling improved emotional and physical health outcomes. Aiming at early intervention and screening can potentially minimize the ill effects of anxiety disorders, ensuring that the development process of the affected children is guided in a positive manner (Amanda et al., 2025) (Figure 7.6).

7.2.1. Types of Anxiety Disorders in Children

Disorders of anxiety in children include a variety of disorders, each of which includes excessive worry or fear that impairs daily functioning. The three most prevalent are generalized anxiety disorder (GAD), social anxiety disorder, and separation anxiety disorder. GAD includes generalized worry across a number of domains that impacts a child's social relationships and school performance. On the other hand, social anxiety disorder involves excessive and intense fear of social interaction, and most often it leads to avoidance behaviors that prevent a child from being able to form friendships and mesh with group activities. Lastly, separation anxiety disorder is marked by excessive and inappropriate fear when the child anticipates or realizes separation from important caregivers, and it can affect both the child's and caregivers' well-being. A knowledge of these specific disorders also better promotes the identification and management of anxiety in pediatric populations. Onset of anxiety disorders in children can occur at various stages of development, which usuallied symptoms for each stage of age. For instance, younger children will manifest behaviorally, such as, such as clinging or tantrums, while older children will be more verbal with their fears and complain about performance or social fears. This line of development highlights the importance of age-specific markers for diagnosis. Untreated childhood anxiety has been demonstrated to have long-term implications, including increased risk for depression and later academic difficulties. Early detection of symptoms lends support to early intervention, which is paramount for effective management. With clinicians noting the developmental context of the anxiety disorders, they can modify interventions that are sensitive to cognitive and affectivto promote better outcomes in children with such disorders. The comorbidity with other diseases, such as, such as headaches, only contributes to the clinical picture. Studies have established a strong correlation between anxiety and migraines in children, with each appearing to exacerbate the other. This comorbidity supports the need for a multi-disciplinary treatment approach. For instance, cognitive-behavioral (CBT) has been useful in alleviating symptoms of anxiety as well as addressing co-morbid issues such as, such as chronic headaches. By impinging on metacognitive processes—strategies for monitoring and the evaluation of one's thoughts—treaters can help children to regulate more effectively anxiety as well as concomitant disorders. Because maladaptive thinking is known to worsen the onset of anxiety as well as headache attacks, treatments aimed at enhancing metacognitiv pivotal in regulating these highly interconnected disorders (Daviss et al., 2017; Calderoni et al., 2017) (Figure 7.7).

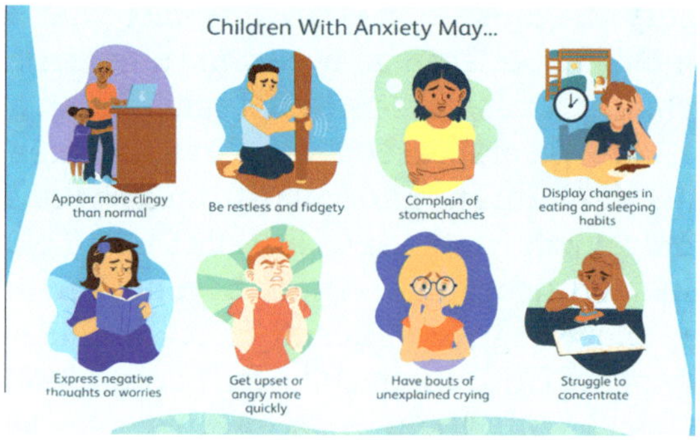

Figure 7.7. Anxiety disorders in children encompass a variety of conditions.

Source: https://s26164.pcdn.co/wp-content/uploads/2022/05/Picture-2.png.

7.2.2. Signs and Symptoms to Recognize

The treatment and detection of early pediatric psychiatric disorders rely on the identification of signs and symptoms of the disorders. Changes in a child's behavior, for example, being more irritable, social withdrawal, or persistently sad, indicate underlying mental health pathology. The behavior is presented with physical signs, for example, appetite or sleep changes, which complicate a child's functioning at home and at school. Experts further underscore the importance of monitoring the behaviors over time rather than forming conclusions based on isolated incidents. Early identification of these signs can lead to consultation with medical professionals at the appropriate time, which could decide the course of the child's mental health and well-being. Pediatric psychiatric disorders also come in various types, based on the type of disorder. For instance, anxiety disorders will present with overanxious worry, restlessness, or avoidance of the feared situation. Mood disorders, however, can manifest pervasive shifts in mood, like mania episodes or extreme depressive periods. Symptoms are relatively dissimilar across developmental phases; young children will express distress through temper tantrums or regression to infantile behavior, while older children will express hopelessness or write about suicide thoughts. Comprehensive assessments are necessary in order to differentiate between normal development and psychiatric disorder, establishing effective treatment strategies. It ought to be remembered also that the manifestation of pediatric psychiatric disorders can differ based on culture and socioeconomic standing. Cultural forces impact perception and symptom expression, such that culturally appropriate means of evaluation and diagnosis are required. For example, in some societies, symptoms of distress will be interpreted in the context of social or family expectations and not in terms of individual psychological problems. Health professionals must observe such differences so that children are not wrongly diagnosed and can be offered proper help. Normalization of mental health conversation and training on symptom recognition among children and caregivers is essential in de-stigmatizing help-seeking for psychiatric disorders, with an eye on better outcomes among children affected (Daniel et al., 2018; Steven et al., 2014).

7.2.3. Therapeutic Approaches and Coping Strategies

Treatment of the complexities of childhood psychiatric disorders typically calls for a mixture of therapeutic interventions and successful coping techniques. Psychosocial therapies play an important role, providing a framework for pediatric patients to control their moods and behaviors. Cognitive Behavioral Therapy (CBT), as a case in point, allows children and adolescents to recognizedify negative patterns of cognition, fostering strength during times of stressors attributed to disorders such as, such as anxiety and depression. Family-focused therapies, on the contrary, not only augment the patients' symptom awareness but also include family members as part of the recovery process, which is highly significant in young populations.

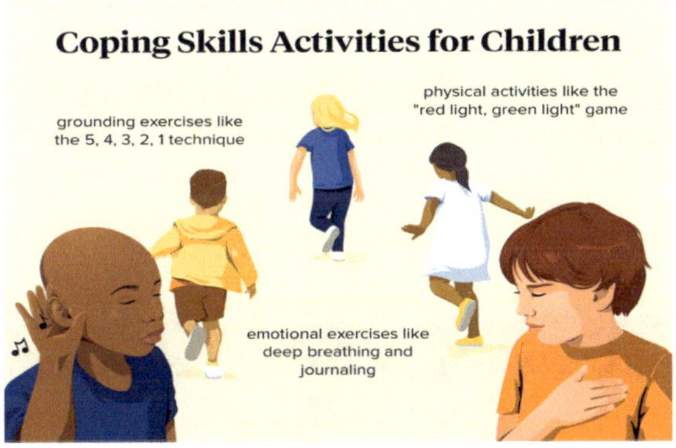

Figure 7.8. The complexities of pediatric psychiatric disorders often necessitates a blend of therapeutic approaches and effective coping strategies.

Source: https://media.post.rvohealth.io/wp-content/uploads/sites/4/2022/06/292262-coping-skills-to-help-kids-manage-stress_1296x1000-1024x790.jpg.

Through communication enhancement and psychoeducation, such therapies solidify the support network needed for achieving outcomes in pediatric patients who are fighting with the load of mental health-related difficulties (Gautam et al., 2019). The use of these modalities in treatment ensures a holistic treatment process, proposing that single use of one modality is insufficient for the treatment of the intricate nature of child psychiatric disorders. Coping skills are ascrucial to help children and adolescents navigate their psyciatric problems. The acquisition of required skills, —i.e., mindfulness, affective regulation, and stress coping, —permits young people to enhance their everyday functioning. Mindfulness therapies are now helpful ways of increasing emotional awareness and decreasing fear so that patients can remain oriented in the here and now. Journal writing, painting, or being physically active may be expressive channels, decreasing symptoms and increasing self-efficing coping skills not only empowers the child but also minimizes the possibility of maladaptive behaviors, such as, such as drug abuse or suicide attempts, emerging as a result of emotional turmoil (Rikinkumar et al., 2018). Additionally, acquiring these skills brings mastery and a sense of responsibility, which contributes to the overall emotional health of the child. While in dire circumstances, pharmacologic treatments can be a necessary intervention, these t utilized when coupled with coping and therapeutic interventions. Treatment most often entails medications such as, such as mood stabilizers or antidepressants, but must be viewed as adjunctive, not single solutions. The risk of side effects and the need for ongoing monitoring are testaments to the need for a balanced treatment plan, in which medication is supplemented by therapy and coping skills. Additional regular monitoring of the efficacy of treatments also allows for prompt revision of individual plans, with maximum therapeutic benefit and minimal risks. Open communication on the part of clinicians with children and families is necessary, with particular significance laid on collaborative treatment decision-making (Gautam et al., 2019). Hence, an integrated model of therapy, coping abilities, and pharmacotherapy ensures that the children not only manage their immediate symptoms but build strengths and functional recovery in order to live a healthier life (Figure 7.8).

Test Your Knowledge

1. What are the main types of anxiety disorders commonly seen in children?
2. What signs and symptoms help in recognizing anxiety disorders in pediatric patients?
3. Which therapeutic approaches and coping strategies are effective in managing childhood anxiety?

7.3. Depression in Children

Learning Outcome

1. Differences between adult and pediatric depression
2. Risk factors and contributing elements
3. Treatment modalities and support systems

Childhood depression, a major etiology of the constellation of common pediatric psychiatric disorders, presents unique challenges both in diagnosis and treatment. Often misdiagnosed or overlooked, childhood depression is marked by many different symptoms including persistent sadness, irritability, and withdrawal from previously pleasurable activities. Interestingly, childhood depression is not merely an extension of adult depression; it is a distinct entity with the capability of hindering cognitive, emotional, and social growth. The etiologic determinants of the disorder range from biological predisposition and environmental influences to psychosocial stressors including family and school pressures. In order to understand these multifaceted aspects is important for both clinicians and caregivers, since early detection and intervention can radically alter the course of the disorder, enabling better outcomes for affected children. Empirical research points out alarming rates of comorbidity between depression and other psychiatric disorders in children. For instance, research indicates that a large proportion of depressed children have co-occurring anxiety disorders, which complicate symptoms and complicate treatment (Amanda et al., 2025). A sleep disorder also frequently co-occurs in pediatric depression, further decreasing overall levels of functioning and quality of life among afflicted children. This synergism again confirms the importance of taking an integrated assessment approach in evaluating children for depression. Clinical researchers are challenged to explore the broad spectrum of mental disorders that may coexist with depression, thereby modifying treatments aimed at both primary and comorbid conditions. Moreover, the chronicity of these comorbidities will prolong suffering, suggesting an interest in mental health care for this vulnerable population. Families and physicians must be made aware of the long-term implications of untreated depression in children. As young people and adults, unresolved depressive symptoms can lead to significant impairment in academic performance, interpersonal relationships, and general level of functioning (Nevra et al., 2024). The chronic course of depression in children not only affects the patient but also families and communitiecally in the form of increased healthcare costs and lost productivity. Interventions targeting depressive symptoms such as, such as cognitive-behavioral therapy and family support, have been shown to prevent such risks effectively. Therefore, community awareness about pediatric depression, in addition to engagement with prevention activities, is very important. Together, the empowerment of mental health care systems can assist in fostering children's resilience in coping with such issues and engendering healthier development patterns (Figure 7.9).

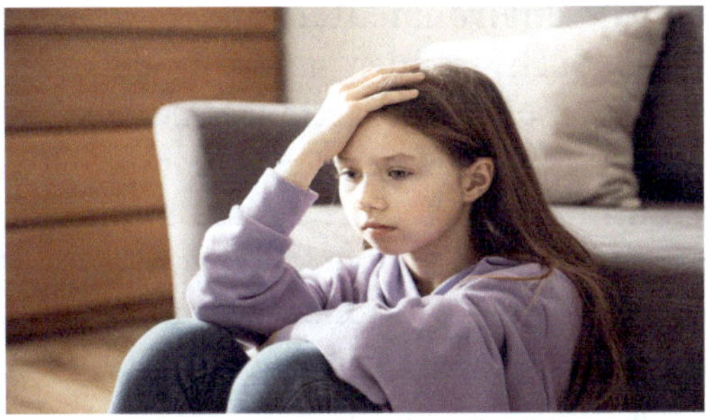

Figure 7.9. Depression in children.

Source: https://external-content.duckduckgo.com/iu/?u=https%3A%2F%2Fwww.news4teachers.de%2Fwp-content% 2Fuploads%2Fshutterstock_2152037855_Depres sion-scaled.jpg&f=1&n ofb=1&ipt=fb043979c74dddd84ab4a9cac9c08c d10ee934fb6650f08c174ef3cf170e637e&ipo=images.

7.3.1. Differences Between Adult and Pediatric Depression

The distinction between child and adult depression reflects significant differences in presentation, diagnosis, and treatment protocols. In adults, depression presents with pervasiveness of sadness, anhedonia, and deficits in cognitive function, with fatigue or insomnia contributing to functional impairment in both work and social fung. Pediatric depression, by contrast, presents with emotional dysregulation, conduct issues, and somatic complaints such as, such as stomachaches or headaches with no medical cause. Children can also present variation in school performance and interpersonal relationships that is different from adult presentation. Such differences in presentation call for adaptable methods of evaluation, given the fact that pediatric patients cannot articulate sadness as adults do, thereby complicating accurate diagnosis and possibly risking missed or misdiagnosed disease (Jacob et al., 2023). Furthermore, the period of development has a determining impact on the aetiology of depression among children versus adults. In adolescence, the develodepression tends to be linked to a complex interaction between biological, environmental, and psychosocial variables, such as, such as hormonal changes and interpersonal interactions. Adults similarly can have an equivalent level of complexity, but contributions of prior life events and situation stressors generally play a larger role. Most important are variations in the expression and elicitation of depressive symptoms, with adults perhaps ruminating on negative thoughts and children displaying irritability, anger, or withdrawal. This diversity calls for context-sensitive intervention. Pediatric models of treatment, including therapy with developmental level adaptations, may be better than the typical adult treatment regimens, particularly calling for age-specific therapeutic interventions (Daniel et al., 2018). Finally, comorbid di are another factor that separates adult and child depression. In adults, there tends to be a comorbid chronic illness such as, such as cardiovascular disease, whereas in children, depression occurs with anxiety disorders, ADHD, or developmental disorders. These disorders complicate treatment and necessitate multidimensional assessment and treatment strategies. Family relationships can also be influenced by child depression, with the pressure placing added burdens upon the child's state. Therefore, valuing these differences is crucial not just for enhanced diagnostic standards but also for enhancement of treatment outcomes and comprehension of the overall implications of depression throughout a person's life. The psychologic and emotional management of families dealing with pediatric depression needs to be included as part of an overall treatment strategy, taking into account the well-being of the child and the caregivers of the child (Jacob et al., 2023) (Figure 7.10).

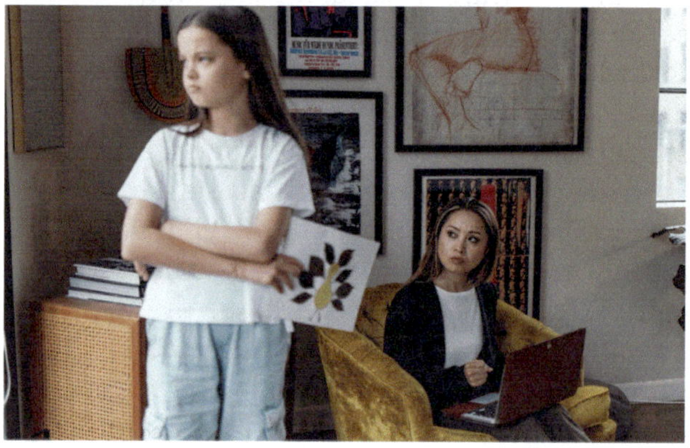

Figure 7.10. Child in a therapy session, highlighting emotional evaluation in pediatric mental health.

Source: https://bhatiapsychology.com/wp-content/uploads/2021/09/Depression-kids-vs-adults.png.

7.3.2. Risk Factors and Contributing Elements

The information regarding pediatric psychiatric disorders is also enhanced by research into causative factors and risk factors that control such disorders. The most important contributors among them are environment poisons, whose harmful effects on mental health are increasingly well established. Heavy metal exposure, including cadmium and lead, is a factor that causes cognitive impairment and behavioral issues in children. These heavy metals have a tendency to settle on land and plants, thereby impacting human systems when ingested, thereby enhancing their ability to induce psychiatric disorders (Alengebawy et al., 2021). How these environmental stressors combine with biological vulnerabilities provides a good starting point for beginning an understanding of the etiology behind psychiatric challenges noticed in children, highlighting the role of critical assessment and intervention strategies. Apart from environmental factors, family and interpersonal relationships play significant roles in the causation of pediatric psychiatric disorders. Children who are raised in less stable family environments, e.g., abuse, neglect, or domestic violence, are at greater risk for developing a variety of psychologic ailments, including anxiety disorders and depression. Social support systems play a role too; those children who do not receive proper emotional and social support can show an enhanced vulnerability to mental health issues. In addition, the effect of social events, including the COVID-19 pandemic, also underlined how stressors in the form of illness and confinement worsened the pre-existing mental health issues of pediatric populations. Children have been found to be particularly vulnerable in states of crisis, where a lack of routine and social interaction can manifest as heightened anxiety and emotional distress (Muller et al., 2020). This speaks to the complexity of risk factors for pediatric mental health. Examination of genetic predisposition further adds one layer of complexity to understanding pediatric psychiatric disorders. Research shows that individuals with a family history of mental illness have a higher chance of also developing such problems. It is possible that genetic factors combine with adversity in the environment, as when a person is exposed to toxicants or there is stress in the home, to give a synergistic effect. This intersectionality emphasizes the importance of understanding both genetic and environmental factors in assessing the development pathways of children. It is essential for effective prevention and intervention to adopt a multi-disciplinary, holistic focus that targets these diverse risk factors. By doing so, clinicians, caregivers, and policymakers can create more effective strategies that consider not only individual vulnerabilities but also the broader social and environmental settings that influence pediatric mental health outcomes (Alengebawy et al., 2021).

7.3.3. Treatment Modalities and Support Systems

The treatment interventions for child psychiatric illness consist of numerous evidence-based interveno deal with the multi-component nature of the illnesses. Behavioral therapy remains a cornerstone and works best with illnesses such as, such as ADHD and the anxiety disorders. Treatment aims at modifying some of the behaviors through reinforcement and modeling. Cognitive-behavioral therapy (CBT) is also highly popular, employing strategies to help children and adolescents recognize and modify automatic thought patterns, ultimately resulting in improved emotional responses. Medication, including stimulants and selective serotonin reuptake inhibitors, may be utilized with some disorders for symptom relief in combination with therapy. Together, these modalities constitute an integrative model that individually targets the personal needs of each child patient, in order to maximize the potential for positive outcomes. Support systems also play a pivotal role in successful management of pediatric psychiatric disorders, extending beyond actual clinical treatments. Family involvement is paramount; for instance, psychoeducation informs families about the nature of the child's disorder, allowing them to support their child effectively. Support groups can also establish coping and resilience in peers with similar issues, enhance social networks and emotional support, support a sense of belonging, and provide a voice to be heard.

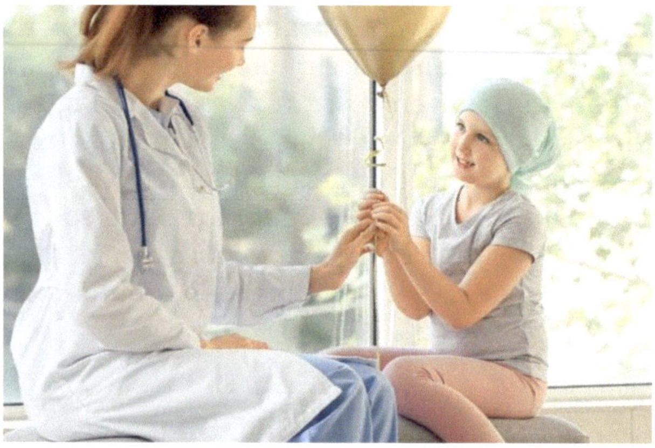

Figure 7.11. Doctor comforting a young pediatric cancer patient during treatment.

Source: https://tischbraintumorcenter.duke.edu/sites/default/files/styles/3_2_small/public/2024-02/hero-child.jpg?itok=tbkbw44t/.

Schools are a part of this network, implementing IEPs and accommodations that address individualized student needs for psychiatric disorders. School programs focusing on mental health awareness and destigmatization can minimize anxiety and encourage students to seek help. These collaborative interventions among schools, mental health professionals, and families target an integratitment approach. Availability of stable treatment modalities as well as systems of support is particularly critical within settings such as, such as pediatric intensive care units (PICUs) where kids are likely to encounter acute psychiatric struggles. Evidence exists for the immense impact of neurological disease on the psychiatric health of children in critical care, with anxiety and depression rates at the time of discharge becoming increasingly alarming (Khanal et al., 2023). Further, those subsets of adolescents involved in the juvenile jsystem have significant levels of psychiatric disorder, wi being highly common and linked to adverse outcomes such as, such as emotional dysregulation (Alengebawy et al., 2021Levenson et al., 2022). Thus, psychiatric treatment of such vulnerable populations needs to be based on a structured system under which proper treatment modalities are integrated with comprehensive support systems so that children not only get clinical care but also emotional and social care so that they can recover and rejoin their communities (Figure 7.11).

Test Your Knowledge

1. How does depression in children differ from depression in adults in terms of symptoms and presentation?
2. What are the major risk factors and contributing elements that lead to depression in children?
3. What treatment modalities and support systems are effective in helping children with depression?

7.4. Autism Spectrum Disorder (ASD)

Learning Outcome

1. Characteristics and spectrum of symptoms
2. Early signs and the importance of early intervention
3. Educational and therapeutic resources available

ASD is a heterogeneous group of neurodevelo pmental conditions that impact the social, communication, and behavioral lives of a child. The prevalence of ASD has been rising steadily, necessitating timely action by families and healthcare providers alike to respond suitably to the special needs of this condition. Assessing such an understanding is central to the importance attached to early diagnosis, ideally at 18 to 24 months of age, since it enables early intervention. According to studies, after an accurate diagnosis is achieved for the child, tailored interventions combining educational, behavioral, and pharmacological approaches can have significant benefits. Prioritizing family-centered care enhances the quality of experience for both the child and the family to have a supportive setting in which the different aspects of ASD-related behaviors can be addressed, hence promoting better integration into society (Bultas et al., 2016). ASD behavioral symptoms can even pose additional challenges in medical encounters. The majority of children with ASD are highly anxious and stressed, particularly when placed in new or overwhelming environments, making it challenging to provide health care. Families and health care providers must be provided with effective strategies to facilitate interaction. An example is prior measures taken that inform anticipated procedures, which can minimize anxiety, allowing children to navigate health care spaces more smoothly. Furthermore, identification of the individual sensory sensitivities prevalent in most instances of ASD enables professionals to create supportive environments, which in turn reduces incidences of challenging behaviors. In creating a hospitable environment sensitive to the needs of individualistic children with ASD, health care professionals enable more positive experience that not only considers medical needs but also respects the emotional and psychological subtleties of the condition (Bultas et al., 2016).

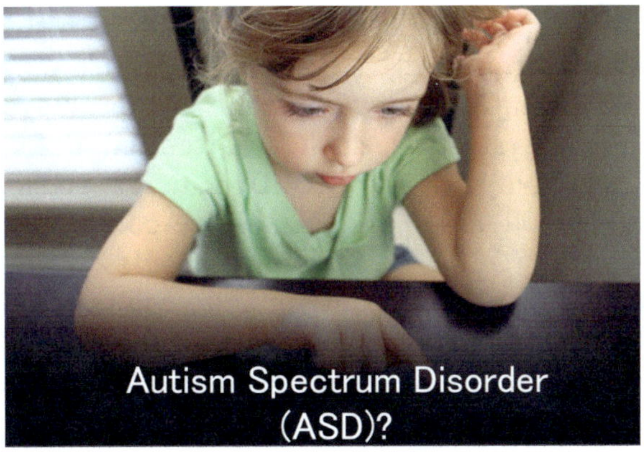

Figure 7.12. Autism spectrum disorder.

Source: https://external-content.duckduckgo.com/iu/?u=https%3A%2F%2Fspeechtherapycentres.com%2Fwp-content%2Fuploads%2F2019%2F10%2Fasd.jpg&f=1&nofb=1&ipt=df6db74a64d0facc67428028cb14bfb47e5916db5a8034e24d7831fe0c172a99&ipo=images.

Recent interventions of the different symptoms of ASD have shown promising outcomes. One of these is the utilization of multi-sensory environments (MSE), which are specially designed to provide individualized sensory experiences that can regulate the levels of anxiety and increase physiological responses among children with ASD. A study demonstrated that MSE was effective in reducing anxiety with evidence indicating that treatment needs to be customized so as to address the diverse needs of each child. The approach highlights the need to accommodate sensory to treatment in consideration of differences, thereby enhancing therapeutic potential. Physiological measures in such interventions, such as, such as electrodermal response, confirm the imperative of creating conducive and engaging environments that trigger healthy neurodevelopmental reactions from ASD children (Figure 7.12).

7.4.1. Characteristics and Spectrum of Symptoms

The characteristics and set of symptoms of common pediaychiatric disorders may be highly varied, significantly impacting children's daily functioning and development. Symptoms of disorders such as, such as attention deficit hyperactivity disorder (ADHD), autism spectrum disorder (ASD), and obsessive-compulsive disorder (OCD) have distinct profiles. ADHD symptoms predominantly manifest in the form of inattention, hyperactivity, and impulsivity, which commonly translate to academic and social problems. Contrarily, ASD is characterized by social communication impairments and the presence of repetitive or restricted behaviors. The symptomatology calls for varied therapeutic intervention according to the needs of each disorder. It is extremely important to understand these differences to enable early intervention and diagnosis that can greatly improve a child's quality of life. The subtle nature of these disorders helps clinicians and caregivers respond to particular needs, creating even more nurturing environments for afflicted children. Additionally, the symptom constellation of pediatric psychiatric disorders generally overlaps, resulting in complicated clinical presentations that destroy diagnostic integrity. Comorbidities are especially common, with children simultaneously harboring multiple disorders complicating the treatment paradigm. For instance, an ADHD-diagnosed child will have symptoms characteristic of anxiety as well, which in turn influence behavioral outcomes and responsiveness to treatments. Effective management of these comorbid symptoms has been proposed through research as a multifaceted process that includes the use of behavioral therapies, social skills training, and pharmacologic interventions when necessary. The intricate interaction of symptoms demonstrates the utility of an integrated assessment process that enables clinicians to differentiate between primary and comorbid conditions efficiently. Such discrimination is at the core of the development of empathetic and effective care plans that will be appropriate for evolving developmental needs of children. Recent evidence has emphasized the influence of environmental and social changes on the worsening of psychiatric symptoms in adolescents. The COVID-19 pandemic id example; it has been associated with a marked increase in sudden onset complex tic-like phenomena in teens, particularly on platforms such as, such as TikTok, in which exposure to the condition can induce mimicry and increased symptom occurrence among vulnerable youths. The implications of this trend extend far beyond tic disorders because it suggests that the media landscape can have an extraordinary influence on the mental health landscape for children. Being aware of these emergent trends is critical for clinicians intent on adapting treatment modalities to effectively respond to emergent happenings. Monitoring the trends and tendencies of pediatric health will allow ccare plans, particularly in the face of a constantly evolving social setting (Alengebawy et al., 2021Pringsheim et al., 2021; Nehme et al., 2020).

7.4.2. Early SIGNs and Importance of Early Intervention

It is crucial in successful intervention and management to detect early signs of pediatric psychiatric disorders. Mood swings, social withdrawal, or sudden changes in school performance could be warning signs for underlying psychological conditions. Current research suggests that early detection, especially during the developmental milestones of childhood and adolescence, permits early intervention, and eventually, better long-term outcomes. It is vital that caregivers and teachers recognize these signs since young children are not necessarily able to communicate their emotions. By creating an open communication environment, adults can facilitate emotional distress to be expressed by children, which usually is experienced behaviorally more than verbally. The failure in early identification will lead to full-blown disorders, making the treatment more complicated and less effective in the reversal of the psychiatric disorders course in children. Early identification intervention strategies can actually reverse the pediatric psychiatric disorders course by far. Early intervention by way of therapy, behavioral modification, and effective medication can reduce the risks of long-term illnesses. For instance, application of combined care models using multidisciplinary teams assures that children are treated as a whole, not only addressing the psychological aspect but also the social and family life engaged. Effective early intervention has the potential to greatly enhance both the quality of family and child life as well as ongoing psychosocial assessment. Screening tests and routine evaluations can be proactive, allowing medical practitioners to monitor not only symptomatology, but also adaptive functioning and family stressors that have the potential to exacerbate mental health disorders. Integration of psychosocial care into routine pediatric practice is important, as it provides the groundwork for more positive outcomes in adolescents who are affected. Lastly, family and caregiver participation is central to early intervention. Inclusion of parents in treatment is important for the acquisition of healthful coping skills and healthy behavioral change in the home setting. Family psychoeducation about signs and symptoms of child psychiatric disorders allows earlier identification and appropriate help-seeking by family members. Home strengthening promotes increasence of children to cope with their problems as well as improved coping skills. Therapeutic interventions that address family functioning, such as, such as treatment interventions that ease the burden on parents, can lead to better overall mental health of the child. It has been established through research that distressed families are less resilient but more capable of providing support towards effective psychiatric treatment in children, hence a bidirectional approach addressing parental and child problems alike being imperative. Incorporating family-oriented models of care is essential to ensure interventions are viable and effective in tial intersection between early signs of distress and the effectiveness of early intervention strategies (Maartje et al., 2022; Marilyn et al., 2022Lopes et al., 2020) (Figure 7.13).

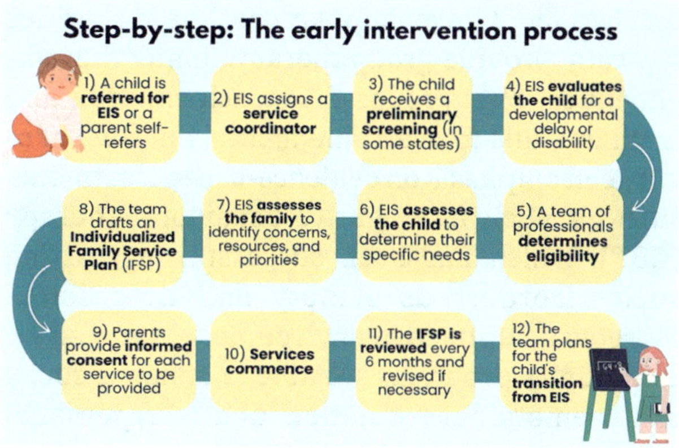

Figure 7.13. Early signs and the importance of early intervention.

Source: https://static.wixstatic.com/media/246537_7c0d285adf2f4a32824e7831910d3160~mv2.jpg/v1/fill/w_980,h_653,al_c,q_85,usm_0.66_1.00_0.01,enc_avif,quality_auto/246537_7c0d285adf2f4a32824e7831910d3160~mv2.jpg.

7.4.3. Educational and Therapeutic Resources Available

Access to educational and therapeutic interventions is critical in managing common pediatric psychiatric disorders. Schools are an essential part of this by integrating mental health professionals into their structures, which enables early identification and treatment of children who are exhibiting psychological distress. These mental health professionals often collaborate with teachers and parents to facilitate supportive schools that enhance child resilience and coping competencies. Moreover, Individualized Education Programs (IEPs) and 504 Plans serve as blueprints to provide individualized accommodations to ensure child with a psychiatric disorder receives the necessary accommodations for academic success. Engaging in school-based mental health care allows for students to access evidence-based interventions and counseling to achieve emotional while facilitating learning simultaneously. Beyond school intervention, community agencies offer extensive therapeutic services for childrenpopulations. These agencies typically provide group therapy, family therapy, ahoeducational groups that teach children and families skills to overcome mental illness. There is a keen emphasis on evidence-based treatments such as, such as cognitive-behavioral therapy (CBT), which has been successful in treating such disorders as anxiety and depression. Moreover, supportive environments created by community programs are able to enhance social skills, emotional regulation, and interpersonal relationships. Interagency coordination between schools, community agencies, and families is essential to ensuring a continuum of care that deals with the complexity of pediatric psychiatric disorders. Finally, the potential of technology to provide teaching and therapy materials should not be overlooked. Telehealth websites have emerged as primary sources for the provision of mental health services, particularly t settings. With the help of online counseling and therapy sessions, children are able to get assistance in time, thereby eliminating constraints such as, such as travel and stigma of seeking assistance. Further, online resources and apps for learning are auxiliary tools for parents and children to educate themselves regarding mental health and acquire coping skills. With continued advancement of digital resources, they create new opportunities for new forms of engaging children themselves in their own mental health treatment, which becomes increasingly consistent with the broader trend toward accessible and individualized treatment methods. This blending of technology ultimately results in a more comprehensive method of treating most prevalent pediatric psychiatric disorders.

Test Your Knowledge

1. What are the key characteristics and range of symptoms seen across the autism spectrum?
2. Why is recognizing early signs of ASD and providing early intervention important for child development?
3. What educational and therapeutic resources are available to support children with Autism Spectrum Disorder?

7.5. Oppositional Defiant Disorder (ODD)

Learning Outcome

1. Definition and key features of ODD
2. Relationship with other behavioral disorders
3. Strategies for management and support

ODD is a prevalent and significant problem in pediatric psychiatric disorders, whose influence extends beyond the individual child to family, school, and social systems. Characterized by a pattern of angry, irritable mood, argumentative and vindictive behavior, and resistance to complying with rules, children with ODD are likely to manifest those challenging behaviors, which disrupt their functioning across settings. The development of ODD is influenced by a complex interaction among genetic, environmental, and psychosocial factors and therefore requires that clinicians and caregivers adopt an integratedstic and intervention approach. Early identification is crucial as untreated ODD can become more severe behavioral disorders or comorbid disorders such as, such as Attention-Deficit/Hyperactivity Disorder (ADHD) or anxiety disorders and therefore the need for multidisciplinary management and treatment. Research indicates that ODD children are likely to display significant deficits in executive functions, as evidenced in research that employed advanced neuroimaging techniques. For example, resting-state fMRI was employed in one study to examine alterations in the brain complexity of ADHD, ODD, and OCD children (Zhang et al., 2025). This research highlighted common impairments of the cool and hot executive function networks, and it revealed that children with ODD exhibited reduced neural complexity in regions typically associated with impulse control and emotion regulation. These results not only inform the neurological underpinnings of ODD but also suggest that treatment approaches focused on enhancing executive functioning can quite effectively assist the afflicted children, ultimately leading to improved social relationships and coping strategies. Secondly, the ecological environment plays a significant role in expressing and developing ODD symptoms. Systematic reviews have indicated that children who come from environments of aggressive communication or parental conflict are at higher risk of developing ODD (Sousa et al., 2024). This relationship highlights the importance of considering system factors when creating intervention strategies. Behavioral therapy programs, parental training, and family therapy have been found to have powerful impact on managing ODD behavior, especially when the entire family is targeted. By developing a stable and safe environment, parents are capable of decreasing considerably oppositional behavior, thereby demonstrating that preventable actions and adaptive interventions can form resilient patterns of children predisposed to developing ODD and other related disorders (Figure 7.14).

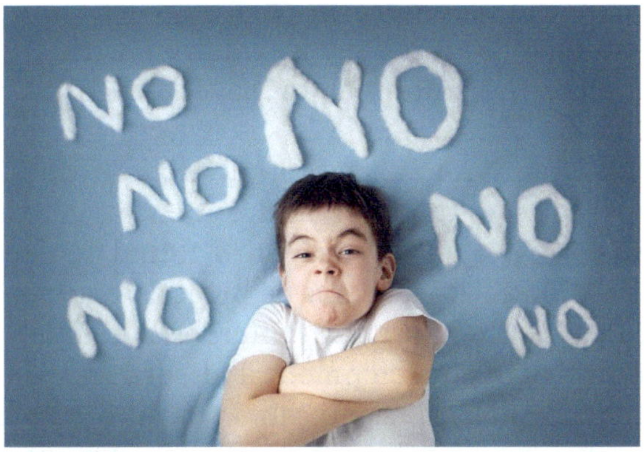

Figure 7.14. Oppositional defiant disorder (ODD).

Source: https://external-content.duckduckgo.com/iu/?u=https%3A%2F%2Fwww.psychologistehsaas.com%2Fwp-content%2Fuploads%2F2022%2F09%2F52382220_m.jpg&f=1&nofb=1&ipt=a84322b84f949c29dbe71fa61c908a7d89b79d4763c93a82a0a43de3500b8d08&ipo=images.

7.5.1. Definition and Key Features of ODD

ODD is a prevalent psychiatric disorder in children with a history of angry, irritable moomentative behavior, and vindictiveness. ODD typically manifests early in childhood and includes impacting a child's function across various settings such as, such as home and school. Defiant behaviors toward authority are typical in children with ODD and can render interpersonal relationships challenging and even lead to academic underachievement. This disorder is not a phase of development but rather a clinical condition that can interfere with social development and individual development. Remarkably, the defining characteristics of ODD can manifest differently in various individuals, which suggests the necessity for exhaustive assessments to identify the level and impact of the disorder on the child's everyday functioning. A complete comprehension of ODD requires a recognition of its co-morbidity with other child psychiatric disorders, in particular irritability. Irritability is prevalent in children with ODD and has the potential to have a significant effect on functioning, just as it does in other conditions, for example, attention deficit hyperactivity disorder and autism spectrum disorder. Irritability has been found to have the potential to become a pivotal feature of ODD, thus complicating differential diagnosis among neurodevelopmental disorders. This intersectionality is significant in terms of raising issues regarding the nature of such symptoms and their implication for treatment strategies. Clinicians should recognize the frequency of irritability in children with ODD, and its trajectory can illuminate risks for anxiety and conduct disorders in adulthood and inform early intervention as well as improve long-term outcomes in targeted children (Leibenluft et al., 2024). Treatment for ODD is typically a combination of behavior treatment and family therapy to reduce oppositional behavior and increase emotional control. Parent management training has been effective, teaching caregivers how to respond to defiant behavior and increase the positive parent-child relationship. Because of the multidimensional presentation of ODD, treatment is formulated based on the individual's needs, considering such factors as co-occurring conditions and specific behavioral challenges. Despite the challenge, effective intervention can decrease symptoms and improve functioning, expanding the child's social and academic possibilities. Ongoing controversy regarding the differences between different neurodevelopmental disorders emphasizes the difficulty in diagnosing and treating ODD and makes evident that additional research and more development of interventions recognizing the overlapping but non-equivalent characteristics of different pediatric psychiatric disorders are required (Bonti et al., 2024).

7.5.2. Relationship with Other Behavioral Disorders

The interaction between general child psychiatric disorders and other behavior disorders is comd bidirectional. For instance, children diagnosed with attention-deficit/hyperactivity disorder (ADHD) are likely to have co-existing behavioral issues such as, such as ODD or CD. Such comorbid conditions may complicate diagnosis and treament because symptoms can overap extensively, leading to misdiagnosis or under-treatment of the primary condition. Since there are so many children with ADHD; —at a rate of 10% of children; —the necessity for full evaluations is important to see if there are any other disorders of behavior. Early intervention and tailored treatment modalities for both ADHD and concomitant behavioral d improved outcomes and life quality for the youth involved, highlighting the necessity to consider these relationships in clinical practice (Maartje et al., 2022Panc., 2020). The overlap between pediatric psychiatric disorders and anxiety disorders is a factor of concern here as well. Children with chronic illnesses, such as, such as diabetes, are more likely to experience high anxiety and stress levels, which may exacerbate any underlying psychiatric conditions or create new behavioral issues. This has placed a significant onus on screening for anxiety in children with established psychiatric diagnoses. Studies have identified that up to 32% of children with diabetes could also exhibit symptoms of anxiety, which would negatively impact their self-management and glycemic control.

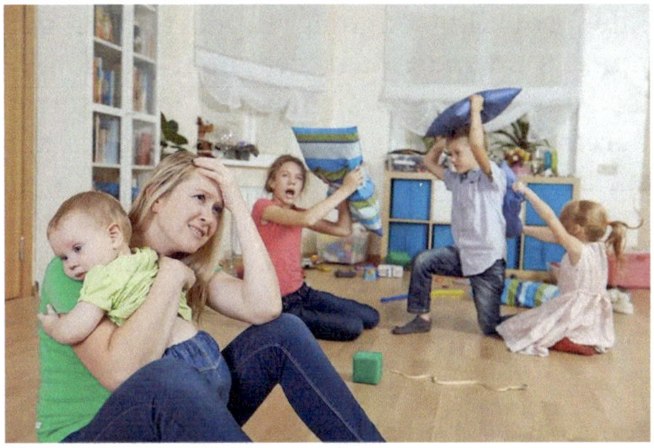

Figure 7.15. The relationship between common pediatric psychiatric disorders and other behavioral disorders is complex and multifaceted.

Source: https://cdn.cdnparenting.com/articles/24207/216207325-1024x700.webp.

Therefore, detecting these interactions becomes crucial in the development of multidisciplinary intervg psychological care along with medical management, ultimately aiming at integrated care centered on both mental illness and chronic disease (Marilyn et al., 2022Lopes et al., 2020). Finally, the tie-in between pediatric psychiatric disease and eating disorders is a significant area of in terms of prevalence and consideration of treatment. Research indicates that diabetic youths and children are at a higher risk of having eating disorders, such as, such as anorexia nervosa or bulimia, particularly when mental health issues, e.g., depression and anxiety, are present. These relationships involve a complex cross-talk of psychosocial processes, including family dynamics, self-concept, and the demands of a chronic disease existence. The consequent disordered eating behavior has the potential to cause significant health issues, including impaired metabolic control and increased risk of diabetic ketoacidosis (DKA). It is thus important that clinicians conduct routine screening for disordered eatingn affected psychiatrically and that medical and psychological management is integrated and responsive to the unique circumstances of each child (Maartje et al., 2022Panchal et al., 2020) (Figure 7.15).

7.5.3. Strategies for Management and Support

A multisystem model of pediatric psychiatric disorder management is paramount in order toto attain the best outcomes for the involved children. Among the fundamental approaches is the coming together of interdisciplinary teams comprising pediatricians, mental health specialists, and relatives. Interdisciplinary working allows for a holistic perspective of the child's condition, tackling biological, psychological, and social concerns in accordance with the biopsychosocial paradigm. Age-appropriate, evidence-based measures in such teams are important to monitor children's quality of life and psychosocial functioning. Regular screening may enable early referral for mental health treatment when needed, particularly in the case of a substantial transition, e.g., diagnosis or adolescence. This anticipatory treatme enhance resilience in children so they are able to successfully overcome complex emotional and behavioral problems associated with their disorders (Maartje et al., 2022Panchal et al., 2020). In addition to clinical interventions, education and support of parents also play a crucial role in the management of pediatric psychiatric disorders. Parents consistently suffer from high degrees of stress as they navigate the intricacies of their children's mental health needs; hence, preparing them with tools and coping mechanisms is paramount. Parent services that offer psychosocial support will decrease parents' stress levels, which will, in turn, have a positive effect on their children's behavioral and emotional outcomes. Parental active engagement in care can also enhance treatment plan compliance and foster a therapeutic home environment. Through the acquisition of adaptive coping mechanisms and the treatmentviors, caregivers are better able to deal with their child's uniqes, towards better clinical compliance and enhanced agency within the family (Marilyn et al., 2022Lopes et al., 2020). The application of evidence-based treatment such as, such as cognitive-behavioral therapy (CBT) and family therapyalso constitutes a critical method in the management of child psychiatric illnesses. These models of therapy not only give children the coping skills they need to survive, but also improve family dynamics through improved problem-solving and communication. Research indicates that therapies that involve working with parents and addressing cithin the household are most likely to produce positive outcomes for children with mental illness. Also, with the addition of the use of technology in the industry, such as, such as telehealth services and mental health apps, can make the treatment more accessible while providing ongoing support. This dual emphasis on individual treatment and family-based interventions signals the impo setting wherein emotional growth and resilience may flourish, ultimately providing youth with the capacity to more effectively manage their conditions (Maartje et al., 2022Panchal et al., 2020).

Test Your Knowledge

1. What is Oppositional Defiant Disorder (ODD), and what are its key behavioral features?
2. How is ODD related to or differentiated from other behavioral disorders such as ADHD or Conduct Disorder?
3. What strategies and support approaches are effective in managing and treating children with ODD?

7.6. Eating Disorders

Learning Outcome

1. Common types of eating disorders in children
2. Psychological and physical implications
3. Treatment approaches and family involvement

Among pediatric psychiatric illnesses, eating disorders represent a complesection of sociocultural, biological, and psychological factors that powerfully affect the quality of life and health of adolescents. The development of eating disorderssuch as, such as anorexia nervosa, bulimia nervosa, and binge eating disorder, is markedly increased in adolescents with chronic illnesses, particularly diabetes. Research indicates that type 1 diabetes subjects have an increased risk for clinical and eating disordered eating disorders, and incidence rates are significantly higher than those in non-diabetic subjects. For instance, data from studies indicate that as high as 30–50% of female young adolescents with type 1 diabetes have the ability to participate in eating disordered behavior, like insulin manipulation as a method of caloric restriction. This intersection underscores the imperative for medical professionals to adopt a vigilant and integrated approach that monitors eating patterns while simultaneously addressing underlying diseases, thereby reaffirming the inseparable link between physical and mental health (Panchal et al., 2020). Adolescence represents a particularly vulnerable period, characterized by profound physiological and psychological changes that significantly contribute to the onset of various psychiatric conditions, including eating disorders.During this phase of transition, adolescents struggle with body development, peer pressure, and internalized societal pressures for body ideal and weight, all of which are variables that can reinforce or precipitate disordered eating behaviors. Notably, the double burden of chronic disease can complicate these already fragile psychosocial processes to produce maladaptive coping processes that include disordered eating. In adolescents with diabetes, the need to manage glycemia imposes further pressure on eating habits, resulting in deleterious practices to achieve perceived beauty standards of slenderness or acceptance. Hence, understanding the excellent interconnection of these factors brings about the need for integrated models of care that address diabetes management and the pogical nature of eating disorders (John et al., 2022). The impact of eating disorders extends further than temporary health effects, with considerable long-term consequences which that could affect physical and emotional well-being. In dren and adolescents, ill-managed eating patave significant complications, including diabetic ketoacidosis and long-term vascular complications. Additionally, the psychologicalpsychological weight of eating disorders — such as, such as body dissatisfaction, low self-esteem, and increased depression and anxiety — contributes to the intricacy of treatment outcomes and quality of life. Multidisciplinary care strategies that include counseling on diet, psychotherapy, and family support are important in managing the complex aetiology of eating disorders in these individuals. By concentrating on a multidisciplinary practice, health practitioners can better screen for and treat mental health problems associated with eating ddevelop healthier coping strategies as well as enhance the resilience of adolescents grappling with the complexities of maintaining their mental and physical health (Maartje et al., 2022Panchal et al., 2020) (Figure 7.16).

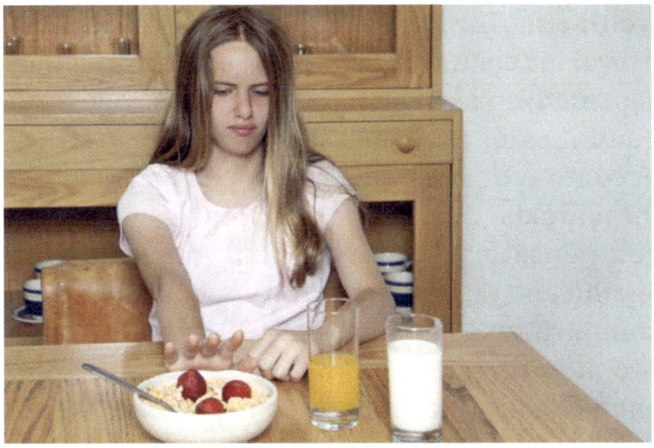

Figure 7.16. Child showing signs of food aversion, indicating a possible eating disorder.

Source: https://external-content.duckduckgo.com/iu/?u=https%3A%2F%2Fwww.indiancrestpeds.com%2Fwp-content%2Fuploads%2F2021%2F04%2FEating-Disorders-in-Kids-scaled-e1617774508653.jpg&f=1&nofb=1&ipt=298c22df2fc240698bfefc36f2a68dffa6580a6f1c087d03586067ece2776829.

7.6.1. Common Types of Eating Disorders in Children

Among pediatric psychiatric conditions, eating disorders are a serious concern, particularly because they are closely linked with physical and mental health. The most prevalent eating disorders among children are anorexia nervosa, bulimia nervosa, and eating disorder with binge. Anorexia nervosa is characterized by morbid fear of gaining weight and distorted body image, which entails extreme avoidance of food. This condition poses significant health risks, causing growth issues and severe malnutrition. Bulimia nervosa, on the other hand, is typified by flip-flopping cycles of purging and bingeing as a means of weight control, with purging activities involving self-induced vomiting or excessive exercise. These conditions not only have physical consequences but also intensely impact mood, with children generally struggling with anxiety and depression, making it critical to identify and treat them to avoid long-term effects on their well-being. Binge eating disorder is another prevalent eat among children, characterized by repeated episodes of eating excessively large quantities of food, marked by a feeling of loss of control. Unlike bulimia, binge eating disorder individuals do not participate in recurrent compensatory behavior and may develop significant weight gain and associated health complications due to obesity. Most importantly, the identification of binge eating disorder should take place early since children can develop shamnd emotional turmoil from their consumption and tend to keep such incidents a secret from caregivers. The rising incidence of these disorders can also be attributed, to a certain extent, by to social and cultural influences, like media portrayal of ideal body image and increased pressure on children to conform to these. Research shows that increased knowledge on eating disorders is needed among parents, educators, and healthcare professionals for early intervention istance. Moreover, co-morbidity of eating disorders with other psychiatric disorders is especially disturbing. Children with eating disorders most often co-exist with other conditions such as, such as depression, anxiety, and attention-deficit/hyperactivity disorder (ADHD)ich makes the clinical picture complex and difficult to treat. The interrelatedness of these conditions emphasizes the need for a combination treatment plan addressing both psychiatric and also someds. Partin pediatric environments need to be highly attentive to the monitoring of indicators of eating disorders, as they may develop alongside chronic diseases such as, such as diabetes mellitus type 1type 1 diabetes mellitus (T1D). As pediatric patients with T1D may also exhibit eating disordered habits, combined care from pediatric practitioners, mental health clinicians beneficial coping abilities further deterioration of physical and mental health, as noth on the emotional impact of chronic illness (Goldstein, 2023; Meadows et al., 2020Lopes et al., 2020).

7.6.2. Psychological and Physical Implications

In researching the psychological and physical impact of common pediatric psychiatric diseases, one must value the interrelatedness of mental and physical health. Teens with diseasess, such as diabetes, depression, and anxiety are likely to experience an additive effect in whichlpsychological stress over physical diseases. Chronically diseased children are at a higher risk of developing psychiatric illness. For example, living with diabetes may generate a constant source of stress, which impacts a child's overall psychosocial health. This stress tends to be compounded through critical changes, like the onset of adolescence or the acquisition of new management habits, making it imperative that care is given through an interdisciplinary approach that considers both medical andlpsychological demands within this group 2Panchal et al., 2020). This interdependence necessitates regular psychosocial assessments to identify and mitigate possible distress in children for better global development and resilience. Moreover, the psychosocial impact of pediatric psychiatric illness manifests itself in detrimental forms in most aspects of a child's life. Depressive and anxiety symptoms may disrupt school functioning, interpersonal relationships, and family relationships, leading to reduced quality of life. Complex anxiety disorders, for instance, can discourage children from social contact, ultimately resulting in isolation and a sufficient lack of social support. Additionally, the emotional burdens experienced by these children are likely to spill over into the caregivers, thereby leading to enhanced family stress and probable maladaptive coping within the home environment. With the use of inclusive and interdisciplinary care models consisting of mental health professionals, primary care providers, and family support, healthcare teams all well-positioned to meet these challenges. These integrated methodologies are critical in facilitating not just affected youth but also their families into healthier coping behavior and overall better family function (Nehme et al., 2020). Lastly, the management of the physical outcomes of untreated mental disorders is at the core of managing common pediatric psychiatric disorders efficiently. There is a robust body of evidence that associatcalpsychological distr as, such as untreated depression, with suboptimal self-management behaviors of chronic diseases like diabetes and consequential adverse health outcomes.

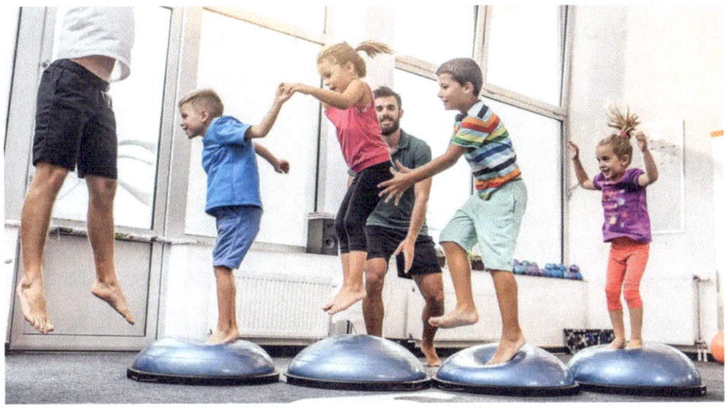

Figure 7.17. The psychologicalpsychological and physical implications of common pediatric psychiatric disorders.

Source: https://i0.wp.com/images-prod.healthline.com/hlcmsresource/images/News/childrens-health/010917_childrenexercise_THUMB_LARGE.jpg?w=1155&h=1528.

For example, children with diabetes and depression or anxiety will more likely exhibit poor adherence to treatment regimens, resulting in poorer glycemic control and increased risk of complications. Further, these mental health issues can lead to physiological consequeh as, such as elevated inflammation or compromised immune status, which, in turn, hasten physical ill health. Hence, the possibility of early detection and the approach of combined treatment strategies involving bicalpsychological therapy and medical management are essential in countering these complications. Prioritizing both mental health and physical health can help healthcare professionals enhance resilience and permit an effective approach towards improved health outcomes for adolescents with psychiatric disor, 2022Panchal et al., 2020) (Figure 7.17).

7.6.3. Treatment Approaches and Family Involvement

Child psychiatric disorders often demand a multi-pch that places strong emphasis on family involvement. Since children and adolescents undergo highly complicated stages of development, families themselves become central to the emotional and psychologicalpsychological well-being of their children. The introduction of family pawithin interventions in treatment adds strength to therapeutic response, since family members can provide central support and context for making sense of a child's behavior. Therapeutic approac, such as family therapy and system interventions highlight the influence of family relationships on mental health. By engaging the family members actively in the treatment process, clinicians are able tocan address family patterns that promote psychiatric disturbances, establishing healthier patterns of communication and interaction. The holistic perspective is useful to tailor specific interventions that address the child's unique environmental and relational context, which ultimately aids in managing pediatric psychiatric disorders more effectively. Secondarily, family-inclusive interdisciplinary treatment models are advances in the understanding of pediatric psychiatric illness. An interdisciplinary staff often employs varied therapeutic methods, including cognitive-behavioral therapy and psychoeducation, to which the input of family members is especially useful. By speaking with parents and brothers/sisters, clinicians can enhance diagnoses of the child's status and adapt treatment protocols that are sensitive to the family's values, beliefs, and functioning. This collaboration not only enriches the therapeutic process bso empowers family members by bestowing them with skills to ensure the recovery of the child. Not only is family involvement crucial fo in the short term, but it also builds resilience and also instructs children on how to navigate adversity in the future. By coordinating treatment goals with family support systems, clinicians are able tocan give children with psychiatric disorders an enduring support system. In addition, psychoeducation becomes a key component of treatment procedures that involve family engagement. By educating families regarding the respective pediatric psychiatric disorders their child is most likely to be struggling with, clinicians promote improved understanding and reduce stigma. Armed witis knowledge, families are empowered to observe stoms, understand treatment options, and actively participate in care plans. An educatedfamily can also provide emotional and practical support that are is critica during times of crisis or adjustment of to treatment. In addition, talking about the family correlates of a child's condition; —e.g., parent-child relationship tal mental health issues, —may uncover some insight into the underlying problems that are distressing the child. The collaborative strategy can facilitate an intervention that can address at the same time the needs of the child and the family environment, with a comprehensive treatment plan. As hrporating clinical objectives with family involvement is critical towards improving treatment outcomes and sustainable changes in pediatric psychiatric disorders (Altunoez et al., 2024; Moretta et al., 2024Panchal et al., 2020).

Test Your Knowledge

1. What are the common types of eating disorders that affect children and adolescents?
2. What psychological and physical implications can result from pediatric eating disorders?
3. How do treatment approaches and family involvement contribute to recovery from eating disorders in children?

SUMMARY

In conclusion, management of common pediatric psychiatric disorders necessitates a better comprehension of the inherent factors driving their occurrence and impact on children. Early detection and intervention are crucial in preventing the long-term consequences of the disorders on a chmic performance, soent, and wellbeing. Evidence has shown that symptoms are likely to manifest in childhood, so parents, teachers, and healthcare providers are required to be observant in order toto detect signs of psychologicalpsychological distress. A labeling ohiatric disorders as actual medical conditions creates a friendly environment that enables children to seek their help and begin their process of treatment and recovery (Panchal et al., 2020Ashish et al., 2020). As such, an assertive strategy toward pediatric mental health can create healthier patterns of growtrovement for the afflicted children. The similarity of pediatric psychiatric disorders to social influences also emphasizes the need for continuous education and advocacy. A variety of external factors, such as, such as the home environment, socioeconomics, and access to mental health care, can exacerbate the issues presented by these disorders in children. It is important stakeholders, including policymakers and mental health clinicians, collaborate to increase resources and access to care for families with these problems. Educational campaigns targeting education on mental health awareness in schools and communities can play an important role in reducing stigma and promoting treatment. Additionally, examination of what makes therapeutic interventions effective goes beyond the field of psychiatric intervention and must encompass wholistic interventions that help the family system deal with these complex conditions (Sara et al., 2020). Emphasis on the importance of social support systems is key in fostering resilience in children who are faced with mental illness. Lastly, long-term success in the treatment of child and adolescent psychiatric disorders is based on a unifying strategy involving education, early intervention, and community-based treatment. As the discipline continues to evolve and grow, it is essential that practitioners keep up with the evolving dynamics of child mental health, applying research to practice through culture-sensitive evidence-ventions that respond to the unique needs of diverse populations. The joint activities of schools, health care systems, and mental health organizations should provide accessible screening and assessment in order toto early identify the children at risk. Giving prominence to mental heale pediatric paradigm will enable society to provide children with psychiatric disease the care, compassion, and intervention they require to construct a better next generation (Panchal et al., 2020Ashish et al., 2020).

In the assess common child psychiatric conditions, there is a need to undestand the multidimensionality of such illnesses and their pervasiveness in the pathways of children's development. The pervasiveness of conditions such as, such as anxiety, depression, ADHD, and ASD makes imperatives meaningful intervention strategies. The clinical setting is also evolving, with increased acknowledgment of alternative therapies above standard pharmacological treatment. The literature has begun addressing other forms of treatment, including massage therapy, which can potentially allevifor anxiety and mood disorders. By the integration of professionals across different therapeutic disciplines, healthcare professionals are able to create more comprehensive treatment plans to treat both psychologicalpsychological and physical well-being in affected children, thereby enhancing their overall quality of life (Rapaport et al., 2018). Another critical component of managing pediatric psychiatric disorders is the advanced understanding of pharmacological therapy. The Clinical Manual of Child and Adolescent Psychopharmacology is a valuable resource for clinicians because it systematically reviews disorders and their corresponding treatment. Each chapter begins with an epidemiologic overview and is accompanied by evidence-based recommendations with the added sophistication of psychiatric presentation among children. This book brings to the limelight the call for making treatment approaches individualized based on the person, particularly when dealing with such serious cases as treatment-resistant depression or the complexity of bipolar conditions in youth populations. The book further critically addresses the issue of off-label prescription and calls for ethics consideration in managing the thorny topic (Panchal et al., 2020Osunsanmi, 2010). Also, management of the interface between psychiatric and physical symptoms is required for total pediatric management. Often seen conditions, like cyclical vomiting and functional abdominal pain, tend to present diagnostic challenges and hence call for an interdisciplinary treatment plan. With an understanding of the importance of co-morbidities, for instance, those seen with Tourettes syndrome and OCD, clinicians can look at things more holistically while developing interventions. The addition of psychotropic medication has improved in relation to its potential side effects as well as meeting the unique needs of children and adolescents, therefore ensuring patient-centered and evidence-based treatment planning. These strategic design factors largely contribute to a better understanding of psychiatric conditions among children and adolescents, an opportunity for improved clinical outcomes and quality of life among the infected children (Osunsanmi, 2010).

KEY TERMS FROM THIS CHAPTER

- Anxiety disorders
- Autism spectrum disorder (ASD)
- Conduct disorder (CD)
- Diagnostic criteria
- Genetics
- Obsessive-compulsive disorder (OCD)
- Pediatric psychiatric disorders
- Psychiatric disorders
- Attention-deficit/hyperactivity disorder (ADHD)
- biological
- Deliberate self-harm (DSH)
- Eating disorders
- Healthcare professionals
- Oppositional defiant disorder (ODD)
- Pharmacotherapy
- Psychologists

CRITICAL THINKING QUESTIONS

1. **Which of the following is NOT a core symptom of ADHD?**
   a. Inattention
   b. Hyperactivity
   c. Impulsivity
   d. Hallucinations
2. **Autism Spectrum Disorder (ASD) is primarily characterized by:**
   a. Persistent sadness and irritability
   b. Social communication deficits and restricted/repetitive behaviors
   c. Aggressive behavior and defiance
   d. Mood swings and euphoria
3. **A commonly used screening tool for ADHD is:**
   a. M-CHAT
   b. Conners' Rating Scale
   c. Beck Depression Inventory
   d. PHQ-9
4. **What is the first-line treatment for moderate to severe pediatric depression?**
   a. Antipsychotic medication
   b. Electroconvulsive therapy
   c. Cognitive Behavioral Therapy (CBT) and SSRIs
   d. Behavioral modification only
5. **Which disorder is most associated with excessive worry about various things in a child's daily life?**
   a. Conduct Disorder
   b. Generalized Anxiety Disorder
   c. ADHD
   d. ASD

Short Answer Questions

1. What are the core symptoms of Attention-Deficit/Hyperactivity Disorder (ADHD)?
2. Define Autism Spectrum Disorder (ASD) and mention two hallmark features.
3. What screening tool is commonly used to assess autism in toddlers?
4. What is the typical age of onset for separation anxiety disorder in children?
5. Name two behavioral therapies effective for managing ADHD in children.
6. How does generalized anxiety disorder typically present in children?

Answer to Critical Thinking Questions

1.(d) 2. (b) 3.(b) 4.(c) 5.(b)

REFERENCES

1. Adamo, E., & Pisano, T. (2024). Exploring the internal medicine comorbidities associated with eating disorders: Correlation between disease severity and cardiac abnormalities in adolescent patients with anorexia nervosa. *Eating Disorders.* https://www.semanticscholar.org/paper/4775b4f8d9124d3e2a45c807f2b448b712623f51 (accessed on 16th June 2025).
2. Alengebawy, A., Abdelkhalek, S. T., Qureshi, S. R., & Wang, M.-Q. (2021). Heavy metals and pesticides toxicity in agricultural soil and plants: Ecological risks and human health implications. *Toxics, 9*, 42–42. https://doi.org/10.3390/toxics9030042 (accessed on 16th June 2025).
3. Bonti, E., Zerva, I. K., Koundourou, C., & Sofologi, M. (2024). The high rates of comorbidity among neurodevelopmental disorders: Reconsidering the clinical utility of distinct diagnostic categories. *Journal of Personalized Medicine, 14*, 300–300. https://doi.org/10.3390/jpm14030300 (accessed on 16th June 2025).
4. Bull, M. J., Trotter, T. L., Santoro, S. L., Christensen, C. K., & Grout, R. W. (2022). Health supervision for children and adolescents with Down syndrome. *Pediatrics, 149.* https://doi.org/10.1542/peds.2022-057010 (accessed on 16th June 2025).
5. Bultas, M. W., Burkett, K., Johnson, N. L., et al. (2016). Translating research to practice for children with autism spectrum disorder: Part I: Definition, associated behaviors, prevalence, diagnostic process, and interventions. https://core.ac.uk/download/213064134.pdf (accessed on 16th June 2025).
6. Chadban, S. J., Ahn, C., Axelrod, D. A., Foster, B. J., Kasiske, B. L., Kher, V., Kumar, D., et al. (2020). KDIGO clinical practice guideline on the evaluation and management of candidates for kidney transplantation. *Transplantation, 104*, S11–S103. https://doi.org/10.1097/tp.0000000000003136 (accessed on 16th June 2025).
7. Chen, J. W., Koester, S. W., Liles, C., Gannon, S., & Bonfield, C. (2024). Evaluating the prevalence of psychiatric comorbidities associated with pediatric scoliosis utilizing Research Match. *Spine Deformity, 12*, 1583–1593. https://www.semanticscholar.org/paper/ca43729640ed49fa2baa48c324755c78bd8412a9 (accessed on 16th June 2025).
8. Daviss, W. B., House, S., Olson, A., O'Neil, M., et al. (2017). Attention deficit hyperactivity disorder (ADHD): Survey report. https://core.ac.uk/download/215540988.pdf (accessed on 16th June 2025).
9. Faraone, S. V., Banaschewski, T., Coghill, D., Zheng, Y., Biederman, J., Bellgrove, M. A., Newcorn, J. H., et al. (2021). The World Federation of ADHD international consensus statement: 208 evidence-based conclusions about the disorder. *Neuroscience & Biobehavioral Reviews, 128*, 789–818. https://doi.org/10.1016/j.neubiorev.2021.01.022 (accessed on 16th June 2025).
10. Jiang, X., Li, H. H., Yu, Z., & Wang, C. (2024). Deliberate self-harm among pediatric psychiatric inpatients in China: A single-center retrospective study. *World Journal of Psychiatry, 14*, 398–408. https://www.semanticscholar.org/paper/57408dfefdad0839dac1800fff542d42de29d000 (accessed on 16th June 2025).
11. Johansen, S. L., Stenhaug, B. A., Robakis, T., Williams, K. E., & Cullen, M. R. (2020). Past psychiatric conditions as risk factors for postpartum depression. *The Journal of Clinical Psychiatry, 81.* https://doi.org/10.4088/jcp.19m12929 (accessed on 16th June 2025).

12. Khanal, S., Singh, S. K., Mishra, R., Kafle, P., & Sharma, M. (2023). Pediatric intensive care unit in a developing nation: Exploring acute neurological illnesses and their clinical course. *Journal of Institute of Medicine Nepal.* https://www.semanticscholar.org/paper/c4b0d86b376a33216c2ca63a583c7b9d23000f2d (accessed on 16th June 2025).

13. Lee, D. W., Santomasso, B., Locke, F. L., Ghobadi, A., Turtle, C. J., Brudno, J. N., Maus, M. V., et al. (2018). ASTCT consensus grading for cytokine release syndrome and neurologic toxicity associated with immune effector cells. *Biology of Blood and Marrow Transplantation, 25*, 625–638. https://doi.org/10.1016/j.bbmt.2018.12.758 (accessed on 16th June 2025).

14. Leibenluft, E., Allen, L. E., Althoff, R. R., Brotman, M. A., Burke, J. D., Carlson, G. A., Dickstein, D. P., et al. (2024). Irritability in youths: A critical integrative review. *American Journal of Psychiatry, 181*, 275–290. https://doi.org/10.1176/appi.ajp.20230256 (accessed on 16th June 2025).

15. Panchal, A. R., Rivard, M. K., Cash, R. E., Corley, J. P., Jean-Baptiste, M., Chrzan, K., & Ristei Gugiu, M. (2020). Methods and implementation of the 2019 EMS practice analysis. *Prehospital Emergency Care, 26*, 212–222. https://doi.org/10.1080/10903127.2020.1856985 (accessed on 16th June 2025).

VACCINE-PREVENTABLE PEDIATRIC DISEASES

8

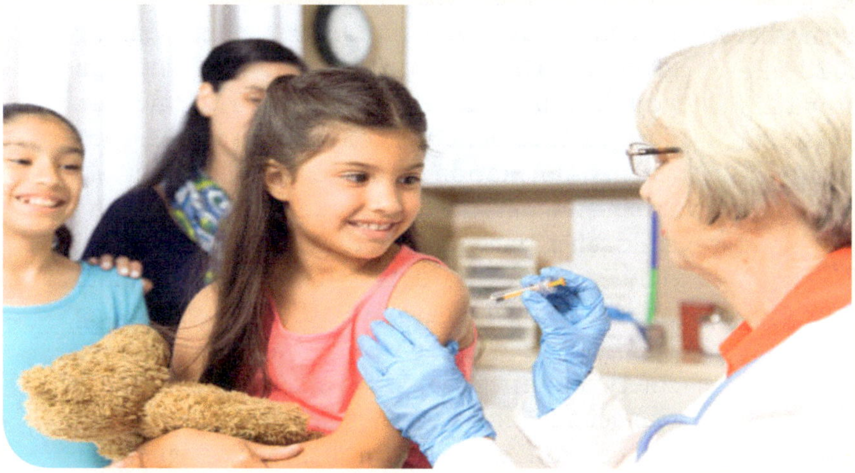

LEARNING OBJECTIVES

After studying this chapter, you will be able to:

1. Offer a summary of vaccine-preventable diseases
2. Stress on immunization schedules and recommendations
3. Explain the barriers to vaccination
4. Explain the role of vaccination in public health

Introduction

Vaccine discovery has, indeed, transformed public health, particularly in the domain of children's illnesses. Through the rollout of immunization programs, numerous diseases that are vaccine-preventable have experienced a record reduction in incidence, paving the way for healthier childhood and reduced mortality. From whooping cough to measles, vaccines are central to safeguarding children against sickness that was formerly endemic and even lethal. Yet, in spite of the overwhelming data on the efficacy of vaccinations, resistance and misinformation persist against public health efforts. In this essay, the background of vaccine-preventable child illnesses will be described along with their history, the science behind immunizations, and the pivotal role of vaccines today. By examining these factors, we can better understand the importance of maintaining htion coverage in order toto protect future generations from the recurrence of preventable diseases (Figure 8.1).

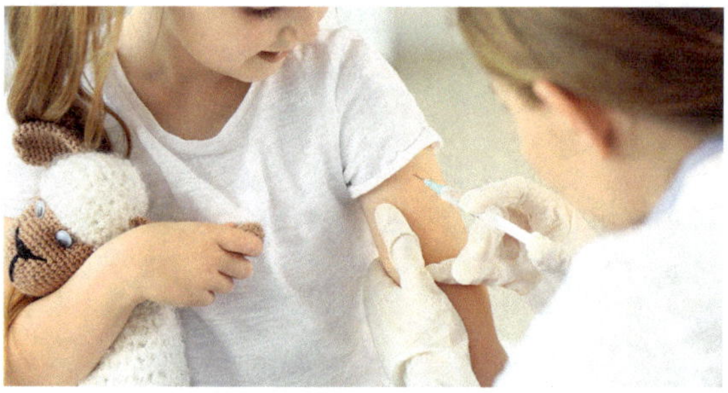

Figure 8.1. Vaccine preventable diseases.

Source: https://external-content.duckduckgo.com/iu/?u=https%3A%2F%2Fwww.kernodle.com%2Fwp-content%2Fuploads%2F2020%2F01%2FKernodle_Vaccine.jpeg&f=1&nofb=1&ipt=c7453b3e8687c187f8fa0e52ed764337a63fa38f9f97c8f871148087f521758a&ipo=images.

Definition of Vaccine-Preventable Diseases

Vaccine-preventable diseases (VPDs) are conditions that can be effectively prevented through immon against pathogens such as, such as viruses and bacteria with the potential to create enormous health risks, particularly to children. Such diseases include, but are not limited to, measles, pertussis, and diphtheria, with a potential to create severe morbidity, mortality, or long-term complications in child populations. Vaccination is a vital public health intervention that enhances herd immunity and minimizes the risk of transmission of such infection within communities. For instance, epidemiological evidence from the Kilifi Health and Demographic Surveillance System indicates the success of vaccination campaigns in stemming childhood morbidity caused by rotavirus and pneumococcal disease (Tsofa et al., 2012). As highlighted by global health organizations, increasing coverage among vaccines like the pneumococcal conjugate vaccine and rotavirus vaccine has been found to decrease significantly the rates of child mortality, making research on VPDs an exceptionally vital field of study in the practice of pediatric medicine (Abigail et al.).

Importance of Vaccination in Pediatric Health

Vaccination is very important in protecting pediatric health by successfully preventing a myriad of contagious diseases that have the capability to affect child morbidity and mortality significantly. For instance, immunization initiatives have enabled the historic reduction of vaccine-preventable disease evident in the laudable increase in children's coverage with immunizations, linked to reduced infant mortality rates and impife expectancy among groups such as, such as the Argentinean population (Malena et al., 2023). However, despitbvious benefits, challenges such as, such as misinformation and vaccine hesitancy do arise and persist, particularly among young children's parents. A study highlighted that only 31.3% of parents intended to vaccinate their children against COVID-19, reflecting deeply seated issues regarding the vaccines safety and effectiveness (Celia et al., 2022). To transcend such challenges, what is required are coordinated public health campaigns that improve comprehension and uptake of the vaccines to enable all children to be included within required medical interventions and live healthy lives within a safe environment.

Overview of Common Vaccine-Preventable Diseases

Immunization is critical in the prevention of numerous infectious conditions with significant impacts on the pediatric health, highlighting immunization as a central focus in public health efforts. Among the most common vaccine-preventable illnesses are measles, mumps, rubella, and pertussis, all of which pose serious complications to children. Measles, a highly contagious viral condition, can result in pneumonia and encephalitis, with outbreaks related to declining vaccination rates. Similarly, mumps causes meningitis and orchitis, while rubella is risky during pregnancy, causing congenital rubella syndrome in infants. Whooping cough caused by the bacterium Bordetella pertussis typically results in excessive spells of coughing, which is not merely painful but potentially life-threatening for infants as well. The immunization campaigns remain vital since they not only vaccinate the particular child but also offer herd immunity, which safeguards populations against these preventable diseases (2024) (Sarya et al., 2023) (Figure 8.2).

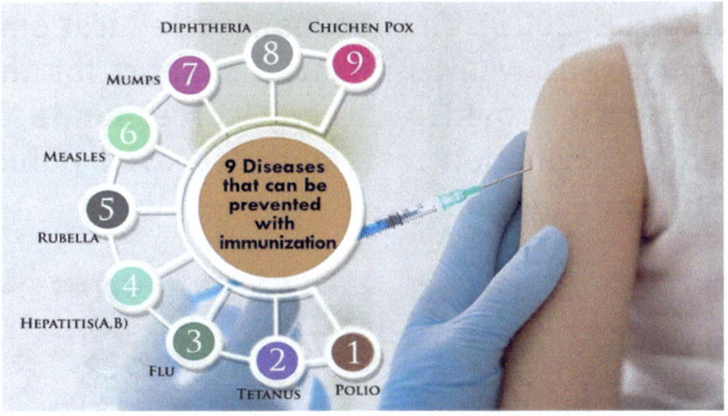

Figure 8.2. Overview of common vaccine-preventable diseases.

Source: https://lh3.googleusercontent.com/proxy/2f3FUD0Cb_RxX1zFCvrKlp3WQyy7mQ9KRtMzIrfP gM20Iny-BjqUBG0J 3U4xTo4oXACVBclfix8vHdNsPeGT ZKCg96kXDa-3i_zU8kgAFaNlBO RSFZh43g1P8Xg2 PHEVsrrmK0ZrVU0.

Historical Context of Vaccination

Historical context on vaccination offers seminal data on its origin and evolution of the public health intervention to avert vaccine-preventable child illnesses. Since the late 18th century, the practice of vaccination has been in a position to look back at its steps, and the pioneering work of Edward Jenner on smallpox was the foundation for immunology. Through the centuries, introducing the vaccines against the diseases of polio, measles, and mumps has wiped out morbidity and mortality rates among children to a significant degree. However, the last few decades have witnessed fluctuating vaccination rates, particularly in nations like Brazil, where declining vaccination levels coincided with the resurgence of disease previously under control. This pattern points to the need for ongoing public health initiatives to maintain high vaccination rates, as neglecting this can compromise not only the health of individual children but also bring about broader outbreaks threatening community health.

Current Vaccination Rates and Trends

Since vaccine coverage is uneven, public health implications become more evident, particularly for vaccine-preventable diseases (VPDs). Recent trends show an alarming rise in personal belief exemptions (PBEs) that have been li outbreaks of once under-control diseases such as, such as measles and pertussis (Boom et al., 2018). The declining vaccination uptake is partly caused bve myths regarding the safety of vaccines, such as, such as the disproven link between autism and vaccines, that have been boosted by misdissemination over the internet (Boom et al., 2018). In California, legislative introduction of Assembly Bill 2109 mandated parents who sought PBEs to be educated in vaccine safety, resulting in a significant decline in exemption requests by app013 and 2016 (Ryan, 2023Goishi-Bessey et al., 2016). This legislative measure is evidence that educational intervention serves to make vaccination efforts more relevant, highlighting the role of community-level immunization programs as the key to eradicating VPDs and protecting public health.

Significance of Public Awareness

Thayed by public enlightenment in combating children vaccine-preventable diseases cannot be overstated, especially during an era marked by mounting vaccine hesitancy. With vaccination coverage among children declining, driven by misinformation and personal beliefs, public education emerges at the forefront in addressing the threine-preventable diseases (VPDs) (Dupel.,

2023Ryan, 2023). Legislative intervention, such as, such as California Assembly Bill 2109 (AB 2109), has played a vital role in solving this issue through the provision that parents seeking exemption from vaccination are provided with crucial information on the safety of f VPDs on children , 2023Goishi-Bessey et al., 2016). This initiative does not only aims at increasing parental education and trust but also underscores the capacity of healthcare providers to provide accurate and full information. Finally, increasing public awareness leads to an enlightened population, thus reducing the risk of outbreaks and providing healthier results for generations to come (Figure 8.3).

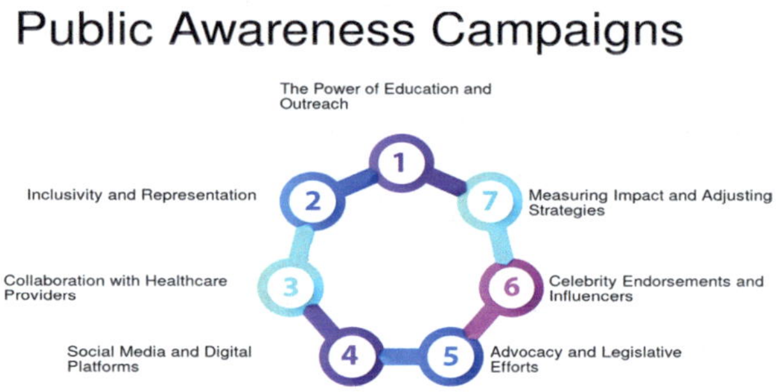

Figure 8.3. The significance of public awareness in combating vaccine-preventable pediatric diseases.

Source: https://fastercapital.co/i/Cord-blood-advocacy-Cord-Blood-Advocacy--Why-It-Matters--Public-Awareness-Campaigns.webp.

Role of Healthcare Providers in Vaccination

Healthcare providers have a central role in promoting and providing vaccinations, especially to pediatric risk groups for vaccine-preventable disease. Not only do they provide vaccines as first contact providers, but because of their position, they are excellent sources of information, responding to parents' queries and addressing their myths and fears regarding immunization. A study found that if healthcare profewere trained in effective communication strategies, such as, such as the use of visual aids within clinics, they can significantly improve vaccination adherence (Hill, 2023). It facilitates the understanding of the immunization schedule by the parents and ensures a conducive environment for evidence-based decision-making. Also, ongoing education on the provider's side of the effectiveness of the vaccines and updated guidelines is important to combat vaccine resistance, which is primarily due to knowledge gaps by the healthcare providers themselves (American Academy of Pediatrics, 2021). Thus, spending on educational resources as well as financial support for the healthcare provider directly corresponds to higher vaccination rates and improved public health in children.

8.1. Overview of Vaccine-Preventable Diseases

Learning Outcome

1. Definition and classification of vaccine-preventable diseases
2. Common vaccine-preventable diseases in children
3. Mechanisms of disease transmission
4. Symptoms and complications of these diseases
5. Impact on public health and community immunity
6. Historical outbreaks and their consequences
7. Role of the immune system in disease prevention
8. Differences between viral and bacterial vaccine-preventable diseases
9. Importance of herd immunity

The prevalence of vaccine-preventable diseases (VPDs) in children presents the extreme importance of vaccination initiatives and evidence-based healthcare practices. Vaccines have successfully lowered the incidence of measles, mumps, rubellaertussis, which, if untreated, can have severe complications such as, such as hospitalization and death. Recent studies identify a bleak decline in immunization coverage due to misinformation and caregiver/caregiver vaccine hesitancy as factors, threhe public health gains. Interventions at the community level, such as, such as reminder messages through electronic media for immunizations, have been observed to raise compliance significantly, indicating the need for ongoing education and active practice within health delivery settings. Therefore, while vaccines are powerful tools in fighting infectious diseases, sustained effort must that children's populations are kept regularly immunized in order toto keep enjoying these life-saving shields, safeguarding public health and future generations (Figure 8.4).

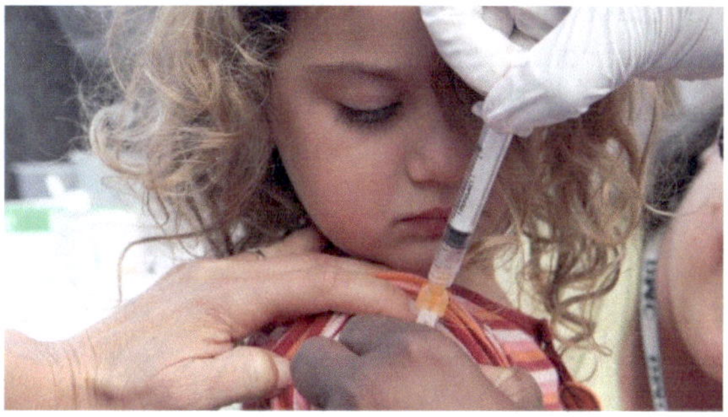

Figure 8.4. Vaccine-preventable diseases (VPDs) in pediatric populations.

Source: https://external-content.duckduckgo.com/iu/?u=http%3A%2F%2Fi2.cdn.turner.com%2Fcnn%2Fdam%2Fassets%2F140630214621-orig-should-i-get-my-child-vaccinated-npr-00003513-story-top.jpg&f=1&nofb=1&ipt=832353d05dd0a2634287211699197a374f99ea2bd4667761f4f9d36524864939&ipo=images.

8.1.1. Definition and Classification of Vaccine-Preventable Diseases

Vaccine-preventable disease is an illness that can be realistically prevented through the utilization of vaccination and reducing morbidity and mortality rates from such illnesses. Vaccine-preventable diseases are classified into different types based on causative, modes of transmission, and hazards posed. For instance, viruses such as, such as measles and rubella infect and are py spread through respiratory droplets, while bacterial infections such as, such as tetanus and diphtheria can be averted by targeted immunization. The effect of these diseases is particularly important among children because of their vulnerability and the prominent public health implications of non-immunization. Specifically, the World Health Organization notes that despite having effective vaccines, the continued incidence of these diseases among unvaccinated populations identifies the urgent need for ongoing vaccination programs and education programs for increased immunization coverage (Asunción et al., 2019; Ugonma et al., 2019).

8.1.2. Common Vaccine-Preventable Diseases in Children

Among the numerous health issues confronting children in the world, vaccine-preventable diseases are a significant public health issue. Measles, mumps, rubella, and pertussis have the potential to trigger severe complications, including neurological damage and respiratory failure, and thereby illustrate the critical importance of immunization. The advent of mass immunization campaigns has dramatically stemmed the outbreak of such conditions; the incidence of measles, for example, has in countries where there is high vaccination coverage (Rebecca et al., 2021Ryan, 2023). Vaccine hesitancy has also emerged as a concerning trend that leads to localized outbreaks and increases the risk for unvaccinated communities. Moreover, the different level of immunity durability across different periods raises queser booster doses for some vaccines are necessary (Ryan, 2023Rita et a 2020). Hence, ongoing public awareness and education on vaccine efficacy is are essential in combating vaccine-preventable diseases and ensuring the health of future generations.

8.1.3. Mechanisms of Disease Transmission

An understanding of disease transmission mechanisms is crucial in the prevention of vaccine-preventable childhood illnesses because the mechanisms of transmission affect outbreak characteristics as well as public health interventions considerably. Influenza and measles are prevalent infectious illnesses that spread predominantly through respiratory droplets, contact via skin with soiled surfaces, or mother-to-child transmission during gesta the variability in how these pathogens transmit (Ryan, 2023Vidya et al., 2024).

In children, their transmission capability is enhanced by their social interaction, unsanitary habits, and immature immune systems, which can facilitate rapid transfer of viruses within groups (Mould-Quevedo et al., 2023). Vaccination is an important intervention, with a significant reduction in the chance of getting infected and spreading it, thereby covering high-risk populations. By revealing these transmission dynamics, public health officials can craft educational programs and vaccine campaigns to optimize community immunity, thus reversing the impact of these diseases on children's health (Figure 8.5).

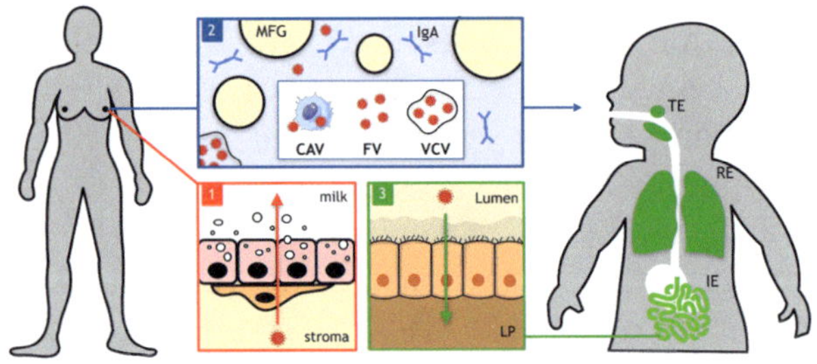

Figure 8.5. The mechanisms of disease transmission.

Source: https://www.mdpi.com/viruses/viruses-13-01312/article_deploy/html/images/viruses-13-01312-g001.png.

8.1.4. Symptoms and Complications of These Diseases

Symptoms and complications of vaccine-preventable child illnen have critical implications on children's health and welfare. Infections such as, such as the flu, which infects 30% to 40% of American children annually, can lead to severe respiratory complications, hospitalization, and even fatalities, particularly among vulnerable populations (Hassan et al., 2009). The flu virus plays a critical role in child fatalities, informing the importance of early vaccination. Despite the clear benefits, the majority of parents fail to vaccinate their kids due to concerns regarding vaccine risk, which can be a result of misinformation and divergent perceptions. Understanding the symptoms and complications helps since it can change the parent's mindset toward vaccination. Large data-based outreach programs are essential in curbing vaccine hesitancy, thus lowering the incidence of such deadly diseases among children.

8.1.5. Impact on Public Health and Community Immunity

The impact of vaccine-preventable childhood diseases on public health and community immunity is vast following the COVID-19 pandemic. The enforcement of strict nonpharmaceutical interventions (NPIs) during the period inadvertently resulted in a reduction in incidence of various infectious diseases, including respiratory syncytial virus (RSV) and influenza, that are significant amog children. These reductions, while helpful in the short term, may build immune debt; —a condition where the children's cohort has reduced exposure to pathogens, thus weakenstem's progression and response to subsequent infections (Ryan, 2023Robert et al., 2021). On the other hand, when the NPIs are lifted, the risk of outbreak of such illness may rise exponentially, undermining not just individual health but also communal immunity (Adva et al.,

2021). Hence, sustaining robust immunization systems is key to rebuilding protective immunity levels and to prevent potential resurgences of such illnesses in children.

8.1.6. Historical Outbreaks and Their Consequences

Historical vaccine-preventable disease outbreaks in the past are a grim reminder of what occurs when under-immunization occurs. For instance, between February 2023 and January 2024, the European region witnessed an increase of over 5,770 cases, especially in Romania, which alone documented over 11,000 and 12 deaths over a period of a few months (Filipa et al., 2024).

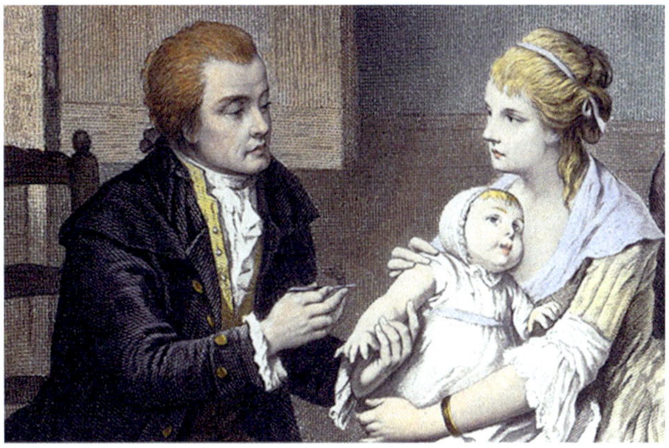

Figure 8.6. Historical outbreaks of vaccine-preventable diseases.

Source: https://assets.mayoclinic.org/content/dam/media/global/images/2025/history-disease-outbreaks-vaccine-timeline/Edward-Jenner-child-smallpox-2208x1472-creativecommons.jpg.

These epidemics are aggravated by low vaccine coverage within the vulnerable and marginalized populations, including prisoners, who are typically left out of immunization campaigns. Additionally, findings from recent research determined that 78% of all confirmed cases of measles in a pediatric population were not vaccinated, once more highlighting the absolute necessity for successful immunization measures (Aslan et al., 2024). Such historical precedents demonstrate the public health necessity of securing high vaccination coverage to prevent the cyclical behavior of such events and safeguard future generations from such outcomes (Figure 8.6).

8.1.7. Role of the Immune System in Disease Prevention

The immune system is key to the prevention of illness, particularly vaccine-preventable childhood illnesses. Immunization is vital as an anticipatory measure, preclinical priming of the immune system to be able to recognize and combat pathogens prior to them having an opportunity to establish an infection. This immunological memory is achieved through the development of antibodies and T-cells specific ase-inducing pathogens and therefore slice the incidence and severity of diseases such as, such as measles, mumps, and whooping cough. Studies have shown that successful immunization campaigns are critical to the attainment of herd immunity, protecting both immunized and unimmunized individuals by discontinuing chains of disease transmission (Adva et al., 2021). The value of robust immune response is particularly apparent in the context of rising vaccine hesitancy, which may jeopardize decades of progress in managing such conditions (Mark et al., 2021). The challenges need to be addressed with aligned public health action to enhance the immune system's critical role in disease prevention through immunization.

8.1.8. Differences Between Viral and Bacterial Vaccine-Preventable Diseases

The distinction between viral and bacterial vaccine-preventable disease is of uevance in the understanding of child health and immunization policy. Viral disease, such as, such as measles and influenza, is caused by pathogens that act within host cells, often triggust immune responses which are characteristically self-limiting. Bacterial disease, such as, such as pneumonia and pertussis, are caused by extracellular bacteria that often live outside the host for occasionally and occasionally for prolonged periods. This intrinsic difference influences vaccine design and delivery; e.g., bacterial vaccines may require boosters to ensure long-term immunity because of the variation in immune response provoked. Additionally, the cross-talk between viruses and bacterial pathogens signals the need for vaccines not just for the protection of an individual but to impact the population; studies have found that viral infection modifies bacterial colonization dynamics, making disease dynamics in children's populations more challenging to control and calling for an integrated vaccination approach (Leigh et al., 2024). It is critical to underso successfully maximize preventive health interventions among children (Christopher et al., 2023Ryan, 2023).

8.1.9. Importance of Herd Immunity

Herd immunity is a core factor in the prevention of child vaccine-preventable diseases, creating aing barrier that guards not just the vaccinated but also those that cannot be vaccinated, such as, such as infants and immunocompromised children. With high coverage of a single population, pathogen tranicularly critical in ensuring optimal high vaccination coverage, as in the recent findings where hesitancy and misinformation have eroded immunization. The COVID-19 pandemic has also shown the direct proportionality between vaccination rates and public health, dem vaccination coverage communities have a larger rate of infections (Ryan, 2023Massimo et al., 2021). Herd imnly achievable through shared accountability; parents must prioritize early vaccination in order toto ensure that communities not only protect vulnerable members but also release health care burdens from preventable diseases (Figure 8.7).

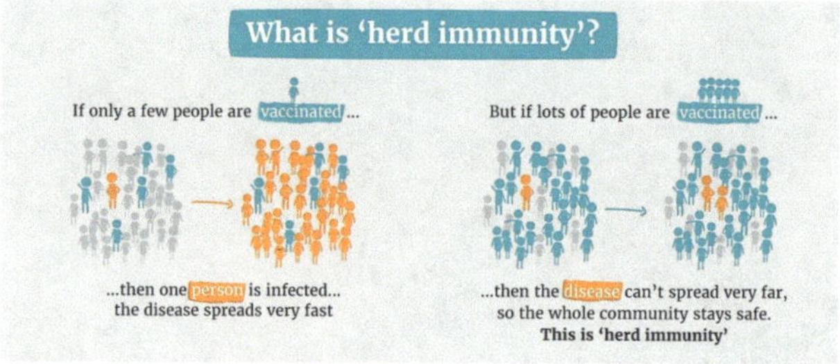

Figure 8.7. Herd immunity plays a pivotal role in the prevention of vaccine-preventable pediatric diseases.

Source: https://www.vpslakeshorehospital.com/uploads/blog/whatisherdimmunity-veY49kYc9E88Odn.jpeg.

Test Your Knowledge

1. What are the common symptoms and potential complications associated with major vaccine-preventable diseases?
2. How do vaccines impact public health and contribute to community (herd) immunity?
3. What are the key differences between viral and bacterial vaccine-preventable diseases?

8.2. Vaccination Schedules and Recommendations

Learning Outcome

1. Recommended vaccination schedules for children
2. Types of vaccines: live, inactivated, and subunit
3. Age-specific vaccination guidelines
4. Catch-up vaccination strategies
5. Role of pediatricians in vaccination education
6. Variability in vaccination schedules across countries
7. Importance of adhering to vaccination schedules
8. Challenges in maintaining vaccination compliance
9. Resources for parents regarding vaccination information

Vaccine schedules and advice are key factors in preventing vaccine-preventable childhood disease, especially if there is a high burden of public health in a specific region. In the Latin American region, the WHO 2030 Immunization Agenda focuses on harmonizing immunization activities at various levels in accine coverage and prevent outbreaks of pertussis and polio, among other diseases (Ryan, 2023Maria et al., 2023). The application and extensive use of combination vaccines are vital in these initiatives because they bring together immunization processes with the target of combating multiple diseases at a time. For instance, the combination of diphtheria, tetanus, and pertussis with other antigens in vaccinationdren has been shown to reduce rates of these ailments among infants substantially (Ryan, 2023 al., 2023). By integrating the recommendations of specialists and surmounting barriers to immunization, such as, such as low coverage and misinformation, the health systems can improve vaccine coverage and significantly decrease the possibility of resurgence among vaccine-preventable diseases in vulnerable populations.

8.2.1. Recommended Vaccination Schedules for Children

Schedules of recommended childhood vaccinations are a central to prevention of vaccine-preventable childhood diseases, and they must be utilized for public health protection. Such schedules are designed to maximize immunity with the minimum risk of adverse effects since extensive research has proved them to be safe and effective within a range of population. For instance.S. Centers for Disease Control and Prevention (CDC) offers a combined timeline with preventable diseases such as, such as measles, mumps, rubella (MMR), and pertussis, which have returned due to declining vaccination rates due to misinformation and fear (Boom et al., 2018). Furthermore, incorporating annual influenza vaccinations into the routine has beparticularly in at-risk groups, as a preventative measure against outbreaks (Ryan, 2023Balaisyte-Jazone et al., 2023). By following these proposed schedules, parents can be confident that their children are free from dangerous diseases and contribute to reaching the shared goal of community immunity (Figure 8.8).

	Birth	2 mos	4 mos	6 mos	9 mos	12 mos	15 mos	18 mos	24 mos	4/5 years	10 years	11 years	12 years	16 years	17 years
Hepatitis B	✓														
Dtap-IPV-HepB		✓	✓	✓											
Pneumococcal		✓	✓	✓		✓									
Rotavirus		✓	✓												
H.influenzae		✓	✓	✓		✓									
MMR							✓								
Varicella							✓								
Proquad (MMRV)										✓					
Dtap							✓								
Hepatitis A						✓		✓							
Dtap-IPV (Kinrix)										✓					
Tdap											✓				
Meningococcal												✓		✓	
HPV 2- 3 doses													✓		
Meningococcal B															✓✓
Influenza				✓	And	every	year	there	after	in	the	fall.			

Figure 8.8. Recommended vaccination schedules.

Source: https://external-content.duckduckgo.com/iu/?u=https%3A%2F%2Fwww.penfieldpediatrics.com%2FImages_Content%2FSite1%2FImages%2FPages%2FImmunizationSchedule.jpg&f=1&nofb=1&ipt=80352f7de354c5c7fa2a9408bee7e12407f8beaf3e6ab8b05a6f174a0f20fd14&ipo=images.

8.2.2. Types of Vaccines: Live, Inactivated, and Subunit

Vaccines play a crucial role in preventing child vaccine-preventable illness, and their classification as live, inactivated, and subunit captures their range of mechanisms and applications. Live vaccines rely on attenuated pathogens to induce a vigorous immune response with prolonged immunity but pose risk in the immunocompromised host. Conversely, inactivated vaccines use killed pathogens, making thr with a known safety and efficacy profile, shown through the development of inactivated vaccines for diseases such as, such as chikungunya, which shows that they are consistent and tried and tested (Kaushik, 2023). Lastly, subunit vaccines aim at specific antigens of pathogens to stimulate immunity without exposing the entire organism, minimizing risk but successfully educating the immune system. It is essential to identify these types of vaccines in selecting the appropriate immunization strategies against infectious diseases among children and hence contributing to the public health outcome (Figure 8.9).

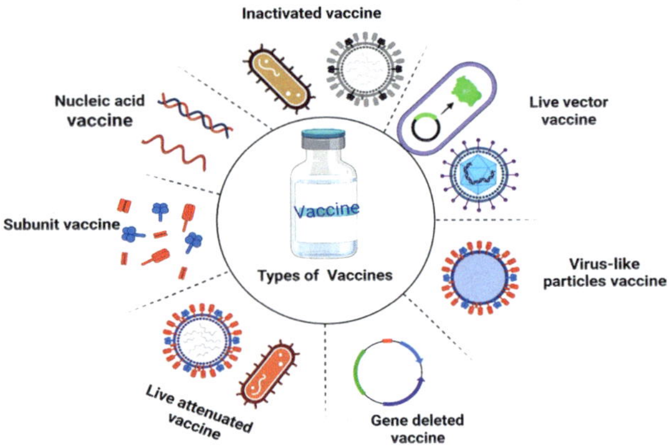

Figure 8.9. Types of vaccines.

Source: Yao Y, Zhang Z and Yang Z (2023) The combination of vaccines and adjuvants to prevent the occurrevets-10-1243835-g001.jpg &f=1&nofb=1&ipt=cbdb6c770c8fbd42423effb 52e9193b59024f1aa6120089bde63316884d3 37f4&ipo=images.

8.2.3. Age-Specific Vaccination Guidelines

Age-specific guidelines for vaccines are important in the prevention of vaccine-preventable illness among children, particularly during the first few years of life when their immune system is still in the developmental process. For instance, Advisory Committee on Immunization Practices (ACIP) strongly recommends pneumococcal conjugate and Hemophilus influenzae type b vaccine administration at the4 months in a bid to avoid high-end risk of disease among younger children. In addition, targeted interventions, such as, such as those emerging from the quality improvement initiative in hematopoietic cell transplantation (HCT), have facilitated the early introduction inations around 6 months post-transplant to boost immunity and decrease vulnerability to infections (Copacia et al., 2023Ryan, 2023). Such an active reaction not only ensures adherence to vaccination calendars but also seeks to break down inequalities in take-up by targeting education and participation strategies among healthcare professionals and families and thus fostering a healthier pediatric population (Bonanni et al., 2023).

8.2.4. Catch-Up Vaccination Strategies

To address the longstanding problem of pediatric vaccine-preventable illnesses, catch-up vaccination interventions have been established as key measures for enhancing vaccination coverage levels among under-vaccinated groups. The interventions are meant to deliver delayed vaccinations to those who have fallen through the cracks of the routine immunization programs and, therefore, preventable conditions like pneumonia and pertussis. Literature indicates that the use of such systems like electronic patient portal reminders yields a dramatic increase in vaccination compliance, with an increase of 2% in fully vaccinated patients in a rural primary care clinic setting (Osbeck et al., 2022). Ultimately, through engagement of under-immunized children through powerful communication and culturally responsive outreach strategies, health workers can ensure that immunization programs not only enhance individual immunity but also facilitate public health goals on a broader level, thereby reducing the social and economic implications of vaccine-preventable diseases (Baldo et al., 2016).

8.2.5. Role of Pediatricians in Vaccination Education

Pediatricians have the important role in vaccinating education, most importantly to prevent vaccine-preventable pediatric diseases. Being trusted sources of health information, pediatricians are best suited to allay the fears of parents towards vaccination by evidence-based facts about their safety and efficacy, according to the American Academy of Pediatrics (AAP) (2021).

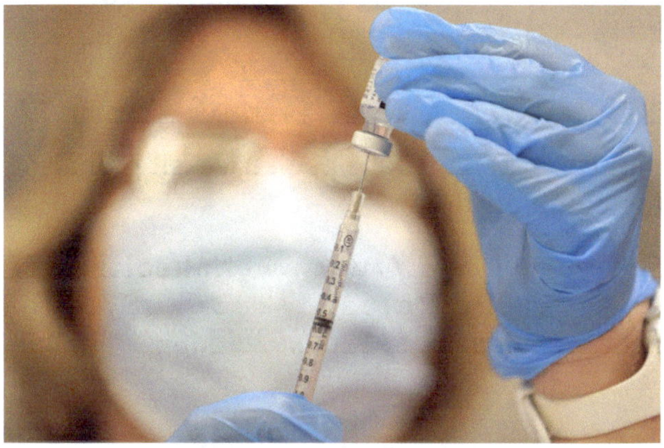

Figure 8.10. Pediatricians in vaccination education.

Source: https://external-content.duckduckgo.com/iu/?u=https%3A%2F%2Fwww.bgsu.edu%2Fcontent%2Fdam%2FBGSU%2Fnews%2F2021%2F03%2Fvaccine%2Fnurse-with-vaccine.jpg&f=1&nofb=1&ipt=71a5fe642aadb45f84a5b8bde05078c7d247878ef5e0079c78bcd4740adb5974&ipo=images.

During routine checkups, pediatricians can capitalize on these interactions to clarifdules and the benefits of immunization, thus discouraging vaccine hesitancy in parents and guardians (Ryan, 2023Angira et al., 2020). They also play an important role in sensitizing populations about new vaccines, including COVID-19 vaccines, so that families are aware of individual as well as population health benefits of immunization. Through open communication, pediatricians are at the forefront of health literacy, allowing families to make well-informed decisions regarding vaccinations and thereby protect the health of children from preventable diseases. Their active participation in the process is important in maintaining vaccination coverages and enhancing community immunization (Figure 8.10).

8.2.6. Variability in Vaccination Schedules Across Countries

The global difference in vaccination schedules reflects the intricate challenges in the battle against vaccine-preventable childhood diseases. Variations in schedules are driven by differences in disease distribution, health systems, and cultural perceptions of vaccination. In regions like Latin America, there are approximately 2.7 million infants with partial vaccination records, particularly in vulnerable environments characterized by restricted access to health services (Avila-Aguero et al., 2024). Besides, evidence reveals that low knowledge among caregivers about vaccination schedules significantly limits immunization processes, which suggests that enhanced communve the potential to reverse misinformation and stimulate mobilization of communities to improve compliance (Ryan, 2023Tripathi et al., 2022). Such discrepancies point towards the utmost priority of context-specific interventions respected by local communities and that promote compliance with evidence-based immunization recommendations. Thus, developing harmonized approaches that are able to meet these gaps is crucial in minimizing the dissemination of vaccine-preventable disease and ensuring equal health returns to children all over the world.

8.2.7. Importance of Adhering to Vaccination Schedules

Compliance with vaccination schedules is essential in the prevention of pediatric vaccine-preventable disease since timely vaccination delivers timely immunity to children and to the population as a whole. Delayed vaccination can cause high susceptibility to outbreaks of the disease, as evidenced by the COVID-19 pandemic, which disrupted routine immunization services and resulted in low vaccine coverage globally. Studies revealed that children skipped vaccinations due to fear of catching the virus in the healthcare setting, leading to the resurgence of infectious diseases that otherwise remained contained (Zoh, 2021). A scheduled vaccination regimen also assists in thimmunity, which protects persons who cannot be vaccinated, such as, such as infants and immunocompromised patients (Ryan, 2023Steven et al., 2020). In light of these dynamics, strict compliance with the vaccintion calendar is essential for families and medical practitioners to secure not only individual protection but public health as well and prevents the recrudescence of outbreaks, which can otherwise impact pediatric populations.

8.2.8. Challenges in Maintaining Vaccination Compliance

Maintaining vaccination coverage poses unprecedented challenges to public health, foremost being the battle against preventable children's diseases caused by vaccines. The greatest challenge is the pervasive influence of misinformation about vaccines, which has grown more rapidly over the past two years, most famously with disproven myths linking vaccines to autism (Boom et al., 2018). Such myths are one of the most important drivers of vaccine hesitancy, causing many parents to delay or decline to give vaccinations to their ch This reluctance not only erodes indiv undermines population immunity, leading to outbreaks of once-contained infections such as, such as measles and whooping cough (Dupervil et al., 2023Ryan, 2023). Access to health care, socioeconomic disparities, and low health awareness of the importance of immunization are some of the barriers that surface. In response to these challenges, health workers must be equipped with accurate, evidence-based information which will help them build trust and facilitate compliance with vaccination in children (Figure 8.11).

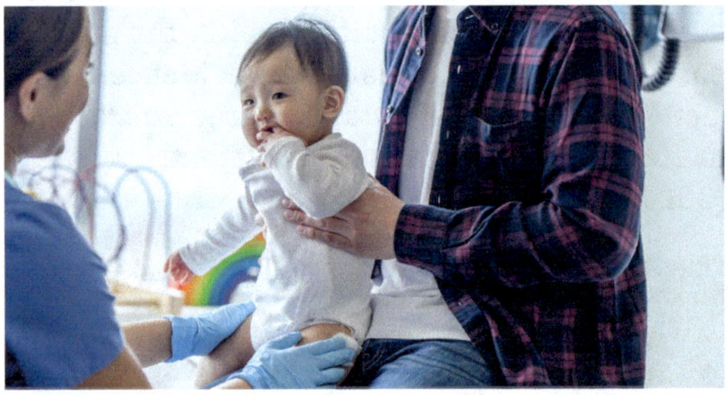

Figure 8.11. Infant at a pediatric visit preparing for immunization.

Source: https://www.weliahealth.org/wp-content/uploads/2024/08/blog-childimmunizations-1200x628-1.jpg.

8.2.9. Resources for Parents Regarding Vaccination Information

Having access to rnformation about vaccination is crucial for parents who must navigate the burden of vaccine-preventable childhood diseases. Education programs, such as, such as California Assembly Bill 2109, have played a central role in arming parents with information about vaccine safety and the risks of vaccine-preventable diseases (VPDs). This legislation calls for parents seeking indins to vaccines to be counseled by a healthcare professional, hence avoiding uninformed choices ae refusal (Ryan, 2023Goishi-Bessey et al., 2016). Furthermore, the position of community health centers is instrumental in embracing visual aids, such as, such as simplified schedules of immunization, in pediatric examination rooms to enhance parental education and compliance with recommended vaccinations (DiCola et al., 2024). By providing readily available and comprehensible information, the resources bridge the gap in knowledge and ultimately result in higher immunization coverage and safeguarding public health against the re-emergence of VPDs.

Test Your Knowledge

1. What are the recommended vaccination schedules for children, and why are they important for disease prevention?
2. How do live, inactivated, and subunit vaccines differ in composition and immune response?
3. What are catch-up vaccination strategies, and how do vaccination schedules vary across different countries?

8.3. Barriers to Vaccination

Learning Outcome

1. Vaccine hesitancy and its determinants
2. Misinformation and myths regarding vaccines
3. Socioeconomic determinants for vaccination coverage
4. Accessibility to healthcare and vaccination services
5. Cultural beliefs and their impacts on vaccination
6. Legislative and policy challenges
7. Social media's role in shaping opinion
8. Measures for overcoming barriers to vaccination
9. Community engagem and education required

Hesitancy in vaccines remains a big barrier to the prevention of spread of vaccine-preventable childhood diseases. Various studies cite as that the most common parental hesitancy driver is fears about vaccine safety and its effects. For example, research on Ohio Amish communities revealed that concerns over potential side effects strongly discouraged parents from vaccinatinulting in outbreaks of diseases like measles, which have the potential to lead to serious health complications and hospitalization (Ryan, 2023Segraves et al., 2015). Similarly, research in Juneau, Alaska, indicated that parents' perceptions of vaccine risk were the only influence on their denial of the influenza vaccine, despite its efficacy to avert severe illness (Leder et al., 2015). The same research emphasizes the requirement for targeted educational programs to refute false beliefs about vaccine safety to enhance vaccination rates and ultimately save children's lives from vaccine-preventable illnesses.

8.3.1. Vaccine Hesitancy and Its Causes

Vaccine hesitancy constitutes a significant hindrance to the achievement of maximum immunization coverage and is a function of numerous factors that are complex in nature and therefore require serious examination. One of the significant reasons is disinformation, particularly enhanced during crises like the COVID-19 pandemic, which has transformed people's attitudes and contributed to vaccine skepticism (Ruth et al., 2024). Parents worry about side effects and safety of immunizations, most often for their children.

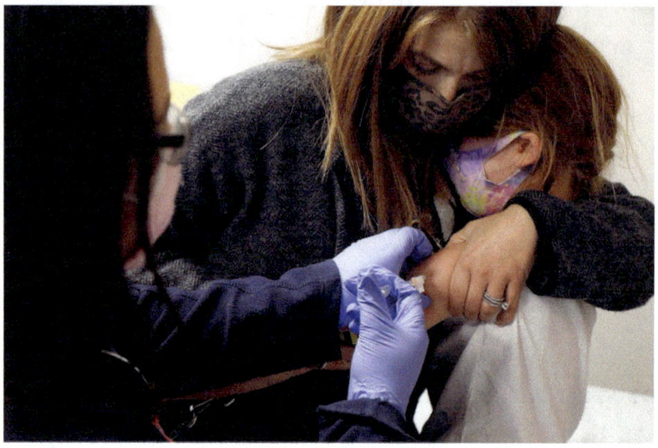

Figure 8.12. Vaccine hesitancy.

Source: https://external-content.duckduckgo.com/iu/?u=https%3A%2F%2Fwww.washingtonpost.com%2Fwp-apps%2Fimrs.php%3Fsrc%3Dhttps%3A%2F%2Farc-anglerfish-washpost-prod-washpost.s3.amazonaws.com%2Fpublic%2F5U4ZPKB5KQI6ZPLP3I3W6RZQJY.jpg%26w%3D1440&f=1&nofb=1&ipt=88efe3b5eabbdfeb910c93d108e2772290bb757625206f597a28c2917175ca83&ipo=images.

A study indicates that while the majority of families are commended vaccination schedules, hindrances to vaccines that are paid for exist, particularly as reluctance tends to be more in such cases (Ryan, 2023Ruth et al., 2024). Besides, socioeconomic status and perceived individual health also influence parental decision-making, leading to delays or denial of vaccinations required for disease prevention among children. Addressing these concerns through targeted education and communication efforts is key to increasing rates of vaccination and safeguarding public health (Figure 8.12).

8.3.2. Misinformation and Myths Surrounding Vaccines

The dissemination of disinformation and myths about vaccines poses a significant public health threat, particularly for vaccine-preventable childhood diseases. Parents are commonly reluctant due to unfounded fears about the safety of vaccines, based on emotive anecdotes that circulate on social media. This reluctance could be driven by anecdotal reports centered on perceived risk, despite the overwhelming evidence attesting to the safety of vaccines. For instance, the dossed that even though there are risks and contraindications, most of the issues circulating in public spaces typically aically not evidence-based. In order toTo overcome such misinformation efficiently, health care professionals should use compassionate communication strategies, such as, such as the C.A.S.E. Model, which enable open dialogue and honest conversations with parents. Trust establishment and open communication of facts can play a significant role in vaccine uptake, which ultimately guards children against preventable diseases.

8.3.3. Socioeconomic Factors Affecting Vaccination Rates

Socioeconomic status is a determining factor in changing vaccination coverage, particularly among children who are vulnerable to vaccine-preventable diseases. Families with lower socioeconomic status usually face barriers in the form of decreased access to care, poor health literacy, and financial barriers that all act against timely vaccinations. Research indicates that parents of premature babies, a group at high risk of vaccine-preventae lower vaccination compared to parents of full-term babies, mainly due to the cost of some vaccines and fear of adverse effects of vaccines (Ryan, 2023Ruth et al., 2024). Furthermore, disadvantaged socioeconomic poputhe appropriate healthcare centers, thus causing loss of parental trust in the healthcare providers as well as the vaccination program itself (Ryan, 2023Ying et al., 2024). Therefore, measures must be taken to diminish such differences by promoting targeted public health interventions to support the acceptance of the vaccine and ultimately minimize vaccine-preventable diseases among vulnerable children.

8.3.4. Access to Healthcare and Vaccination Services

Health and access to immunization are central health determinants of vaccine-preventable child illness. There are inequalities in immunization coverage within marginalized communities, where socmic status and belief are critical factors influencing participation in the vaccine program.

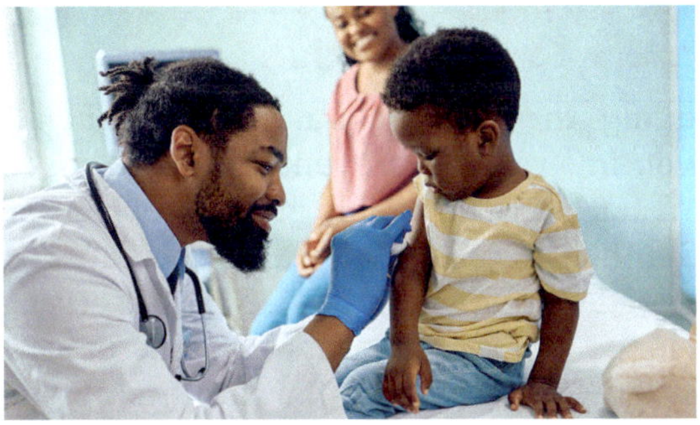

Figure 8.13. Pediatrician administering a vaccine to a young child.

Source: https://www.cdc.gov/hepatitis-a/media/images/2024/04/hepatitis-a-vaccine-administration-thumbnail.jpg.

For instance, a study of the Indigenous Batwa in Uganda presents bch as myths about the safety of vaccines, faith in traditional medicine, and physical distance, which discourage visits to healthcare providers (Ryan, 2023Eustes et al., 2024). Similarly, South African mbarriers in language difference and interpersonal connection with health providers, which affect their ability to navigate immunization systems (Ryan, 2023Stephan et al., 2023). Identification and mitigation of these access barriers through culturally sensitive interventions will enhance trust and facilitate increased vaccine acceptance, ultimately resulting in the prevention of vaccine-preventable disease in risk groups (Figure 8.13).

8.3.5. Cultural Beliefs and Their Impact on Vaccination

Cultural beliefs play a pivotal role in shaping attitudes toward vaccination, particularly within diverse populations. For example, the Nomadic Fulani communities, who adhere strongly to traditional practices, often exhibit suspicion toward modern medical interventions, including vaccination (Fulton et al., 2018). Limited understanding of vaccine benefits and mechanisms, coupled with the absence of tailored health communication, contributes to low vaccination uptake and heightened vulnerability to vaccine-preventable diseases. Similarly, parental perceptions of vaccine safety may discourage immunization, as demonstrated in a study from Juneau, Alaska, where concerns about potential risks were the primary reason for refusal (Leder, 2015). These examples highlight the necessity of culturally sensitive public health strategies that directly address community-specific beliefs and concerns, thereby improving vaccination coverage and overall child health outcomes.

8.3.6. Legislative and Policy Barriers

Legislative and policy challenges significantly impede the effective administration of vaccines in pediatric populations, thereby increasing the incidence of vaccine-preventable diseases. State-level vaccination law inconsistencies have the potential to create zones of vaccine incompleteness, as shown through variations in mandate enforcement and parental opt-out policies, frequently resulting in increased rates of vaccine hesitancy (Olufunto et al., 2021). Besides, socio-ecnants influence access to healthcare, particularly among marginalized populations wh already be experiencing social determinants of health inequalities (Ryan, 2023Jennifer, 2019). Such are further worsened by the lack of a proper public health infrastructure to make ensure complete vaccination initiatives, particularly in times of public health emergencies. As adherence to vaccination is based on legal support and the effectiveness of health policy, there should be a reform in the currently existing laws as well as enhanced community outreach programs so that immunizations are equally provided. Addressing these systemic barriersmes an issue of paramount concern for ensuring public health and preventing outbreaks of entirely preventable illnesses.

8.3.7. The Role of Social Media in Shaping Public Opinion

The sSocial media has been increasingly playing a role in public opinion, specifically concerning vaccine-preventable childhood diseases. With Facebook, Twitter, and Weibo becoming crucial channels of health information, online engagement with medical content shapes attitudes and trends towards immunization. A recent review found that medical bloggers can have a substantial influence on public health through advocacy of d vaccine awareness among their audience, with the evidence noting that around 61.8% of social media users acknowledge their power in preventing disease (Ryan, 2, 2024). Social media further provides an interesting perspective whereby public perception regarding certain vaccines changes, indicating that user-generated content has ability to inform and mislead the public. As demonstrated in research into HPV vaccination controversy on Weibo, opinion generated from social media is valuable information for the overcoming of existing challenges and the maximization of vaccination strategies (Yinqi, 2024). Social media thus performs two functions in that it not only transmits valuable health information but also influences child vaccination public opinion (Figure 8.14).

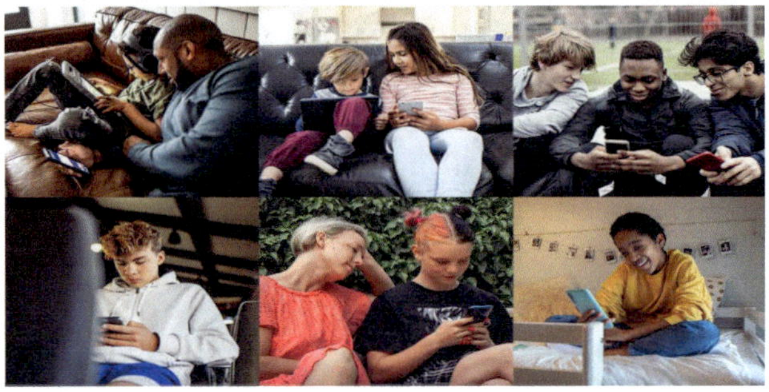

Figure 8.14. The role of social media in shaping public opinion.

Source: https://sachishiksha.com/wp-content/uploads/2025/03/Social-Media-in-Shaping-Public-Opinion-in-2.

8.3.8. Strategies to Overcome Barriers to Vaccination

Bridging the vaccine barriers is crucial in preventing vaccine-preventable child disease, particularly in vulnerable groups such as, such as Southeast Kansas. It was illuminated in a recent study that vaccine safety myths arreatest barrier to compliance, and concerns being the most powerful barrier for parents (Bennett et al., 2022). Overcoming such resistance has proven successful through intervention such as, such as enhancing parental knowledge with the utilization of visual aids. Implementing an efficient immunization schedule in pediatric patients' exam rooms not only heightens awareness but also promotes healthy dialogue among healthcare workers and parents (DiCola et al., 2024). Moreover, engaging community stakeholders in the planning and execution of vaccination efforts provokes a collective sense of endeavor to boost the vaccination rate. Through addressing the issues directly and improving access to educational content, healthcare systems can greatly improve the compliance with vaccination requirements and prevent children from vaccine-preventable diseases through timely vaccination. Such coordinated efforts are important in filling the gap in vaccination and safeguarding public health.

8.3.9. Importance of Community Engagement and Education

Education and community participation are central to vaccine-preventable children's illnesevention, particularly among disadvantaged populations. As a study among Uganda's Indigenous Batwa has confirmed, misconceptions surrounding the safety of vaccines inherent perceptions of the distrust of Western medicine strongly impede vaccination efforts (Eustes et al., 2024). Cultural values and health behavior knowledge amonopulations play the a basis for the development of patiently attuned educational programs that will gaincy with local cultures. Additionally,tives led by medical associations, such as, such as Latin America's, focus on having the requirement to meet up and address vacc. Such as, such associations propose measures such as, such as improving vaccine education and community trust building in a bid to boost immunization program enrollment (Ryan, 2023Maria et al., 2023). By bridging the gap between healthcare professionals and the community through information exchange and reassurance, such efforts can ultimately provide higher vaccination rates and, thereby, prevent outbreaks of vaccine-preventable illnesses among high-risk populations.

Test Your Knowledge

1. What are the common barriers that prevent children from receiving timely vaccinations?
2. How does accessibility to healthcare and vaccination services affect immunization rates?
3. In what ways does social media influence public opinion and attitudes toward vaccination?

8.4. The Role of Vaccination in Public Health

Learning Outcome

1. Historical success of vaccination programs
2. Vaccination and economic benefits
3. Vaccination and reducing health spending
4. Global vaccine programs and their impact
5. For instance, WHO and CDC and their role
6. Future challenges to vaccine development
7. Requirement for continuous research and innovation
8. Vaccine policy and ethics
9. Vaccination and better global health equity

Vaccination is the pillar of public health since it effectively prevents vaccine-preventable childhood disease outbreaks, hence saving community health. Disinformation regarding vaccines has led some parents to postpone or skip routine vaccinations, thus bringing about the resurgence of diseases like pertussis and measles.

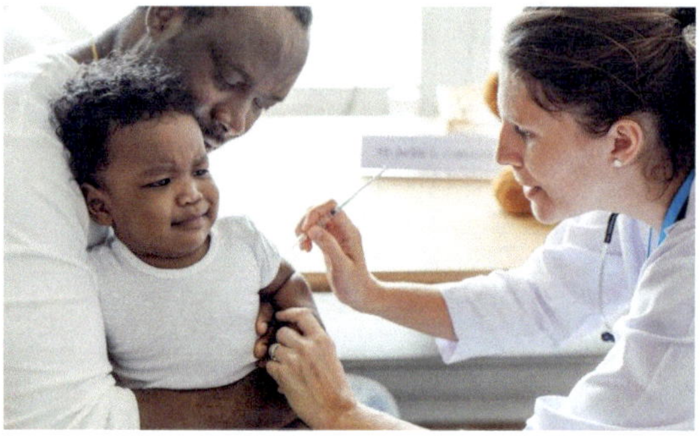

Figure 8.15. The role of vaccination in public health.

Source: https://www.nursinginpractice.com/wp-content/uploads/2022/10/Measles-outbreaks-are-almost-innevitable-say-early-years-vaccination-experts.jpg.

In America, the vaccine-preventable diseases have re-emerged as severe public health concerns in the unvaccinated population, hence the necessity of vaccination. The efforts of public health must tackle the myths surrounding the vaccines and emphasize their safety and effectiveness and the concept of herd immunity which will protect vulnerable individuals who are unable to be vaccinated. Through raising awareness of such issues, health professionals can facilitate informed decision-making among families on immunization, thus enhancing the overall public health outcomes and limiting the spread of infectious diseases among communities (Figure 8.15).

8.4.1. Historical Successes of Vaccination Programs

The history of past success of immunization campaignident in their unprecedented contribution to public health, notably reducing morbidity and mortality caused by vaccine-preventable childhood disease. Vaccines have profoundly lowered the spread of disease such as, such as smallpox, measles, and polio for over two centuries, and in so doing, safeguature generations.

The World Health Organization estimates that vaccines already save 3.5 to 5 million lives each year, pointing to the profound difference they make in the health of children. Achievements such as, such as the global eradication of smallpox and near-eradication of polio illustrate the potential of vaccination campatop infectious diseases. Further, historical evidence shows that vaccination not only enhanced individual health outcomes but also facilitated socioeconomic advancement and community resilience (Ryan, 2023Amy, 2024). Amidst the tide of skepticism towards vaccines, such successes can be recalled to revive confidence in vaccination as an essential instrument for public health.

8.4.2. Economic Benefits of Vaccination

Vaccination campaigns not only are a useful public health measure but also have significant economic benefits, particularly in the context of vaccine-preventable childhood diseases. The economic rationale in favor of expanded coverage with vaccination is compelling, as studies have established that vaccination can avert major healthcare costs of treatment and lifelong disability. For instance, the Hib vaccine has been shown to reduce healthcare expenses, decrease parental absence from work, and prevent productivity losses from child morbidity (Abigail et al.). Moreover, successful vaccination is likely to stimulate economic growth by preventing child mortality, which in turn can influence fertility decisions and labor market performance. Investing in vaccinations by policymakers would enable them to expect lower economic costs of disease outbreaks, eventually leading to healthier populations and overall economic stability. It is therefore essential to address vaccination reluctance and ensure sufficient coverage to help optimize overall health and economic gain for society.

8.4.3. Vaccination and The Reduction of Healthcare Costs

The impact of vaccination programs to decrease healthcare costs of vaccine-preventable illnesses, particularly in children, has been well documented. A case in point is the unprecedented reductions in the incidence of varicella and related hospitalizaGermany following the introduction of universal varicella vaccination (UVV) programs, as highlighted by a systematic review that highlighted the economic importance of employing such intervention (Ryan, 2023Angela et al., 2020). The economic effects go beyond the expense of hospitalization; routine immunization can prevent the costly interventions engaged in during outbreaks, thereby saving healthcare resources. Furthermore, this advced by findings that increased provider training in vaccination practices considerably increases immunization levels among kids, closing knowledge gaps that often result in suboptimal immunization coverage (Dupervil et al., 2023Ryan, 2023). Thus, a harmonized approach in immunization programs not only better enhances the health status of the population but also is a strategic way of reducing economic burdens on healthcare systems (Figure 8.16).

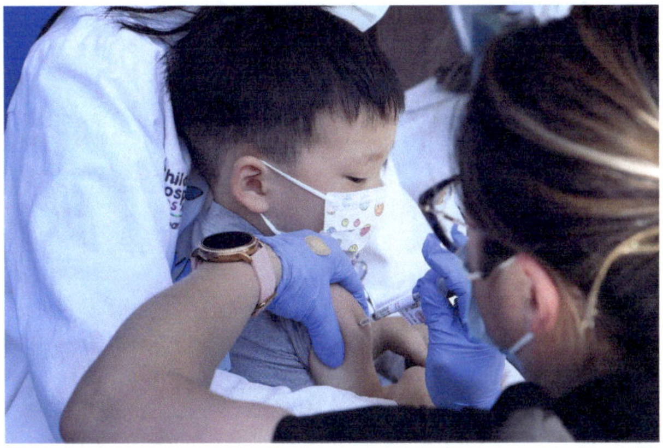

Figure 8.16. Child receiving a vaccine while being comforted by a caregiver.

Source: https://www.americanprogress.org/wp-content/uploads/sites/2/2023/06/GettyImages-1241629425.jpg?w=1680.

8.4.4. Global Vaccination Initiatives and Their Impact

The rollout of global immunization programs has had a profound effect on the profile of child health, markedly reducing the number of vaccine-preventable illnesses. Vaccinations given to children save an estimated three million lives annually, illustrating the imperative of these programs in fostering child survival worldwide. Despite all this progress, infectious illnesses like measles, tetanus, and whooping cough remain some of the leading causes of child mortality, particularly in low-resource settings, and represent lingering inequalitiemunization coverage (Lepage, 2006). Also, advances in vaccination against rotavirus, the cause of severe diarrhea with an estimated annual 440,000 deaths worldwide in developing nations, has been highlighted through efforts such as, such as the European PROTECT program aimed at raising awareness and increasing immunization uptake (Lepage, 2006). All these efforts show the significance of continued activism and advocacy in bringing vaccination benefits to all children across the globe, ultimately improving health and quality of life (Figure 8.17).

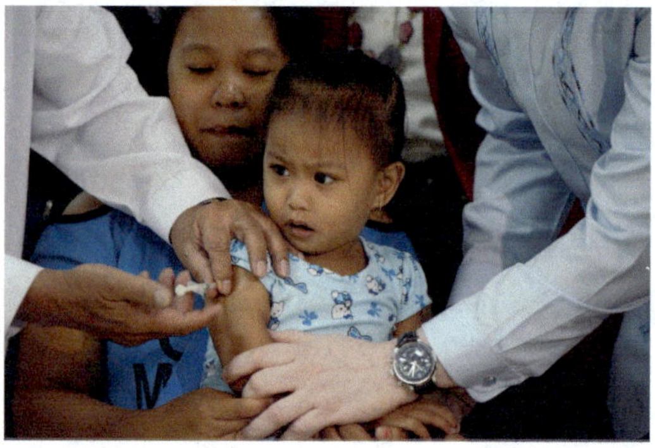

Figure 8.17. Global vaccination initiatives.

Source: https://external-content.duckduckgo.com/iu/?u=https%3A%2F%2Fstatic01.nyt.com%2Fimages%2F2015%2F07%2F22%2Fbusiness%2Fiional%2F22db-kk%2F22db-kk-superJumbo.jpg%3Fquality%3D90%26auto%3Dwebp&f=1&nofb=1&ipt=87dd1eedfd85b68ed5f8ea2f44f90ac7d224916c2acb7f82238da809865af3ce&ipo=images.

8.4.5. The Role of Organizations Like WHO and CDC

Organizations such as, such as the World Health Organization (WHO) and the Centers for Disease Control and Prevention (CDC) play a central role in combating vaccine-preventable childhood diseases through comprehensive public health initiatives and education programs. These agencies provide guidelines for immunization and policy recommendations to help ensure that children are up-to-date on their vaccinations and do not experience disease outbreaks, including measles, which is a threat even though it is preventable with vaccinations. For example, the CDC informs us of alarming rises in cases of measles, predominantly caused by under-vaccination in specific populations, which indicate the urgent necessity of targeted educational campaigns targeting parents and guardians (Price, 2020). Moreover, the WHO mobilizes global efforts to raise vaccination rates, reporting that well-implemented vaccine programs can potentially save millions of lives each year, confirming their function in maintaining herd immunity and protecting vulnerable populations (Megana et al., 2024). Hence, the collective action of these organizations is essential for safeguarding children's health against preventable diseases.

8.4.6. Future Challenges in Vaccine Development

While vaccine research goes on, the problems of the future have to be addressed so that the efficacy and acceptability of vaccines for childhood diseases remain constant. One of the biggest challenges is growing skepticism regarding vaccination as a result of ignorance of faith in medical authority. This has been seen to create a paradox between parental personal choice and public health requirements, where personal choice immediately influences public health. Also, recruiting specific vaccines, such as, such as bacterial meningitis ones, onto mandatory school schedules has been controversial, particularly in regions of weak legislative support, as has been the case with recent proposals in Alaska for awareness and policy initiative. Hence, vaccine development initiatives in the future should not only advance science but also maintain inclusive public education and ethical standards that contribute to community trust building and collaborative efforts for increased pediatric vaccination coverage within a rapidly evolving health landscape.

8.4.7. Importance of Continuous Research and Innovation

The significance of continuing reseh annovation in the field of vaccine-preventable diseases in children cannot be overemphasized. Over the past 50 years, immunization efforts have helped to avert an estimated 154 million deaths globally, making the continued support to of the vaccination programs essential (Baidya et al., 2024). Research is essential in the creation of new vaccines and the improvement of existing vaccines, particularly against the backdrop of the new pathogens that are challenging public health eradication of diseases like measles. For instance, recent research noted that 78% of unvaccinated confirmed cases of measles, demonstrating the direct correlation between vaccination snd disease severity (Ryan, 2023Aslan et al., 2024). Moreover, new diagnostic strategies, e.g., concurrent utilization of ELISA and RT-PCR, have proven to facilitate early detection of infections, improving clinical outcomes. Instances such as, such as these demonstrate that research and innovation remain essential in overcoming the impacts of vaccine-preventable diseases and ensuring community health security (Figure 8.18).

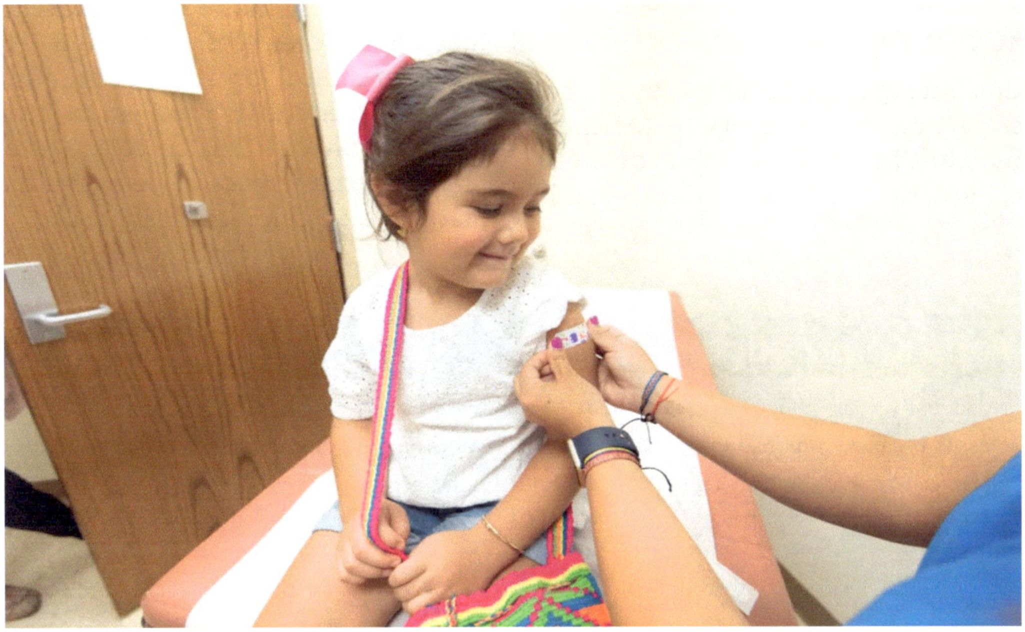

Figure 8.18. Child receiving a bandage after vaccination at a pediatric clinic.

Source: https://pedsav.com/wp-content/uploads/2024/02/innovations-in-pediatric-care-new-treatments-and-technologies-jpg.webp.

8.4.8. Ethical Considerations in Vaccination Policies

The ethical consideration of immunization policies is of top priority, particularly in the case of vaccine-preventable childhood illnesses. Not only does vaccination play an individual protective function in each child, but it also has a societal mandate to ensure the well-being of the population.

Ethical considerations have put forward a two-prong approach: the necessity to safeguard the children and the advancement of ty to vaccinate is partially based on the need for herd immunity; by permitting personal concerns to overrule the well-being of society, the threat of outbreak grows, undermining public health programs (Chukwueke & Wen, 2019Bilgrien et al., 2018). Therefore, policies should include mandatory vaccination with educational intervention to alleviate parental fears and establish confidence and informed choice. Significantlylike Catholic social teaching principles emphasize human dignity and the common good and prefer a middle path between the rights of individuals and community responsibilities in vaccination policy debates (Chukwueke & Wen, 2019Bester et al., 2020).

8.4.9. The Impact of Vaccination on Global Health Equity

Immunization is a key impetus for health equity worldwide, particularly in terms of vaccine-preventable childhood diseases. Provision of vaccines greatly reduces morbidity and mortality rates from infectious diseases, enhancing the health of vulnerable groups of people worn program delivery through sysmatic administration, as per the Advisory Committee on Immunization Practices, not only addresses the epidemiologic disease burden but also fosters equity in healthcare access (Chukwueke & Wen, 2019Murthy et al., 2024). Inequities persist, however; , low-income countries are likely to have issues of vaccine supply logistics and healthcare infrastructure and therefore suffer from unequal vaccination coverage and resulting health inequities. Global immunization efforts must be intensified through collective action to eliminate such obstructions so that all children get vaccinated irrespective of geographical or socio-economic position. Ultimately, equitable vaccination strategies can achieve universal health coverage as well as minimize the impact of pediatric diseases on marginalized communities globally.

Test Your Knowledge

1. How have global vaccine programs contributed to reducing infectious diseases worldwide?
2. What roles do organizations like the WHO and CDC play in promoting and coordinating vaccination efforts?
3. How doetion contribute to achieving better global healty and access to healthcare?

SUMMARY

The statistics regarding vaccine-preventable childhood diseases illustrate the substantive impact of immunization campaigns on population health. Evidence, such as, such as the evaluation of the effectiveness of Italyunization Program (Italy), suggests that benefits decisively outweigh costs, with estimates referencing the averted 1.8 million cases and thousands of lives saved and a benefit-cost ratio of 5.6 at the societal level (Chukwueke & Wen2024). Similarly, Belgium's childhood immunization system demonstrates a principal return on investment, wherein for every €1 invested in childhood vaccines, approximately €3.2 in cost savings to society is achieved (Chukwueke & Wen, 2019Carrico et al., 2023). Such evidence shows the essential contribution vaccines make in averting children's morbidity and mortality as well as easing economic burdens on healthcare systems. Thus, investing in vaccination strategies in the long term is not merely a necessity for individual health results but also a key to effective public health policy.

In vaccine-preventable childhood disease research, some major findings emerge that emphasize the role of vaccine strategies in the protection of child health. Recent studies havat 4-component recombinant protein-based (4CMenB) vaccination is over 90% effective at preventing serogroup B meningococcal disease in children below six years of age in Italy, particularly when early immunization occurs (Chukwueke & Wen, 2019L., 2023). This suggests the hope of age-targeted intervention among p younger age groups that are not yet vaccine-eligible, thus reducing the burden of disease significantly. In addition, the discovery of mechanisms of pediatric allergic disease, such as, such as asthma, highlights the significance of biological pathways such as, such as Wnt signaling, in their pathogenesis ancidence of vaccine efficacy and disease pathogenesis stresses the imperative of ongoing research as well as the adjustment of immunization procedures to further enhance protective interventions for childhood diseases (Chukwueke & Wen, 2019Nooralam et al., 2022).

KEY TERMS FROM THIS CHAPTER

- Chronic infections
- Efficacy
- Immunizations
- Misconceptions
- Morbidity
- Pertussis
- Public health
- Society
- Vaccination
- Diseases
- Herd immunity
- Immunology
- Misinformation
- Pediatric health
- Pregnancy
- Rubella
- Transmission
- Vaccine-preventable diseases (VPDs)

CRITICAL THINKING QUESTIONS

1. **Which of the following vaccines protects against a disease caused by Hemophilus influenzae type b?**
   a. DTP
   b. MMR
   c. Hib
   d. IPV
2. **What does the "MMR" vaccine protect against?**
   a. Measles, Mumps, Rubella
   b. Meningitis, Malaria, RSV
   c. Mumps, Measles, Rotavirus
   d. Measles, Mumps, Rabies
3. **Which of the following is a live attenuated vaccine?**
   a. Hepatitis B
   b. DTaP
   c. MMR
   d. Hib
4. **At what age is the first dose of the Hepatitis B vaccine typically given?**
   a. At birth
   b. 2 months
   c. 6 months
   d. 1 year
5. **The DTaP vaccine protects against which of the following diseases?**
   a. Diphtheria, Tetanus, Pertussis
   b. Diphtheria, Typhoid, Pneumonia
   c. Dengue, Tetanus, Polio
   d. Diphtheria, Tuberculosis, Pertussis

Short Answer Questions

1. Explain the importance of childhood immunization programs in the prevention of infectious diseases. How do vaccine-preventable diseases impact pediatric health globally?
2. Describe the mechanism of action, schedule, and common side effects of the DTaP vaccine. What diseases does it prevent, and why is each significant in pediatrics?
3. Discuss the role of the MMR vaccine in controlling outbreaks of measles, mumps, and rubella. Include transmission, complications, and public health strategies.
4. Outline the causes, clinical features, and complications of poliomyelitis in children. How has the introduction of OPV and IPV impacted the global incidence of this disease?
5. Compare and contrast the rotavirus vaccine and influenza vaccine in terms of disease burden, target populations, administration methods, and outcomes.
6. What is the significance of the Hepatitis B vaccine in newborns? Describe the transmission of the virus, its long-term effects, and the recommended vaccination schedule.

Answer to Critical Thinking Questions

1.(c) 2. (a) 3.(c) 4. (a) 5.(a)

REFERENCES

1. Alves da Costa, F., & O' Moore, E. (2024). Preparing for outbreaks of vaccine preventable diseases: Why are prisons invisible? *Health Promotion International, 34*. https://www.semanticscholar.org/paper/d088fcace8ec58643bcb2886968398e57af6ad39 (accessed on 16th June 2025).
2. Antônio Rosa, S. S. S., Prereia Júnior, A., Pontes, A. N., & Bichara, C. C. (2024). Mandatory childhood vaccination coverage and notifications of vaccine-preventable diseases in a municipality in the Eastern Amazon. *Revita Pan-Amazonia de Saude*. https://www.semanticscholar.org/paper/f9970be08e7c6e03556f8e0a1c7235cae4bba064 (accessed on 16th June 2025).
3. Avola, G. M., & Lyon, J. A. (2012). Understanding caregiver factors influencing childhood influenza vaccination. *University of New Hampshire Scholars' Repository*. https://core.ac.uk/download/72047940.pdf (accessed on 16th June 2025).
4. Bechini, A., Kauffmann, F., Casabona, G., Bonanni, P., & Wutzler, P. (2020). Varicella vaccination in Italy and Germany–Different routes to success: A systematic review. *Human Vaccines & Immunotherapeutics*. https://core.ac.uk/download/589962371.pdf (accessed on 16th June 2025).
5. Bennett, D. (2022). Factors influencing vaccination rates in children under two in Southeast Kansas. *Pittsburg State University Digital Commons*. https://core.ac.uk/download/543565433.pdf (accessed on 16th June 2025).
6. Bharati, K. (2023). Development and evaluation of an inactivated Chikungunya virus vaccine. *Journal of Medical Virology*. https://www.semanticscholar.org/paper/188c0c1eb6bed7d17cc37127c9addccc051811f5 (accessed on 16th June 2025).
7. Chukwueke, U., & Wen, P. Y. (2019). Use of the Response Assessment in Neuro-Oncology (RANO) criteria in clinical trials and clinical practice. *CNS Oncology, 8*. https://doi.org/10.2217/cns-2018-0007 (accessed on 16th June 2025).
8. Connors, M., Graham, B. S., Lane, H. C., & Fauci, A. S. (2021). SARS-CoV-2 vaccines: Much accomplished, much to learn. *Annals of Internal Medicine, 174*, 687–690. https://doi.org/10.7326/m21-0111 (accessed on 16th June 2025).
9. Copacia, J., Danino, D., Taylor, K., Sanborn, P., Abu-Arja, R., & Ardura, M. (2023). Optimizing vaccine delivery among pediatric allogeneic hematopoietic cell transplant recipients: A quality improvement initiative. *Journal of Pediatric Hematology/Oncology*. https://www.semanticscholar.org/paper/0d56535cd76fcded863afd5de040aac04479e416 (accessed on 16th June 2025).
10. Elil, J. (2019). Barriers to hepatitis A vaccination in homeless populations: A narrative literature review. *Journal of Public Health and Epidemiology*. https://www.semanticscholar.org/paper/1e877398414da23b9564cfb253e8f8b7e5357459 (accessed on 16th June 2025).
11. Fisher, C. B., Bragard, E., Jaber, R., & Gray, A. (2022). COVID-19 vaccine hesitancy among parents of children under five years in the United States. *Vaccines, 10*, 1313–1313. https://doi.org/10.3390/vaccines10081313 (accessed on 16th June 2025).

12. Huang, Z. (2024). The evolution and impact of animal vaccines: Advancements, applications, and future directions. *Vaccine Research Journal*. https://www.semanticscholar.org/paper/d325c9bb6e2f4ca846d940ab1ce9038641943bc1 (accessed on 16th June 2025).

13. Hulstine, A. (2017). Vaccine implementation: Alaska 2017. *University of Alaska Anchorage*. https://core.ac.uk/download/286607590.pdf (accessed on 16th June 2025).

14. Kasavaraju, M., & Gowda, M. (2024). Patterns of vaccine titers after childhood leukemia treatment. *Journal of Pediatric Hematology/Oncology*. https://www.semanticscholar.org/paper/a6370abfbd608c58fde4002c63093aedbdf9254b (accessed on 16th June 2025).

15. Kigongo, E., Opollo, M. S., Nalwoga, V., Musinguzi, M., Kwizera, G., & Kabunga, A. (2024). Perspectives of pediatric vaccination among the Batwa community in Western Uganda: A qualitative study. *Journal of Public Health in Africa, 11*. https://www.semanticscholar.org/paper/91dd4250252d4c1cead4886720787e15851f8df0 (accessed on 16th June 2025).

16. Leder, L. (2015). *Vaccination Hesitation: Investigation Why Parents Decline Pediatric Influenza Vaccines in Juneau, Alaska*. University of Alaska Anchorage. https://core.ac.uk/download/162577318.pdf (accessed on 16th June 2025).

17. Lepage, P. (2006). Rotavirus infection in Europe: Time for effective prevention? *Vaccine, 25*, 5–6. https://www.semanticscholar.org/paper/ef7c8ed909927ff01edfc02bae1281a9da6bd115 (accessed on 16th June 2025).

18. Maldonado, Y. (2002). Current controversies in vaccination: Vaccine safety. *JAMA, 288*(24), 3155–3158. https://www.semanticscholar.org/paper/0ecbb3a8ff02e849c6f8286756b5e56e2551eabf (accessed on 16th June 2025).

19. Mejías, A., Rodríguez Fernández, R., Peeples, M. E., & Ramilo, O. (2019). Respiratory syncytial virus vaccines. *The Pediatric Infectious Disease Journal, 38*, 266–269. https://doi.org/10.1097/inf.0000000000002404 (accessed on 16th June 2025).

20. Murthy, N., Wodi, A. P., McNally, V. V., Daley, M. F., & Cineas, S. (2024). Recommended adult immunization schedule, United States, 2024. *Annals of Internal Medicine, 177*, 221–237. https://doi.org/10.7326/m23-3269 (accessed on 16th June 2025).

21. Olusanya, O. A., Bednarczyk, R., Davis, R., & Shaban-Nejad, A. (2021). Addressing parental vaccine hesitancy and other barriers to childhood/adolescent vaccination uptake during the coronavirus (COVID-19) pandemic. *Frontiers in Public Health, 12*. https://www.semanticscholar.org/paper/3e6a587fc84580882a01b9a271e3e32e3111b7b4 (accessed on 16th June 2025).

22. Rai, N., & D'Armiento, J. (2022). Wingless/integrase-1 signaling in allergic asthma and pediatric lung diseases. *Pediatric Pulmonology, 34*, 572–579. https://www.semanticscholar.org/paper/9a387d5c7346f206ca2e618e86a851f6a41d92db (accessed on 16th June 2025).

23. Ryan, E. (2023). *Mandates, Mistrust, and Misconceptions: An Overview of Vaccine Hesitancy*. Scholars Crossing. https://core.ac.uk/download/568250035.pdf (accessed on 16th June 2025).

24. Siegel, R. L., Miller, K. D., Fuchs, H. E., & Jemal, A. (2021). Cancer statistics, 2021. *CA: A Cancer Journal for Clinicians, 71*, 7–33. https://doi.org/10.3322/caac.21654 (accessed on 16th June 2025).

25. Vijayan, V. K. K., & De Paris, K. (2024). Nonhuman primate models of pediatric viral diseases. *Vaccine Research Journal*. https://www.semanticscholar.org/paper/5de46778b0e7010de2689acab0019592f18227dc (accessed on 16th June 2025).

PEDIATRIC SURGERY: COMMON PROCEDURES AND EMERGENCIES

9

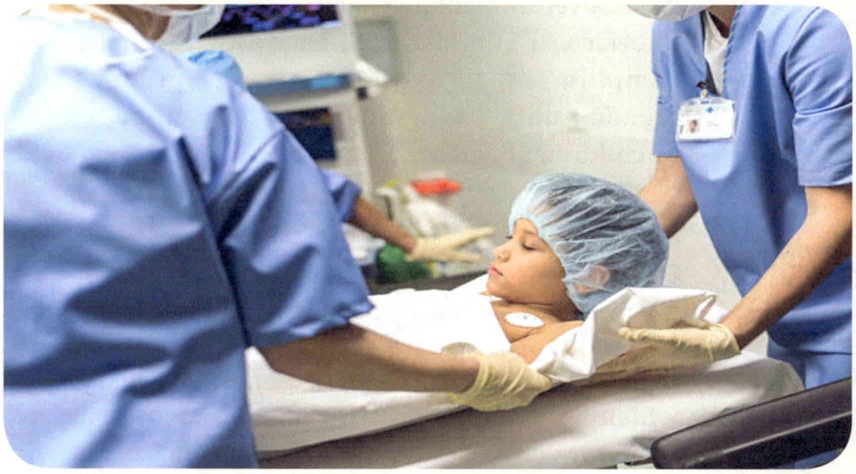

LEARNING OBJECTIVES

After studying this chapter, you will be able to:

1. Enumerate the most frequent pediatric surgical procedures
2. Describe pediatric surgical emergencies
3. Describe preoperative considerations
4. Highlight postoperative care
5. Recognizalpsychological impact on pediatric patients
6. Describe advances in pediatric surgery

Introduction

In children's surgery, the sophistication of children's process and emergency has to be thoroughly understood. Pediatric patients present a distinct set of physiell as psychologicalpsychological problems that are unlike those presented by adults. Such disparity necessitates specialized surgical techniques considering the development phases of children, in addition to a specialist's awareness of their transforming anatomy. According to the reports, pediatric surgery is not just a branch of general surgery but rather a separate discipline involving expertise from various areas of medicine to provide the best results and deal with possible complications optimally (John et al., 2020). The most common procedures in pediatric surgery, including hernia repairs and appendectomies, are important interventions that can significantly impact the course of a child's life and quality of life later on. Pediatric surgical emergencies demand fast and precise action due to the vulnerability of younger patients. Obstruction of the intestine, traumatic injuries, and appendicitis typically require immediate surgery, and therefore prompt diagnosis and assessment are essential skills for pdiatric surgeons. Patients size, anatomical quiddities, and potential comorbidities also complicate such emergencies, which can vary significantly in children. An in-depth understanding of airway management and sedation procedures is crucial in such cases, with the inability to prepare adequately havnces (Charles et al., 2019Abib et al., 2022). Pediatric surgeons must not only be technically competent but also possess the ability to manage the psychosocial aspects of treatment, providing a supportive environment to cir families in the midst ofduring anxious medical situations.

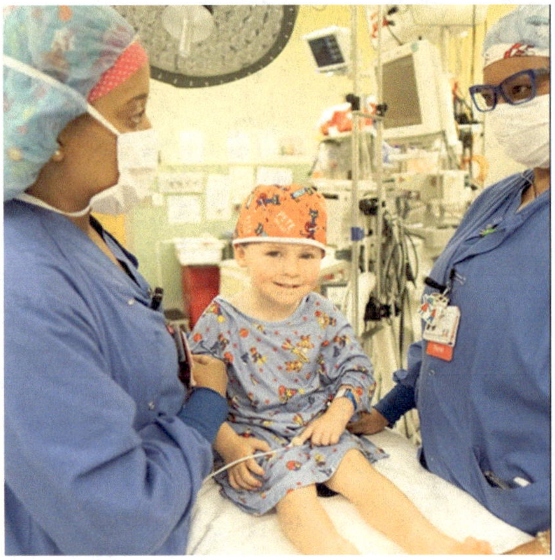

Figure 9.1. Pediatric surgery: common procedures and emergencies.

Source: https://www.choa.org/-/media/Images/Childrens/global/highlight-pods/medical-services/surgery/surgery-small-boy-in-operating-room-surgeons-475x475.ashx.

Implementation of new technology and techniques in pediatric surgery has contributed to progress in elective as well as emergency surgery. New techniques of surgery, like minimally invasive surgery, enhance recovery times and reduce days in the hospital, but require advanced training and experience that is specialized to the child population. Additionally, as healthcare systems evolve, coupled with evidence-based interventions and multidisciplinary practice, it is paramount in developing procedures that address the unique needs oft al., 2022John et al., 2020). The ongoing challenges posed by conditions like COVID-19 also underscore the necessity ofptable protocols in order toto maintain surgical care at minimal risks. Overall, pediatric surgery is an intensive interface of surgical skill, emergent care, and commitment to patient-centered practice founded on a commitment to the well-being of children (Figure 9.1).

Definition of Pediatric Surgery

Pediatric surgery is a specialty of medicine that is entirely involved in diagnosis and operative treatment of disorders in children, adolescents, and infants. In contrast to general surgery, which is concerned with adults, pediatric surgery considers unique aspects in terms ofphysiological, and psychologicalpsychological distinctions between children and adults. This specialty embraces a wide variety of conditions ranging from congenital malformations, injury due to trauma, to neoplasms. Pediatric surgeons do not only require surgical expertise but also the skill to manage the special requirements of pediatric patients, which in most cases means personalized techniques of anesthesia, care following surgery, and counseling of parents. Because the population of pediatric patients has specific health concerns, pediatric surgery is all about understanding these differences and using surgical treatments that yield the best outcomes for children. The ASA physical status classification system also illustrates the challenges of pediatric surgery. The system, originally developed for use with adults, is widely applied to assess perioperative risk in children and is seriously tested in accurately representing the health status of children.

The critical analysis of ASA-PS in children's surgery reveals a tendency to minimize chronic disease loads according to standardized characterizations, which can then influence surgical decisions, risk stratification, etc. As pediatric surgery evolves with advancements in medical technologies and technics, practitioners need to adapt and modify existing classification systems to incorporate the pediatric anatomy and pathophysiology specifics. These changes will ensure that surgical operations not only are appropriately relevant but also safe and effective in children receiving surgical operations (Leahy et al., 2018). Apart from complex physical status assessments,eatment of congenital disorders such as, such as congenital adrenal hyperplasia and gastrointestinal abnormalities needs special surgery. The conditions often arise at birth and necessitate immediate surgical and ongoing medical care. Pediatric surgeons must address the intricate nature of these conditions, extending beyond the surgical correction to include long-term effects on growth, development, and quality of life. With increasing understanding of congenital conditions, the function of pediatric surgery becomes increasingly critical in delivering holistic multidisciplinary treatment beyond the time of surgical involvement. By aligning surgery with changing clinical guidelines, pediatric surgeons can improve patient outcomes while reducing unique safety and quality of life concerns in the treatment of chronic disease in thn (Abib et al., 2022Speiser et al., 2018).

Importance of Pediatric Surgery in Child Health

The contribution of pediatric surgery to promoting child health cannot be exaggerated as it involves a wide array of interventions whose purpose is to repair congenital malformations, trauma, and other potentially life-threatening abnormalities among children. Pediatric surgery plays an important role repair of developmental anomalies such as, such as congenital cardiac anomalies and gastrointestinal anomalies so that children can lead healthier lives. Finally, early surgery can eliminate suffering and restore function, which is most important to a child's physical and emotional development. Increasing understanding of the unique differences in pediatric anatomy and physiology has led to modified surgical techniques that enhance outcomes and minimize complications and attests to the need for experienced pediatric surgical capabilities within the healthcare system. In the emergency setting, pediatric surgery is crucial in stabilizing life-threatening states that require immediate attention. Pediatric Emergency Departments are found to be effective overall and associated with their readiness to treat pediatric cases, as presented in recent studies that show primary factors of emergency department (ED) pediatric readiness affecting survival rates of children with injuries. Specifically, developments in policy and hardware regulating pediatric treatment significantly enhance patient outcomes for surgical emergencies. For instance, the application of certain pediatric guidelines and protocols in trauma centers has been linked to improved survival rates, demonstrating just how crucial such procedures are in maintaining children's health in situations of medical emer et al., 2023). Moreover, the psychologicalpsychological well-being aspect of pediatric surgical intervention is a significant factor to consider. Children who must be operated on typically experience anxiety and distress; therefore, managing preoperative anxiety is at the center of child practice. Studies have shown that addressing the mental status of a child can lead to better experind outcomes during surgery. Methods such as, such as iatrosedation and hypnosis have been found to be effective non-pharmacologic anxiety reduction interventions in pediatric patients, with a balanced concept of health focusing on both somatic aacco & Zanette, 2017Abrahamsson et al., 2017). As the character of pediatric surgery evolves, the emphasis on general straoster surgical preparedness and psychologicalpsychological well-being highlights the ongoing importance of pediatric surgery in improving the overall health and welfare of children (Figure 9.2).

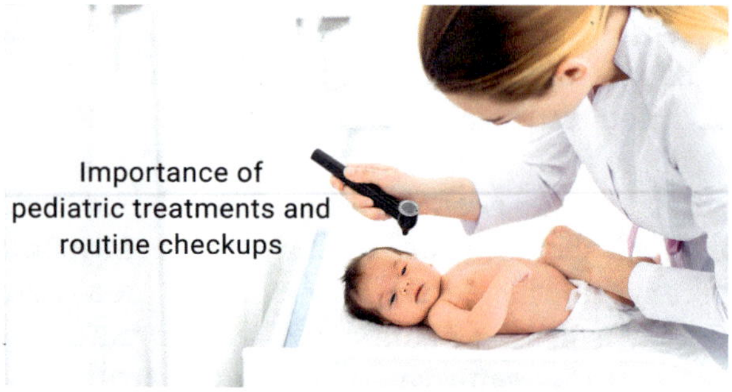

Figure 9.2. Importance of pediatric surgery in child health.

Source: https://www.eternalhospital.com/uploadedfiles/gallery/1669380294_Importance-of-pediatric-treatments-and-routine-checkups1.jpg.

Overview of Common Procedures and Emergencies

In pediatric surgery, it is vital to be profhe normal procedures and emergencies in order toto offer the patient the best possible outcome. Appendectomies, herniorraphies, and circumcisions are among the most frequently performed surgeries in the pediatric operating room. The appendectomy, which is often necessary for appendicitisne in an attempt to prevent complications such as, such as perforation, which can lead to life-threatening infections. Similarly, inguinal hernias which are normally encountered in children and infants must be operated on early to avoid incarceration or strangulation of the bowel tissues. Such interventions with general anesthesia entail skilled techniques and post-operative care to avoid any complications and bring about healing. The availability of such interventions highlights the importance of pediatric surgical expertise in dealing with common but severe childhood conditions. Pediatric surgical emergencies require immediate and effective resp prevent serious complications. Emergencies such as, such as traumatic injuries, bowel obstructions, and acute abdomen require immediate assessment and intervention. Trauma cases, most often due to accidents or falls, can require operation to diagnose and repair the internal injuries. Obstructions in the intestine can be due to congenital conditions or acquired disorders and require emergency operation to relieve the obstruction. Surgical teams are educated to recognize such emergencies rapidly, following a systematic assessment and management approach. Effective communication between surgical teams and emergency medical services is critical to guarantee prompt and life-saving treatment to children in distressing conditions, avoiding rm impairments or death. New training methods such as, such as simulation-based training (SBT), play a crucial role in preparing surgical teams for handling emergencies. Such a training methodology allows surgeons and allied healthcare workers to develop their capacity in a secure manner within a simulated setting, navigating sophisticated circumstances. As one example, extracorporeal membrane oxygenation (ECMO) is an aggressive procedure typically required during severely acute cardiac or respiratory collapse in pediatric patients. Utilizing an ECMO simulator allows clinice prepared for such life-threatening situations, such as, such as those related to cannulation, which is the diversion of blood flow for oxygenation. Through collaborative efforts like those with Hamad Medical Corporation (HMC), such simulators look to enhance actual decision-making and procedural realism. By mimicking possible complications, like low pressure flow or mispositioned cannulas, SBT not only enhances the education of clinicians but also has a significant role in increasingoverall patient cencies (NAbib et al., 2022/A, 2008; Abdallah et al., 2019).

9.1. Common Pediatric Surgical Procedures

Learning Outcome

1. Appendectomy
2. Hernia Repair
3. Circumcision

One of the most common pediatric surgical procedures is the appendectomy, or the removal of the appendix for appendicitis. Appendicitis is a frequent pediatric emergency with pain and inflammation in the abdomen. The indication for an appendectomy is primarily based on the risk of perforation, which can lead to peritonitis and severe morbidity. Studies have indicated that appendectomy procedures for appendicitis are well-outcome in children, though there are potential complications like unplanned return to operating room (uROR). Surprisingly, appendectomies accounted for a sizeable percentage of uROR cases examined in a recent case series. The findings revealed error in surgical technique was prevalent, hence necessitating enhanced surgical protocol in the pediatric setting, primarily to prevent risk in emergency operations, which have shown a higher level of complications compared to elective operations (Juki et al., 2022). Correcting congenital anomalies, e.g., inguinal hernias and congenital diaphragmatic hernias, is another key procedure in pediatric surgery. Inguinal hernias are typically diagnosed in infancy and must be repaired to prevent complications like strangulation or incarceration of the herniated tissue. Repair in the outpatient setting includes reinforcement of the abdominal wall, which prevents recurrence. Congenital diaphragmatic hernia repairs are more complex, typically performed shortly after birth for relief of respiratory distress secondary to the hernia impeding lung development. These procedures require multidisciplinary collaboration between pediatric intensivists and surgeons to ensure optimal perioperative management. Inability to manage potential postoperative complications, i.e., infection or respiratory failure, underscores the necessity of customized surgical care in infants and neonates to ensure optimas well as quality of life (Abib et al., 2022Gregory et al., 2019).

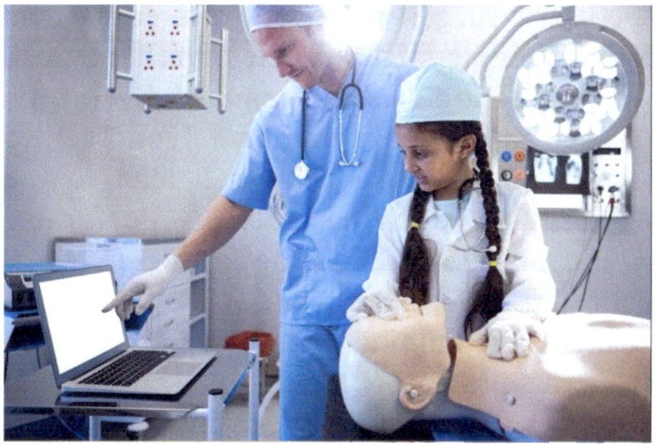

Figure 9.3. A common pediatric surgical procedure is the appendectomy.

Source: https://www.vachhanihospital.com/blog/wp-content/uploads/2024/02/Understanding-the-Most-Common-Pediatric-Surgical-Procedures.jpg.

Traumatic injuries of children often require urgent surgery, particularly fractures of the cervical spine. Such fractures have been noted to become more common, and their effect on patient management and surgical outcome is significant. Usually resulting from motor vehicle crash or sports injury, these fractures may need extensive surgical intervention to stabilize the cervical spine and avoid complications, including SCI. Data suggest predictors of surgical intervention are the degree and nature of injury, as well as the presence of concomitant injuries complicating treatment for the patient. According to the expanded understanding of complications for these procedures, pediatric surgeons are warned to maintain heightened vigilance on a perioperative basis. This focus can enhance patient safety and align treatment strategies with contemporary best practices in pediatric trauma care to supterm outcomes for children (Abib et al., 2022Gregory et al., 2019) (Figure 9.3).

9.1.1. Appendectomy

Appendectomy is a routine surgical procedure in pediatric surgery, primarily offered for acute appendicitis. It is the result of inflammation of the appendix, usually caused by luminal obstruction of the appendix. Prompt inton is necessary because delay can lead to fatal complications such as, such as perforation and peritonitis. Pediatric appendectomies are performed either by conventional open surgical procedures or minimally invasive laparoscopy, with the latter becoming increasingly favored due to benefits that involve reduced postoperative pain and faster recovery rates. Selection of surgical technique frequently depends on the specific situation of the patient and the competence of surgeons in pediatric surgery. Appendectomy, however, is not riskless. Among the pertinent issues is the unplanned 30-day return to the operating room (uROR) after the initial surgery. Through research, it has been discovered that one of the reasons for this occurrence is appendectomies, and the reason pinpoints procedural difficulty and potential surgical error. In a thorough analysis, the most common cause of uROR was attributed to technical errors in surgery, which emphasized the importance of regular training and vigilance among child surgeons (Juki et al., 2022). Thus, surgical outcomes following appendectomy can be an essential quality indicator in pediatric surgery, providing feedback on the effectiveness as well as safety of operations. Where resources are scarce, as in most low-to-middle-income countries, appendicectomy capability can make a large contribution towards pediatric surgical provision. Despite difficulty through limited availability of highly skilled surgical teams, attempts at upskilling rural general practitioners so they can perform such important procedures as appendectomies have proven that they can indeed do so very effectively. A Nepalese retrospective analysis found that general practitioners conducted a lot of surgeries, including appendectomies, successfully, enhancing surgical availability among communities. This is a significant shift in healthcare delivery and draws attention to training and resource allocation in pediatric surgery (Dangal et al., 2021). Subsequently, access to appendectomy can enhance clinical outcomes and contribute towards aggregate surgical capacity in poor regions.

9.1.2. Hernia Repair

In children's surgery, hernia repair is a frequent procedure, particularly in infants and young children. It is largely for inguinal hernias, which occur when abdominal contents, such as bowel or omentum, protrude through a weakness in the abdominal wall at the inguinal canal.. Althrequently discovered at birth, en left untreated for many times years until complications occur, such as, such as incarceration or strangulation. These emergencies may result in major morbidity if left untreated. Surgical intervention typically involves a herniotomy, in which the sac is removed and the defect in the abdominal wall is repaired. Elective repairs, if done early, can ensure better outcomes with minimal complications, underlining the significance of strong health systems that support early detection and management of pediatric hernias (Naluyimbazi et al., 2024). Availability of the resources for surgery is key to successful hernia repair in children, especially in low- and middle-income countries (LMICs). Most systems face issues with inadequately available mesh for repairs, leading to increased rates of complications and recurrences, especially in emergency situations. Children in these regions also present late due to access barriers to early care, leading to preventable complications. Empirical evidence suggests that bolstering local surgical capacity through the training of general practitioners would do a great deal to address such issues and improve child health outcomes (Dangal et al., 2021). Such taskg not only enhances local capties but also guarantees that key surgery surgeries like hernia repair is are being done safely and efficiently in rural hospitals.

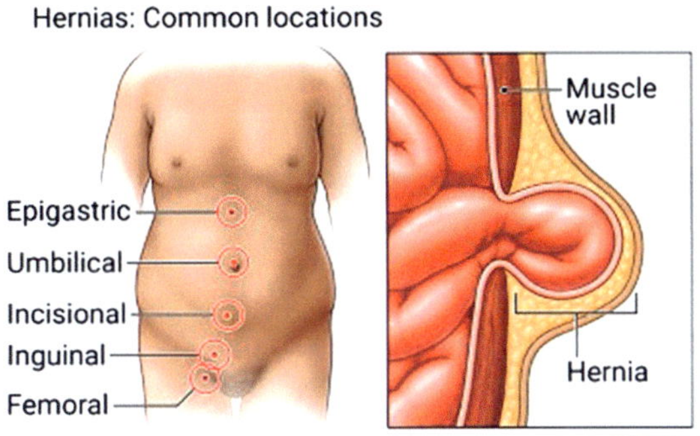

Figure 9.4. In the realm of pediatric surgery, hernia repair is a prevalent procedure.

Source: https://ixbapi.healthwise.net/Resource/14.5/en-us/media/medical/hw/aci3786_368x240.jpg.

Ultimately, successful hernia repair holds far-reaching consequences that extend beyond isolated patient outcomes, as a reflection of health systems' overall surgical capability. The success of care for pediatric hernias can be used as a measure of the availability of and quality of surgical care provided throughout an arther, as evident from existing studies, availability of materials such as, such as hernia mesh is increasingly being recognized as a crucial component for the success of surgical interventions across various settings (Naluyimbazi et al., 2024). By taking hernia repair as a representative operation and a bellwether for the provision of surgery into account, sytems can identify the highest-priority areas for improvement and resources development, and impose a proactive approach to the children's surgical requirements in different economic contexts (Figure 9.4).

9.1.3. Circumcision

Circumcision is a standard pediatric surgical procedure commonly performed for both medical and nonmedical reasons. Circumcision is a surgical procedure where the foreskin, or skin fold that covers the Glan of the penis, is removed. Phimosis, which is when the foreskin is unretractable over the glans and can lead to infection or the inability to urinate, is a primary medical indication for circumcision. In addition to this, frequent urinary tract infections (UTIs) are also linked with non-circumcised men, so parents are inclined towards getting circumcision done as a preventive measure. Balancing risks against advantages like reduced infection rates for some and enhancing personal hygiene are the guidelines that decide whether one should get this surgery performed. Even though circumcision is safe by general criterion, physicians need to discuss it time and again with parents to make consensual choices. The age at which circumcision is performed varies, with some being done shortly after birth and others when they are older in childhood. Neonatal units are usually the place where early circumcision is performed because of the presence of senior staff who are qualified to handle any arising issues. Circumcision as an older child, however, has additional complications in that older children may require more prolonged anesthetic and pain relief measures. Circumcision customs can vary tremendously across cultures and socioeconomic environments, and culturally aware medical practice is therefore indicated. For instance, certain communities may favor circumcision as a rite of transition or for religious reasons, whereas others may not follow this tradition at all. Pediatric surgeons should be aware of the common perception of circumcision when advising families on whether to perform the procedure or not. Complications of circumcision, while for the most part rare, include bleeding, infection, and injury to the glans. Complications are estimated to occur in about 1% of cases, placing emphasis upon the place of skill ethod as well as post-operative care. In addition, emotional and psychologicalpsychological effects of circumcision cannot be excluded; some studies indicate possible long-term effects on body image and sexual function. In pediatric surgery, it is crucial todisciplinary approach encompassing not only the physical but also psychologicalpsychological and social aspects of the decision-making process. As outlined in the literature, the landscape of pediatric emergency surgery, which may include emergent circumcision procedures in cases of acute diests an imperative to continue education in pediatric surgical care in order toto enhance the outcomes of children (Aisuodionoe-Shadrach et al., 2011; Firomsa et al., 2018).

Test Your Knowledge

1. What are the main indications and steps involved in performing an appendectomy in children?
2. How is hernia repair carried out in pediatric patients, and what are the common postoperative considerations?
3. What are the medical and cultural reasons for performing circumcision, and what care is required after the procedure?

9.2. Pediatric Surgical Emergencies

Learning Outcome

1. Intestinal Obstruction
2. Trauma and Injury
3. Testicular Torsion

Pediatric surgicies are a broad spectrum of conditions that must be addressed promptly in order toto avoid fatal complications. Such types of emergencies often manifest as gastrointestinal and abdominal pathology, foreign bodies, and injuries resulting from trauma. In a retrospective analysis at Tikur Anbesa Hospital, abdominal emergency accounted for 46.3% of pediatric cases, indicative of the high need for specialized surgery within this area. Moreover, foreign body ingestion as a condition, with 29.3% of reported cases, proves that pediatric populations are very vulnerable to such incidents. Early identification and treatment are essential because delayed presentation is common; over 40% of the patients within the research presented over five days following the onset of illness, it further underscores the critical need for heightened awareness among caregivers and healthcare providers regarding the timeliness of pediatric surgical conditions (Firomsa et al., 2018). In low-resource areas, pediatric surgical emergencies can be exacerbated by systemic issues to cause substantial delays in treatment. For instance, in Uganda, 15% of children have been projected to be fighting with un-treated surgical conditions due to economic considerations, beliefs, and ineffective healthcare infrastructure. Dependence on traditional community healers usually puts off patients from accessing proper medical care, and those who do access health facilities are usually overwhelmed by overcrowding and unavailability of resources that make their treatment complicated. Consequently, pediatric surgery in such environments is not only a question of qualified professionals but also ongoing measures to expand access to services through improved infrastructure, greater training for local healthcare staff, and mobilization for shifting healthcare culture to support timely intervention (Alberti et al., 2024). Despite the issues that contribute to pediatric surgical emergency care, significant progress has beed in improving children's outcomes in various settings.

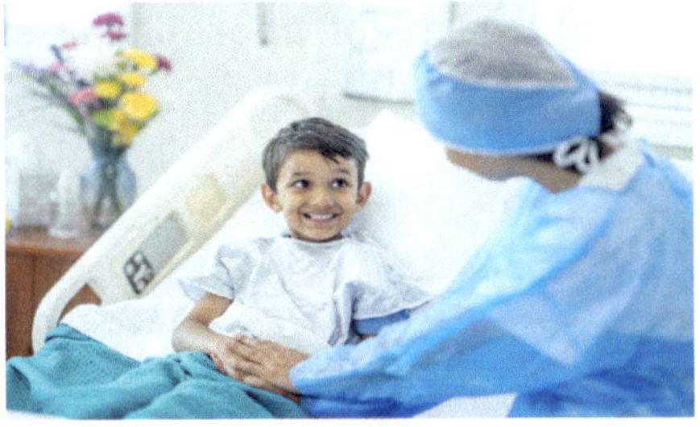

Figure 9.5. Smiling child interacting with a healthcare provider during hospital recovery.

Source: https://jamaicahospital.org/newsletter/wp-content/uploads/2025/04/GettyImages-1500142631.jpg.

Proactive measures, such as, such as the establishment of specialist pediatric theatres and surgical fellowship training programs, are aimed at increasing the quality of care offered to children. In Uganda, the introduction of specialized surgery facilities in Mulago National Referral Hospital is an essential step toward meeting unmet surgical requirements, allowing for an environment where pediatric emergencies may be addressed effectively. Additionally, the organization of surgical camps and courses dedicated to the management of pediatric surgical emergencies has the potential to upgrade the technical skills of healthcare providers, ultimately delivering better patient care in needy areas. As the pediatric surgery fraternity continuously adapts and keeps up with the needs of the times, the future of pediatric emergency care is increasingly brighter, with far brighter outlooks for the most helpless members of society (Alberti et al., 2024) (Figure 9.5).

9.2.1. Intestinal Obstruction

Small bowel obstruction is a significant pediatric surgical emergency that presents severe challenges to clinicians. Intestinal obstruction may be caused by a myriad of etiologies, including congenital illness, adhesions, or tumors, and may lead to extreme complications like bowel ischemia or perforation if promptly managed. Pediatric are known to present with unique symptoms compared to their adult counterparts, such as, such as abdominal distension, vomiting, and altered bowel habits. Prompt diagnosis, using imaging modalities like abdominal X-rays or ultrasonography, is crucial to the establishment of the obstructions presence and cause. Additionally, the urgency of operation significantly affects outcomes because delayed operation can exacerbate the risk of potentially life-threatening complications. Familiarity with the special aspects of pediatric intestinal obstructions is crucial in management and improved survival in children. Surgical intervention of intestinal obstruction is usually directed at relieving the obstruction and its cause. The operation varies immensely with the etiology of the obstructions, ranging from as minimal as decompression to more than that with extensive resections. For instance, the etiology of congenital anomalies like intestinal volvulus typically involves resection of portions of non-viable bowel to prevent further complications. Postoperative care is also a critical part oment, and vigilant monitoring must be carried out for infections or complications such as, such as anastomotic leaks. Recent studies have found that the majority of surgical emergencies in children are gastrointestinal emergencies, and this puts a focus on pediatric surgeons becoming well versed in handling such cases (Firomsa et al., 2018). With an expansive surgical strategy, including preoperative optimization and postoperative management, health care providers can maximize recovery and support long-term outcomes in these children. In pediatric surgery, intestinal obstruction not only requires emergency treatment but also helps to demonstrate prevention and patient education for caretakers. Most obstructions can be prevented by early intervention and management of risk factors in a manner that is timely, therefore, reducing the presentation time for surgery. Parents and guardians are also important players in the surveillance of their children's health, and education on early signs can greatly change presentation time for surgical management. Further, the surgeons must be updated on evolving treatment modalities and pediatric surgery procedure advancements that can provide quicker recovery times and improved patient outcomes. Incorporating these into routine pediatric practice can lead to an active approach in treating intestinal obstructions and preventing long-term complications among children (Beekley et al., 2018).

9.2.2. Trauma and Injury

Injury and trauma are both parts of pediatric surgery as crucial challenges, which could involve urgent intervention. These injuries are usually part of the course of everyday life and accidents and are thus unpredictable and prevalent. For instance, ear, nose, and throat (ENT) injuries are prevalent among the pediatric population, where children might unknowingly get in contact with foreign bodies or experience trauma as a result of falls and impacts. A study of 456 patients reported that foreign bodies were the most common cause of ENT trauma, with 61.8% of the cases, and followed by road traffic accidents with 22.4% of the cases (Okoye et al., 2013). The foregoing illustrates not only how common such events aalso the exigency for early management interventions to prevent additional conditions such as, such as suppurative otitis media and traumatic epistaxis. Chest trauma is another serious concern in children following trauma, and this has primarily been attributed to road traffic accidents (RTCs). A prospective study involving 150 patients confirmed that 72.7% had blunt injuries and that RTC was the leading cause, which affected 50.7% of the study sample (K et al., 2011). The impacts of these injuries are severe, often leading to conditions such as, such as hemothorax and rib fractures necessitating complex interventions. Treatment outcomes are variable, with the majore cases being managed on a non-operative basis; however, the fact that complications, such as, such as wound sepsis, do occur underscores the emergent nature of appropriate surgical and medical interventions.

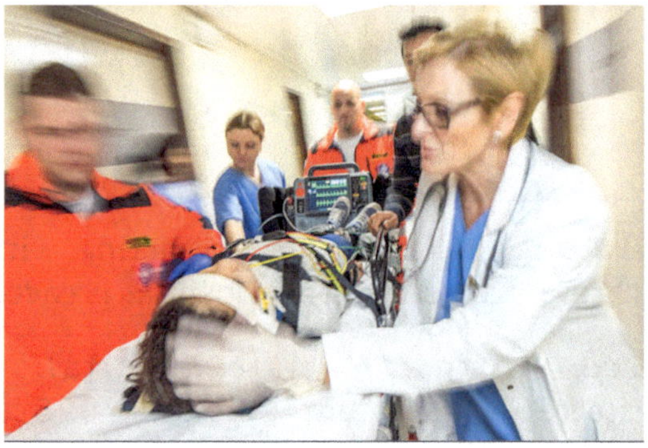

Figure 9.6. The trauma and injury represent critical challenges that can necessitate urgent intervention.

Source: https://uwnewsroom-prod-backend.parallelpublicworks.com/sites/default/files/child-ed-head-trauma.jpg.

The prevalence of concomitant injuries, especially to the musculoskeletal system and head, adds to the complexity of care and underscores the significance of global care strategies in pediatric trauma management. Injury and trauma management among children entails a wide-ranging approach encompassing prevention, emergency treatment, and chronic care. The apparent high levels of morbidity related to injuries call for both clinical adjustments and public health initiatives aimed at reducing the frequency of accidents, particularly RTCs. Schools and other institutions can conduct public information campaigns among parents and caregivers, with a focus on safety habits in whatever environments children engage in activities. Operating teams must also be prepared for a multitude of routine procedures that address the acute effect of injuries but also for possible long-term consequences of unresolved trauma. By facilitating an interdisciplinary understanding of these dynamics, healthcare practitioners are able to significantly enhance pediatric outcomes in patients with traumatic injury (Figure 9.6).

9.2.3. Testicular Torsion

Among the numerous emergencies encountereatric surgery, torsion of the testis stands alone in its potential for severe damage, such as, such as repeated loss of the affected testis. This surgical emergency typically presents suddenly, almost exclusively in adolescent males between 12 and 18 years of age, but can present at any age. The primary pathology is rotation of the spermatic cord, which causes compromise of the blood supply to the testis. The clinicians must act promptly, as ischemia will be established within hours and can lead to necrosis or permanent damage. A high index of suspicion is required for prompt diagnosis when a child develops an acute scrotum, vomiting, or nausea. It is the challenge to differentiate from testicular torsion from other etiologies like epididymitis, which is similar in presentation but has a different effect on the pediatric age group. Management of testicular torsion is predominantly surgical, encompassing detorsion and stabilization of the testis in the scrotal sac to prevent recurrence. The surgery, referred to as orchidopexy, aims to reestablish blood flow early and fix the testis to the scrotal wall, thus removing the potential for future torsion. Surgical examination has also been good if undertaken early, and evidence has indicated that the optimal window for testicular salvage is within six hours of the onset of symptoms (Simone et al., 2022). Postoperative care is portant since the child will be in discomfort and should be monitored for complications such as, such as infection or recurrence of torsion. In addition, family education regarding the symptoms and signs of testicular torsion is important, as early diagnosis significantly enhances prognoses and diminishes long-term morbidity. Aside from surgery, understanding the epidemiological determinants of testicular torsion will also enhance outcomes in pe populations. The condition is more common among men with some anatomical predilections such as, such as the bell clapper deformity, wherein the testis has no normal fixation to the scrotum. These risk factors underscore the need for preventive education and awareness among parents and medical staff. Furthermore, the inclusion of ultrasound technology as an aid to diagnosis offers non-surgical approaches to determining scrotal pain, which will aid in the differentiation between torsion and pathology (Hoppmann et al., 2022). Overall, treatment of testicular torsion in the broad range of pediatric surgery involves both initial treatment and ongoing education to ensure that early and effective intervention is delivered to affected children.

Test Your Knowledge

1. What are the common causes, symptoms, and management approaches for intestinal obstruction in children?
2. How should pediatric trauma and injury be assessed and managed in surgical emergencies?
3. Why is early recognition and prompt treatment critical in cases of testicular torsion in children?

9.3. Preoperative Considerations

Learning Outcome

1. Assessment and Diagnosis
2. Parental Ivolvement and Consent
3. Anesthesia in Pediatric Patients

Preoperative considerations in pediatrics surgery play a critical role in ensuring the safety and effectiveness of procedures. They involve careful evaluation of the child's general health status, including a comprehensive medical history, physical assessment, and necessary diagnostic workup. The anesthetic risk must also be evaluated, particularly in pediatric patients, as they can have physiological differences that influence drug metabolism and action. Pediatric patients require a customized approach that accounts for age-based complications that may not be encountered in adults. For instance, congenital abnormalities or disorders of development need to be taken into account while designing the surgical plan and the anesthesia plan. Effective communication with parents is required to minimize fear and establish a clear perception of procedural risk versus benefit associated with surgery, thus establishing trust with the healthcare team. One of the most important parts of pediatric preoperative surgical planning is the recognition of patients at high risk for postoperative complications. Adherence to guidelines for the prevention and management of specific issues can go a long way in enhancing patient outcomes. Guidelines, for instance, emphasize the need to recognize risk factors for postoperative delirium in children, although less common than among adults. Early identification of such risks, along with proper intraoperative management, is important to prevent untoward effects. Mciplinary teams need to cooperate to ensure that medical as well as surgical needs are met before the procedure. This approach not only streamlines the preoperative process but also secures ensures that intensive preoperative assessment is re-established as a major consideration in improving general preparation for surgery and lowering perioperative complications, as stressed in surgical practice guidelines (César et al., 2017). Parental involvement is also still among the cornerstones supporting preoperative variables in children. Including parents in dialogue about the proposed surgical procedure, anticipated outcomes, and potential risks fosters a climate of collaborative decision-making and reassurance.

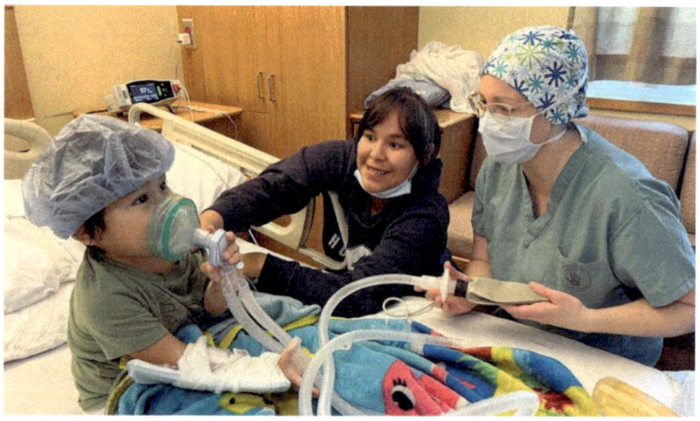

Figure 9.7. The preoperative considerations.

Source: https://media.oralhealthgroup.com/uploads/2023/02/1a-1-e1675365018428-1024x576.jpg.

This partnership is particularly significant since parents have the potential to be strong allies to their child's comfort and care. During preparation for surgery, educational materials must be provided to prepare parents to know what to expect preoperatively, intraand postoperatively. In addition, the application of measures in managing any form of psychologicalpsychological distress among the child and caregivers yields better overall perioperative results. Lastly, these preoperative factors optimize not just communication but also the opportunity for positive surgical results, streang the larger objective of pediatric surgery: health and well-being of the smallest patients (Eric Abib et al., 2022) (Figure 9.7).

9.3.1. Assessment and Diagnosis

In pediatric surgery, the diagnosis and evaluation phase is pivotal in making patient management a success. The initial step of this process involves careful examination of the child's history, physical, and use of diagnostic aids. Pediatric patients present with non-specific signs and symptoms, hence the process of diagnosis very challenging. Incorporation of the diagnostic imaging modalities such as, such as ultrasonography and MRI, is important in establishing underlying pathologies. The systematic process cannot be overemphasized, since the accuracy and timing of the diagnosis allow for timely surgical intervention, while tremendouslng the prognosis in children. Moreover, the application of standardized reporting guidelines, such as, such as the TRIPOD Statement, can increase transparency in predictive model research, such that clinicians can analyze the risk versus benefits of surres accordingly (Moons et al., 2015). Proper assessment also involves understanding the psychologicalpsychological profile of the pediatric patients since their age of development can indeed influence symptom presentation as well as compliance with tests. Pediatric surgeons must apply child-centered communication techniques to elicit proper feedback from their young patients, an essential component of appropriate diagnosis. Involvement of care partners, typically parents or guardians, in discussions of the symptoms and child's history is often beneficial in offering background information that is helpful in constructing a whole clincal picture. This multidisciplinay approach keeps in mind the multiple facets of the child's health, —physical, emotional, and social, —throughout the process of diagnosis. Because pediatric surgeries are generally so different from those of adults, having a clear understanding of the child's overall health is critical to tailor treatment accordingly. Quick diagnosis and evaluation in certain emergency conditions can be a matter of life and death. Intussusception or appendicitis must be treated promptly with appropriate surgery within a timely manner to prevent complications. Under such circumstances, pediatric surgeons utilize a combination of clinical presentation, laboratory workup, and imaging results to diagnose a child rapidly. Recombinant factor VIIa (rFVIIa) use, though typically off-label, has been a valuable hemostatic agent in the management of uncontrolled bleeding disorders in children, particularly in surgical contexts (Revel et al., 2013). By ensuring a timely diagnosis, one can take proactive measures, i.e., preparing for potential surgical or postoperative complications. Hence, the underpinnings of pediatric surgery are directly founded on streamlining assessment methods, which in turn have direct implications for patient safety and clinical results.

9.3.2. Parental Involvement and Consent

Parental participation is of utmost significance in pediatric surgery, especially when making surgical interventions for their children. Parents are significant advocates of their child's health, and they contribute knowledge on their child's specific needs and tastes. The decision-making process is often challenging, and there should be good communication between healthcare providers and parents. This discussion then takes on a unique importance in gender allocation in ambiguous genitalia or sexual developmental disorders, as outlined in the parent counseling guidelines. Parents must be enabled to provide their opinions but must also be educated concerning potential future results and dangers associated with different methods. Inclusive sessions with the local multidisciplinary committee (LMDC) are intended to improve this communication in order for parental concerns to be integrated into the decision-making process, thus providing a more personalized response to the child's care (Sarin et al., 2onsent is also a vital element of pediatric surgery, particularly when addressing sensitive issues such as, such as surgical treatment for differences in sex developmentrocess of informed consent must be approached in a sensitive manner with consideration of the psychologicalpsychological and emotional dimensions involved in such decisions. In the management of children with DSD, medical staff must provide parents with an extensive briefing on the impact of surgery and level of family care. This implies consideration of the potential for gender dysphoria and whether or not to factor in long-term implications of isions on the child's well-being. A child psychologist can be especially valuable at this stage in order toto assist in mediating between healthcare providers and families to make sure tof them have ice, thus providing an open forum through which informed consent can be attainedt al., 20182022). Moreover, the issue of consent by parents has to be addressed carefully in the event thatf a child's capacity to provide assent is age-dependent. Parents would normally make decisions on behalf of children in the event of pediatric surgery, but with advancing age, children's choices and opinions must increasinglyo the decision-making process. This shift is most relevant where surgical interventions have the capacity tocan cause substantive changes to a child's identity or quality of life. For kids at and over the age of 12 years, written assent is required since this is a reflection of eloping autonomy and capability for participation in the surgical process. This multi-dimensional aspect to of consent ensures that not only parental wishes but also the voices of the children are heard, thereby complementing an integrated model of pediatric surgical care thats the nuanced relationship between parental involvement and the child's emerging identity and rights (Sarin Abib et al., 2022) (Figure 9.8).

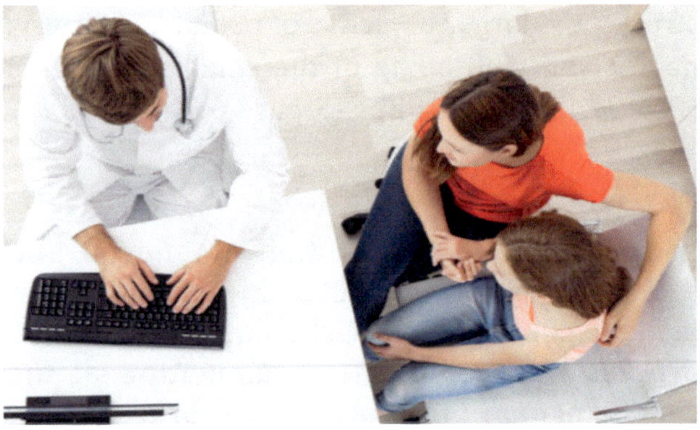

Figure 9.8. Parental involvement and consent.

Source: https://www.wcgclinical.com/wp-content/uploads/2020/02/doctor-consultation-child-parent.jpg.

9.3.3. Anesthesia in Pediatric Patients

The anesthetic management of children presents unique challenges that must receive serious attention from medical practitioners. Children are physiologically different from adults, and this makes it necessary to approach anesthetic management on an individual basis. Pediatric anatomy and anesthetic drug pharmacodynamics vary, which affects drug absorption, distribution, metabolism, and elimination. The differences indicate the necessity of dosing the child based on age, weight, and clinical condition. In addition, developmental levels and emotional reactions need to be taken into account, as children are unable to express their fears or discomfort clearly, making anesthesia difficult. By recognizing such complexities, anesthesiologists are able to reduce risks and achieve better outcomes, bettering the experience for patients and caregivers alike in the operating room. Recent studies suggest that adequate anesthesia management can also be a crucial component in reducing unplanned reoperations in pediatric surgery and is therefore an integral part oe overall surgical plan (Juki et al., 2022). One of the extremely crucial aspects of pediatric anesthesia are is risk factor considerations that can impact the success of surgery. The American Society of Anesthesiologists (ASA) classification is also frequently utilized to assess the global state of health in a child prior to surgery. Children with ASA class three or worse, for instance, are known to experience greater postoperative complications and longer hospital stays. This has specific relevance in the context of emergent surgeries, where unplanned reoperation risks can be considerable. It has been proven based on evidence that emergency operations of pediatric patients have much higher unplanned reoperation rates compared to elective operations, what anesthetic planning and management play a significant role in emergencies (Abib et al., 2022Juki et al., 2022). As such, awareness of these risk factors can help anesthesia providers develop well-informed care plans to achieve better results for children. The emergence of the COVID-19 pandemic has complicated pediatric anesthesia, requiring practice adjustments. Anesthesiologists must now weave through greater precautions to avoid viral spread as they provide timely and effective surgical care. The implementation of preoperative screening protocols, re-scheduling of surgeries based upon community infection rates, and the use of telemedicine for preoperative visits have all become standard practice elements. Being able to transform surgical workflows, as demonstrated through COVID-19, is essential to effectively coping with the changing nature of threats from public health crises. Also, as the pediatric population is largely asymptomatic carriers, stringent infection control measures are necessary during anesthesia induction and recovery. This evolving situation demands resilience and adaptability in pediatric anesthesia, with the safety of the patient being of paramount importance in the presence of unprecedented challenges.

Test Your Knowledge

1. What key factors are evaluated during the assessment and diagnosis before pediatric surgery?
2. Why is parental involvement and informed consent essential in the preoperative process for children?
3. What special considerations are required when administering anesthesia to pediatric patients?

9.4. Postoperative Care

Learning Outcome

1. Pain Management
2. Monitoring for Complications
3. Nutritional Needs

Postoperative care is an essential component of pediatric surgery, significantly affecting the patient's outcome and recovery. Postoperatively, infants and children can have unique issues, including control of pain, prevention of infeand support for emotional well-being. Medical caregivers will be required to monitor closely for complicationssuch as, such as infection or exsanguination by observing the vital signs as well as incision sites. Pain relief is also of utmost importance, using age-dependent analgesio ensure comfort. Also, postoperative space requires a healing space that supports physical comfort and psychologicalpsychological confidence, especially among young patients who may be anxious or scared of undergoing surgery. This integrated approach of postoperative care is essential to maximize the quality of recovery and speed up the return to normalcy among pediatric patients. Good communication among healthcare providers, families, and patients is key postoperatively. The caregivers and parents need to be well informed regarding the specific care needed after surgery, including drug administration, restriction of activity, and identification of potential complications. Evidence identifies families who are included in the care process as potentially being able to improve compliance with postoperative instructions in patients and to achieve better outcomes, reduced hospital readmissions.

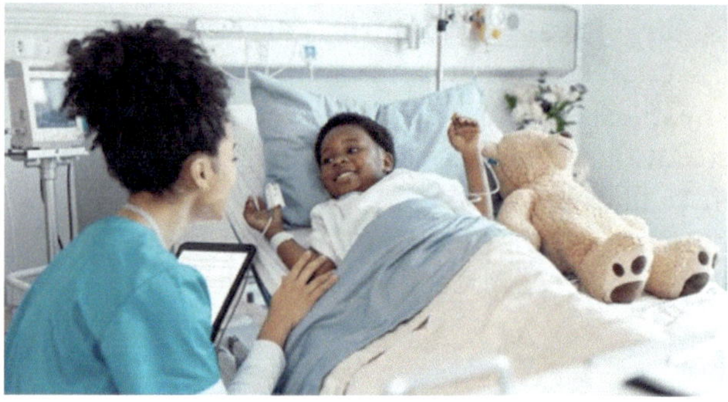

Figure 9.9. Postoperative care is a critical component of pediatric surgery.

Source: https://www.shutterstock.com/image-photo/tablet-nurse-black-child-patient-260nw-

9.4.1. Pain Management

Ideal pain management in children undergoing surgery is central to the avoidance of desired outcomecomplications and the promotion of recovery in children. Pain, if not adequately controlled, can have many undesired consequences, including increased anxiety, longer hospital stays, and even a possible risk of chronic pain syndromes. The current recommendations favorably emphasize the use of a multi-modal pain management plan comprising pharmacologic interventions combined with non-pharmacologic measures in the form of behavior therapy and physical therapy. This interdisciplinary method is especially relevant in the pediatric patient, in which the developmental considerations need to inform treatmerence to individualized pain management strategies that are relevant to each patient's unique needs can enhance significantlysignificantly enhance the worldwidocedure and healing, ultimately manifesting improved patient outcomes and satisfaction (Dean et al., 2016). The psychologicalpsychological aspect of pain management cannot be overlooked, particularly with children presenting for surgery. Children cannot communicate about their discomfort and therefore, are a priority to be evaluated using age-related instruments for ascertaining the degree of pain. Utilization of self-reporting instruments and observation will be helpful in the accurate appraisal of children's pain. In addition, the implementation of family values based on care, where parents and caregivers are actively engaged in reporting pain and pain management planning, is useful in providing an improved healing environment. This multimodal strategy not only ensures that pain is under controlparental anxiety, providing a better perioperative course for the child and the family (Abib et al., 2022Barbara et al., 2014). Moreover, the outcome of ineffective pain management extends beyond immediate post-operative recovery and may affect long-term health outcomes. Evidence indicates that, if pain in pediatric patients is not treated effectively, patients become increasingly sensitive to pain in their next medical visits and are at greater risping anxiety disorders. Hence, it is crucial to incorpordence-based practices in pain management guidelines in order toto minimize these risks. Empirical results consistently revise inform clinicians with the best methods of various surgical interventions so that they can successfully address the complications related to pediatric pain management. By adopting continuous learning and using integrated pain management strategies, medical practitioners can play a dramatic role in steering the course of recovery and long-term health for pediatric surgical patients (Dean et al., 2016).

9.4.2. Monitoring for Complicans

In pediatric surgery, complication monitoring is as crucial to maintaining patient safety and surgical quality as it is to in adult surgery. Due to the wide variability of children from adults in physiology, the danger of unexpected complications necessitates a careful monitoring protocol. This includes not only observation of vital signs but careful monitoring of pain management and postoperative status. Effective monitoring requires careful attention to the child's normal general health and any pre-existing conditions that place them at risk of complications. For instance, children with respiratory issues or those who need a procedure under sedation should be checked for airwa of respiratory distress, pointing to the need for tailored monitoring strategies in this high-risk group (Charles et al., 2019Abib et al., 2022). In addition to physiological monitoring, clinicians are also vigilant for specific complications that are related to various surgical interventions. General development of infective endocarditis is a good illustration of the complexity of postoperative surveillance. Based on the changing epidemiology and relative preva causal pathogens with this illness, a multidisciplinary type of monitoring is required. Pediatric surgery that is associative associated with vascular anatomy modification or extended residence may predispose to the development of this life-threatening infection. Hence, there should be a teamwork strategy among pediatric professionals and surgical teams with the objective of early detection and management of such complications. Evidence-based guidelines in implementing protocols assist in lifting the level of care, and there will be greater possibilities of favorable outcomes while minimizing the intrinsic risks associated with pediatric surgery (Larry et al., 2015). Finally, the recovery room after surgery is a crucial time during which monitoring for complications occurs, and this requipped environment as well as experienced staff. Recovering children following surgery must be carefnitored in order toto help them regain the pre-sedation state of awareness, as well as manage any emergent complications such as, such as bleeding and infection. This also means monitoring this time not only within the hospital setting but extending into the home situation on discharge. Parents and caregivers must also be appropriately taught about signs to recognize and when to re-present to medical attention, with a focus on maintaining continuity of care beyond the operating department. Family preparation for effective monitoring can emerge as a significant consideration in maximizing recovery andtions, setting the worth of detailed discharge instructions and post-operative visits in pediatric surgery (Charles et al., 2019Abib et al., 2022) (Figure 9.10).

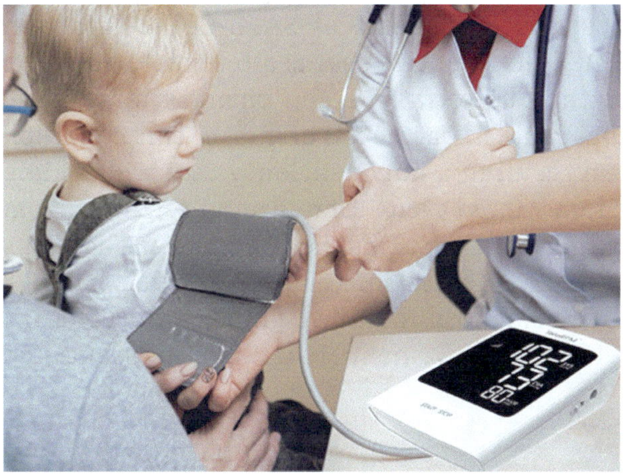

Figure 9.10. Monitoring for complications.

Source: https://www.transtekcorp.com/uploads/image/20240523/ensuring-accuracy-in-blood-pressure-monitoring-for-children-small-arm-circumference-solutions.jpg.

9.4.3. Nutritional Needs

In pediatric surgery, it is necessary to consider the nutritional needs of children, especially in the perioperative period. Good nutrition not only assists with healing but also plays a vital role in preventing complications post-surgery. Operative children may be at varying degrees ritional deficiency depending on underlying medical illness, type of surgical operation, and their developmental ageof development. Pediatric patients can experience metabolic changes that would elevate their caloric and protein requirements, hence the need for the healthcare workers to assess and address these requirements adequately. For instance, pediatric patients who are recovering from surgeries would require greater levels of proteins for repairing tissues and immune functions, and there is a requirement for personalized nutritional protocols designed particularly for pediatric patients who are undergoing surgeries (Laura et al., 2022). Included in the nutritional blend is the recent peak of cases pertaining to the COVID-19 pandemic, which has compounded challenges. Children with post-acute sequelae of SARS-CoV-2 infection (PASC) may require special attention to nutrition status due to fatigue and changes in appetite that could impact levels of intake. This condition can result in a nutr deficiency that will initiate an unwanted cycle, complicating recovery from surgery and exposing the child to complications such as, such as infection or delayed healing. Involvement of multidisciplinary interventions with the involvement of dietitians is essential to meet the individual nutritional needs of these children. Adequate nutritional intervention can contribute importantly to successful surgeries, thus emphasizing the importance of maximizing such factors in clinical practice (Leahy et al., 2018). Also, pediatric surgical patients can respond differently to different types of nutrition, making a full understanding of proper dietary care indispensable. Enteral feeding via the use of feeding tubes may be required in others when oral intake is unsafe or insufficient, especially among patients who are young or have certain chronic diseases. Enteral formulas that are suitable for pediatric energy and nutrient requirements can be utilized to deliver adequate caloric and ontent while minimizing gastrointestinal complications. Moreover, respect for the role of psychosocial factors on nutrition, such as, such as stress from hospitalization and surgery, can promote better compliance and results. Customized nutrition intervention to every patient's tolerance, need, and preference can finally result in recovery and reduced lengthting the critical role nutrition plays in the overall management of pediatric surgical patients (Abib et al., 2022Laura et al., 2022).

Test Your Knowledge

1. What are the most effective methods for managing pain in children after surgery?
2. Which signs should be monitored to detect potential postoperativens in pediatric patients?
3. How do nutritional needs change during the recovery period following pediatric surgery?

9.5. PsychologicalPsychological Impact o Patients

Learning Outcome

1. Anxiety and Fear of Surgery
2. Coping Mechanisms for Children
3. Role of Child Life Specialists

The psychologicpsychological impact of surgery on children is profound and multifaceted, influencing both the short- and long-term status of children. Preoperative expectation can produce anxiety and far, in effect stimulated by unfamiliarity with the procedure and the outcome. Preoperative fear is found in the majority of children, as a reflection of limited experience with such medical interventions. Primary caregivers are also instrumental in alleviating such feelings with reassurance and communication, paving the way to emotional safety. Potoperative recovery can also heighten anxio physical pain, hospitalization, and lack of knowledge about future health; —each a source of emotional challenge. Tlogicalpsychological impact is not fully transient; if it is not treated, it can continue as long-term psycders, such as, such as post-traumatic stress disorder or generalized anxiety disorders, further confirming the place of psychologicalpsychological support in and following surgical intervention. This foresight in pediatric surgery extends beyond the individual child to the family and extended support network. The family also goes through a process of emotions, some of which are fear and stress and do not necessarily help avoid child anxiety. Research has noted that when family members react positively and in a composed manner, the child follows the same suit and thereby contributes to more overall outcomes. The role of siblings cannot be neglected either; they, like others, may go through anxiety or distress regarding their brothers or sisters' medical condition. Instructing and providing families with information about expected outcomes of surgery and the recovery process instills a sense of group resilience, which is paramount in alleviating emotional distress. This blended approach allows families to be navigated through the surgical process as a whole, minimizing stress and fostering a positive environment critical to the emotiof the pediatric patient. Moreover, involving mental health clinicians in the operating team is cruciressing the psychologicalpsychological impact of pediatric surgery. Clinicians are able to provide personalized interventions, such as, such as cognitive-behavioral therapy, to enable children to cope with their experience and acquire coping skills for anxiety, pain management, and adjustment to physical state changes.

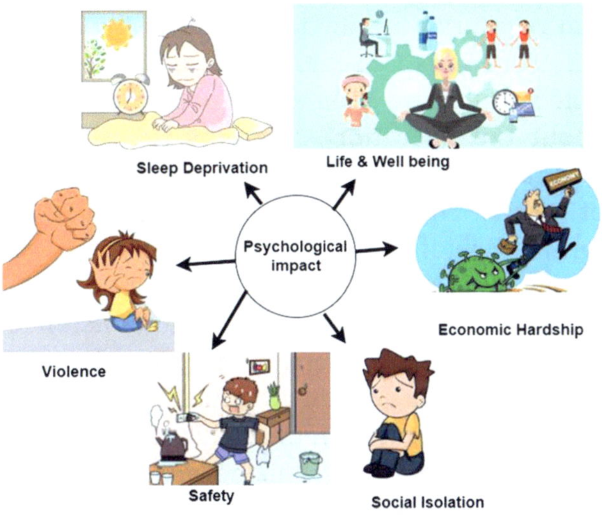

Figure 9.11. The psychologicalpsychological impact of surgery on pediatric patients is profound and multifaceted.

Source: https://media.springernature.com/lw685/springer-static/image/art%3A10.1186%2Fs43045-022-00256-3/MediaObjects/43045_2022_256_Fig4_HTML.pnxiety and Fear of Surgery

Similarly, educational courses that explain surgical procedures in terms of the developmental level of a child can de-mystify the experience and reduce anxiety. As more pediatric patients' management comes to acknowledge the interconnectedness of physical and menta creating care plans that include mental health support is imperative. This holistic strategy not only addresses immediate psychological needs but also fosters resilience, which may strengthen children and their families to manage potential long-term psychologicalpts after medical intervention, as exemplified in complex results of PASC patients in recent studies (Abib etl., 2022) and other conditions like cenal hyperplasia featured in updated guidelines (Abib et al., 2022Speiser et al., 2018) (Figure 9.11). Surgery fear and anxiety are prevalent problems in pediatric surgical patients, with significant psychologicalpsychological health and recovery outcome implications. Children's emotional response to surgical procedures tends to be based upon a paucity of information about the operation, unfamiliarity with the hospital, and apprehension about pain or loss of control. This fear can express itself in many forms, including crying, withdrawal, or even physical responses like a rising heart rate. These fears need to be addressed for the provision of an emotionally supportive environment that ensures positive surgical outcomes. Preoperative education at the level of the child's development plays a vital role in minimizing anxiety through providing the patient with information as to what can be expected and, therefore, reducing fear and ensuring cooperation with the surgery. Furthecaregivers can enhance comfort and security of the child during this vulnerable time. Along with educational interventions, psychologicalpsychological therapy plays a crucial role in treating anxiety and fear in children undergoing surgery. CBT can provide children with coping skills to overcome their fears effectively. CBT is aimed at altering negative surgery-relought patterns and behavior, providing the young patients with a sense of confidence and control. Moreover, relaxation techniques such as, such as deep breathing or guided imagery can be taught to children in a way to minimize anxiety in the hours leading up to the procedure. More significantly, intervention into the psychosocial components of surgery may yield improved post-surgical outcomes sincth lower levels of anxiety tend to be more likely to comply positively with their recuperation. Finally, the integration of psychologicalpsychological support into surgical treatment must be provided to optimize both emotional and physiological responses of pediatric patients. Family systems also come into play in shaping a child's experience of anxiety from surgery.

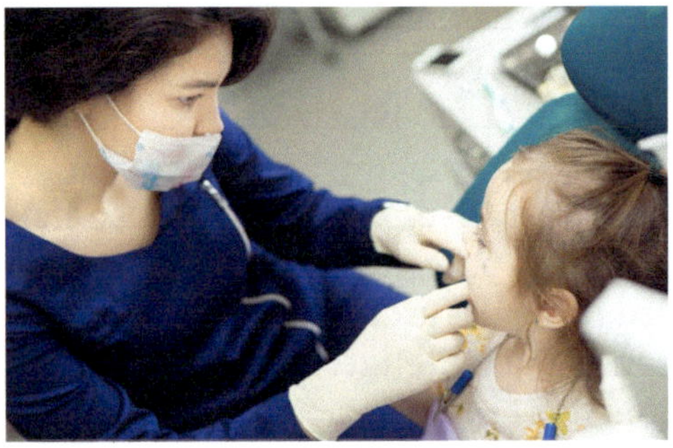

Figure 9.12. Dentist examining a young child's teeth during a dental visit.

Source: https://cliftonandmauney.com/wp-content/uploads/2023/10/How-To-Manage-Anxiety-in-Children-Undergoing-Anesthesia-1024x683.jpg.

Anxious parents tend to project their concerns on children and thus end up perpetuating what already is a stressful situation for children. Hence, it is imperative that parents also be educated and assisted in recognizing and managing their emotions towards their child's operation. Open lines of communication between healthcare professionals, children, and their families can contribute to ensuring comprehension as well as provide emotional support networks that are helpful for pediatric patients. Also, integrating psychosocial assessment into preoperative consultations will allow us to identify families that require additional support resources, and this will enable us to initiate a patient-tailored anxiety management strategy. Creating a family-centered care model will not just enhance the experience of the individual child but also optimize the overall emotional strength of the family as a whole in relation to operative events (Figure 9.12).

9.5.1. Coping Mechanisms for Children

Pediatric patients who are waiting for surgery are likely to go through an immense range of emotions that range from anxiety to fear. oTo deal with these, some good coping mechanisms are required. One such way is the use of distraction, where the child can be involved in playing games, reading books, or drawing pictures prior to surgery. All these help to shift the focus away from the upcoming procedure and decrease tension. Furthermore, the utilization of age-appropriate information regarding what to expect can empower children, transforming their anxiety into a sense of consciousness. Research indicated that when children are informcd about how the surgery is carried out, their anxiety levelsobefore being operated on considerably decrease, thereby enabling them to cope with their overall state of mind throughout the procedure. Through these actions, the medical team, as well as parents, can empower the child's coping mechanism greatly throughout the surgical procedure. Besides distraction and education, emotional support is also important in helping children cope with the stress of surgery. The presence of caregivers, family members, or specially trained pediatric nurses may provide valuable comfort to a child having the procedure done on the day of surgery. These individuals provide not only physical presence but also exhibit coping strategies for the child to follow. Basic acts of reassurance, cuddling, or communication of fears verbally give a child's emotional expression, their feelings being legitimized and enabling them to employ anxiety constructs efficaciously. Additionally, the employment of known objectss, such as a favorite toy or blanket, can give a sense of security in the clinic. Thelpsychological benefit of support systems is key, since mental illness often accompanies surgery, pointing to the importance of a supportive environment within children's hospitals (Ogundele, 2018). Lastly, application of mindfulness training has also been shown to be an effective coping mechanism among children who are undergoing surgery. Mindfulness, or the practice of focusing on the present moment and accepting things as they are without judgment, could be very effective in reducing anxiety levels. Techniquess, such as deep breathing, guided imagery, and simple meditation can educate children to regulate their emotional response to stressful situations. These procedures facilitate the child to stay relaxed and calm, which is not only essential for their emotional well-being but also for post-surgical recovery. Furthermore, the incorporation of pleasurable mindfulness activities in the pre-operative process can facilitate the acquisition of relaxation and enjoyment responses related to health care environments, which are more acceptable to child patients. With mental health professionals working with children as their recommenders, these coping behaviors can be utilized to decrease immediate and post-surgical delayedlpsychological impact of surgery, highlighting their importance in an integrated care for children (Abib et al., 2028).

9.5.2. Role of Child Life Specialists

Incorporafe Specialists into pediatric surgery is vital in ensuring that young patients not only get medical care but also emotional and psychologicalpsychological support during their hospital stay. The specialists are also trained to become familiar with children's developmental stages and customize interventions accordingly, making them capable of calming fears and anxiety about undergoing a surgical procedure. By utilizing therapeutic play, preparation, and education, Child Life Specialists can deconstruct complex medical procedures into language understandable by children, thus enhancing their knowledge and sense of control. Proactive in this way is especially crucial in children's environments, where fear can be debilitating due to unknown spaces and procedures. Consequently, kids are better ready for what transpires, and that helps foster cooperation with processes, reduced distress, and quy, all of which serve to optimize the quality of patient outcomes in pediatric surgery (Laura et al., 2022). Besides preparation psychologicalpsychologically, Child Life Specialists also help optimize family-centered care. They work closely with parents to empower and assist them during stressful times so that families feel capable of advocating the needs of their child. This kind of assistance is particularly vital in pediatric surgery settings, where parents often find themselves grappling with anxiety and helplessness. Child Life Specialists also facilitate communication among medical staff and families, describing procedures, assuaging fears, and reminding them of the value of emotional support during their child's hospitalization. Evidence points to families well-informed and emotionally supported during medical encounters being reported as more satisfied and less anxious. Hence, the contribution of Child Life Specialists not onlyen but is also significant in enhancing the overall experience of the family under surgical interventions (Abib et al., 2022Neunert et al., 2019). As hospitals increasingly emphasize comprehensive care, the contribution of Child Life Specialists is increasingly expanding, particularly in facilitating children to undergo normal surgical procedures and emergent care. These experts perform interventions which are specifically designed to teach and empower childreents who are going through surgery. By the giving of coping skills and emotional expression, Child Life Specialists counteract the psychologicalpsychological impact of surgical experience, encouraging a resilient and adaptive spirit among young patients. The incorporation of child life practices into the preoperative process is increasingly intended as best practice, allowing for smoother transitions before and after surgery. Apart from that, constant collaboration between medical staff and Child Life Specialists ensures that psychosocial issues become a part of the treatment plan and posty, which subsequently translates into better results and greater well-being for children undergoing surgery (Abib et al., 2022Laura et al., 2022) (Figure 9.13).

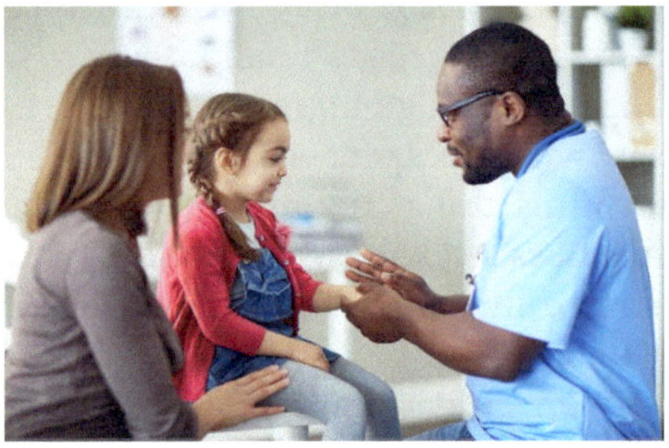

Figure 9.13. Role of child life specialists.

Source: https://www.gebauer.com/hubfs/2016/child-life-specialist-with-patient.jpg.

Test Your Knowledge

1. What factors contribute to anxiety and fear of surgery in pediatric patients?
2. What coping mechanisms can help children manage stress before and after surgery?
3. How do Child Life Specialists support the emotional and psychological well-being of children undergoing medical procedures?

9.6. Advances in Pediatric Surgery

Learning Outcome

1. Minimally Invasive Techniques
2. Robotic Surgery
3. Innovations in Surgical Tools and Technology

Pediatric surgeryperienced unprecedented expansion during the last few years, greatly enhancing the treatment option offered to children. New technologies such as, such as minimally invasive surgery have gained popularity to such an extent that recovery time is shorter and there are fewer problems after surgery. A good example is laparoscopic surgery, which allows surgeons to perform complex procedures using small incisions, leading to minimal pain and scarring compared to open surgery. This trend is part of a larger movement in medicine toward less invasive methods, supporting the belief that children can derive benefit from surgical procedures that consider their unique physiological needs. Additionally, the inclusion of advanced imaging technologies, including MRI and 3D reconstruction, has enhanced planning and outcomes for surgery. These technologies enable pediatric surgeons to visualize complicated anatomical structures more colorfully, thus facilitating precision in delicate procedures that are pivotal for achieving maximum long-term well-being in children. In addressing specific conditions requiring surgery, the management of disorders of sex development (DSD) has been particularly revolutionized by recent innovations. The intricacy surrounding DSD has become better understood, allowing healthcare providers to modify their approach to each individual case. Multidisciplinary teams of pediatric surgeons, endocrinologists, and gencombined care for children who are affected. Given increased awareness of underlying developmental etiology, as reported by Ahmed et al. (2017), clinical practice is more and more directed by evidence-based advice that considers both acute s and broader societal context, including evolving perspectives on gender identity. This general strategy embraces the physical and psychologicalpsychological dimensions of care so that the resulting health for the children with abnorgenitals is optimized in the short term as much as in the long term. Moreovees to enlarge through the advances in research in the various subspecialties (Caffarelli et al., 2019), as documented in Bernasconi et al. (2019). Advances in surgery for congenital heart disease, gastrointestinal disease, and oncology have required the development of standardized guidelines that enhance the quality of patient care across all clinical settings. For example, improved surgical approaches in congenital heart disease have promoted better survival rates and quality of life for children. Surgical teams are better and better prepared to deal with the complexities of such conditions, thanks to greater training and use of advanced technology. Continued research continues to raise the chances of innovative treatments, eventually resulting in a more effective and compassionate healthcare system unique to the health needs of children. Developments underscore the importance of continuing education and communication among caregivers in facilitating further pediatric surgical treatment (Abib et al., 2022).

9.6.1. Minimally Invasive Techniques

Minimally invasive surgery has revolutionized pediatric surgery with dramatic improvement in outcome and postoperative recovery. Minimally invasive surgery, e.g., laparoscopic and robotic-assisted surgery, has many advantages over open surgery, including reduced postoperative pain, shorter length of stay in the hospital, and quicker return to normal activity. Pediatric patients also are very well matched for these techniques since their smaller body anatomy and softer physiology are able to utilize the precision provided by such minimally invasive techniques. Second, these techniques have the potential to minimize the risk of infection and scarring, which are very significant factors to take into consideration when treating children. The application of such technologies demands a high level of surgical skill and training, creating an evolving setting that necessitates advanced education in pediatric surgery. The integration of minimally invasive techniques into standard pediatric procedures has been showove the delivery of surgery while maintaining safety and effectiveness. For example, laparoscopic forms of procedures to address gut issues, such as, such as appendectomies or fundoplications, have been increasingly used in place of the conventional methods with minimal incisions and less trauma to surrounding tissues. There is evidence that the use of such techniques results in better pain control and shorter hospital stays, allowing children to return to normal life in no time (Rhodes et al., 2017). Additionally, as additional pediatric practitioners adopt these methods, there is a new emphasis on improving training and establishing protocols so that advanced techniques will be utilized in a safe and effective way in diverse healthcare settings. Clear training and practices will offer confidence in routine use and improved general quality of pediatric surgical care. Despite the numerous advantages associated with minimally invasive techniques, adoption and implementation issues exist. Significant disparities in exposure to advanced technologies and training abound, especially in resource-limited environments where children's surgical problems are likely to be severe. ial implications of installing robotic surgical systems and training personnel can be a hurdle to extensive use (Abib et al., 2022Larry et al., 2015). Ongoing technological advancements are likely to relieve some of the concerns, but addressing the issues of equity in access and training are still essential to make sure that all pediatric patients have access to the best quality of surgical care. With ongoing research and practice, emphasis should be placed on partnership arrangements that promote innovation while considering the individualistic needs of pediatric patients, ultimately leading to better outcomes across a variety of healthcare settings (Figure 9.14).

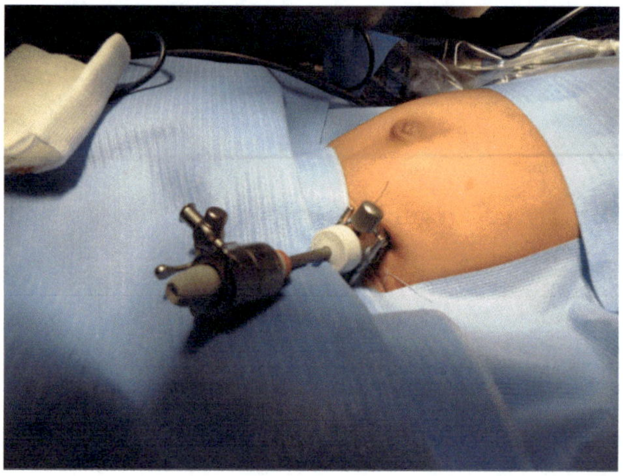

Figure 9.14. Pediatric patient undergoing minimally invasive laparoscopic surgery.

Source: https://www.drnadachildsurgeon.com/wp-content/uploads/2019/09/Screen-Shot-2019-09-25-at-11.04.04-AM-1024x770.png.

9.6.2. Robotic Surgery

The addition of robotic surgery to pediatric surgery has revolutionized the practice of many standard procedures. Robotic systems provide accuracy and dexterity in addition to that of the standard laparoscopic techniques, allowing surgeons to perform complex procedures with more control. This is especially helpful in pediatric surgery, where the anatomic variation and lower operative fields present unique challenges. With the help of robotic surgery systems, surgeons are able to carry out intricate maneuvers without much trauma to surrounding tissuprecision not only serves to improve clinical results but also shortens recovery for children and makes operations less invasive and acceptable (Jarosław Abib et al., 2022). As more hospitals adopt this technology, the level of pediatric surgical care increases by leveraging advancements with direct implications on the pediatric patient population's health. Robotic surgery further facilitates enhanced preoperative planning and intraoperative simulation, both critical in pediatric settings. Preoperative visualization and manipulation of 3D patient anatomy models allow surgeons to virtually plan and rehearse procedures. This approach is invaluable since it equips medical practitioners with the necessary tools to address potential complications that may arise during surgery, thus building a safer surgery experience for children (Bansal et al., 2022). The impact of robotic systems is not limited to surgical performance since they provide learning opportunities. Experts in novels can be trained on simulators that replicate robotic surgery exactly, allowing training to keep up with technological progress hand-in-hand. This innovation, therefore, is not only an instrument but a revolutionary element in surgical practice and training. Despite the many advantages associated with robotic surgery among children, there are many obstacles lying ahead before embracing it at a universal level. These are cost barriers, with the cost of robotic technology having the potential to render some healthcare institutions inaccessible. Moreover, surgeons' adaptation to robotic technology involves the use of a lot of training and practice, which would be an enormous investment of resources. Reimbursement for robot-assisted procedures versus standard surgery also influences the cost-benefit ratio of adopting robotic systems (Jarosław Abib et al., 2022). Thus, as impressive as the potential of robot surgery to improve the outcomes of pediatric surgery is, meeting these logistical, economic, and educational challenges will be key in deciding its future place in pediatric surgery. Collaboration among healthcare professionals, lawmakers, and educators will be necessary to overcome these challenges so that innovation benefits children who are being operated on in different healthcare settings.

9.6.3. Innovations in Surgical Tools and Technology

Theof pediatric surgery has come a long way with advances in surgical technology and equipment, enhancing the safety and efficacy of operations. Advances such as, such as minimally invasive surgical procedures have transformed the traditional methods of performing operations, reducing patient recovery times and complications. Laparoscopy equipment, equipped with high-definition cameras and fine instruments, allows surgeons to make much smaller incisions, with less damage to the body of the child. This is particularly important in children, who often have unique anatomical problems. Furthermore, the addition of robot-assisted surgery has made new possibilities for precision in delicate procedures become available, and for improved results, enabling surgeons to perform high-level maneuvers with greater control and dexterity. Such developments are indicative of continued attempts at enhancing the quality of pediatric surgical care, ultimately leading to improved patient experiences and results. In addition to that, pediatric surgery is significantly aided by the development of sophisticated imaging technologies. Advanced imaging technologies like intraoperative ultrasound and augmented reality provide the surgeon with real-time visual cues during procedures. The technologies provide enhanced anatomical visualization along with facilitating accurate navigation, particularly in complicated surgical settings. Through the incorporation of imaging solutions into the surgical process, surgeons are provided with the necessary information that can minimize the risk of errors and optimize surgical techniques. Such innovations underscore the importance of technology as it boosts surgical practices and provides pediatric patients with effective and safe care. Last but not least, the combination of superior surgical technology with superior imaging technology is proof of how continuous innovation is changing the face of children's surgery. To add to that, patient safety has driven the evolution of surgery equipment especially designed for children. Technology that considers the unique physiological characteristics of children is a key factor in reducing risks in surgery. For instance, machines intended for smaller body stature and having protection against unintentional harm are a necessity in a pediatric setting. Strategies outlined in existing case studies suggest the need for feedback from clinical teams and healthcare organizations that aspire to establish safer environments for children (Blumenthal et al., 2006). By being exposed to concepts from effective innovations and collaborative undertakings, the occupation has all the equipment required to be constantly readjusting and perfecting its practices. As these technological advances continue to progress, they not only enhance results for surgery but also provide patients and their loved ones with greater assurance of what otherwise may seem to be an impossible endeavor (Figure 9.15).

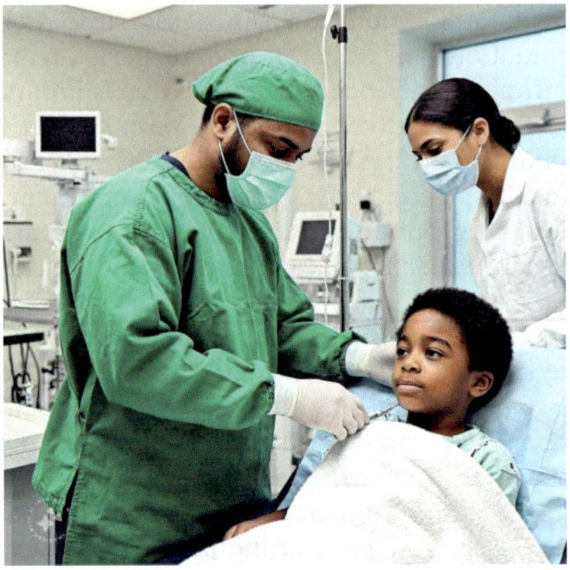

Figure 9.15. The field of pediatric surgery has significantly benefited from innovations in surgical tools and technology.

Source: https://www.hi-techhospital.in/blogs/wp-content/uploads/2024/11/WhatsApp-Image-2024-11-29-at-4.52.52-PM.jpeg.

Test Your Knowledge

1. How have minimally invasive surgical techniques improved outcomes and recovery times in pediatric patients?
2. What are the benefits and challenges of using robotic surgery in pediatric procedures?
3. How are innovations in surgical tools and technology transforming the field of pediatric surgery?

SUMMARY

It is critical to value the urgent balance between surgical treatment and non-surgical care in the management of common pediatric emergencies. Surgical procedures, ranging from appendectomies to complex congenital repair, are drastic procedures that have a significant impact in improving the health outcome of a child. Such procedures are necessary because of the acute illnesses that require immediate attention. Thus, awareness of the intricacies of such procedures enables the surgical team to understand the complexities of pediatric care. Preoperative assessment and thorough evaluation play a central role, as these elements not only minimize risks but also acclimatize the child and family to the impending surgery. A proper understanding of the intricacies of pediatric anatomy and physiology is imperative for any practitioner working with such high-risk cases. Furthermore, the integration of modern sedation techniques into pediatric surgery significantly enhances procedure safety and comfort for patients. Current evidence demonstrates varying effectiveness between intermittent bolus and continuous infusion sedation techniques, suggesting important implications for practice settings where pediatric patients could receive a variety of procedures. For example, findings indicated no statistical difference in vital parameters among sedation techniques but indicated that recovery times can be significantly reduced with cusion techniques. Such adaptability in recovery allows for an easier transition to normalcy in children and minimizes interruptions in their physical and psychologicalpsychological well-being. Further research on sedation protocols in other pediatric uses, including the treatment of dental anxiety, points toadjustment to the particular needs of child patients, as evident in consideration of treating dental anxiety in children (Facco & Zanette, 2017Abrahamsson et al., 2017). Ultimately, the practice of pediatric surgery is characterized by ongoing advances and commitment to quality improvement. As demonstrated in various environments of surgery, the incorporation of evidence-based practices ensures practice is responsive to family and patient needs. Further, an understanding of pediatric emergencies and operation details allows healthcare providers to maximize interdisciplinary collaboration and communication to provide an integrated care strategy. Ongoing education and compliance with protocols based on clinical evidence open the door to better outcomes and fewer complications in this vulnerable group. More than ever, it is imperative to cultivate a culture that encourages growth and inon in pediatric surgical techniques, thus ensuring that children are provided with the best possible level of care along their medical journeys (Ahmed & Markosyanet al., 2017).

The landscape of pediatric surgery encompasses a vast array of procedures designed specifically for children from treating congenital abnormalities to emergent situations. The main routine operations include appendectomies, hernias, and circumcisions, which are done to excise symptoms of gastrointestinal and urogenital diseases. Pediatric surgeons need specialized training to grasp differences in anatomy and physiology in children compared to adults. It cannot be overstressed how central proper preoperative assessment and postoperative management are, as these factors are pivotal in avoiding complications and ensuring an uneventful course of recovery. Coupled with this, advances in minimally invasive techniques are constantly altering pediatric surgical practice, allowing for quicker recovery times and improved results. This once again highlights the need for surgeons working within this specialty to keep abreast of evoethodology in an effort to provide optimal management. In pediatric emergency situations, swift and accurate decision-making is of utmost value. Triage conditions such as, such as traumatic injury, torsion of the testis, and acute surgical abdomen, can present with subtle and diverse symptomatology in children that could hamper appropriate diagnosis. Additionally, good communication with families is also important since anxious parents may affect a child's behavioral approach towards surgery. Pediatric pharmacology knowledge is also essential, as the dosages of adult medications are considerably different and must be computed with delicate care to avoid risk. Furthermore, the impact of implicit bias on healthcare professionals can affect racial and ethnic minority patients' care, potentially leading to disparities in emergency departments. Overcoming these prejudices is crucial to ensure equity to pediatric surgery so that children of all demographics receive quality medical attention. Evidence-based practice in pediatric surgery is required to better educate clinical decision-making and ensure outcomes. Continuing education through systematic review and trial data will warn surgeons of the latest advancements and possible treatment options. The relationship between implicit bias and clinical decision-making, while still under discovery, raises significant questions about the manner in which such unconscious biases indirectly influence the treatment process and patient relationship in pediatric care. For example, studies have shown evidence of implicit physician preferences to inform decisions despite stated preference for fair treatment. Thus, an understanding of these dynamics will encourage pediatric surgeons to examine their practice and strive towards improved standards of care provision. By focusing on technical proficiency as much as empathetic, non-prejudiced care, pediatric surgery can be developed to meet the multiple requirements of diverse child populations, a move towards healthcare equity to be welcomed.

KEY TERMS FROM THIS CHAPTER

- Anesthesia
- Appendectomy
- Emergency department (ED)
- Extracorporeal membrane oxygenation (ECMO)
- Pediatric patients
- Pediatric surgern
- Rapid assessment
- Anesthesiologists
- Circumcision
- Emergent care
- Hernia repairs
- Pediatric surgeons
- PsychologicalPsychological wellness
- Simulation-based training (SBT)

CRITICAL THINKING QUESTIONS

1. **Which of the following is the most common surgical cause of vomiting in infants?**
   a. Intussusception
   b. Hirschsprung's disease
   c. Hypertrophic pyloric stenosis
   d. Gastroesophageal reflux
2. **What is the hallmark radiological sign of intussusception on ultrasound?**
   a. Double bubble sign
   b. Air-fluid levels
   c. Target (or donut) sign
   d. Ground-glass appearance
3. **The most appropriate initial management for suspected testicular torsion is:**
   a. Analgesia and observation
   b. Ultrasound with Doppler
   c. Immediate surgical exploration
   d. Antibiotic therapy
4. **What is the primary diagnostic tool for Hirschsprung's disease?**
   a. Barium enema
   b. Rectal suction biopsy
   c. Abdominal X-ray
   d. Ultrasound
5. **A "double bubble" sign on abdominal X-ray in a newborn is most indicative of:**
   a. Meconium ileus
   b. Duodenal atresia
   c. Intussusception
   d. Pyloric stenosis

Short Answer Questions

1. Describe the clinical presentation, diagnosis, and surgical management of hypertrophic pyloric stenosis in infants. Why is early recognition crucial?
2. Explain the pathophysiology, types, and surgical approaches to the management of congenital diaphragmatic hernia.
3. Discuss the causes, diagnostic steps, and emergency surgical treatment of intussusception in children.
4. How does appendicitis commonly present in young children versus adolescents?
5. What is Hirschsprung's disease? Describe its etiology, clinical features, diagnostic approach, and surgical treatment options.
6. Explain the surgical management of undescended testes (cryptorchidism) in children.

Answer to Critical Thinking Questions

1.(c) 2.(c) 3.(c) 4.(b) 5.(b)

REFERENCES

1. Abib, S. C. V., Chui, C. H., Cox, S., Abdelhafeez, A. H., Fernández-Pineda, I., Elgendy, A., Karpelowsky, J., et al. (2022). International Society of Pediatric Surgical Oncology (IPSO) surgical practice guidelines. *ecancermedicalscience, 16*. https://doi.org/10.3332/ecancer.2022.1356 (accessed on 16th June 2025).
2. Facco, E., & Zanouse-Green, S., Andrews-Hanna, J., et al. (2017). The odyssey of dental anxiety: From prehistory to the present. A narrative review. https://core.ac.uk/download/84923580.pdf (accessed on 16th June 2025).
3. Ahmed, S. F., & Markosyan, R. (2017). Sex assignment in conditions affecting sex development. https://core.ac.uk/download/150597685.pdf (accessed on 16th June 2025).
4. Ahmed, S. S., Hicks, S., Nitu, M., Slaven, J., et al. (2017). Intermittent bolus versus continuous infusion of propofol for deep sedation during ABR/nuclear medicine studies. https://core.ac.uk/download/227054213.pdf (accessed on 16th June 2025).
5. Aisuodionoe-Shadrach, O. I. (2011). Range of urologic surgical procedures in two district tertiary care hospitals in Abuja, Nigeria. https://core.ac.uk/download/478294052.pdf (accessed on 16th June 2025).
6. Alberti, P., & Kisa, P. (2024). Pediatric surgery in Uganda: Current challenges and opportunities. https://core.ac.uk/download/613842991.pdf (accessed on 16th June 2025).
7. Ames, S. G., Auerbach, M., Babcock, S. R., Bailey, B., et al. (2023). Emergency department pediatric readiness among US trauma centers: A machine learning analysis of components associated with survival. https://core.ac.uk/download/617033722.pdf (accessed on 16th June 2025).
8. Assimos, D. G., Krambeck, A. E., Miller, N. L., Monga, M., Murad, M. H., Nelson, C. P., Pace, K. T., et al. (2016). Surgical management of stones: American Urological Association/Endourological Society guideline, PART I. *The Journal of Urology, 196*, 1153–1160. https://doi.org/10.1016/j.juro.2016.05.090 (accessed on 16th June 2025).
9. Baddour, L. M., Wilson, W. R., Bayer, A. S., Fowler, V. G., Tleyjeh, I. M., Rybak, M. J., Baršić, B., et al. (2015). Infective endocarditis in adults: Diagnosis, antimicrobial therapy, and management of complications. *Circulation, 132*, 1435–1486. https://doi.org/10.1161/cir.0000000000000296 (accessed on 16th June 2025).
10. Caffarelli, C., Santamaria, F., Mastrorilli, C., Santoro, A., Iovane, B., Petraroli, M., Gaeta, V., Di Pinto, R., Borrelli, M., Bernasconi, S., & Corsello, G. (2019). Report on advances for pediatricians in 2018: allergy, cardiology, critical care, endocrinology, hereditary metabolic diseases, gastroenterolreditary metabolic diseases, gastroenterology, infectious diseases, neonatology, nutrition, respiratory tract disorders and surgery. https://core.ac.uk/download/286528671.pdf (accessed on 16th June 2025).
11. Blumenthal, D., & McCarthy, D. (2006). Committed to safety: Ten case studies on reducing harm to patients. https://core.ac.uk/download/71350251.pdf (accessed on 16th June 2025).
12. Coté, C. J., & Wilson, S. (2019). Guidelines for monitoring and management of pediatric patients before, during, and after sedation for diagnostic and therapeutic procedures. *Pediatrics, 143*. https://doi.org/10.1542/peds.2019-1000 (accessed on 16th June 2025).
13. Dangal, B., Ng, J., Gauchan, B., Khadka, M. B., & Pathak, M. (2021). Role of general practitioners

in transforming surgical care in rural Nepal–A descriptive study from eastern Nepal. *Journal of General Practice and Emergency Medicine of Nepal, 8*, 5–9. https://doi.org/10.59284/jgpeman70 (accessed on 16th June 2025).

14. Dehon, E., Weiss, N. H., Jones, J. S., Faulconer, W., Hinton, E., & Sterling, S. M. (2017). A systematic review of the impact of physician implicit racial bias on clinical decision making. *Academic Emergency Medicine, 24*, 895–904. https://doi.org/10.1111/acem.13214 (accessed on 16th June 2025).

15. Firomsa, T., Tadesse, A., & Teferra, M. (2018). Trends and outcomes of emergency pediatric surgical admissions from a tertiary hospital in Ethiopia. https://core.ac.uk/download/478439504.pdf (accessed on 16th June 2025).

16. Isselbacher, E. M., Preventza, O., Black, J. H., Augoustides, J., Beck, A. W., Bolen, M. A., Braverman, A. C., et al. (2022). 2022 ACC/AHA guideline for the diagnosis and management of aortic disease: A report of the American Heart Association/American College of Cardiology Joint Committee on Clinical Practice Guidelines. *Circulation, 146*. https://doi.org/10.1161/cir.0000000000001106 (accessed on 16th June 2025).

17. Meyer-Szary, J., Luis, M. S., Mikulski, S., Patel, A., Schulz, F., Tretiakow, D., Fercho, J., et al. (2022). The role of 3D printing in planning complex medical procedures and training of medical professionals—Cross-sectional multispecialty review. *International Journal of Environmental Research and Public Health, 19*, 3331–3331. https://doi.org/10.3390/ijerph19063331 (accessed on 16th June 2025).

18. Moons, K. G. M., Altman, D. G., Reitsma, J. B., Ioannidis, J. P. A., Macaskill, P., Steyerberg, E. W., Vickers, A. J., et al. (2015). Transparent reporting of a multivariable prediction model for individual prognosis or diagnosis (TRIPOD): Explanation and elaboration. *Annals of Internal Medicine, 162*, W1–W73. https://doi.org/10.7326/m14-0698 (accessed on 16th June 2025).

19. Naluyimbazi, R., & Fitzgerald, T. N. (2024). Hernia repair as a tracer for elective surgical care. *The Lancet Global Health, 12*, e1069–e1070. https://doi.org/10.1016/s2214-109x(24)00214-6 (accessed on 16th June 2025).

20. Neunert, C., Terrell, D. R., Arnold, D. M., Buchanan, G. R., Cines, D. B., Cooper, N., Cuker, A., et al. (2019). American Society of Hematology 2019 guidelines for immune thrombocytopenia. *Blood Advances, 3*, 3829–3866. https://doi.org/10.1182/bloodadvances.2019000966 (accessed on 16th June 2025).

21. Ogundele, M. (2018). Behavioural and emotional disorders in childhood: A brief overview for pediatricians. *World Journal of Clinical Pediatrics, 7*, 9–26. https://doi.org/10.5409/wjcp.v7.i1.9 (accessed on 16th June 2025).

22. Pandiaraja, J., Chakkarapani, R., & Arumugam, S. (2021). A study on patterns, indications, and complications of an enteric stoma. *Journal of Family Medicine and Primary Care, 10*, 3277–3282. https://doi.org/10.4103/jfmpc.jfmpc_123_21 (accessed on 16th June 2025).

23. Poorman, G. W., Segreto, F. A., Beaubrun, B. M., Jalai, C. M., Horn, S. R., Bortz, C., Diebo, B. G., et al. (2019). Traumatic fracture of the pediatric cervical spine: Etiology, epidemiology, concurrent injuries, and an analysis of perioperative outcomes using the Kids' Inpatient Database. *The International Journal of Spine Surgery, 13*, 68–78. https://doi.org/10.14444/6009 (accessed on 16th June 2025).

24. Revel-Vilk, S., Cox, P. N., Robitaille, N., & Blanchette, V. S. (2013). Hematological problems in pediatric intensive care. *Pediatric and Adolescent Medicine.* https://doi.org/10.1159/000350346 (accessed on 16th June 2025).

25. Yawn, B. P., Buchanan, G. R., Afenyi-Annan, A., Ballas, S. K., Hassell, K. L., James, A., Jordan, L., et al. (2014). Management of sickle cell disease. *JAMA, 312*, 1033–1033. https://doi.org/10.1001/jama.2014.10517 (accessed on 16th June 2025).

26. Young-Hyman, D. L., de Groot, M., Hill-Briggs, F., Gonzalez, J. S., Hood, K. K., & Peyrot, M. (2016). Psychosocial care for people with diabetes: A position statement of the American Diabetes Association. *Diabetes Care, 39*, 2126–2140. https://doi.org/10.2337/dc16-2053 (accessed on 16th June 2025).

PEDIATRIC PULMONOLOGY

10

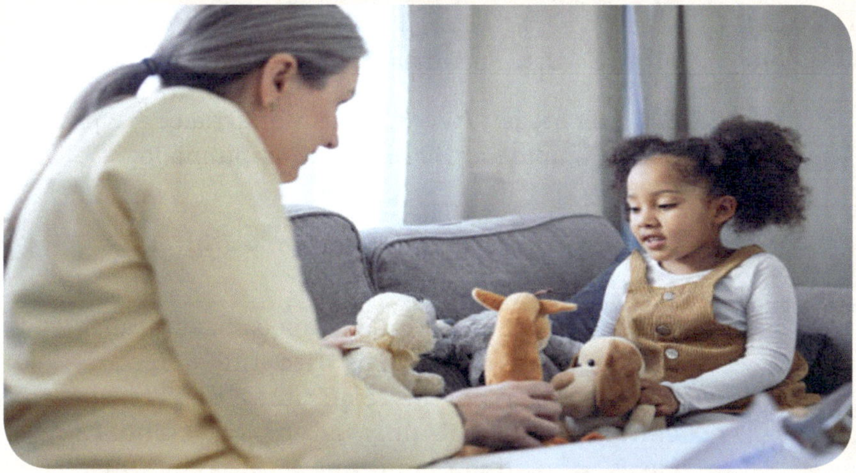

LEARNING OBJECTIVES

After studying this chapter, you will be able to:

1. Discuss the anatomy and physiology of the pediatric respiratory system
2. Describe common pediatric respiratory disorders
3. Highlight diagnostic approaches in pediatric pulmonology
4. Identify treatment modalities in pediatric pulmonology
5. Discuss the role of the pediatric pulmonologist
6. Be aware of current research and developments in pediatric pulmonology

Introduction

Pediatric pulmonology is a subspecialty medical practice that specializes in the diagnosis and treatment of diseases of the respiratory system of infants, children, and teenagers. The subspecialty manages a variety of disorders, including asthma, cystic fibrosis, respiratory infections, and congenital lung disease. Due to the unique physiological characteristics of children, pediatric pulmonologists must consider growth factors that differentiate from adult systems entirely. For instance, lung development in childhood patients is gradual throughout childhood and may potentially influence diagnostic and therapeutic approaches. Pediatric pulmonologists try to improve the quality of life in childhood patients with respiratory disorders by capitalizing on advances in clinical techniques and technology. Greater understanding of such diseases directs clinicians in navigating the complexities of treatment, and knowledge of both medical and psychosocial determinants of young patients and families is necessary. One of the largest parts of pediatric pulmonology is applying sophisticated diagnostic technology and management techniques to properly evaluate and treat young patients successfully. With advancements in non-invasive imaging technology and complex laboratory tests, including pulmonary function tests and genetic tests, the field has undergone phenomenal leaps. Simulation technologies, for example, have helped better prepare healthcare professionals to learn to conduct clinical procedures, having a generation of healthcare professionals learn to provide pediatric care both safely and effici009Dietrich et al., 2022). These developments allow for treatment plans to be tailored to the specific needs of every patient, with greatly enhanced outcomes. As pediatric pulmonology evolves, ongoing research and education are necessary to address new challenges and increase the quality of care, particularly in treating chronic respiratory disease and uncommon genetic diseases that occur exclusively in children. Collaboration and emphasis on the multidisciplinary nature are highly essential in pediatric pulmonology because the management of respiratory conditions often incorporates the intervention of multiple healthcare professionals. Specialists, like allergists, immunologists, and nutritionists, play specific roles to optimize patient careermore, initiatives such as, such as the initiative on rare and undiagnosed diseases (IRUD) are excellent examples of how collaborative communities can aid in diagnosing difficult cases, enhance diagnostic accuracy, and promote research into underlying genetic etiologies of pediatric respiratory conditions (Yūji et al., 2022). Besides providing valuable information regarding patient diagnostics, these collaborations also enhance management strategies based on the particular difficulties of pediatric patients. Lastly, the coordination of diverse expertise forms an integrated strategy consisting of medical, educational, and emotional support, reiterating the central position of cooperation in ensuring the best care possible in pediatric pulmonology (Figure 10.1).

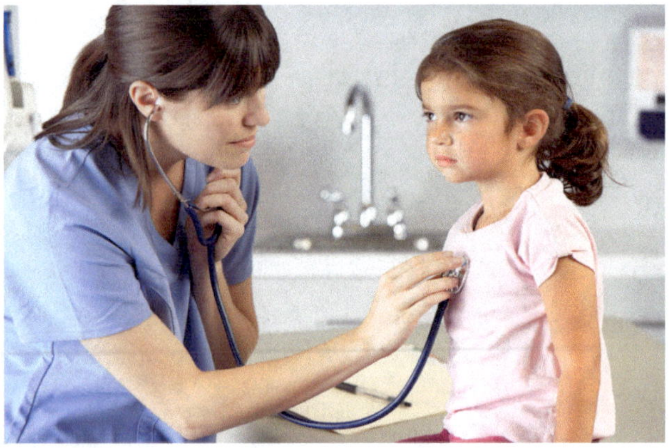

Figure 10.1. Pediatric pulmonology.

Source: https://www.sitarambhartia.org/wp-content/uploads/2018/10/peds-pulmo.jpg.

Definition and Scope of Pediatric Pulmonology

Pediatric pulmonology is a specialized branch of medicine concerned with the diagnosis and management of respiratory diseases of childhood. It not only addresses standard cases of asthma and pneumonia but also addresses more complex congenital anomalies and long-term lung diseases, including cystic fibrosis and interstitial lung disease. Pediatric pulmonologists play a vital role in managing such intricate illnesses, both through treatment modalities and preventive care to maintain lung health from infancy through adolescence. Pediatric pulmonology is not just a clinical pursuit; it involves continuous research to understand the onset of respiratory illness, that of the pediatric patient in particular, thus involving subspecialist expertise in this field. The integration of investigation and clinical methods is a fundamental element of pediatric pulmonology to form effective treatment plans that are tailored specifically to children. Recent advancementoccurred via initiatives such as, such as the human phenotype ontology (HPO), which categorizes phenotypic manifestations that are involved in respiratory disease. Clinicians and researchers are able to engage in genomic diagnosis and enhance understanding of the genetic underpinnings of lung disease through this resource. Absence of a framework for such a classification risks losing the nuances of pediatric pulmonary disease in the process, leading to ineffective interventions. Ongoing efforts at increasing the HPO corroborate the need for phenotypic characterization in ensuring effective and precise care in pediatric pulmonology and thereby merging clinical practice and translational research (Gargano et al., 2023). The more collaborative nature of pediatric pulmonology is evidenced by ration of other specialties, such as, such as immunology and cardiology, in the treatment of lung-related conditions in children. As lung health affects the overall pediatric condition, there is a demand for a multidisciplinary practice for proper care. Furthermore, initiatives to harmonize methta gathering and management, such as, such as represented by attempts to integrate the HPO into electronic health records, allow for enhanced efficiency and efficacy in treatment protocols. Coordination is also essential in solving the broader implications of respiratory disease, including their long-term impact on quality of life and use of health care resources. As the practice matures in investigation and improved clinical methods, pediatric pulmonology presents as a vibrant specialty with a solid commitment to developing patient care (Hayes et al., 2019).

Importance of Respiratory Health in Children

The significance of respiratory well-being during childhood cannot be overstressed, as it has a direct impact on the child's health and development. Respiratory illnesses become evident early in life, thus highlighting the need for thorough assessments and interventions at this growth stage. Children are particularly v to environmental pollutants, such as, such as tobacco smoke and airborne allergens, which have the potential to exacerbate underlying lung disease or establish new respiratory illness. Effective management of child respiratory health is thus necessary not only for the relief from acute conditions, but also for overall long-term health. Detection and intervention strategies, including vaccines and public health initiatives, can be very effective in reducing the prevalence of respiratory conditions, and therefore reinforce the significance of respiratory health to pediatric practice. In pediatric pulmonology, an understanding of child respiratory health also entails an appreciation for the interplay between genetic predisposition and environmental factors. Children who have asthma or some other respiratory disease in their family, for example, are more likely to develop the same. This calls for customized treatment that takes into account hereditary factors as well as environmental toxins children are subjected to throughout their lie. Pediatric pulmonologists bill with for keeping an eye on the development a function, utilizing equipment such as, such as spirometry to measure the capacity of the lungs and assess if there are gaps. This broad spectrum strategy will ensure that children receive personalized attention as guided by their personal health histories, leading to improved respiratory outcomes and an improved quality of life for kids. The persistent burden of respiratory disease in children emphasizes the need for multidisciplinary collaboration between health professionals, families, and communities. Community awareness campaigns about the importance of respiratory health are crucial in educating parents and caregivers on prevention, including healthy nutrition, refusing second-hand smoke exposure, and ensuring maximum indoor air quality. Additionally, the integration of respiratory health assessment in the care of children can lead to earlier diagnosis and treatment of asthma and allergy conditions. Some evidence suggests that the human phenotype ontology (HPO) has potential to be a rich resource for clinicians to standardize the examination of respiratory conditions and thereby improve communication and outcome of care across tDoug et al., 2009Sebastian et al.,

2020). Such inter-professional collaborations enhance the provision of pediatrics pulmonology and also provide an environment that honors and safeguards the respiratory well-being of children (Salvatori et al., 2020) (Figure 10.2).

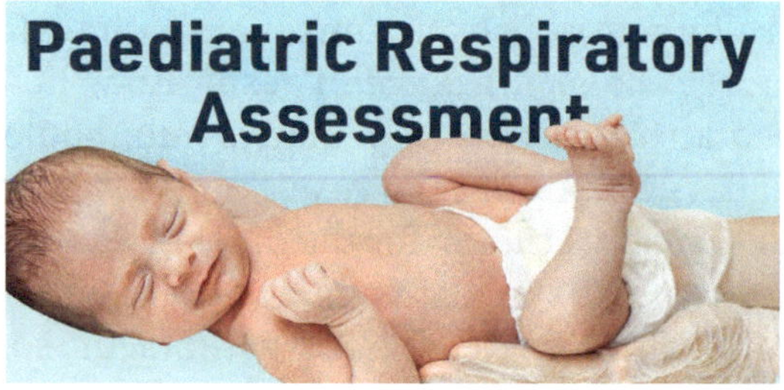

Figure 10.2. Importance of respiratory health in children.

Source: https://cdn-images.ausmed.com/ausmed-articles/20151202_cover_v3.jpg.

Overview of Common Pediatric Respiratory Conditions

Pediatric respiratory diseases describe a range of illnesses that affect children, asthma and pneumonia being two of the most common. Asthma is an inflammatory disease of the respiratory system and is characterized by wheeze, breathlessness, and cough, with allergens, respiratory tract infections, or environmental exposures as triggering agents. Though asthma can be managed using medication and lifestyle modifications, the disease remains a very common cause of morbidity among children. Unlike, however, is pneumonia, an infection of the lungs that is a more pressing danger, especially for young children who have underdeveloped immune systems. Since pneumonia moves so rapidly important to recognize symptoms such as, such as fever, cough, and difficulty breathing for prompt treatment, including antibiotics and supportive care. Another frequent respiratory disease in children is bronchitis, either acute or chronic. Acute bronchitis, often of viral origin, is characterized by cough and inflammation of bronchial airways, typically secondary to upper respiratory infections. Chronic bronchitis in children is, however, ofanifestation of underlying causes such as, such as exposure to tobacco smoke or air pollution. The illness has long-term health risks and needs to be treated with cautious consideration, often with measures of avoidance and symptomatic management. Furthermore, of respiratory support equipment, such as, such as nebulizers and inhalers, cannot be overrated when it comes to treating acute exacerbation of these conditions. Parents and guardians must receive appropriate education on symptoms that demand immediate medical attention to prevent complications. In more complex cases, icians typically handle disorders such as, such as sleep-disordered breathing (SDB) and their associated complications. SDB, potentially inclusive of obstructive sleep apnea, tends to occur in children with comorbid underlying health conditions, including neuroongenital anomalies. Fauroux et al. (2024)Research highlights that interventions like non-invasive ventilation (NIV) and continuous positive airway pressure (CPAP) can significantly reduce symptoms in the affected child, enhancing quality of sleep and reducing dyspnea. Additionally, underlying conditions that complicate respiratory health, particularly among immunocompromised populations, need in the acute caresetting. Kegel et al. (2024) Studies postulates that a large number of children undergoing intensive treatment receive numerous interventions at the time of death, which stresses the need for the integration of palliative care. Overall, it is essential to know these diverse pediatric respiratory conditions to effectively devise treatment protocols and enhance patient care (Doug et al., 2009).

10.1. Anatomy and Physiology of the Pediatric Respiratory System

Learning Outcome

1. Differences between pediatric and adult respiratory systems
2. Developmental stages of the respiratory system in children
3. Impact of growth on respiratory function

Pediatric respiratory anatomy varies from that of adults because children have varying physiological demands. Newborns come into the world with a fairly increased airway resistance and reduced airway caliber and are more prone to respiratory distress. Infant bronchi and tracheae are less in diameter, with the average tracheal diameter ranging from 4–5 mm, and therefore it becomes crucial to factor in this anatomical feature while diagnosing and managing respiratory diseases. Having compliant chest walls due to pliable rib cages impacts ventilation mechanics, requiring pediatric health care professionals to employ specialized tests and interventions unique to the pediatric population. Appreciation of these anatomical differences in the airway is crucial in the delivery of therapeutic care, especially where surgical treatment is an option for conditions like subglottic stenosis, where geometric evaluation can play a significant role in therapy determination, as outlined by the exciting findings of the recent pediatric airway investigation (Davis et al., 2015). Physiologically, the child's respiratory system operates with varied parameters from adults due to varying lung volumes and rates of respiration. Respiratory rate is increased in infants with a rate typically greater than 40 per minute to meet their oxygen demand, always greater than that for older children and adults. Also, pediatric patients have lower functional residual capacity and tidal volume relative to their body size, thus they are more prone to oxygen desaturation in the presence of respiratory compromise. Pulmonary system compliance and the increased diaphragm position also influence respiratory patterns. These physiological characteristics necessitate an alternative method of performing pc pulmonology, particularly interventions such as, such as non-invasive ventilation and airway administration that require adjustment to address these ynamics (Doug et al., 2009College and System, 2020). Furthermore, the relationship between anatomical and physiological characteristics within the pediatric respiratory system underscores the necessity for integrative diagnostic devices in ag airway function and integrity.

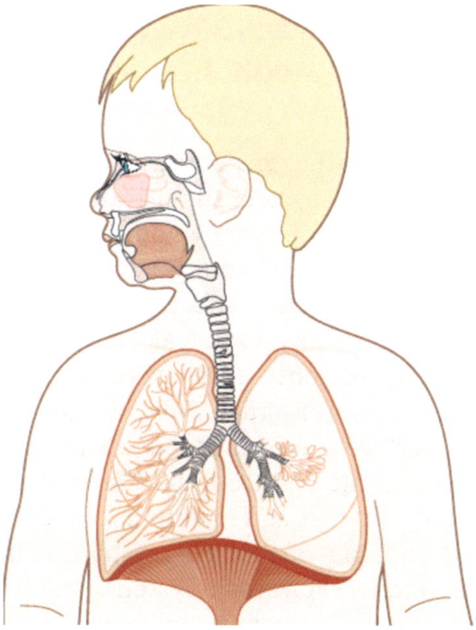

Figure 10.3. Anatomy and physiology of the pediatric respiratory system.

Source: https://dm3omg1n1n7zx.cloudfront.net/rcni/static/journals/ncyp/aop/ncyp.2020.e1246/graphic/ncyp.2020.e1246_0001.jpg.

Techniques such as, such as computed tomography and computational fluid dynamics models have shed the light to improve understanding of pediatric airway pathologies, especially in illnesses like subglottic stenosis. These new techniques allow geometric size and airflow dynamics to be evaluated, which are crucial for defining successful treatment strategies. The ability to visualize and measure airway structure not only enhances diagnostic accuracy but also allows for the creation of objective standards to direct surgical treatment against conservative management. As science unravels, future advances in these diagnostic methods will continue to advance pediatric pulmonary medicine so that the nuances of the pediatric respiratory system get the attention they deserve in clinical application (Davis et al., 2015) (Figure 10.3).

10.1.1. Differences Between Pediatric and Adult Respiratory Systems

The understanding of pediatric compared to adult respiratory system distinctions is critical in an attempt to adequately address the health care requirements of young patients. One of the most significant differences lies in the anatomical and physiological content of the lungs. Young patients have narrower airways, elevated respiratory rates, and a less mature alveolar surface area compared to adults. These factors make the children more susceptible to respiratory distress and infection, as their lungs are less capable of resisting extrinsic injury. The neonatal respiratory system only serves to complicate this dynamic further. The infants also have greater dependence on the diaphragm for breathing; any impairment in diaphragmatic function can lead to very accelerated decompensation, and hence interventions should be initiated in a timely manner. Furthermore, the immunological pattern differs significantly between the two populations, and this determines the manifestation of respiratory disease and its progression, necessitating certain clinical approaches in pediatric pulmonology. Aside from anatomical difference, physiological reaction to respiratory pathology is significantly different in children compared with adults. For instance, the pediatric respiratory apparatus exhibits a higher metabolic rate as well as oxygen usage, necessitating effective and efficient gas exchange. Also, children have a very limited set of compensatory mechanisms in response to hypoxia, i.e., they can deteriorate very rapidly when there is respiratory pathology. The prevalence of some of these respiratory diseases is also highly variable, and the children are more prone to asthma and viral infections that are less apparent in adults. All these variations in the presentation of disease mean that it is crucial to stress preventative medicine and early detection in the children. Besides, treatment strategies would need to be adjusted based on developmental phases, underlining the importance of a specialty practice of pediatric pulmonology (Lee et al., 2018). Furthermore, developmental influences play an important role in pediatric variations in the respiratory system. Lung maturation in neonates can be influenced by several factors including prematurity, where there is r production of surfactant, leading to complications such as, such as respiratory distress syndrome (RDS). Conversely, adult respiratory disease is more of an environmental and physiological deterioration due to age. The long-term effects of diseases like chronic obstructive pulmonary disease (COPD) or lung cancer make adult respiratory care different from children, who are more involved with acute infection or congenital anomdiatric pulmonology must consider such unique aspects, such as, such as family-centered care and genetic counseling in conditions like cystic fibrosis or dyskinetic cilia syndromes. In the long term, the identification of these differences not only leads to successful diagnosis and treatment but also enhances the care management and qualie in pediatric patients (Doug et al., 2009Richard et al., 2017).

10.1.2. Developmental Stages of the Respiratory System in Children

The emergence of the respiratory system in kids is a multifaceted phenomenon that starts in embryonic life and extends well into early childhood. As early as around the fifth week of pregnancy, the foundation of the respiratory system forms with the development of the trachea and bronchial tree. This complex airway network undergoes extensive growth with bifurcation into primary, secondary, and tertiary bronchi that act as very important structures for efficient gas exchange. These structures are necessary for proper gas exchange. During fetal development, the production of surfactant is stimulated around the 24th week of pregnancy, which is the key to respiratory maturity. The lack of mature surfactant in preterm infants is one of the primary causes of Neonatal Respiratory Distress Syndrome (NRDS), a pediatric pulmonology challenge, and this underlines the importance of monitoring lung development during pregnancy and early life. After birth, the respiratory system undergoes some necessary changes that allow for independent respiration. The lungs of neonates change from fluid-filled organs to air-filled organs at their first breath, which reflects the role of extrinsic factors in respiratory adaptation. Lung development is hastened by six months of age, making the lung volume and surface area double, which is necessary for effective gas exchangering this phase that breathing patterns in children also undergo a change, from predominantly abdominal (diaphragmatic) to an adult-type thoracic pattern. All such changes are imperative as faulty development of lungs will cause respiratory complications in the long run, and it becomes crucial for pediatric healthcare practitioners to assess the lung function and screen for any indication of breathing complications in follow-up visits. As children develop during early childhood, the respiratory system matures in various stages parallel to the general development and activity of the children. While the children are three years old, airway resistance reduces and thus the respiratory capacity becomes more effective. Children also begin to exhibit greater respiratory reserve with better muscular strength as they can perform more physically demanding tasks. But along with this development comes a higher rate of respiratory infections through ed contact with pathogens, particularly in group environments such as, such as daycare. The pediatric pulmonology must fise to some extent, particularly in children with comorbidities such as, such as asthma or in cases of families with a history of respiratory illness as these will go a long way to influence lung health for the rest of the child's life (Figure 10.4).

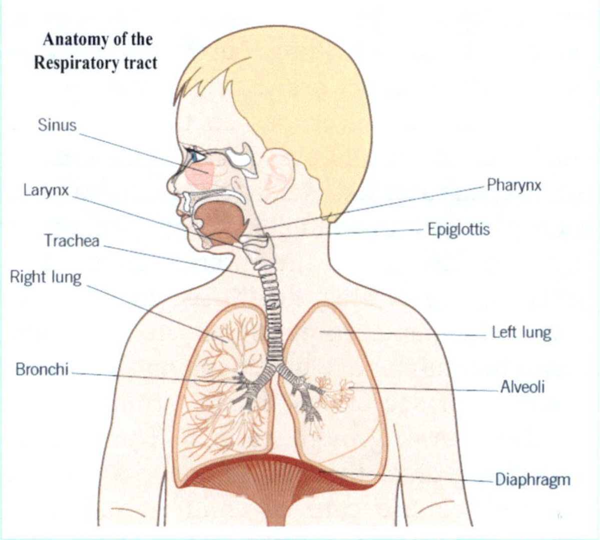

Figure 10.4. Developmental stages of the respiratory system in children.

Source: https://dm3omg1n1n7zx.cloudfront.net/rcni/static/journals/ncyp/23/7/ncyp2011.09.23.7.25.c8684/graphic/ncyp_v23_n7_8684_0003.jpg.

10.1.3. Impact of Growth on Respiratory Function

Child development plays a vital role in the growth and normal functioning of the respiratory system. While developing from infancy through childhood and well into adolescence, there are dramatic changes in physiology that influence respiratory health. Development is marked by increased lung volume, compliance of the chest wall, and airway maturation. Growth spurts can lead to enhanced pulmonary function, as children develop more respiratory muscle strength and efficiency. The enlarging alveoli also increase in quantity and size, which results in increased gas exchange capacity. Pediatricians and pulmonologists must appreciate these growth-related changes to appropriately assess respiratory function and intervene when necessary. For instance, defective lung formation at critical stages of development predisposes the child to chronic respiratory disease and close monitoring and control measures to prevent sequelae of long standing. Furthermore, some conditions which are prevalent in children may exert significant influences on the manner in which growth will affect respiratory function. For instance, diseases like ataxia telangiectasia (A-T) leading to immunodeficiency and pulmonary complications depict the interdependence of growth and respiratory health. A-T children will also exhibit impaired pulmonary function due to chronic pulmonary infections and impaired clearance of secretions, further contributing to their overall growth pattern. This unique synergy predicts the necessity for a holistic approach to the care of children in which respiratory health is monitored in parallel with measurements of growth. The ability to monitor over time allows medical providers to identify any divergence from normal growth patterns that would signal underlying pulmonary disease. Personalized treatment schedules can be designed to treat both the respiratory and growth needs, thereby enhancing the quality of lirticipating children (Rothblum et al., 2016). Additionally, psychologicalpsychological and social dimensions of growth and respiratory function must also be treated in pediatrics. Growth is not merely a physical process; it encompasses emotional and developmental factors that contribute to a child's assessment of their own health. Children with chronic respiratory conditions are likely to develop anxiety and reduced self-esteem regarding their illness, predisposing them towards worsening their attitude towards physical exercise critical to normal growth. Stigma of hospitalization or respiratory limitation could further result in social isolation. Psychiatric support measures must, therefore, become an integral part nagement in pediatric pulmonology. Multidisciplinary integration, such as, such as pulmonologists, nutritionists, and mental health professionals, may facilitate a culture that supports optimal growth and respiratory function and fosters a balanced method of approaching pediatric well-being, especially in the case with complex disorders (Kurland et al., 2013).

Test Your Knowledge

1. What are the key anatomical and physiological differences between pediatric and adult respiratory systems?
2. How does the respiratory system develop through the various stages of childhood?
3. In what ways does growth affect respiratory function and efficiency in children?

10.2. Common Pediatric Respiratory Disorders

Learning Outcome

1. Asthma: prevalence and management
2. Cystic fibrosis: genetic implications and treatment
3. Bronchopulmonary dysplasia: causes and long-term effects

Pediatric respiratory illness is a significant field of attention in pediatric medicine that requires a sensitive understanding of several underlying pathologies. Of all the respiratory illnesses, asthma remains among the most frequent chronic illnesses of childhood, consisting of reversible airway obstruction due to inflammation and hyperreactivity. Asthma can present very variably, with wheeze, cough, and breathlessness commonly presenting, particularly with exertion or at night. Treatment of asthma typically requires a careful history and physical, and, as mentioned, pulmonary function tests. Pediatric pulmonology plays a role in the management of asthma as well by using pharmacologic treatment, lifestyle modifications, and patient education to optimize patient outcomes and quality of life. Early diagnosis and treatment are important, as poorly controlled asthma may lead to exacerbations, loss of lung function, and may significantly impact a child's daily life. Apart from asthma, other common childhood respiratory illnesses are various forms of interstitial lung disease (chILD), a heterogeneous group of disorders of the lung interstitium. Characterized by impaired gas exchange at the alveolar-capillary level, chILD can exhibit varying degrees of severity and varied symptoms. Infants typically present with tachypnea as a prominent symptom, while older children may have more subtle symptoms such that early diagnosis becomes difficult. As chILD is susceptible to complications, patients should be referred to pediatric pulmonologists so can be appropriately evaluated and managed. An orderly structure, such as, such as the Delphi method, has been developed to systematize treatment protocols for such illnesses so that better patient outcomes may be achieved through best-available therapeutic strategies (Fenu et al., 2023). Apart from asthma and chILD, other illnesses, like cystic fibrosis (CF), are also of fundamental importance in pediatric pulmonary morbidity. CF is caused by mutations in the CFTR gene, leading to the secretion of dehydrated, stickiest mucus, blocking the airways and making the patient prone to chronic respiratory infection. It leads to chronic lung damage over years and typically needs an international approach with respiratory and nutritional interventions. Technology innovations and the application of the human phenotype ontology (HPO) have facilitated the sophisticated comprehension and management of phenotypic manifestations associated with CF and other child respiratory disorders, allowing health care workers to provide more precise diagnoses and treatment. By taking advantage of databases like the HPO, physicians can better track phenotypic abnormalities and streamline treatment plans according to individual patient requirements, emphasi specialized pediatric pulmonology (Doug et al., 2009Sebastian et al., 2020) (Figure 10.5).

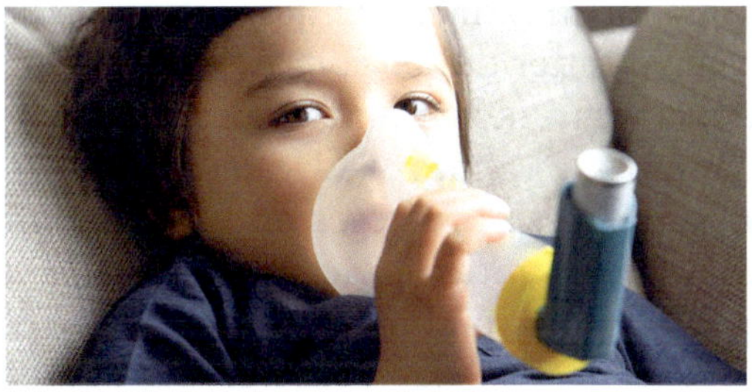

Figure 10.5. Common pediatric respiratory disorders.

Source: https://cdn.prod.website-files.com/5ee7039040ea6efb80d7521c/66c992c3d97ecbeee3e90362_5feda59391f4633785fa3c6d_Breathing-Bothers-1400x700.jpeg.

10.2.1. Asthma: Prevalence and Management

The health burden of asthma globally is mostly predominant in low and middle-income countries (LMICs). The most noticeable trend among such populations is the rising incidences of asthma in children, obviously a grim public health concern. This trend in population is alarming since children represent a greater proportion of the population pyramid in LMICs. Ineffective asthma control in such areas is compounded by the reality that health systems are largely engaged in controlling acute and infectious conditions and not controlling chronic conditions like asthma. Inevitably, poor asthma control leads to higherand mortality levels among children who suffer from the disease. In order toTo address the issue, e effort to increase the availability of essential controller drugs, such as, such as inhaled corticosteroids, combined with systemic reform with the goal of placing chronic disease treatment at the center of healthcare policy (Lachner et al., 2024). The inclusion of mental health care in the management of asthma has increasingly been seen as valuable, particularly in children. Recent studies highlight the interplay between asthma and mental health in high-risk groups, showing that asthma children are more prone to developing mental illness. By integrating clinical psychology into multidsthma treatment clinics, doctors are able to manage better the psychologicalpsychological burden in chronic asthma. This approach not only offers an improved care support for children but also promotes an integrated form of care. Early intervention in mental health care is vital in reinforcing overall results, as other recent studies attest to supporting a positive correlation between mental health intervention and the success of asthma care (Aver 2023). Further study of new approaches to asthma care is needed in order toto further treat pediatric patients. Solutions will have to be found for environmental and health care obstacles that prevent successful asthma control. Encouraging commitments from local governments and health care providers may lead to policies that become models of asthma care, emphasizing consistent access to needed medicines. Additionally, public health measures to edcate healthcare providers and the general population as a wholeon asthma, —along with measures to limit smoking and air pollution levels, —can greatly contribute to improving the quality of life for affected children. To ensure that these strategies asful, ongoing research and collaboration among various stakeholders, such as, such as public health organizations and local governments, are essential for creating environments with asthma care and services for pediatric populations (Lachner et al., 2024).

10.2.2. Cystic Fibrosis: Genetic Implications and Treatment

Cystic fibrosis (CF) is a genetic disease caused by mutations in the gene that encodes the cystic fibrosis transmembrane conductance regulator protein. The role of this protein is to regulate chloride ion transport across epithelial membranes and thus modulate secretions in a number of organs, including the lungs, pancreas, and intestines. The most common mutation, F508del, results in abnormal folding and function of the CFTR protein, forming thick, sticky mucus that leads to plugged airways and repeated infections. The genetic impact of CF is relevant, in that it is inherited in an autosomal recessive pattern, with both parents having to donate the affected gene for the child to be affected. Genetic counseling and carrier screening should be done for prospective parents to identify their risks and potential effect on offspring. Proper management of cystic fibrosis requires a multidisciplinary treatment approach to manage the symptoms and improve the quality of life. Pancreatic enzyme supplements, nutritional supports, and aggressive airway clearance therapies which enable the removal of mucus from the lungs form the regular care. Furthermore, the patients require antibiotics for treating and preventing respiratory infections, particularly those occurring from opportunistic pathogens like Pseudomonas aeruginosa. The advent of CFTR modulators marks a milestone in the treatment regimen, targeting the source genetic defect rather than just addressing symptoms. These therapies, ivacaftor and lumacaftor, have proved promising in preserving lung function and reducing hospitalization in appropriate patients by mahe dysfunctional CFTR protein. Despite the advances in treatment, psychologicalpsychological and emotional distress to families with cystic fibrosis cannot be overestimated.

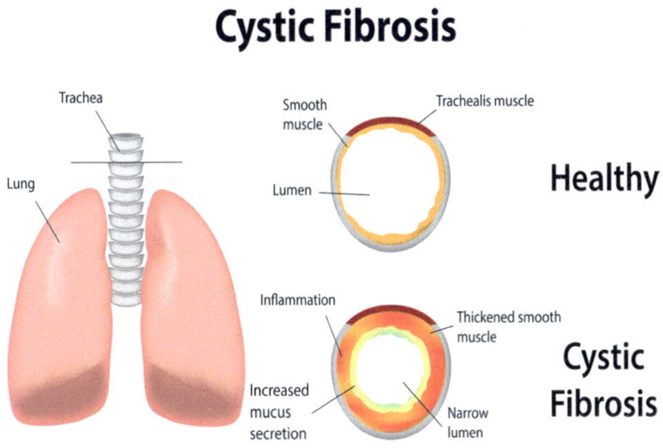

Figure 10.6. Cystic fibrosis: genetic implications and treatment.

Source: https://www.yashodahospitals.com/wp-content/uploads/2024/11/cystic-fibrosis.jpg.

Parents of chronically ill children most often report lower quality of life for their children compared to healthy children, primarily due to the challenges and burdens involved in caring for them. Coping strategies play an important role in moderating such problems and can significantly affect the health of both the parents and the child. established that adaptive coping mechanisms correlate with better psychologicalpsychological results, whereas maladaptive ones have been known to compound stress and negatively influence the quality of life. Knowledge and optimization of such coping mechanisms are essential in developing interventions that enable cystic fibrosis families to actter outcomest just for the patients but also for their caregivers (Fairfax Doug et al., 20192009) (Figure 10.6).

10.2.3. Bronchopulmonary Dysplasia (BPD): Causes and Long-Term Effects

The pathogenesis of BPD is typically linked with a variety of interconnected etiologies that are typically observed among preterm babies. BPD typically occurs in infants who require mechanical ventilation or oxygen supplementation for the purpose of immature lungs. The causes of lung damage characteristic of this condition include being exposed to oxidative stress, inflammation, and mechanical damage due to the application of invasive ventilation techniques. These become compounded by the prematurity and low birth weight of the infants, which make them susceptible to respiratory problems. Additional risk factors like infection and the need for prolonged supplemental oxygenation contribute to the severity of BPD, bringing about an intricate interplay between environmental and biological determinants of lung maturation. The determination of these causes is crucial to the development of preventive interventions, as corroborated by ongoing studies calling for prenatal consultation and controlled delivery processes to neutralize such pervasive causes (Miyoshi et al., 2005). The long-term effects of bronchopulmonary dysplasia vastly surpass the temporary respiratory issues experienced in neonatal age, impacting predominantly neurodevelopment and quality of life. Children with BPD experience a range of chronic complications, including recurrent respiratory infections, asthma, and reduced exercise capacity, as per research. Cognition and motor development could also be impaired due to the interaction of environmental stressors and the inherent pathophysiological alterations of BPD. These long-term outcomes cause heavy loads on health care systems, as children with BPD require constant medical care, respiratory therapy, and schooling interventions. Their health course is further influenced by socio-economic factors and the quality of follow-up care they get, necessitating a powerful multidisciplinary treatmetimize their lopmental course and address their multifaceted needs (Bentsen Doug et al., 20182009). The effective treatment of bronchopulmonary dysplasia involves the use of both preventive and therapeutic strategies preceded by the knowledge of causes and long-term effects of the conditions. Prevention strategies like prenatal administration of corticosteroids and surfactant therapy aim at enhancing the functioning of the lung and minimally decreasing the occurrence of BPD among high-risk individuals. Postnatally, a co-ordinated approach by a multi-disciplinary team can provide inclusive care, which includes individualized management plans in consideration of the unique challenges faced by ent. Research into new non-invasive methods for measuring lung function, such as, such as electromagnetic inductance plethysmography, holds out the promise to allow early intervention and optimal follow-up care in infants with BPD. Finally, the development of pediatric pulmonology knowledge on BPD will not only inform clinical practice but also enhance the quality of life of affected individuals through targeted prevention and treatment (Miyoshi et al., 2005).

Test Your Knowledge

1. What is the prevalence of asthma in children, and what are the key strategies for its management?
2. How does cystic fibrosis develop genetically, and what treatments help manage its symptoms?
3. What causes bronchopulmonary dysplasia, and what are its potential long-term effects on respiratory health?

10.3. Diagnostic Techniques in Pediatric Pulmonology

Learning Outcome

1. Pulmonary function tests: purpose and methodology
2. Imaging studies: X-rays and CT scans in diagnosis
3. Bronchoscopy: indications and procedures

The emerging field of pediatric pulmonology is more reliant on advanced diagnostic techniques, which are needed to accurately classify respiratory diseases in children. Among the top methods is through the use of molecular testing to detect respiratory viruses, an important role that is especially crucial in the management of bronchiolitis. A study of 723 previously healthy infants hospitalized with bronchiolitis identified fourteen respiratory viruses by nasopharyngeal aspirate and identified the most prevalent as the respiratory syncytial virus (RSV). The ability to detect specific viral agents is an improvement over clinical practice with certain management strategies that are able to make a difference in morbidity and use of healthcare resources. Additionally, epidemiologic features analysis may uncover variability in clinical presentations and hence improve diagnostic accuracy and predictability of seasonal epidemics that occur to thousands of infants annually (Antonelli et al., 2016). Imaging modalities likewise find their niche in pediatric pulmonology, notably in the assessment of pneumonia that remains the most frequent cause of morbidity in children. Chest X-rays and other imaging modalities like computed tomography (CT) may aid in the evaluation of the presence and extent of pneumonia, supporting further treatment regimens. Not only do these imaging modalities aid in the detection of pneumonia, but also in the evaluation of complications like pleural effusion or abscesses. Certain challenges arise when diagnosing pneumonia in children because they are different and share similar clinical presentation with other respiratory infections. For instance, viral versus bacterial pneumonia is significant, as treatment regimens are very different.

As highlighted in recent literature, differences need to be realized to further improve outcome and avoid long-term pulmonary sequelae in children (Chang et al., 2013). In addition to conventional imaging and molecular techniques, bronchoscopic investigations are now increasingly relevant in pediatric pulmonology. This invasive but often needed diagnostic tool allows one to see directly down the bronchial tree and readily obtain samples, which may be of utmost value in making complex respiratory illness diagnoses. For instance, in the case of suspected infect non-infectious disease, bronchoscopy can shed light on underlying etiologies such as, such as aspiration, anatomical defects, or presence of a foreign body. Moreover, the facility to perform bronchoalveolar lavage with the help of this procedure has the capability to yield individual microbial cultures or cytological examination, thereby yielding valuable information regarding chronic respiratory disease. Nevertheless, careful consideration towards the risk vs. benefits of carrying out such procedures in children is paramount and demands efficient pre-procedure assessment and experienced clinical staff to ensure patient safety and effective diagnostic outcomes (Figure 10.7).

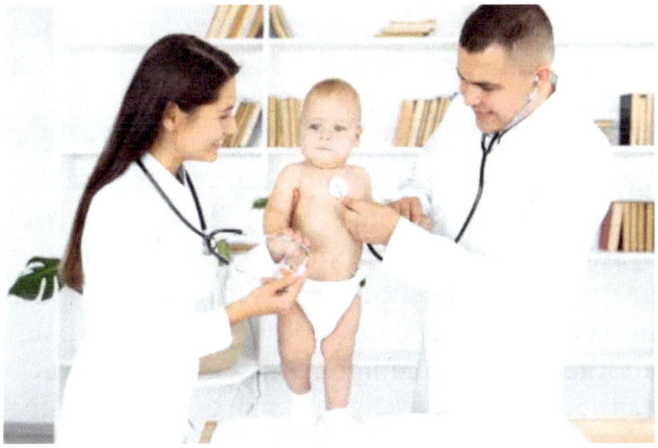

Figure 10.7. Diagnostic techniques in pediatric pulmonology.

Source: https://www.medicusunion.com/_next/image?url=https%3A%2F%2Fapi.medicusunion.com%2Faws-s3%2Ffile%2F1713777492657-Pediatric_pulmonology_1.png%3Fsize%3D150&w=3840&q=75.

10.3.1. Pulmonary Function Tests (PFTs): Purpose and Methodology

PFTs are an essential pediatric pulmonology tool having both diagnostic and monitoring roles in many lung diseases. PFTs measure lung volumes, flow of air, and the capacity for gas exchange, providing useful information regarding the integrity and function of the respiratory system. Initiation of PFT in children should be followed by precise consideration of their level of development and ability to understand the testing process required to provide accurate results. Children aged five can, on certions, be encompassed in simple spirometry tests, while more intricate techniques, such as, such as body plethysmography and diffusing capacity tests, may be suitable in older adolescents. With appropriately selected methods, the clinical practitioners can ensure the validity of the test r, which makes it easier for proper treatment and planning of respiratory diseases (AmorimLucas et al., 2019). The method applied in PFTs is often a combination of various procedures, each measuring a unique aspect of pulmonary function. Spirometry, for instance, is a fundamental test that measures the of air and rate of air flow on inhalation and exhalation and provides parameters such as, such as Forced Vital Capacity (FVC) and Forced Expiratory Volume in one second (FEV1). In patients with cystic fibrosis and asthma, these interventions are crucial in quantifying disease severity and in treatment decisions. Body plethysmography, another essential component, quantifies thoracic gas volume and airway resistance, detailing lung mechanics in-depth.

Further, test outcomes can enlighten the healthcare providers regarding the dynamics of chronic disease, enabling timely interventions and adjustments in therapy (Tomlinson et al., 2019). PFT result interpretation requires a refined understanding of pediatric norms and the impact of all types of pathophysiologic diseases. Because children's lungs have unique anatomical and physiological characteristics, their pulmonary function parameters are very different from those of adults.

This necessitates age-specific reference values when interpreting test results. For istance, in primary ciliary dyskinesia diseases, a clearly defined pulmonarerbations on the basis of PFT information refines disease complication management (AmorimLucas et al., 2019). With pediatric pulmonologists developing more precise strategies for determining children through the use of PFTs, studies and consensus building continue to harmonize methods and improve accuracy in assessments, resulting in improved patient outcomes through customized treatment regimens.

10.3.2. Imaging Studies: X-Rays and CT Scans in Diagnosis

Imaging tests are central to the diagnostic workup in pediatric pulmonology, especially X-rays and computerized tomography (CT) scans. X-rays become the initial imaging tool because of their accessibility, quickness, and efficiency in detecting prevalent pulmonary ailments like pneumonia or bronchial blockage. Their capacity to give quick information on lung structures makes them particularly useful in pediatric patients since they might need to be evaluated instantly. Pediatric anatomy may be particularly difficult due to varying development, so precise X-ray interpretation is important. When X-rays show indefinite findings, or where more detailed visualization is desired, CT scans are a highly useful means. They provide superior imaging to enable doctors to examine intricate lung morphology and make it easier for them to diagnose complicated diseases in pediatric patients. CT scans have greater resolution and three-dimensional imaging, both of which are critical in the assessment of children with pulmonary disease. The high-resolution cronal images are able to detect abnormalities that can be occult on standard X-rays, such as, such as diffuse pulmonary nodules, vascular malformations, or bronchiectasis. However, the increased radiation exposure from CT scans is a concern, especially taking into account the augmented risk to children from the effects of radiation. Accordingly, clinicians must carefully weigh the benefits of obtaining more precistic information against the hazards of radiation exposure. Enhanced CT technology, such as, such as reduced-dose methods and iterative reconstruction algorithms, can minimize certain risks, allowing for safer imaging with retained diagnostic efficacy. These considerations speak to the need for a thoughtful approach to imaging in pediatric pulmonology. The use of both CT and X-ray scans within the diagnostic workup significantly enhances the ability to provide accurate and timely diagnoses in pediatric patients with respiratory disease. Despite the advantage that each of these imaging methods offers, it is wise for clinicians to remember the ever-evolving setting of imaging practice. Recommendations continue to be provided, not only for appropriate use but also in ensuring optimization of patient safety. In addition, the collaboration of the disciplines of oncology, pulmonology, and radiology enhances the optimal application of these imaging tools in the identification of those diseases that can stimulate immune-related side effects in therapies like immune checkpoint inhibitor therapy, especially among children. By continuous renewal of guidelines and protnclude the latest research and technological advancements, pediatric pulmonology is able tocan offer children access to the most effective andable, thus improving patient outcomes (Jarosław Meyer-Szary et al., 2022; Bryan et al., 2021Lucas et al., 2019) (Figure 10.8).

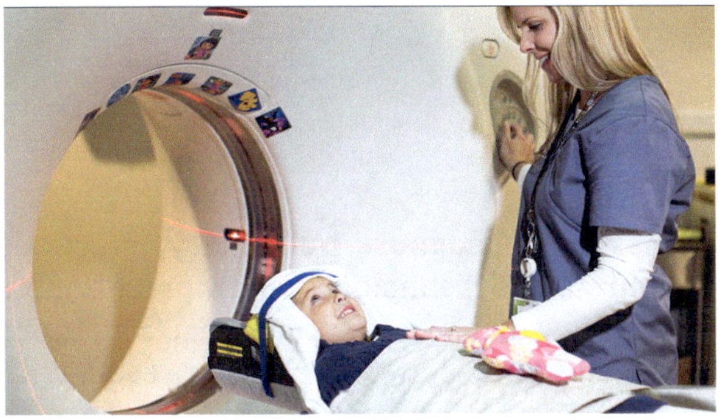

Figure 10.8. Imaging studies: X-rays and CT scans in diagnosis.

Source: https://childrenswi.org/-/media/chwlibrary/newshub/2018/xray-ct-scan/child-imaging-exam.jpg?h=514&mw=900&w=900&hash=286C831AA485C11CAD1A6C38346EFCBA.

10.3.3. Bronchoscopy: Indications and Procedures

Bronchoscopy is an effective tool in pediatric pulmonology, as it enables diagnosis and treatment to be carried out in children with breathing problems. Bronchoscopy enables physicians to visualize the adirectly and obtain valuable specimens, which is crucial for diagnosing some diseases such as, such as infection, anomalies of the airway, and chronic cough. As stated earlier, diagnostic presentations of bronchoscopy include repeated presentations of symptoms like stridor, wheezing, and pulmonary hemorrhage, and conditions like atelectasis that are likely to be challenging to manage via standard evaluation avenues (Moslehi, 2022). Prompt diagnosis of these complications will have a significant effect on management avenues and outcomes for the patients, thereby pre-empting the need for more invasive procedures. The amenability of bronchoscopic equipment to varying anatomical and physiological characteristics in children is indicative of the dynamic versatility of pediatric interventional pulmonology and the necessary personalization in treatment. The two principal types of bronchoscopes, rigid and flexible, offer different benefits depending on the clinical scenario encountered. Rigid bronchoscopes, though also the gold standard in some circumstances, necessitate deep anesthesia and are usually utilized in the operating room setting. Flexible bronchoscopes can be with light sedation and allow for the execution of procedures in several environmenas, such as at the bedside (Moslehi, 2022). Greater flexibility of the approach paths, such as, such as through the nostrils or endotracheal tubes, enhances diagnostic and therapeutic performance with fewer difficulties. Flexibility of the bronchoscopes guarantees versatility in intervention of congenital and acquired conditions, highlighting their importance in pediatrics. Aside from this, technological advances in bronchoscopy further guarantee that physicians gain new techniques to manage hard-to-treat respiratory conditions. Despite challenges presented by the COVID-19 pandemic, pediatric pulmonology faces, the contribution of bronchoscopy also remains imperative despite reported declines in procedure during this period. With th outbreak of the pandemic, clinical visits and laboratory testing, —even flexible bronchoscopy, —were greatly minimized, emphasizing the need for prompt utilization of this technique in diagnosed conditions. The ability to respond quickly in addressing acute airway obstruction secondary to foreign bodies or inflammatory processes emphasizes the need for available and proficient staff within pediatric pulmonology departments. As evidence mounts, preventing complications of bronchoscopy is achievable through judicious selection and expert technique, underpinning ongoing education and training for pediatric bronchoscopy experts. Addition of multi-center studies and development of professional communication can serve as further pillars to secure foundations for safe and effective practice within this important arena of pediatric healthcare.

Test Your Knowledge

1. What is the purpose of pulmonary function tests in children, and how are they performed?
2. How are imaging studies such as X-rays and CT scans used in diagnosing pediatric respiratory disorders?
3. What are the main indications for performing bronchoscopy in children, and what does the procedure involve?

10.4. Treatment Approaches in Pediatric Pulmonology

Learning Outcome

1. Pharmacological treatments: inhalers and nebulizers
2. Non-pharmacological interventions: physiotherapy and education
3. Surgical options: when and why they are considered

Treatment in pediatric pulmonology is continually being improved through biomedical technological advancements and a better understanding of respiratory disease. A significant improvement is the application of artificial intelligence and digital image processing to diagnose pulmonary infections in children. The technologies allow practitioners to accurately diagnose and categorize conditions like pneumonia and tuberculosis, even with limited medical resources. For instance, a reliable deep transfer learning solution has excelled at explaining pediatric chest X-ray scans, accurately classifying them. Not only does this innovation enhance diagnostics, but it reduces morbidity and mortality rates in pediatric patients, allowing for more successful interventions in a health care system that demands precision and safety (Marvin et al., 2022). Moreover, the given treatment setting for pediatric respiratory diseases is hupplemented by incorporating standardized phenotypic examination, particularly through resources such as, such as the Human Phenotype Ontology (HPO). The extended framework rigorously recruits many phenotypic abnormalities in an open and periodic manner so that illnesses of children's respiratory systems can be described in a better manner. As the HPO was extended to include multiple medical specialties, including pulmonology, it enables clinicians to diagnose and treat complex cases with improved contextual representation of symptoms. Not only does this information integration across multiple ontologies enhance the trustworthiness of clinical practice, but it also promotes inter-professional con, resulting mproved diagnostic and therapeutic approaches tailored to children's needs (Sebastian Lucas et al., 20202019). Finally, pediatric pulmonology treatment regimens must also incorporate prevention interventions and patient education to successfully treat chronic disease.

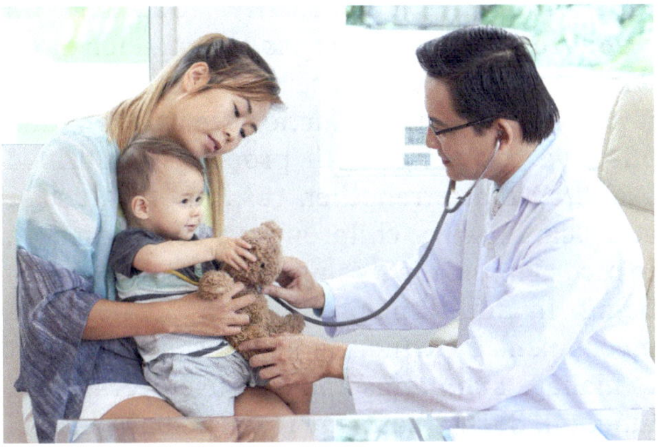

Figure 10.9. Treatment approaches in pediatric pulmonology.

Source: https://thehospitalatmaayo.com/wp-content/uploads/2022/03/baby-visiting-hospital-with-mom.jpg.

Asthma treatment, for example, often involves not only pharmacological management but also lifestyle modification and tailored action plans. Through education of families in the avoidance of precipitants and self-management techniques, health care providers can empower patients and reduce the use of emergency care. Apart from that, collaboration between pulmonologists and multidisciplinary teams like allergists and nutritionists is crucial for complete treatment. Emphasis on preventative methods along with newer treatment strategies not only improves the quality of life in the patient but also public health objectives of reducing hospitalization and healthcare costs. Ultimately, a multifaceted approach combining technological advancements, standardization of phenotypic data, and patient-centered care will define pediatric pulmonology's future (Figure 10.9).

10.4.1. Pharmacological Treatments: Inhalers and Nebulizers

Inhalers and nebulizers are two important modalities of pharmacological treatment of pediatric respiratory diseases. Both devices are employed to deliver medicines to the lungs where their action is felt almost immediately, providing rapid relief of obstructive symptoms of such diseases as asthma and chronic obstructive pulmonary disease (COPD). Inhalers are used most frequently for convenience and portability, with the majority preferring the use of metered-dose inhalers (MDIs) that can be utilized with spacers to enhance drug delivery and eliminate oropharyngeal deposition. Nebulizers, however, which deliver aerosol medication through the use of a machine, are especially convenient for very young patients or those with overwhelming respiratory distress, as they are less patient labored than inhalers. Continual evaluation and comparison of such delivery systems emphasize the importance of the right piece of equipment appropriate to the clinical setting and patientlity. Pharmacologic agents used on inhalers and nebulizers are generally comprised of bronchodilators such as, sua-agonists, corticosteroids, and anticholinergics, with varied therapeutic activities. Beta-agonists, such as, such as albuterol, have a key function in quickly relaxing bronchial smooth muscle and thus decreasing acute bronchospasm. Additionally, systemic corticosteroids may be used for their powerful anti-inflammatory effects, particularly in managing asthma attacks. Evidence supports the success of these medications in both chronic and acute management settings in children. When one considers the prevalence of respiratory diseases in children, especially in light of today's COVID-19 pandemic, the use of these medications becomes incry vital. Current studies sest the potenial benefits of nebulized medications for viral infections such as, sucS-CoV-2, and it they indicates that their administration could be extended beyond conventional uses (Kaufman Lucas et al., 2022).

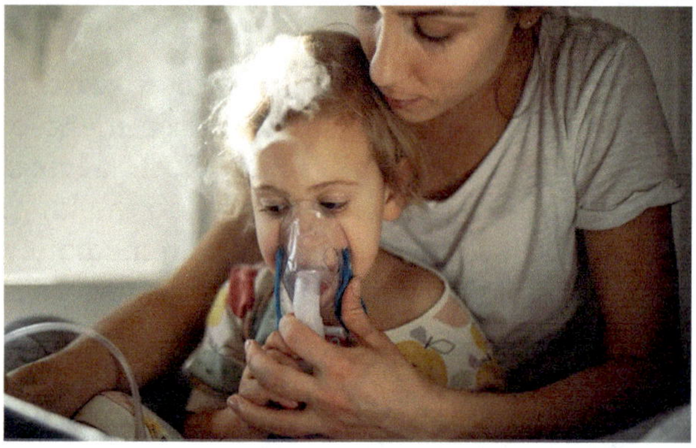

Figure 10.10. Mother assisting child with nebulizer therapy for respiratory relief.

Source: https://www.grxstatic.com/4f3rgqwzdznj/4fgu6P6z80VGxcCuc63GCq/a83a7a9455450d60bd3ea30301d745c4/mother_helping_daughter_with_nebulizer-1372188657.jpg?format=pjpg&auto=webp&width=704.

The choice between nebulizer and inhaler also relies on some factors which are the age of the patient, severity of the illness, and ease of use. Current literature emphasizes a strong preference for MDIs in the outpatient environment because they are efficient and convenient, particularly when used with spacers that maximize aerosol dispersion (Amantea et al., 2007). Nonetheless, nebulizers remain highly valuable in the acute care environment since they can administer higher doses of medication more easily. Pediatric pulmonology decision-making typically depends on a subtle recognition of pharmacologic properties, device capabilities, and patient characteristics for modulating proper treatment regimens. Clinicians ought to understand these dynamics in the attempt to optimize therapeutic responses and optimize the management of pediatric pulmonary conditions (Figure 10.10).

10.4.2. Non-pharmacological Interventions: Physiotherapy and Education

The use of non-pharmacological treatment, such as, such as education and physiotherapy, is an integral component of pediatric pulmonology. Physiotherapy, specifically focusing on respiratory physiotherapy, is essential for those with chronic respiratory conditions because it can improve lung function, ventilation, and effective coughing. With properly prescribed exercises that strengthen respiratory muscles and clear airways, children have been observed to record impressive gains in their general well-being. In addition, physiotherapy offers the mechanism by which children can be taught to manage symptoms and improve overall lung function. Such treatment is particularly useful where drug therapy is not available or will have ide effects, allowing for a more holistic way of caring that prioritizes the child's physical and psychologicalpsychological requirements. Education is also a significant component of non-pharmacological management in pediatric pulmonology. Educating families and children about their respiratory disease has the potential to improve self-management and medication compliance. Education activities may include a variety of topics, from an understanding of the disease process through to following medication and how to manage exacerbations. Furthermore, educating carers on early warning signs allows for medical intervention at an early stage, possibly preventing crisis development. By establishing an open environment within which the families feel engaged and informed, healthcare professionals can enhance the overall management of respiratory disorders in children, ultimately leading to improved health reduced hospitalization. Apart from education and physiotherapy, a multidisciplinary approach with psychologicalpsychological support and social services can also enhance the effectiveness of non-pharmacological interventions. Children with chronic respiratory issues are likely to have associatend behavioral issues, making overall care andf the child more complex. Integration of psychologicalpsychological support not only addresses the psychologicalpsychological needs of the child but also instills coping and resilience. Creation of a holistic care plan with education, physiotherapy, and emotional support can cause major improvements in long-term outcomes in pediatric respiratory patients. With icknowledgment of the beneficial impacts of such comprehensive methods, ongoing research is necessary in order toto optimize these interventions as part of the overall treatment system in pediatric pulmonology so that children receive the highest quality and kind treatment.

10.4.3. Surgical Options: When and Why They Are Considered

Surgery is generally reserved in pediatric pulmonology when medical therapy by itself cannot repair respiratory disease. Bad asthma, bronchopulmonary dysplasia, repeated pneumonia, and congenital defects can all necessitate surgery. For instance, congenital malformations of tracheoesophageal fistulas are occasionally managed with corrective surgery to achieve successful airway management and respiratory function. Similarly, thus, in unresponsive severe asthma, therapies like bronchial thermoplasty can be used to suppress airway hyperresponsiveness. These surgical procedures are pivotal not only in alleviating relief for acute respiratory distress but also in improving the quality of life in the long run in children, thus underlining the significance of exploring the option for surgery as a part of the complete therapeutic plan. Timing of surgical intervention in pediatric pulmonology is crucial and will have to be determined by the severity of the child's state, health status, and risk factors associated with surgery. For example, children presenting with poor growth, severe respiratory compromise, or frequent hospitalization due to their condition can be ideal candidates for surgical intervention. Furthermore, surgical intervention may require multidisciplinary consultation involving pulmonologists, surgeons, and critical care physicians to ensure a balanced approach in the management of the child's lungs.

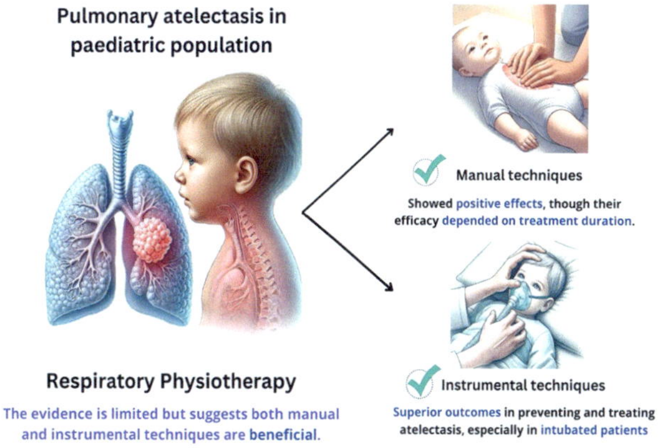

Figure 10.11. In pediatric pulmonology, surgical options are often considered when medical management alone fails to adequately address respiratory issues.

Source: https://pub.mdpi-res.com/children/children-11-01364/article_deploy/html/images/children-11-01364-ag.png?1731685787.

Ascertaining the probability of benefit through surgery against its negative consequences is important, as inappropriate timing or unjustified surgery can lead to complications that complicate the underlying pulmonary diseases, thereby necessitating caution. Additionally, off-label drug use occurs frequently in pediatric patients, as suggested by a study that refers to off-label prescribing being prevalent in neonatal intensive care. Reliance on such drugs often calls for cal interventioo manage complications due to ineffective pharmacological control of respiratory diseases (Jain Morris et al., 20232022). This is a prime consideration in the pediatric pulmonology model, where surgery may be required as a component of a broad plan to prevent the deleterious effects of these medications and optimize respiratory capacity. Moreover, the evolving nature of pediatric pulmonology indicates that surgery, when appropriate, can have a significant beneficial effectutcome in children and hence remain part of being an integral treatment regimen (Morris et al., 2022Network LVH, 2013) (Figure 10.11).

Test Your Knowledge

1. How are pharmacological treatments such as inhalers and nebulizers used to manage pediatric respiratory conditions?
2. What role do non-pharmacological interventions like physiotherapy and patient education play in improving respiratory health in children?
3. When are surgical options considered necessary in the treatment of pediatric pulmonary disorders, and what are their goals?

10.5. Role of Pediatric Pulmonologists

Learning Outcome

1. Training and qualifications required
2. Collaboration with other healthcare professionals
3. Importance of family involvement in treatment plans

The pediatric pulmonologists play a vital function in the care of diverse respiratory illnesses in children, with additional skills and knowledge that set them apart from adult practice. They are specifically trained to handle the anatomical and physiological differences atrics so that they can provide focused diagnosis and therapy. Pediatric pulmonologists use advanced techniques such as, such as bronchoscopy, and this can be achieved with flexible bronchoscopes, minimizing the need for sedation and allowing for procedures to be performed closer to the patients bedside.

Flexibility is required with the difficulty of working with the pediatric patient population, including variations in airway anatomy and responses to anesthetic agents. Increasing complexity and variety in pediatric pulmonary diseases once more illustrate the need for specialized care and underlie the highly valuable contribution of the specialists towards ensuring the maximum respiratory wellness for children (Moslehi, 2022). In addition to the basic clinical management experediatric pulmonologists are also critical components of the multidisciplinary care approach for complex diseases such as, such as cystic fibrosis (CF). CF, an illness caused by mutations in the gene encoding the CF transmembrane conductance regulator (CFTR) protein, necessitates interdisciplinary coordination of more than one specialty, including gastroenterology, nutrition, and psychology, for effectiveric pulmonologists generally manage these multidisciplinary teams to provide respiratory, nutritional, and psychologicalpsychological care. Their understanding not j in monitoring and managing pulmonary features but even in detection and screening for associated complications, such as, such as cystic fibrosis-related liver disease. As understanding on CF continues to advance, pediatric pulmonologists are at the forefront of implementing emergapy and ensuring that affected children are given proper and timely interventions (Morris et al., 2022Ayoub et al., 2019). Also, the rapid growth of interventional pulmonology tailored to accommodate pediatric patients is a huge revolution in pediatric pulmonology. Pediatric pulmonologists are presently busily involved in minimally invasive procedures, employing the newest technologies to correct airway blockage, foreign body removal, and other forms of therapeutic treatment with minimal risk. As evidenced by ongoing improvements in equipment and methodology, the demand for pediatric interventional bronchoscopists grows, which is an indication of growing recognition of the necessity of specialized education within this field. This field not only enhances diagnostic potential but also achieves optimal therapeutic results for complex pulmonary disease in children. Therefore, continued education and collaboration across disciplines by pediatric pulmonologists and specialists from other disciplines are needed in an effort to stay current with developments, ultimately improving care delivery and patient outcomes in pediatric pulmonology (Moslehi, 2022).

10.5.1. Training and Qualifications Required

The pediatric pulmonology specialty must be trained and qualified apart from the rest so that medical doctors are able to properly diagnose and treat respiratory conditions in children. Pediatric pulmonologists typically pursue a three-year residency in pediatrics after medical school that gives them the foundation of general pediatric treatment. Next, they pursue an additional two- to three-year fellowship in specifically pediatric pulmonology. This advanced training exposes them to a wide range of respiratory diseases, ranging from cystic fibrosis and asthma to congenital respiratory tract abnormalities. With such extensive training, pediatric pulmonologists develop the skills and expertise required to manage cases of complexity and synchronize their level of expertise with children's developmental and physiological needs. This rigorous educational pathway eventually equips practitioners with training to manage pediatric respiratory health complexities. Combined with academic education, field experience proves crucial in the professional upgradation of pediatric pulmonologists. Through their fellowshi practitioners have clinical rotations which include hands-on interaction with pediatric patients in various places, such as, such as hospitals and outpatient clinics. This experience-based learning plays a vital role in developing clinical judgment and decision-making competencies for the management of respiratory disease. Furthermore, pediatricians usually practice in multidisciplinary teams, which could consist of respiratory therapists, physiotherapy technicians, and other health care professionals to devise overall management for children with chronic pulmonary diseases. As highlighted by recent cystic fibrosis multidisciplinary team debates, there is a need for increased physical activity and exercise intervention standardizations, an indication of the push towards improved training and teamwork within the specialty (Barker et al., 2019). Such teamwork has heightened the importance of coordinated care strategies, enhancing the effectiveness of treatment interventions. Along with that, continuous professional education is an integral component of maintaining pediatric pulmonology certification because of the dynamic developments in the technology of medicine and therapeutic options.

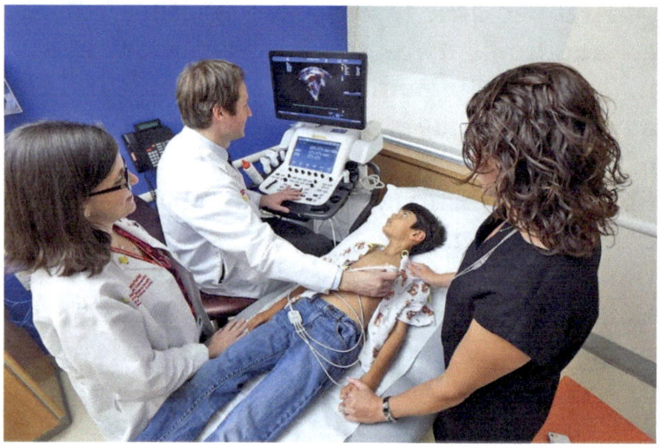

Figure 10.12. The field of pediatric pulmonology requires.

Source: https://static.wixstatic.com/media/f4a4c6_ff7d98e49dfd40f39f5a3ebc52ff60b8~mv2.jpg/v1/fill/w_980,h_653,al_c,q_85,usm_0.66_1.00_0.01,enc_avif,quality_auto/f4a4c6_ff7d98e49dfd40f39f5a3ebc52ff60b8~mv2.jpg.

Professionals are encouraged to engage in continuous learning by attending workshops, conventions, and access to new research work on pediatric respiratory therapy. Staying updated on such new learning is essential because pediatric pulmonology is also rapidly changing with the introduction of new therapies and diagnostic tools. Moreover, professional bodies and societies help significantly in providing resources, guidelines, and information related to best practice within the field. For instance, the creation of standardized guidelines will improve the quality of part of cystic fibrosis treatment, which will lead to improved training outcomes (Morris et al., 2022Court U of Appeals, 2008). Together, these aspects of training, experience, and ongoing education form a comprehensive foundation for pediatric pulmonologists, one that equips them to provide top-notch care to patients (Figure 10.12).

10.5.2. Collaboration with Other Healthcare Professionals

Interdisciplinary teamwork is essential in pediatric pulmonology, as it allows for worldwide care for the child with disease of the lung. Optimal treatment of pediatric pulmonary diseases will frequently involve a coordination effort by physicians, nurses, respiratory therapists, and allied health professionals. Each of these professions contributes expertise that is valuable to overall consciousness of a child's complex health concerns. For instance, asthma can be diagnosed by a pediatric pulmonologist, but patient management is also highly reliant on the guidance of a respiratory therapist who provides good education to the family. By ensuring open communication lines between members of staff, healthcare providers are able to better guarantee treatment protocols which are best practice-oriented and cohesive in children's care. This collaborative care not only optimizes therapeutic interventions but also improves better health outcomes in pediatric patients with respiratory conditions. The incorporation of telemedicine in pediatric pulmonology is a significant advancement in collaborative care, particularly for patients with chronic respiratory disease. Telemedicine allows health professionals to connect with patients and their caregivers remotely, promoting ongoing management without the need for frequent clinic visits. This approach not only enhances availability of advanced care but also ensures that child patients receive timely assessment and interventions. For example, the patients can be evaluated in follow-up remotely, and the respirators and pediatricians can collaborate to monitor symptoms and modify treatment plans effectively. Telemedicine tools enable effective interprofessional collaboration, which enhances continuity of care. Additionally, healthcare professionals can access the knowledge of public experts beyond their immediate geographic regions, expanding the pool of accessible resources and information to better serve pediatric patients, ultimately leading to greater patient ction and outcomes. Alongside this, successful implementation of collaborative models is oftentimes supported by resources such as, such as the Human Phenotype Ontology (HPO), which supports improved clinical diagnosis in pediatric pulmonology. The HPO serves to normalize pediatric respiratory nomenclature, thus facilitating better collaboration among healthcare professionals. With a common vocabulary, clinicians can work more efficiently together, increasing the prospect of diagnosing and treating complex cases. For instance, this ontology has the potential to facilitate beneficial sharing of information among pulmonologists, geneticists, and other allied professionals, resulting in better patient evaluation. With pre-emptive utilization of co-operation tools and protocols, healthcare practitioners create a cooperative foundation for pediatric pulmonology that is rooted in child-oriented approach. This cooperative pr aspect of an individual's care is discussed, thereby leading to optimal pediatric care (Gargano et al., 2023; Esposito et al., 2023).

10.5.3. Importance of Family Involvement in Treatment Plans

Involvement of families in treatment planning is a critical part of good pediatric practice, particularly in specialty fields like pediatric pulmonology. Families' involvement entails that the treatment plans not only are comprehensive but also tailored to the child's individual needs and preferences. By engaging family members in discussions about the child's health, clinicians are able to gain a lot about the child's day-to-day life, preferences, and problems that are not apparent on clinical visits. By this participatory method, the relationship of trust between families and healthcare providers is enhanced, therefore optimally increasing the overall efficacy of the treatment regimen. When patients' families feel engaged, they are more likely to adhere to prescribed care, monitor symptoms, and notify caregivers of changes in the child's health, which consequently leads to better health outcomes. Family involvement is also vital in ensuring the transition from pediatric to adult medical care. During this stage of this vital transition, adolescents with chronic illness are struggling most with the issues that can have a significant influence on healthcare outcomes.

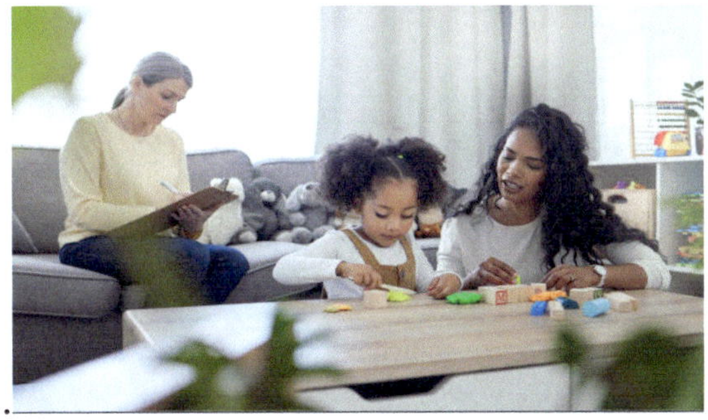

Figure 10.13. Importance of family involvement in treatment plans.

Source: https://media.istockphoto.com/id/1388592712/photo/shot-of-a-mature-therapist-observing-how-a-young-mother-interacts-with-her-daughter.jpg?s=612x612&w=0&k=20&c=EGskL_bnGqjgdXcpqK7vCLl W6tO53295Nk9DWLhRBGI=

A systematic review that analyzed transition models highlighted the significant role played by families in facilitating effective care for young people with chronic conditions. Family engagement can help overcome effective transition barriers by making young patients well-educated, competent in self-management, and endowed with psychosocial support. Also, by fostering collaboration between pediatric and adult caregivers, families can fill in gaps of continuity in care and therefore make the transition experience less stressful. This thus underscores the fact that family participation is not an add-on but a central component in formulating effective treatment plans, especially for pediatric patients who require specialt in pulmonology. Family involvement is not only limited to the coordination of healthcare; it extends to emotional and psychologicalpsychological care, which is required in pediatric patients with chronic respiratory conditions. Families come to play pivotal roles as advocates and caregivers, helping in the alleviation of stress and anxiety toward illness. Family involvement enables healthcare professionals to empower them to function as assistants to the child's emotional and physical health. Studies have shown that families involved in the care process have children who exhibit higher levels of resilience and coping, leading to improved compliance with treatment. Also, recognizing the family as one of the main determinants of healthcare empowers the family to take a more active role in decision-making, hence their ownership of the long-term health and well-being of the child in pediatric pulmonology clinics, where management of chronic illness is an everyday practice (Figure 10.13)

Test Your Knowledge

1. What training and qualifications are required to become a pediatric pulmonologist?
2. How do pediatric pulmonologists collaborate with other healthcare professionals to provide comprehensive care?
3. Why is family involvement essential in developing and implementing treatment plans for children with respiratory disorders?

10.6. Current Research and Advances in Pediatric Pulmonology

Learning Outcome

1. Innovations in treatment modalities
2. Genetic research and its implications for future therapies
3. The role of technology in monitoring respiratory health

Recent research in pediatric pulmonology has introduced significant innovations in the management of cystic fibrosis (CF), which has transformed treatment concepts and outcomes for affected children. Cystic fibrosis transmembrane conductance regulator (CFTR) modulators have transformed life expectancy, going beyond the traditional management paradigms. These utic advances necessitate a shift of focus towards management of complications that are typically observed in elderly CF patients such as, such as CRC with early onset. There is evidence that the absence of functional CFTR gene expression augments the risk of CRC due to inflammatory alterations and microbial dysbiosis in the gut. Thus, the Cystic Fibrosis Foundation encourages a systematic approach to screening, recommending that patients undergo colonoscopies at the age of 40 years, or at the age of 30 if they have already had transplant, calling for the importance of increased vigilance and prevention among this vulnerable population (Raza et al., 2024). Simultaneously, there has been enhanced knowledge of rare and diffuse lung disease in children that has prompted unprecedented expansion of the science of pediatric pulmonology. As research continues to illuminate us about entities like interstitial lung disease, noncystic fibrosis bronchiectasis, and primary ciliary dyskinesia, these disorders continue to become more complex. Notably, research focuses on delineating genotype-phenotype correlations and pathophysiologic mechanisms behind these disorders that render them unique. New research highlights the importance of multicenter studies and registries that contribute to a more in-depth understanding of these rare disorders. The findings of many research studies in high-impact journals highlight theeased awareness among researchers and clinicians to stimulate ongoing research and enhance therapy (Morris et al., 2022Daniel et al., 2024). With the evolving pediatric pulmonology, sophisticated research techniques become the solution to the particular issues posed by pediatric lung illnesses. Present studies aim to introduce new diagnostic techniques and therapy interventions specially developed for children. Coordination among healthcare professionals in multidiscs is becoming increasingly prevalent, which promotes an integrated therapeutic regimen that treats not only physical but also psychologicalpsychological elements in lung illnesses. Moreover, the development of targeted therapies emphasizes the importance of personalized medicine, which is crucial in the treatment of the diverse presentation of pediatric pulmonary disease. By fostering a culture of collaborative research and clinical practice, the field of pediatric pulmonology not only enriches the patient outcomes but also paves the way for future research that holds the potential for innovative breakthroughs and improved quality of life among children.

10.6.1. Innovations in Treatment Modalities

The field of pediatric pulmonology has undergone a tremendous revolution in the past few decades, with numerous advancements in therapeutic modalities leading to better patient outcomes. Extracorporeal membrane oxygenation (ECMO) is a revolutionary technology that supports life in life-threatening conditions of respiratory or cardiac failure. The technique has been extremely successful in children, and the survival rate has reached up to 80% in children requiring prolonged support. As the technology of ECMO becomes more advanced, its future use may even extend outside of intensive care units, and home management of patients with chronic respiratory illnesses becomes a realistic option. This signals a more patient-centered practice, focusing on comfort and quality of life after convalescence from a critical illness. As clinicians integrate these innovations into practice, the general outlook for kids with severe respiratory complications is considerably better than it was in the past, redefining treatment outcomes and recovery expectations. In addition to ECMO, advances in telemedicine and digital health platforms are revolutionizing pediatric pulmonology by the method of livery. These modalities allow remote monitoring and real-time interventions, most useful in children with chronic respiratory illness such as, such as asthma or cystic fibrosis. By allowing healthcare providers to access real-time information on patient health parameters, these technologies allow for proactive control of symptoms and compliance with treatment regimens. Further, the presence of mobile health applications allows patients and families to track symptoms, medication regimens, and triggers more effectively. As this integration of technology into clinical care becomes increasingly prevalent, not only does it improve health outcomes but also patient education and participation. Through ongoing innovation, pediatric pulmonary care will beesponsive and adaptive to the unique needs of each patient. Ongoing education andch within the discipline will be necessary in order toto carry forward the momentum of these innovations. Continuing education courses such as, such as the American Thoracic Society Pediatric Core Curriculum play a significant role in keeping clinicians current with fresh practices and creating therapeutic options.

The yearly courses update healthcare providers with the most recent advancements in pediatric pulmonary disease, maintaining a learning cycle that improves standards of care. Secondly, participation in such conferences as ECMO technology conferences encourages collaboration among experts to share best practices and ideas based on evidence. Not only are treatment methods enlightened but also advancements within populations are made possible, especially in the third world. As more pediatric pulmonology experts embrace such state-of-the-art techniques, the future of respiratory therapy is bright, with improved outcomes and an enhanced quality of life for children worldwide (Figure 10.14).

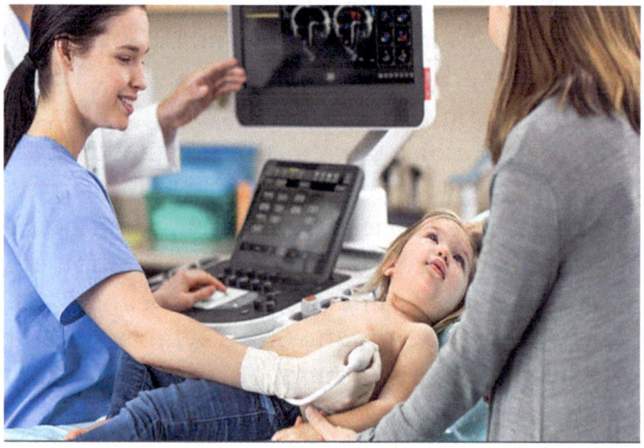

Figure 10.14. Innovations in treatment modalities.

Source: https://www.philips.com/c-dam/corporate/innovation-and-you/global/jun-2021/teaser-child-being-scanned.jpg.

10.6.2. Genetic Research and Its Implications for Future Therapies

As pediatric pulmonology continues to advance, genetic research stands at the forefront of leadure interventions in children with respiratory disease. Genetic discovery has enabled researchers to learn more about pulmonary diseases such as, such as CF and primary ciliary dyskinesia (PCD). Not only do these discoveries allow for targeted interventions, but they hold out the prospect of personalized therapies tailored to each individual patient. For instance, the Swiss cystic fibrosis registry highlighted the importance of high-quality data for the detection of the prevalence and impact of single genetic variants, which, when accurately detected, e treatment options aimed at the management of the symptoms and improvement of lung function as a whole (Morris et al., 2022Collaud et al., 2023). Thus, the progression of genetic investigation is essential since it is a foundation for new therapeutic strategies within pediatric pulmonology. Also, genetic variationpopulations is quite influential on disease presentation and response to treatment in children. Evidence shows that genotypes of diseases such as, such as PCD vary geographically, with different populations possessing different founder variants (Amirav et al., 2024). This has a direct effect on the clinical phenotype, e.g., respiratory symptoms and lung function tests. For pediatric pulmonologists, it is essential to recognize these genetic variations to maximize diagnostic approaches and select treatments that work. The genotype-phenotype correlation places importance on a personalized care paradigm, with the ultimate result being enhanced treatment efficacy through therapy matched to a child's unique genetic profile. With the development of genetic research, it provides doctors with the ability to design multidisciplinary treatment plans combining genetic testing with therapeutic management. Lastly, the therapeutic environment of pediatric pulmonary diseases is to be transformed through the convergence of genetic knowledge with new technologies like gene therapy and precision medicine. Recent breakthroughs in the field of genetic editing, including the CRISPR-Cas9 technology, offer new possibilities for the repair of underlying genetic abnormalities of conditions like CF and PCD. By targeting the specific genes that are responsible for these diseases, not only can it be prevented from worsening but also reversed normal function in the diseased population. As highlighted by registry research today, the connection between genetnical presentation can allow for anticipation of response to treatment, resulting in proactive management (Morris et al., 2022Amirav et al., 2024). Pediatric pulmonologists' future treatment strategies, founded on robust genetic studies, have the potential to revolutionize the manner in which practitioners approach these complex respiratory diseases (Figure 10.15).

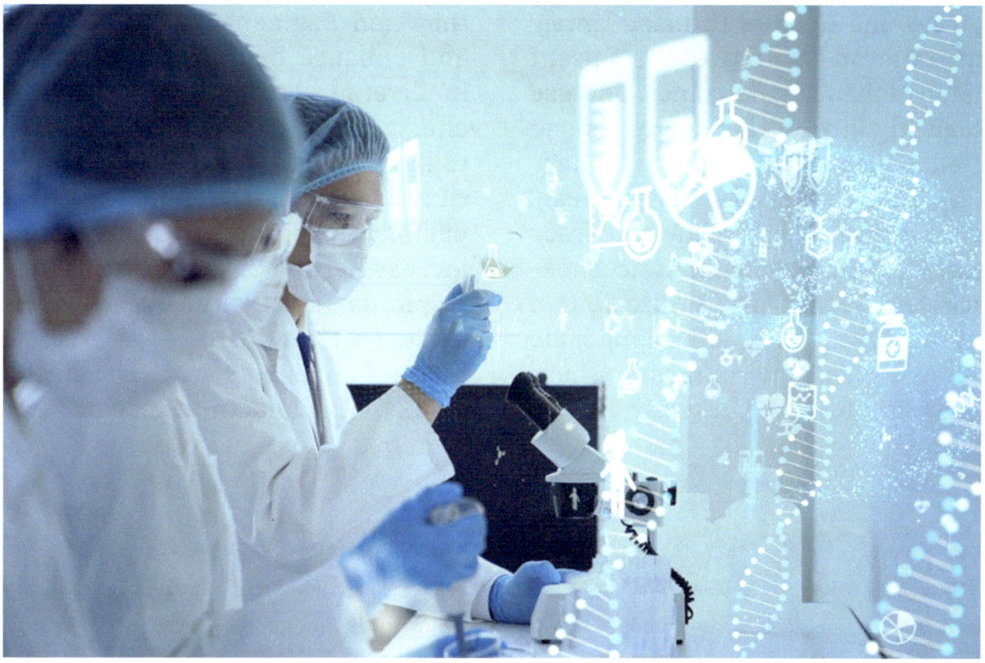

Figure 10.15. Scientists conducting gene therapy research in a laboratory.

Source: https://insights.ibx.com/wp-content/uploads/2023/01/gene-therapy-research.jpg.

10.6.3. The Role of Technology in Monitoring Respiratory Health

The development of technology has dramatically reshaped the field of pediatric pulmonology, especially in the surveillance of respiratory function. New tools, like wearable technologies, have become invaluable assets, which enable caregivers to monitor key respiratory parameters in children round the clock. These innovations allow for continuous real-time monitoring of pulmonary function, heart rate, and respiratory rate so that healthcare professionals can act swiftly on any worsening situation. The use of these devices in clinical practice, beyond enhancing patient involvement and treatment adherence, ensures early detection of respiratory distress in children, from reactive to proactive care level. This shift is significant considering the high prevalence of respiratory diseases in children, which increases the demand for creative methods specifically tailored for such vulnerable patients. Application of artificial intelligence (AI) in the monitoring of respiratory health is only to emphasize the significant connection between health and technology. Through the application of sophisticated algorithms, AI can scan through vast amounts of data obtained from monitoring devices to identify patterns and predict potential health crises early. For instance, the use of AI has been successfully applied in a number of animal disease models and established a very high correlation between environmental factors and endpoints in the pulmonary that could be translated into human medicine environments. This prediction allows caregivers and doctors to make timely interventions tailored to individual patient needs, ultimately enhancing outcomes. The use of machine learning in wearable devices is one such cutting-edge step in pediatric pulmonary health, as these devices can learn continuously from new data and improve predictive accuracy with time, thus strengthening clinical decision-making processes. Technology utilization in monitoring breathing health is most applicable in resource-constrained environments where advanced diagnostic technologies may not be available. For instance, wearable technology has proved highly promising in low- and middle-income environments, enabling continuous physiologic monitoring of respiratory-sick children. In these environments, such technology can be a valuable asset for health workers, enabling early detection of sepsis and other respiratory complications without the need for substantial laboratory facilities. That such devices are even possible is proof they can augment existing healthcare needs and enhance pediatric pulmonology capacity in diverse settings. With scientists ongoing efforts to upgrade smartphone-based systems to have the ability to offer both telemetry and clinical alert features, implications for expanded pediatric respiratory health monitoring become increasingly apparent. The capacity to track respiratory health in an effective manner enables health systems to provide interventions on time, thereby enhancing pediatric health outcomes globally (Bachmann-Gagescu et al., 2019).

Test Your Knowledge

1. What recent innovations in treatment modalities are improving outcomes for children with respiratory disorders?
2. How is genetic research contributing to thopment of new therapies in pediatric ?

SUMMARY

In pediatric pulmonology, it is important to know the complexities of conditions such as, such as acute chest syndrome (ACS) in order toto successfully treat patients. According to recent studies, ACS is a leading cause of morbidity and mortality in cith sickle cell disease (SCD), often necessitating hospitalization for acute pain crisis management. The employment of innovative strategies, such as, such as the use of Bi-level positive airway pressure ventilation (BiPAP), has emerged as a critical add-on in managing respiratory complications of ACS. The incorporation of BiPAP into standard care on general pediatric wards has been recommended by clinicians with a dramatic increase in prevention of respiratory decompensation and enhancement of successful patient outcomes. The evidence regarding the positive effect of BiPAP provides a compelling case for the widespread application of BiPAP (Burrowes et al., 2024) and calls for ongoing evaluation of its use in varied clinical settings. Moreover, the multi-center study has opened doors towards broader understanding of facilitators and barriers to the use of new interventions like supportive non-invasive ventilation for prevention of acute coronary syndromes (SNAP). Healthcare team interviews pinpoint safe implementation, good communication, multidisciplinary support, and cultural acceptance in institutions as critical for effective implementation. Most importantly, the consensus on the effectiveness of BiPAP demonstrates its potential for being safely incorporated into pediatric practice without the need for intensive care unit transfers. Identifying such contextual influences allows for context-relevant strategies targeted at unique inswhich is crucial when broadening the applicability of such interventions in pediatric pulmonology (Bachmann-Gagescu et al., 2019Burrowes et al., 2023). With changes in healthcare systems, embedding learning from qualitative studies can underpin the efficacy of respiratory therapy for children in hospitals. With advancing research, addressing the complex issues that impact patient experience with treatments like BiPAP remains crucial. Though healthcare practitioners appreciate the life-saving potential of these technologies, individual patient situations cannot be overemphasized in their intricacy. Facilitating patients' comfort while on BiPAP and promoting effective team member, patient, and caregiver communication are central to successful implementation. Feedback mechanisms and iterative refinement, based on qualitative comprehension, may facilitate greater flexibility in the utilization of BiPAP for children at risk for ACS. The collaborative efforts and results of recent studies are providing a foundation for future studies for the establishment of protocols for multicenter trials. These protocols will not only study sustainable pediatric pulmonology practices with patient-centeredness (Bachmann-Gagescu et al., 2019Burrowes et al., 2024; Burrowes et al., 2023).

Pediatric pulmonology encompasses a broad range of conditions and interventions affecting the respiratory systemren. Certain of the most significant aspects of discussion within the specialty tend to be associated with the management of chronic conditions, such as, such as asthma and cystic fibrosis, which require continued surveillance and specific interventions. Asthma, for instance, is unique in its etiologic multifactorality and variability in severity in children. Research highlights an interdisciplinary approach involving families and healthcare providers for enhancing adherence to treatment protocols and optimal patient outcomes. Additionally, the transition period from children's to adult services for patients with chronic illness has been of particular concern, pointing towards the necessity of planned transition programs that can ensure continuity of care. In pediatric pulmonology, the evaluation of treatment modalities' effectiveness has become essential with the evolving therapeutic methods. Specialists frequently consult evidence-based practices to revise their approach, which may include pharmacological treatments or new methods of treatment. The need for strong clinical guidelecomes apparent in studies indicating the non-uniform quality of existing transition programs without standardizing treatment for some conditions (Adi etDoug et al., 2009). The evidence is that whi of programs, including notably those used to treat cystic fibrosis, have sufficient empirical support, others lack enough robust evaluations in order toto determine their effectiveness. Such disparity reflects a pressing need for health systems to build more universal transition approaches to be applied to a variety of pediatric pulmonary conditions, thereby improving patient care overall as young adults transition from childhood into adult healthcare settings. The integration of technology and data analysis into pediatric pulmonology presents challenges and opportunities. With constant advances in monitoring equipment and data acquisition techniques, clinicians must be able to manage efficiently the noise in physiological signals. Careful efforts to enhance datare critical because noise signals can overwhelm critical patient data and hamper diagnosis and treatment (Bachmann-Gagescu et al., 2019Abbott et al., 2004). Through the adoption of novel noise reduction methods and further enhancement of patient information clarity, pediatric pulmonologists have the ability to significantly improve their know-how of respiratory disease. The new technique not only has the capability of enhancing clinical outcome but also enhances a paradigm change in the mode by which pediatric respiratory health is known and addressed in upcoming healthcare systems.

KEY TERMS FROM THIS CHAPTER

- Adolescents
- Continuous positive airway pressure (CPAP)
- Human phenotype ontology (HPO)
- Initiative on rare and undiagnosed diseases (IRUD)
- Non-invasive ventilation (NIV)
- Pediatric well-being
- Respiratory conditions
- Collaboration
- Holistic approach
- Immune systems
- Medical community
- Pediatric respiratory system
- Pulmonology
- Respiratory disorders

CRITICAL THINKING QUESTIONS

1. **What is the most common chronic respiratory disease in children?**
   a. Pneumonia
   b. Asthma
   c. Bronchiectasis
   d. Tuberculosis
2. **Which of the following is a hallmark symptom of bronchiolitis in infants?**
   a. Productive cough
   b. Stridor
   c. Wheezing
   d. Pleuritic chest pain
3. **The most common caommunity-acquired pneumonia in children under 5 is:**
   a. Mycoplasma pneumoniae
   b. Streptococcus pneumoniae
   c. Hemophilus influenzae
   d. Staphylococcus aureus*Staphylococcus aureus*
4. **A barking cough and inspiratory stridor in a toddler are characteristic of:**
   a. Asthma
   b. Foreign body aspiration
   c. Croup (laryngotracheobronchitis)
   d. Epiglottitis
5. **Which test is commonly used to assess lung function in children with asthma?**
   a. Chest X-ray
   b. Peak Expiratory Flow Rate (PEFR)
   c. CT scan
   d. ABG (Arterial Blood Gas)

Short Answer Questions

1. Discuss the pathophysiology, clinical presentation, diagnosis, and management of asthma in children. How is asthma severity classified and what are the long-term goals of therapy?
2. Describe the etiology, symptoms, and treatment of bronchiolitis in infants. What is the role of supportive care, and when is hospitalization indicated?
3. Explain the causes, clinical features, diagnostic approach, and treatment of pediatric pneumonia. How does the management differ based on age and causative organisms?
4. What is cystic fibrosis? Discuss its genetic basis, pulmonary manifestations, diagnostic methods, and multidisciplinary management in children.
5. Describe the presentation, complications, and emergency management of foreign body aspiration in children. What diagnostic tools and surgical interventions are commonly used?

Answer to Critical Thinking Questions

1.(b) 2.(c) 3.(b) 4.(c) 5. (b)

REFERENCES

1. Doug, M., Adi, Y., Williams, J., Paul, M., Kelly, D., Petchey, R., & Carter, Y. H. (2011). Transition to adult services for children(2009). Transition to adult services for children and young people with palliative care needs: A systematic review. https://core.ac.uk/download/44454.pdf (accessed on 16th June 2025).

2. Akil, N., Benscoter, D., Blatter, J. A., Boyer, D., et al. (2019). American Thoracic Society 2019 Pediatric Core Curriculum. http://deepblue.lib.umich.edu/bitstream/2027.42/152541/2/ppul24482.pdf (accessed on 16th June 2025).

3. Amirav, I., Athanazio, R., Olbrich, H., Pennekamp, P., et al. (2024). Analyses of 1236 genotyped primary ciliary dyskinesia individuals identify regional cstant, S., et al. (2019). Pulmonary exacerbations in patients with primary ciliary dyskinesia: An expert consensus definition for use in clinical trials. Lucas, J. S., Gahleitner, F., Amorim, A., Boon, M., Brown, P., Constant, C., Cook, S., Crowley, S., Destouches, D. M. S., Eber, E., Mussaffi, H., Haarman, E., Harris, A., Koerner-Rettberg, C., Kuehni, C. E., Latzin, P., Loebinger, M. R., Lorent, N., Maitre, B., Moreno-Galdó, A., ... Carr, S. B. (2019). Pulmonary exacerbations in patients with primary ciliary dyskinesia: an expert consensus definition for use in clinical trials. *ERJ open research*, *5*(1), 00147-2018. https://doi.org/10.1183/23120541.00147-2018 (accessed on 16th June 2025).

4. Antonelli, G., Cangiano, G., Capocaccia, P., Evangelisti, L., et al. (2016). Bronchiolitis. Analysis of 10 consecutive epidemic seasons. https://core.ac.uk/download/74319410.pdf (accessed on 16th June 2025).

5. Ayoub, F., Li, H., Blay, C., Trillo-Alvarez, C., Lascano, J., & Morelli, G. (2019). Multidisciplinary care for cystic fibrosis liver disease: Where does the adult hepatologist fit in? *Clinical Liver Disease, 14*, 187–190. https://doi.org/10.1002/cld.845 (accessed on 16th June 2025).

6. Bachmann-Gagescu, R., Dempsey, J. C., Bulgheroni, S., Chen, M. L., D'Arrigo, S., Glass, I., Heller, T., et al. (2019). Healthcare recommendations for Joubert syndrome. *American Journal of Medical Genetics Part A, 182*, 229–249. https://doi.org/10.1002/ajmg.a.61399 (accessed on 16th June 2025).

7. Bagnall, A., Day, R., & Kime, N. H. (2013). Systematic review of transition models for young people with long-term conditions: A report for NHS Diabetes. https://core.ac.uk/download/29018738.pdf (accessed on 16th June 2025).

8. Barker, A. R., Denford, S., Oades, P. J., Shelley, R., et al. (2019). Promotion of exercise in the management of cystic fibrosis–Summary of national meetings. https://core.ac.uk/download/186332829.pdf (accessed on 16th June 2025).

9. Bentsen, M. H. L. (2018). Tidal breathing parameters in extremely premature infants: Feasibility and clinical utility of electromagnetic inductance plethysmography. https://core.ac.uk/download/544027821.pdf (accessed on 16th June 2025).

10. Chang, A. B., Grimwood, K., Ooi, M. H., Perera, D., et al. (2013). Improving the diagnosis, management, and outcomes of children with pneumonia: Where are the gaps? https://core.ac.uk/download/47201185.pdf (accessed on 16th June 2025).

11. Collaud, E., Derkenne, M.-F., Fischer, R., Hensen, J., et al. (2023). Data accuracy, consistency and completeness of the national Swiss cystic fibrosis patient registry: Lessons from an ECFSPR data quality project. https://core.ac.uk/download/592040677.pdf (accessed on 16th June 2025).

12. Davis, B., Davis, S., Fine, J., Fordham, L., et al. (2015). Quantitative assessment of the upper airway in infants and children with subglottic stenosis. https://core.ac.uk/download/84832065.pdf (accessed on 16th June 2025).

13. Fenu, G., Astori, C., & Lombardi, E. (2023). Childhood interstitial lung disease: When to suspect and what to do. *Global Pediatrics, 8*, 100110–100110. https://doi.org/10.1016/j.gpeds.2023.100110 (accessed on 16th June 2025).

14. Gargano, M., Matentzoglu, N., Coleman, B., Addo-Lartey, E. B., Anagnostopoulos, A. V., Anderton, J., Avillach, P., et al. (2023). The Human Phenotype Ontology in 2024: Phenotypes around the world. *Nucleic Acids Research, 52*, D1333–D1346. https://doi.org/10.1093/nar/gkad1005 (accessed on 16th June 2025).

15. Ggaliwango, M., & Alam, M. G. R. (2022). Explainable augmented intelligence and deep transfer learning for pediatric pulmonary health evaluation. *2022 International Conference on Innovations in Science, Engineering and Technology (ICISET)*. https://doi.org/10.1109/iciset54810.2022.9775845 (accessed on 16th June 2025).

16. Kaufman, J. (2022). The use of nebulizer medications as a possible treatment for COVID-19. https://core.ac.uk/download/520100997.pdf (accessed on 16th June 2025).

17. Lee, S. B., Oh, J. H., Park, J. H., Choi, S. P., & Wee, J. H. (2018). Differences in youngest-old, middle-old, and oldest-old patients who visit the emergency department. *Clinical and Experimental Emergency Medicine, 5*, 249–255. https://doi.org/10.15441/ceem.17.261 (accessed on 16th June 2025).

18. Miyoshi, M. H., Monte, L. F. V., Rozov, T., Silva Filho, L. V. F., et al. (2005). Bronchopulmonary dysplasia. https://core.ac.uk/download/37705844.pdf (accessed on 16th June 2025).

19. Morris, E. A., Hauer, J., & Bogetz, J. F. (2022). Asset-based health care for children with severe neurologic impairment. *Pediatrics, 150*. https://doi.org/10.1542/peds.2021-055654 (accessed on 16th June 2025).

20. Moslehi, M. A. (2022). Interventional pulmonology: The new horizon in pediatric pulmonology. *Pediatric Respirology and Critical Care Medicine, 6*, 63–64. https://doi.org/10.4103/prcm.prcm_24_22 (accessed on 16th June 2025).

21. Rothblum-Oviatt, C., Wright, J., Lefton-Greif, M. A., McGrath-Morrow, S. A., Crawford, T. O., & Lederman, H. M. (2016). Ataxia telangiectasia: A review. *Orphanet Journal of Rare Diseases, 11*. https://doi.org/10.1186/s13023-016-0543-7 (accessed on 16th June 2025).

22. Salvatori, G., De Rose, D. U., Concato, C., Alario, D., Olivini, N., Dotta, A., & Campana, A. (2020). Managing COVID-19-positive maternal–infant dyads: An Italian experience. *Breastfeeding Medicine, 15*, 347–348. https://doi.org/10.1089/bfm.2020.0095 (accessed on 16th June 2025).

23. Şıklar, Z. (2023). Management of endocrinological problems in children on home invasive mechanical ventilation. *Authorea (Authorea)*. https://doi.org/10.22541/au.168907865.52915909/v1 (accessed on 16th June 2025).

24. Tomlinson, O. W. (2019). Cardiopulmonary exercise testing in the assessment and treatment of young people with cystic fibrosis. https://core.ac.uk/download/186332807.pdf (accessed on 16th June 2025).

25. Touro College & University System. (2020). *2020 Touro College & University System Faculty Publications*. https://core.ac.uk/download/482149446.pdf (accessed on 16th June 2025).

PEDIATRIC PSYCHIATRY AND BEHAVIORAL HEALTH

11

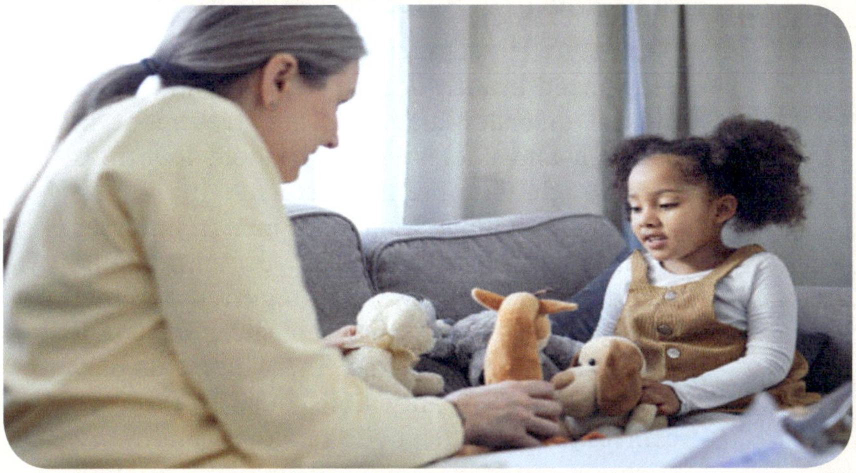

LEARNING OBJECTIVES

After studying this chapter, you will be able to:

1. Discuss the historical context
2. Explain the common pediatric mental health disorders
3. Have an emphasis on assessment and diagnosis
4. Be aware of the treatment approaches
5. Understand the role of pediatricians
6. Know the impact of social factors

Introduction

Pediatric Psychiatry and Behavioral Health is a critical field of study focusing on the complex relationship between mental illnesses and children's behavioral complications. As human understanding of such diseases expands, it becomes increasingly clear that early detection and intervention are vital for enhancing long-term possibilities for target groups. Mental illness, left untreated, will exacerbate other learning and developmental challenges, forming a never-ending cycle of dysfunction. Integration of mental health into pediatric practice not only validates discussion of such conditions but also provides preventive interventions for detection and control. It is a matter of significance that the plans of the future are directed at evolving integrated frameworks in the service of clinical practice and policy-making for pediatric mental health. At the heart of quality pediatric mental health care is a recognition of adverse childhood experiences (ACEs) and the profound and long-lasting impact they have on a child's overall health. While research has conclusively demonstrated the short- and long-term implications of ACEs and social determinants of health (SDOH) on child health and well-being,. Identification and mitigation of these factors need to be coordinated and systems-focused with pediatric primary care leadership of these efforts. As more community partners, including school districts and non-profit organizations, become involved in mitigating ACEs and SDOH, pediatric healthcare providers should have the training and tools available to identify these experiences and respond appropriately. In so doing, the structure of improved mental health outcomes can be established.

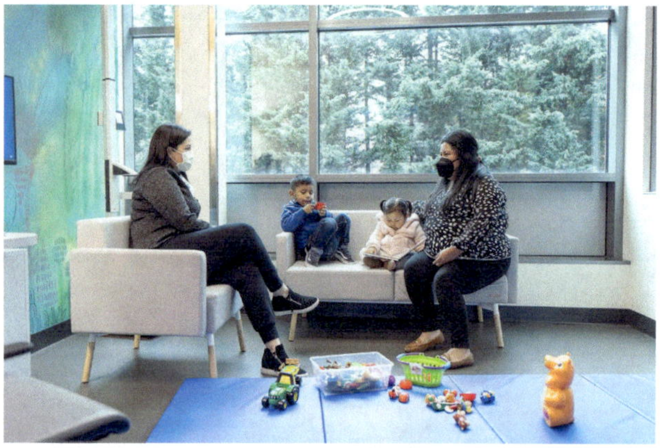

Figure 11.1. The field of pediatric psychiatry and behavioral health.

Source: https://www.seattlechildrens.org/globalassets/images/clinics/psych/magnuson_observationroom_drminjarez-3500-alt-callout.jpg.

Moreover, where child health behavioral health intersects wironmental factors such as, such as the child welfare system, there are unique challenges and complexities. Figures indicate that children in the child welfare system have increased rates of psychotropic medication use than their peers in the general population. This lack of congruence emphasizes the need for child welfare professionals, particularly rural professionals, to vigilantly track medication use. Furthermore, understanding pediatric medication decision-making is still crucial to optimizing care. Professionals must monitor not only clinical guidelines but also community norms and unique patient circumstances. As the field of Pediatric Psychiatry and Behavioral Health continues to advance, consideration for these complicated concerns will be required in the service of an integrated approach to meeting the mental health requirements of children and adolescents (Figure 11.1).

Definition of Pediatric Psychiatry

Pediatric psychiatry encompasses the specialized branch of medicine that addresses mental disorder diagnosis and treatment in children and adolescents. The field identifies unique development patterns in young patients and understands that mental illnesses manifest differently than they do with adults. Pediatricians employ an integrated mbined biological, psychologicalpsychological, and social factors to comprehend how these elements play out in a child's reality. Consequently, they are confronted with diagnode range of conditions, such as, such as mood disorders, anxiety disorders, and behavioral issues, which need to be viewed with a special clinical perspective appropriate for the pediatrician. Since the research into the child mental illness goes on to unravel the complexities of the problem, pediatric psychiatry plays the key role in formulating interventions that can effectively address the problem and bring about healthier outcomes for children. These challenges are compounded by the growing incidence of mental illness among children, driven in part by rising levels of exposure to factors including digital technology and socio-economic stressors. Research suggests that overuse of the Internet by teenagers, for example, is associated with greater symptoms of somatic and depression, as well as behavioral issues (Cerutti et al., 2017). This relationship emphasizes the importance of pediatric psychiatrists adjusting their treatment and diagnosis methods against evolving pressures in society. Further, detection of delayed development early on is necessary; primary care physicians are often likely to miss such problems, which can hinder early intervention and support (Sices, 2007). Therefore, pediatric psychiatry not only deals with treating already established disorders but also emphasizes prevention and early detection, offering families and communities ways to foster children's mental well-being. Moreover, pediatric psychiatry emphasizes a multidisciplinary approach, consultation with teachers, families, and other physicians to offer integrated care. This collaboration is critical to address the complexity of children's mental health, as therapy success depends on the engagement of various stakeholders in a child's life. Pediatric psychiatrists are able to employ behavioral therapies, medication, and psychoeducation to create customized care plans that address specific needs. It cannot be overemphasized how critical it is to establish supportive settings, as children thrive in settings that promote emotional regulation and resilience. At its very essence, pediatric psychiatry is a commitment not only to treating mental illnesses but to fostering overall development and well-being during the pediatric age span, toward healthier living as they face the difficulties of contemporary life.

Importance of Mental Health in Children

The significance of children's mental health is increasingly being recognized as an integral aspect of theirevelopment of physical psychologicalpsychological attributes at an early stage paves the way for emotional health, social functioning, and academic performance throughout life. Mental illness in young people can manifest in various forms, including anxiety, depression, and behavioral disorders. These issues not only hinder a child's unique development but haasting effects in adulthood, such as, such as increased risk of continued mental health problems. Pediatricians and clinicians working with mental health must become acquainted with these issues because identification and intervention early on greatly affect a child's trajectory. Furthermore, the COVID-19 pandemic has intensified pre-existing risks, and it is of urgent necessity to have extensive mental health treatment delivered in pediatric contexts, a point raised by recent studies that single out heightened symptoms of mental health in childrghton et al., 2014Douglas et al., 2021). Additionally, the home environment is a central component in managing children's mental health. Family functioning, including parental mental health, socioeconomic status, and social support, is a strong predictor of children's management of stressors and affective difficulties. Treatment that engages the family in mental health intervention not only enhances outcomes but also provides caregivers with skills to promote their children's emotional development. A coordinated treatment approach provides increased resilience and improved mental health outcomes by establishing an empowering home environment. The call for a collaborative strategy in redressing mental health disparities emphasizes social commitment, particularly following the disruptions caused by the COVID-19 pandemic. Putting priority on families mental health needs alongside those of children will help foster a robust support system (Hoagwood et al., 2020). Alongside talking about the importance of children's mental health, solving its significance also means tackling systemic barriers influencing accessibility to care. Prior to the pandemic, the system for children's mental health services was already fragmented and it became challenging to offer integrated care. The urgent need is to establish a strategic plan with equal access to mental health treatment, particularly for vulnerable populations. Based on research, disparities in healthcare access can exacerbate mental health issues, necessitating increased interventions that are sensitive to socio-economic as well as racial disparities. A paradigm shift to all-policies-for-children would, in opinion leaders' views, actually aid in improving policy-making and resource allocation to meet children's mental health demands. Community empowerment and inter-stakeholder coordination are essential in creating a seamless system for improved management of pediatric mental health (Hoagwood et al., 2020) (Figure 11.2).

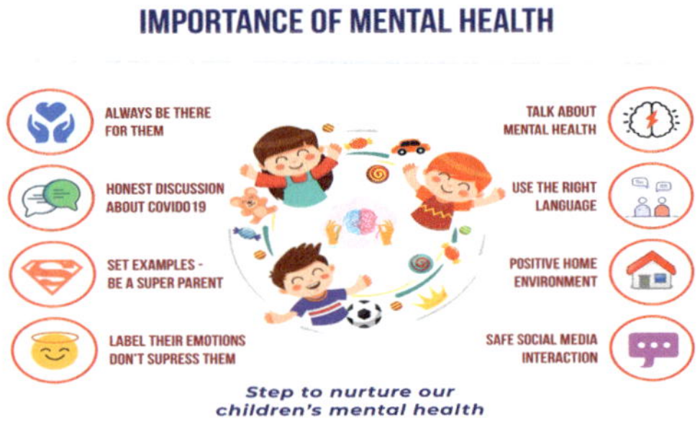

Figure 11.2. The significance of mental health in children.

Source: https://www.vega.edu.in/vega-blog/wp-content/uploads/2023/08/635e3717ec74e7b476da2ab9bfd8e246.jpeg.

Overview of Behavioral Health in Pediatric Populations

Pediatric behavioral health encompasses a wide array of mental health problems that can significantly affect the quality of life and development of children. During childhood and adolescence, people go through essential developmental milestones, which are often preceded by stressors with manifestations in terms of behaviors. These problems range from anxiety and depression to more complicated disorders like Attention-Deficit/Hyperactivity Disorder (ADHD) and autism spectrum disorders. Early identification and treatment are critical in optimizing the management of these conditions, thereby minimizing long-term consequences of untreated mental illness on children's academic school performance, socialization, and relationships within the family. Enhanced access to behavioral health care is crucial among pediatric populations because many of these children go undiagnosed and untreated despite available resources. The intersection of child populations and behavioral health has been an increasing area of emphasis over the past decade, leading to the creation of numerous evidence-based treatments specifically for children. Cognitive-behavioral therapy, family therapy, and pharmacologic treatment have been applied at both the clinical and community levels to address mental health problems. Besides, teamwork between pediatricians, mental health workers, and educators is necessary in coming up with a child-friendly environment for children presenting with behavioral health concerns. Present research indicates that the integration of behavioral health services into regular pediatric practices can facilitate better delivery of services and avoid the stigma associated with using mental health services. By encouraging such multidisciplinary collaboration, communities can position themselves to address the growing needs of youth and adolescents with behavioral health issues most optimally (Troyanskaya et al., 2023). Treatment of pediatric populations with behavioral health disorders not only includes effective treatment strategies but also preventive strategies that are aimed at reducing the incidence of these disorders. Interventions that promote resilience, social-emotional learning, and coping skills have been successful both in schools and community programs. The programs focus on equipping children with the ability to endure difficulties in life and establish strong support structures. Parents' participation and education cannot be overstated as family life has been found to impact a child's behavioral health outcomes. Offering supportive home contexts with open communication and empathy are at the heart of risk-reduction for developing mental health problems. Ongoing research and advocacy are essential in shaping policies that place children's behavioral health at the forefront, enabling all young people access to the appropriate resources and supdevelopment pathw(Angélica Torres-BerríoDeighton et al., 20222014).

11.1. Historical Context

Learning Outcome

1. Evolution of pediatric psychiatry
2. Key figures in the development of the field
3. Changes in societal attitudes towards children's mental health

The practice of pediatric psychiatry and behavioral health cannot be understood in its entirety without reference to the historical background that has moulded its growth over decades. In the past, children's mental health disorders tended to be misinterpreted, and hence underwent intense stigmatization as well as the lack of proper treatment. It is remarkable that, until the 20th century, children showing behavioral disturbances were largely subjected to punitive interventions instead of empathetic care. As socigly understood that children's psychologicalpsychological needs are qualitatively distinct from adults', the tide in favor of more empathetic models of care increased. The process was fueled by a series of children's rights and mental health consciousness movements, which laid the groundwork for pediatric psychiatry as a specialty devoted to improving the emotional well-being of young people. Knowledge of this historical context is invaluable for an understanding of the field's evolution and its present-day relevance. The establishment of scientific inquiry in the second half of the 20th century further fueled the developments of pediatric psychiatry. This era witnessed the introduction of developmental psychology, which stressed the significance of emotional and cognitive phases of child development. Researchers began employing more sophisticated methodologies to understand psychiatric illness in adolescents so that clinicians may formulate effective intervention strategies. Furthermore, growing attention to the impact of childhood trauma—spurred by studies linking poor experiences with later mental illness created greater focus on prevention and early intervention. This information was essential in guiding reasonable approaches that would ultimately contribute to children's mental well-being. With pediatric psychiatry embracing evidence-based treatment, more and more essential to complete care and the treatment of intricate conduct disorders in children became standard in the modern day. Through the last decades, technology incorporation in pediatric psychiatry has reflected ongoing socio-cultural progress and has influenced treatment methods.

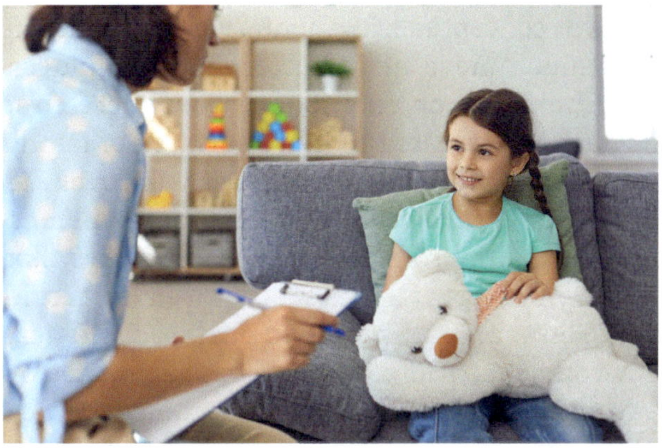

Figure 11.3. The field of pediatric psychiatry and behavioral health cannot be fully understood without considering the historical context that has shaped its development over the decades.

Source: https://www.metropediatrics.com/wp-content/uploads/2023/09/pediatric-mental-health.jpg.

Telemedicine, driven particularly by the COVID-19 pandemic, has opened new avenues for access that cross geographic and socioeconomic lines previously making access to child mental health care difficult. The ability to offer therapeutic services remotely has made possible extended services for vulnerable populatioch is important in addressing situations such as, such as anxiety and depression among youths. This change reflects broader cultural trends toward technological solutions in health and also chronicles differences in technology access among demographically varied groups. As pediatric psychiatry and behavioral health look to the future, the preceding history of such advances, coupled with the present shortcomings, continues to influence practices that act touths (Rashid et al., 2020; Gausman et al., 2020Deighton et al., 2014) (Figure 11.3).

11.1.1. Evolution of Pediatric Psychiatry

Pediatric psychiatry has also changed a lot since its inception, progressing from being stigmatized towards conceptualizing mental health in children as a much more multifaceted entity. Children with behavior or emotional issues were first neglected or treated as mere surfaces of family dysfunction. But as studies began to uncover the complexities involved in children's development, mental health professionals became aware that there were special ways orequired to tackle children's unique psychologicalpsychological environments. This movement was augmented by advances in neuroscience and psychology, which placed emphasis on early intervention. Thus, pediatric psychiatry began introducing models of development in understanding and treating child mental illness in a bid to move towards a more integrated and beneficial model of care. The realization of the significance of childhood mental health as a whole towards long-term well-being over the last few decades has also propelled the practice of pediatric psychiatry. The integration of neurodevelopmental processes and behavioral expressions in children has been elucidathe help of sophisticated imaging techniques, such as, such as magnetic resonance imaging (MRI). MRI has thrown significant light on how environmental and genetic factors interplay to orchestrate cognitive and affective well-being in stages of critical development. For instance, developmental changes of the cerebral cortex have been followed in a detailed manner and revealed how macro- and microstructural characteristics affect cognitive abilities as well as vulnerability to mental illness (Linn et al., 2021). Such evidence points to the significance of child professionals adopting an educated approach that not only addresses immediate behavioral problems but also considers the associated neurobiological and psychosocial determinants of emotional health. Also, the maturation of pediatric psychiatry as a specialty has hastened the integration of interdisciplinary models focusing on holistic behavioral health care. Organizational sites have extended beyond traditional psychiatric clinics to include schools, primary care practices, and community-based settings, expanding the reach of mental health care. Such an evolution reflects heightened awareness of the multidisciplinary nature of child and adolescent mental health, encompassing social, emotional, and cognitive domains. While medical professionals strive to screen, diagnd treat illness in a holistic way, modalities such as, such as heart rate variability (HRV) testing are increasingly at the forefront for their non-invasive capacity to quantify autonomic modulation and stress responses in children (Qin et al., 2021). These advances underscore the interdependent nature of body and mind within pediatric psychiatry, calling for an integrated model of behavioral health.

11.1.2. Key Figures in the Development of the Field

The development of pediatric psychiatry and behavioral health has been shaped significantly by pioneers whose own research laid the groundwork for the core tenets of the field. Such a pioneer is Mary Ainsworth, whose attachment theory and infant-caregiver interaction research has significantly influenced ideas about child psychology. Ainsworth's work established the importance of emotional relationships in early life, a finding since followed in subsequent therapeutic treatment of children with behavioral and emotional problems. Ainsworth was able to distinguish among various attachment patterns in her research that have been employed by clinicians and researchers in identifying children's mental health problems. This theory system not only teaches diagnostic standards but also assists in crafting effective interventions designed to specifically improve parent-child relationships, as is the practice today in pediatric psychiatric treatment that values relational processes as critical to emotional well-being. Another key figure in child psychiatry is Benjamin Spock, whose highly popular book, The Common-Sense Book of Baby and Child Care, revolutionized the raising of children and demanded a less strict, more compassionate style of bringing up children. Spock challenged the authoritarian, strict parental styles prevalent at the start of the 20th century, demanding an awareness of children's feelings and a nurturing atmosphere. His advocacy for parents' emotional intelligence has reached throughout the field of pediatric psychiatry by highlighting the role of parental behavior in child development and mental health outcomes. Spocks writings further legitimized the acknowledgment of early years' importance to mental health, which raised awareness and improved intervention behaviors in the pediatric setting emphasizing emotional care and family involvement in the treatment of mental health. With the development of the field, technological advancements have introduced new ways of comprehend treating child mental health issues. Pioneers such as, such as in the case of artificial intelligence (AI) and machine learning (ML) have opened up new battlefronts for treatment and risk assessment. A systematic review stated the utilization of antenatal AI in predicting suicidal behavior among children and adolescents, revealing the capability for near-perfect accuracy in risk classification modeling as well as outcomes prediction, with greater% accuracy in modg among various studies (Rebecca Deighton et al., 20202014). They also enable advanced data analysis but bestow clinicians with extremely sophisticated tools for assessing risk as well as strategizing intervention measures. As pediatric psychiatry integrates these technologies, continued contributions of historical and contemporary leaders continue to shape the landscape of children's mental health treatment, underscoring the necessity for ongoing investigation and practice evolution (Figure 11.4).

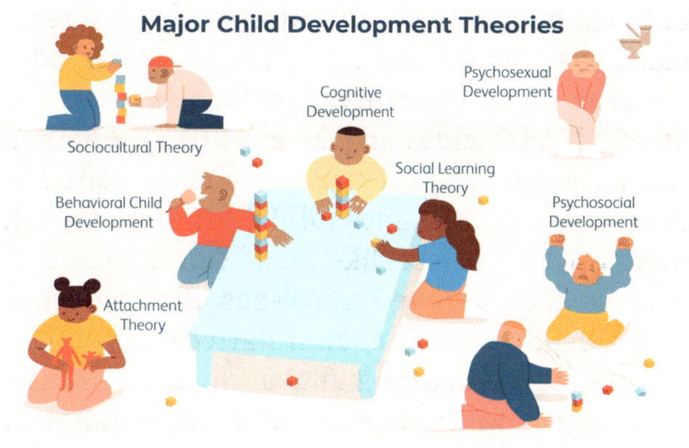

Figure 11.4. The development of pediatric psychiatry and behavioral health has been significantly shaped by pioneering figures whose work laid the foundational principles of the field.

Source: https://www.verywellmind.com/thmb/FhY7F2-ZFQD3D1MOOCahyppulv8=/1500x0/filters:no_upscale():max_bytes(150000):strip_icc()/child-development-theories-2795068-final-b0d7a20d00274f2cbc51b5d51d2169cd.png.

11.1.3. Changes in Societal Attitudes Towards Children's Mental Health

With the developments of society, perceptions of children's mental health have shifted significantly, from stigmatization to the more comprehensive realization of mental wellbeing. Previously, child mental illnesses were often refused or attributed to behavioral problems, mainly due to ignorance and poor information. Contemporary developments in pediatric psychiatry, however, have directed attention to etervention as well as the discovery of disorders such as, such as Attention-Deficit/Hyperactivity Disorder (ADHD). The greater understanding that mental health is part of general child development has generated a culture in which parents, educators, and doctors are more attuned to look for help for children demonstrating signs of mental distress. This shift reflects a burgeoning understanding not only of the incidence of mental health disorders but also of what, left untreated, their long-term consequences will be, and that has informed a broader social tolerancepsychiatrically (Moore et al., 2011Chakrabarti et al., 2015). Further, recent initiatives have prioritized interventions that can address mental health for at-risk populations. Projects like the Children's Ground project have adopted place-based approaches that respond to the cumulative social and environmental determinants of children's health. In foregroundingrdependent determinants of children's development, such as, such as socio-economic status and social support networks, these projects foreground an integrated concept of mental well-being. This paradigm shift emphasizes responding to children's mental health through an integrated response that not just addresses therapeutic interventions but also builds community capacity. Evidence-based practices outlined through these initiatives reflect a concern for enhancing child and family outcomes and a demand for systemic reforms that ze mental heals well as physical health care (Lorains Moore et al., 20252011). Parallel to these transformations in society, grassroots movements have been crucial in reformulating discussion around children's mental health. Public campaigns, awareness-raising activities, and advocacy campaigns have been a major force in de-stigmatizing mental illness and encouraging once forbidden discussions. Parents and communities are now playing a more active role in advocating for their children as champions, advocating for increased accessibility of mental health facilities and services. This increasing awareness has also influenced policymakers, with funds being pumped into mental health programs and research, particularly for disorders like ADHD. By holding spaces in which mental health topics are on the table, communities are able to better serve children to reach their full potential. Ultimately, these changes in public opinion reflect not only growing recognition of children's mental health needs but also a commitment to creating an environmen et al., 2011Chakrabarti et al., 2015; Lorains et al., 2025).

Test Your Knowledge

1. What major developments have shaped the growth and recognition of pediatric psychiatry as a medical field?
2. Why is early identification and treatment of mental health issues in children increasingly emphasized in modern psychiatry?

11.2. Common Pediatric Mental Health Disorders

Learning Outcome

1. Anxiety disorders
2. Attention-deficit/hyperactivity disorder (ADHD)
3. Depression and mood disorders

Prevalence of pediatric mental disorder ranks top in contemporary health care. Anxiety disorders, depression, and attention-deficit/hyperactivity disorder (ADHD) are but some of the most common among children and youth. They have an overarching impact on not just the patients but also their families and schools. Anxiety disorders, characterized by excess fear and anxiety, are often manifested in restlessness and avoidance behaviors. On the other hand, depression in children may manifest as persistent sadness, irritability, and withdrawal from social contacts. Empirical observations suggest that these disorders can be reduced by early interventions involving therapeutic and educational support, leaving an improved long-term prognosis for such affected children. Newer approaches to managing these pediatr illnesses have emerged over the last decade or so, such as, such as using mobile technology for promoting mental well-being. Although such apps have potential, their effectiveness and quality have to be rigorously examined. A systematic review of mental health apps for adolescents and children revealed that very few among the available apps were scientifically backed and of good quality. Of the 3806 identified apps, only 15 met the high-stakes eligibility criteria directed towards anxiety, depression, or post-traumatic stress disorder (PTSD) in adolescents. These findings emphasize the importance of science-based research into the development and testing of mental health technologies, especially since the current market fails to feature science-based ones that clinicians and families trust to use in the healing process (Domal., 2021). Besides, specific high-risk populations, such as, such as children undergoing cancer treatment, offer unique mental health challenges. These children not only endure the physical effects of their illness and its treatment but also endure increased vulnerability to mental illness, don particularly being prevalent. Effective treatments such as, such as expressive group art therapy have been found effective in reducing depression levels among child patients. As per studies, structured therapeutic interventions can promote emotional resilience and allow stability of mind state throughout critical patment. Thus, the integration of evidence-based psychologicalpsychological treatments within pediatric oncology practice highlights the growing recognition of the interdependence between physical and mental health in providing holistic care for this high-risk group (Naveed et al., 2021) (Figure 11.5).

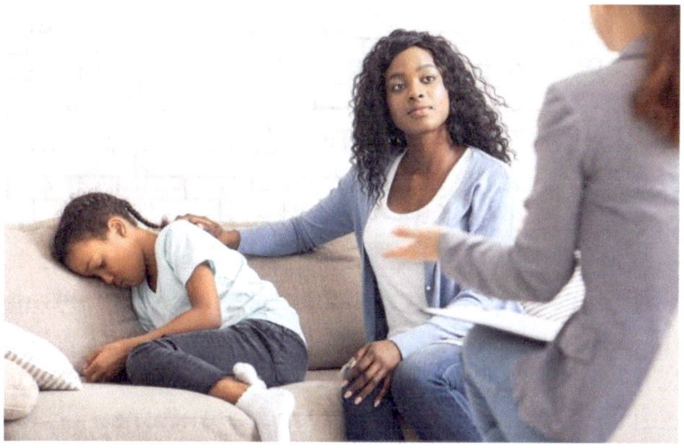

Figure 11.5. Child and parent in a counseling session addressing mental health concerns.

Source: https://s3.amazonaws.com/utep-uploads/wp-content/uploads/online-regis-college/2020/11/17034153/Parental-mental-health.jpg.

11.2.1. Anxiety Disorders

Anxiety disorders are an important aspect of pediatric psychiatryal health that interfere with the emotional and psychologicalpsychological development of children. The disorders consist of generalized anxiety disorder, social anxiety disorder, and separation anxiety disorder that may appear in numerous adverse forms. Children with anxiety disorders may exhibit excessive worry, fear, or avoidance behaviors that interfere with normal function and interpersonal relationships. Prevalence of such disorders in the pediatric age group necessitates early detection and interveeir untreated form can develop into more serious psychologicalpsychological problems in adolescence and adulthood. Furthermore, understanding the nuances of every disorder is crucial when devising suitable treatment regimens personalized to meet, which can involve behavioral interventions, medication, or both. The therapeutic environment for childhood anxiety disorders has changed considerably, with cognitive behavioral therapy (CBT) becoming a top intervention. Meta-analyses reveal that between 60% of children can be recovered from anxiety disorders after CBT, although recovery can differ extensivetain diagnostic criteria (Moore et al., 2011Cooper et al., 2017). This discrepancy underscores the challenge of measuring treatment efficacy since results could depend on whether children are being tested for one solitary primary condition or on whether many anxiety disorders exist. The necessity of standard diagnosis reporting in clinical trials becomes evident, allowing for more successful data synthesis and more clarity into the effect of interventions. Thus, practitioners need to exercise prudence in the application of evidence-based therapies as well as consider the individual contexts and situations of their pediatric patients. Neuroimaging studies have greatly assisted in elucidating the neurobiological underpinnings of anxiety disorders and has learned things that can be applied in the formulation of treatment plans. Neurodevelopmental disorders, including obsessive-compulsive disorder (OCD), have been studied to show potential changes in structural and functional characteristics of the brain associated with anxiety (Arnold et). The partnership of international research consortia, such as, such as the ENIGMA project, is the worth of sharing resources and capability to bolster sample size and analytic power. Early results from these investigations reveal important information regarding brain connectivity and neurodevelopmental timing of changes that can be credited to anxiety disorders. Because these studies support the neurobiological models of anxiety, they are of significant importance to the construction of targeted therapeutic interventions in pediatric populations, ultimately enhancing the overall understanding of pediatric psychiatry and behavior.

11.2.2. Attention-Deficit/ Hyperactivity Disorder (ADHD)

ADHD is a prevalent neurodevelopmental disorder that poses significant challenges within the domain of pediatric psychiatry and behavioral health. Involving inattention, hyperactivity, and impulsivity, ADHD holds the ability to immensely impact not only a child's performance at school but also onships and emotional weg. Both organic and psychologicalpsychological illnesses such as, such as anxiety, depression, and learning disability often coexist with ADHD, making it hard to diagnose and manage. It is essential for practitioners to understand the multidimensional nature of ADHD. Effective management involves comprehensive assessment that identifies the child's individual problems, including any co-morbid conditions, thereby enabling individualized interventions aimed at optimizing cas well as behavioral functioning. Co-morbid conditions, such as, such as Tourette's Disorder (TD), have been found to complicate the clinical presentation of ADHD children. A neurocognitive functioning study found that the teens who exhibited both ADHD and tics had impaired working memory and motor inhibition compared with those in the tics-only group. These deficits in cognition indicate that clinicians should use a holistic method for evaluating treatment. This also holds true in the growing literature, which indicates that effective treatment strategies need not only to correct for the core symptoms of ADHD but also for the impacted cognitive processes due to comorbid illness. The role of behavioral therapies, i.e., the Comprehensive Behavioral Intervention for Tics, is focused on the potential for concomitant treatment plans depending on the individual neth such comorbid diagnoses (Moore et al., 2011Chang et al., 2018).

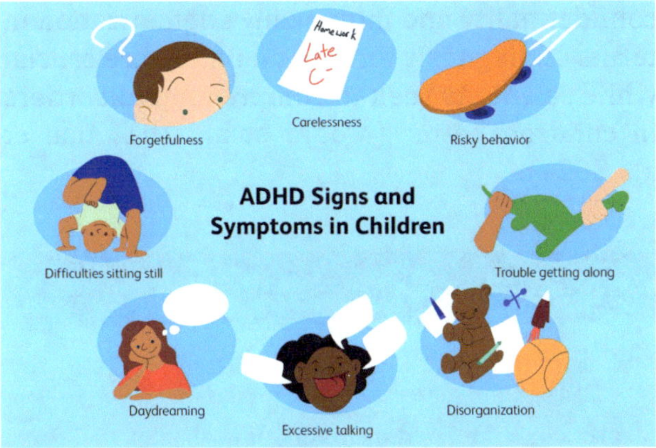

Figure 11.6. Attention-deficit/hyperactivity disorder (ADHD).

Source: https://www.verywellhealth.com/thmb/zeZQkVPST5khjvEmDpoW4KxpWGk=/1500x0/filters:no_upscale():max_bytes(150000):strip_icc()/adhd-attention-deficit-hyperactivity-disorder-included-definition-symptoms-traits-causes-treatment-5084784_final-bc92546bc9df465ea7f13fc423c2085b.jpg.

ADHD treatment must be tailored, including taking into account comorbid disorders that may affect the treatment outcome. Contemporary guidelines propose a concomitant decision-making process involving medical professionals, caretakers, and the patients themselves. Such an interactive strategy guarantees that several treatment modalities—varying from behavioral therapies to pharmacotherapy—are taken into account in addition to the patient's overall mental health status and cognitive ability. For example, regular reevaluation of the efficacy of treatment is important, particularly in children with both tic disorders and ADHD. The use of psychoeducation with caregivers and teachers, coupled with ongoing communication and care across treatment, is consistent with best practice in pediatric psychiatry, enhancing a nurturing environment conducive to a child's success and well-being (Cavanna et al., 2019) (Figure 11.6).

11.2.3. Depression and Mood Disorders

Depression and mood disorders in children have increasingly come to be understood in the field of psychiatry. These disorders, typically characterized by persistent sadness, irritability, and loss of interest in activities once found pleasurable, can significantly affect a child's social and academic function. In the majority of cases, these issues occur during critical developmental stages, so early identification and treatment arel. As highlighted in the existing literature, conditions such as, such as trichotillomania and body dysmorphic disorder tend to co-exist with mood disorders, hence complicating clinical presentations and treatment. This is a demonstration of the significance of the presence of a multidisciplinary team comprising mental health practitioners and pediatricians to ensure various needs of the involved children are addressed holistically, as recommended by existing evidence-based practice guidelines in childhood psychiatry (Leonard B Goldstein, 2024). Pathbreaking research in the field of pediatric psychiatry has also indicated the intricate biological mechanisms of mood disorders from an epigenetic point of view. Epigenetic mechanisms, wherein gene expression is modified but the DNA sequence remains unchanged, are environmentally sensitive, including stress and trauma. Knowledge of these mechanisms is crucial since they play an important role in deciding the mode of treatment in juvenile patients. For instance, DNA methylation differences associated with depression reveal potential targets for antidepressant therapy. Through the study of how genes interact with the environment, doctors will be able to better narrow their approaches so that therapy not only succeeds but also is tailored to the individual child's specific requirements. This new research field places the primacy of personalized medicine at the forefront of the treatment of mood disorders and has the potential to transform intervention in pediatric psychiatry (Alaa et al., 2024). With these developments, the translation of epigenetic data into practice has the potential for yet more creative and compassionate care in pediatric psychiatry. As child mental health clinicians examine the impact of genetic profiles on treatment results, specific therapeutic interventions can be designed to optimize effectiveness and maximize results for adolescents with mood disorders. Early detection of depressive symptoms, combined with access to individualized treatment protocols, can help limit long-term outcomes of these disorders in substantial ways. Furthermore, as mental health awareness grows, so does the necessity of addressing the moral concerns involved with using epigenetic information. Maintaining patient confidentiality and minimizing stigmatization in terms of diagnosis for mental illness are crucial while scientists seek to comprehend disorders in children better (Moore et al., 2011Alaa et al., 2024).

Test Your Knowledge

1. What are the common types and symptoms of anxiety disorders in children?
2. How does Attention-Deficit/Hyperactivity Disorder (ADHD) affect a child's behavior and learning?
3. What are the main causes and treatment approaches for depression and mood disorders in pediatric patients?

11.3. Assessment and Diagnosis

Learning Outcome

1. Tools and methods for assessment
2. Role of parents and caregivers in diagnosis
3. Challenges in diagnosing pediatric mental health issues

Pediatric psychiatric diagnostic evaluation and diagnosis need a sequential and comprehensive process according to the symptoms complexity exhibited in children. Because children will not likely express their experience or feelings suitably, observation and interaction are important in information gathering. Clinicians utilize standardized measures of assessment and parent interviews to gather multidimensional feedback regarding a child's behavioral habits. In addition, assessments need to consider developmental and environmental factors that may influence a child's mental health condition. An ongoing assessment process allows for the identification of specific disorders but also facilitates the creation of individually tailored treatment plans that can be tailored to comply with the child's unique needs and circumstance, makle for targeted interventions that target the child's psychologicalpsychological well-being in their own environment. The incorporation of telephonic clinical and psychiatric consultation into the assessment process is a significant step forward for pediatric mental health treatment. By virtue of this new model, primary care providers are afforded access to specialist consultation concurrent with their contribution to the evaluation of the individual needs of the child. By generating an interface between pediatrics and mental health personnel, clinicians are able to offer in-person evaluation, transitional therapies, or connection to community services as needed. The coordination provided by this system improves the quality of care delivered to children with mental health problems, facilitating smoother movement through treatment stages. With mental health problems growing among adolescents, effective operation of such programs is a testament to the potential of increased integration in pediatric psychiatry (Holt et al., 2010). Effective management of pediatric bipolar disorder (PBD) is essentially aimed at emphasizing the necessity to combine psychopharmacotherapy with psychotherapy during the assessment and diagnosis process. The definite psychopathological traits of childrluding severe irritability and occurrence of co-morbidities such as, such as attention deficit hyperactivity disorder, necessitate a delicate diagnostic approach that is specifically formulated to counteract the challenges posed by such features. There is empirical support for the use of combined treatment modes, indicating combination therapy with second-generation antipsychotics and mood stabilizers is superior to monotherapy. The incorporation of family-based and cognitive behavioral therapies also enhances treatment, indicating the usefulness of psychosocial treatments in the overall treatment of PBD. Knowledge of such treatment dynamics is crucial for clinicians with the aim of providing optimal therapeutic services to adolescents with PBD and highlighting the interface betwesment and optimal intervention (Moore et al., 2011Mani et al., 2005) (Figure 11.7).

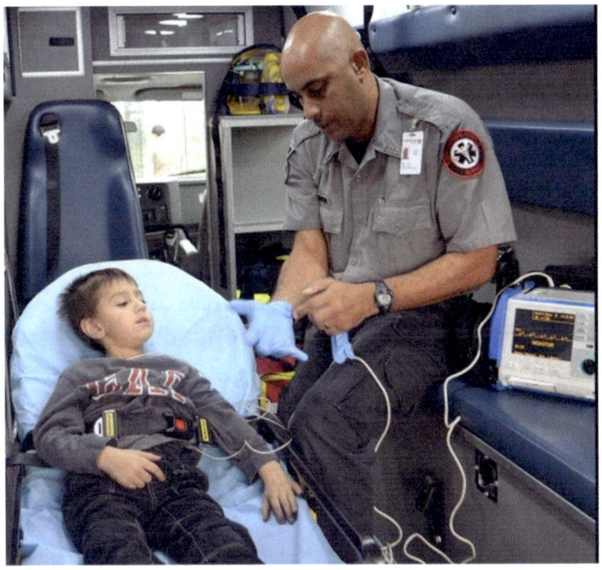

Figure 11.7. The assessment and diagnosis of pediatric psychiatric conditions.

Source: https://s3.us-east-2.amazonaws.com/medictests-production/ckeditor_assets/pictures/1248/content_Community-Involment.jpg.

11.3.1. Tools and Methods for Assessment

The assessment of children's psychiatric and behavioral well-being requires an holistic approach that utilizes several instruments and techniques, allowing for accurate diagnosis and best treatment planning. One of the significant developments in the field has been the development of standardized assessment devices that quantify children's mental health and behavioral problems on a numerical scale. These measures come in the form of clinician ratings and self-report questionnaires, which can measure a wide range of issues includinssion, anxiety, and behavior difficulties. Applying measures such as, such as the Strengths and Difficulties Questionnaire and the Pediatric Symptom Checklist, clinicians have a greater capacity to ascertain the severity of disorders and changes over time. This systematic evaluation facilitates informed clinical decisions, enhancing the quality of clinical practice for vulnerable children. The psychometric properties of these measurement tools are essential to their application in practice. The review of broadband measures for children reveals that although numerous have been applied widely, there are inherent limitations and strengths in each in terms of reliability and validity. For instance, while the Achenbach System of Empirically Based Assessment is appreciated because it provides a large framework, it lacks sufficient psychometric data to measure change over time across some populations. This lac ongoing development and validation of these instruments in order toto satisfy the special needs of different pediatric populations.

Thus, practitioners must thoroughly examine such measures against certain criteria for determinacy to ascertain that chosen tests not only provide pertinent informatilso facilitate interactions with families during treatment (Brown etDeighton et al., 2014). Beyond this, early screening and developmental monitoring are imperative components of pediatric psychiatric assessment. The presence of unrecognized developmental delays among children highlights the importance of primary care providers in identifying vulnerable populations. By improving developmental monitoring through structured screening tools and routine follow-up, clinicians can refine early intervention activities, significantly enhancing long-term results in children who suffer from mental health problems. Recommendations from the literature underscore the importance of proper training for primary care clinicians to recognize such delays early on and therefore enhance overall health surveillance in pediatric practice. As technology evolves and evaluation should be updated, it is important that the health systems continue to evolve to include these methods properly (Sices, 2007).

11.3.2. Role of Parents and Caregivers in Diagnosis

Parent and caregiver participation are of critical value in pediatric psychiatry and behavioral health diagnosis. Parents are the first reporters of a child's behavioral patterns, emotional state, and developmental milestones and, therefore, contribute significant information that informs healthcare providers. Parent descriptions allow for complete comprehension of the child's symptoms, generating a context that has a significant influence on diagnosis. The American Academy of Pediatrics emphasizes the importance of these histories provided by parents for appropriate assessment and management of conditions apt to affect child and adolescent mental health (Laura et al., 2022).

In another respect, the involvement of parents in diagnosis facilitates a collaborative partnership with practitioners that is essential to the creation of effective treatment plans particular to the needs of the individual child. In the households whose existence has been challenged by the new challenges posed by the COVID-19 pandemic, parents and caregivers are even more vital. Mental health issues have risen as a result of economic and social stressors, and it is thus essential that the caregivers not only observe but also articulate their children's issues. Parents can be confronted by challenges that may potentially exclude them frong early intervention for their child's mental health issues, such as, such as economic hardship or unavailability of services (Yoshikawa et al., 2020).

In addition, caregivers will naturally perceive their child's challenges in accordance with their mental and emotional structures, which may influence the accuracy of symptom reporting. Therefore, parents must be empowered with resources and capacity to facilitate them in articulating their findings so that a more accurate and efficient diagnosis can be established for the children. Besides, the various impacts of parents' mental health on the diagnostic process cannot be overlooked. The studies indicate that parents themselves having mental health issues fail to identify and report the symptoms of their child proped to misdiagnosis or undiagnosis (Moore et al., 2011Laura et al., 2022). Transgenerational effects of mental health explain why clinicians need to assess not only the child but the family dynamics as well. Creating an environment of support in which parents feel comforted is crucial to correct diagnosis and subsequent treatment. Additionally, health systems can focus on programs that equip parents with educational materials and mental health services, regarding them as valuable partners in the health journey of their children. All of these can bridge disparities in diagnosis and treatment, ultimately improving pediatric psychiatry and behavioral health outcomes (Figure 11.8).

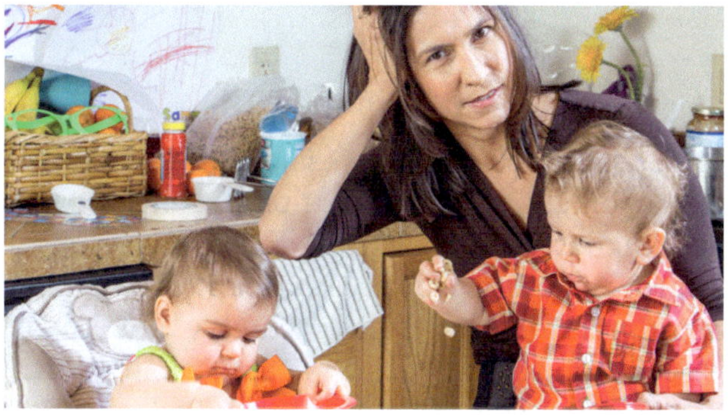

Figure 11.8. Role of parents and caregivers in diagnosis.

Source: https://learnbehavioral.com/wp-content/uploads/2021/05/on-stress-and-parenting-kids-with-autism.jpg.

11.3.3. Challenges in Diagnosing Pediatric Mental Health Issues

Pediatric mental illness diagnosis is beset with a range of difficulties that can undermine intervention and treatment. One of the primary challenges is symptom presentation diversity among children, which will differ from that of adults. Emotionalms, for instance, can present themselves as behavioral disorders such as, such as aggression and tantrums, leading to potential misdiagnoses. The subjectivity of parent and teacher observation also complicates this process further because biases and varied perception can warp a child's mental state evaluation. The New Hampshire Pediatric Improvement Partnership (NHPIP) survey pinpoints such concerns, with clinicians themselves reporting feeling poorly equipped to properly assess and manage issues like Attention Deficit Hyperactivity Disorder (ADHD) because they have a low rate of responding to their inquiry about how they approach diagnosing (Daviss et al., 2017). Such findings point to the utmost need for standardized diagnostic criteria and training to enable proper assessment. Another factor that contributes to the diagnosis of mental illness in children is stigma that discourages help-seeking. Parents may avoid visiting healthcare professionals for fear of stigmatizing their child or of social repercussions from admitting that their child has mental issues. The situation is compounded by the lack of resources, including access to specialist healthcare professionals. The majority of primary care practitioners report not having enough confidence in dealing with such cases if not given adequate support. Telehealth programs that encompass the provision of psychiatric and clinical guidance to primary care providers are highly suited responses to addressing this issue. The projects not only aid in the early diagnosis but also encourage family models for accessing help without the stigma of the face-to-face clinical encounter. By integrating these services, early identification and intervention (Holt, 2010) could be improved. Last, children's dynamic nature adds one more layer of challenges to diagnosing mental health. Signs which can show a specific disorder may evolve as a child grows, both complicating diagnosis and treatment in the future. In addition, pediatric mental health issues tend to co-occur or overlap with each other, and it is difficult for clinicians to settle on one diagnosis. This complexity necessitates the utilization of a multi-faceted approach considering the child's development, family environment, and surroundings. Otherwise, multi-faceted problems are at risk of being oversimplified, and the treatment process is ineffective. Continuous education of healthcare providers is, therefore, necessary. This includes not only understanding the nuances of children's mental health but also employing collaborative care principles, thus ensuring that the unique needs of individual children are met at each point along their development trajectory.

Test Your Knowledge

1. What tools and methods are commonly used to assess mental health disorders in children?
2. How do parents and caregivers contribute to the diagnosis and understanding of a child's mental health condition?
3. What challenges are often faced in accurately diagnosing mental health issues in pediatric patients?

11.4. Treatment Approaches

Learning Outcome

1. Psychotherapy and counseling techniques
2. Pharmacological interventions
3. Integrative and holistic treatment options

Treatment modalities for children and adolescents in child and adolescent psychiatry are a variety of methodologies that address an extensive set of mental health needs. The historic standard of care for therapy has been traditional in-office psychiatric treatment. With the recent technological developments, the new and rapidly emerging alternative is telepsychiatry. A randomized trial comparing the efficacy of both approaches demonstrated telepsychiatry to be able to produce similar clinical outcomes to regular face-to-face sessions, with clinical improvement from evaluations replicated for both modes. Results identified significant clinical improvements for both treatment groups and demonstrated that telepsychiatry effectively meets the required need for accessible mental health services in this present digital age (Pak et al., 2024). This availability is particularly significant because the prevalence of mental health issues among children and adolescents is continually on the rise, which requires versatile intervention approaches. Another central treatment approach within pediatric psychiatry is also that of the incorporation of behavioral health services within primary care environments, which focuses on prevention efforts rather than remedial interventions. Interventions like the Integrated Behavioral Healt (IBH-P) intervention demonstrate the potential for incorporating psychologicalpsychological support within routine well-child visits. This pilot study demonstrated that delivering preventive behavioral health interventions effectively encourages positive parenting practices among low-income mothers of infants. Although early findings showed no difference in maternal attunement or caregiving behavior between groups, secondary analysis identi-efficacy in intervention-exposed mothers (Moore et al., 2011Robert et al., 2024). These findings demonstrate the benefits of early recognition and treatment of mental health requirements through integration with primary care, eventually resulting in more healthy developmental outcomes in children. The two treatment models, telepsychiatry and integrated behavioral health services, indicate a shift in paradigm in child mental health care, with a focus on prevention and accessibility.

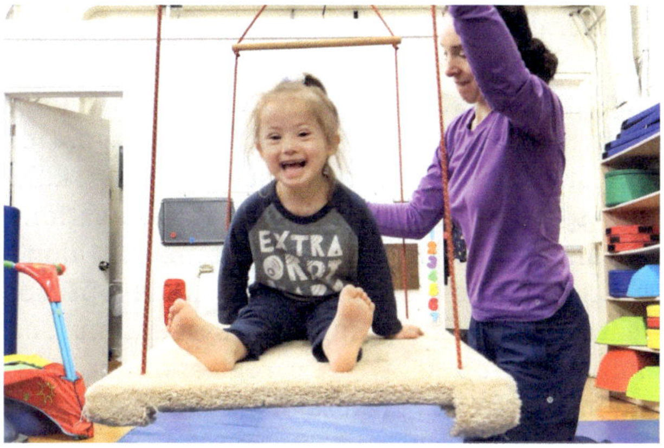

Figure 11.9. Treatment approaches.

Source: https://paediatricphysiotherapy.com/wp-content/uploads/2023/06/FullSizeRender-3-copy-1-2048x1365-1-1024x683.jpg.

As the healthcare profession keeps evolving, the need to adapt to novel practice cannot be overstated. Telepsychiatry offers unmatched access for services, effectively bridging geographical barriers and reducing obstacles that most often prevent young patients from accessing early intervention. Concurrently, the integration of mental health interventions into general pediatric practice allows for early identification and treatment of behavioral difficulties, avoiding the dismal long-term outcomes of unattended mental illness. By embracing these comprehensive approaches, pediatric psychiatry can significantly enhance patient outcomes and offer children and adolescents the broad care they require in a welcoming environment (Figure 11.9).

11.4.1. Psychotherapy and Counseling Techniques

The present situation with psychotherapeutic and counseling interventions in pediatric psychiatry is famplementing efficient interventions aimed at the special emotional and psychologicalpsychological requirements of children and adolescents. One of these interventions, trauma-focused cognitive behavioral therapy (TF-CBT), is an outstanding one, particularly applicable to adolescents and children with post-traumatic stress disorder (PTSD). Evidence indicates that single-site implementations of TF-CBT have been demonstrated to be highly effective in reducing symptoms of PTSD significantly than the effects of waitlist control groups. The approach includes elements such as, such as cognitive restructuring and narrative exposure that allow children to confront and speak directly about their traumatic experience. Considering the high rates of exposure to trauma among adolescents, the incorporation of TF-CBT into treatment plans is crucial for enhancing the mental health of this vulnerable group (Mavranezouli et al., 2019). In addition, depression management among adolescents using evidence-based guidelines igthening mental health care in primary care (Moore et al., 2011Petersen et al., 2019). The updated clinical practice guidelines recommend universal screening for depression in adolescents 12 years and above on health maintenance visits. By taking such a proactive approach, not only is early identification of at-risk individuals made easier but systematic assessment strategies can also be guided using valid scales of depression and structured interviews. These best practices highlight the importance of achieving a broad knowledge of the specific context of every adolescent and encouraging open communication among families, patients, and clinicians. These guidelines have the potential to improve access to mental health care while providing a framework for effe in managing adolescent depression as a whole (Moore et al., 2011Rachel et al., 2018). Finally, inclusion of a variety of therapeutic modalities extends the range of usefulness of psychotherapy and counseling techniques beyond TF-CBT and depanagement protocol. Encouraging findings suggest that adjunctive treatments, such as, such as mindfulness meditation and child-parent psychotherapy, may yield beneficial effects in children with a variety of psychiatric disorders. Though effectiveness for these treatments is still to be studied, early reports demonstrate favorable effects on emotional regulation and behavioral function in children. With practitioners trying to individualize treatment plans, such consideration of personal preferences and the unique needs of children and families is increasingly important. Taking a multimodal approach that includes traditional and innovative therapies can eventually lead to more comprehensive and tailored care for those who have to deal with the challenges of pediatric mental health (Mavranezouli et al., 2019).

11.4.2. Pharmacological Interventions

Pharmacologic management in child psychiatry and behavioral health is a focus of managing most neurodevelopmental and psychiatric disorders in childrenolescents. These medications are intended to diminish symptoms of conditions such as, such as ATTENTION-deficit/hyperactivity disorder (ADHD), autism spectrum disorder (ASD), anxiety disorders, and depression. Current guidelines highlight the importance of careful clinical assessment, a thoughtful weighing of the child's developmental level and individual background before the advent of any drug treatment. This serves to emphasize the overriding significance of individualized treatment plans that are compounded of both pharmacological and non-pharmacological intervention. As pediatric practitioners navigate these complex treatment paradigms, the application of pharmacotherapy always entails balancing effectiveness against potential side effects so that not only do children experience remission of symptoms but are also endy to thrive in their everydronments (Deighton et al., 2014Gausman et al., 2020). Atypical antipsychotics such as, such as risperidone and aripiprazole have proven useful to treat irritability and emotional dysregulation in children with ASD specifically. These medications are specific to specific behavioral presentations, a significant departure from earlier methodologies of giving unilateral emphasis on symptom attenuation alone. Second, as indicated by drug therapies, they work best in conjunction with ongoing behavioral treatment, which has the goal of providing adolescents with essential coping skills. This synergy acknowledges that medications can ameliorate transient symptoms but don't constitute a sole solution. To achieve optimal treatment outcomes, supportive systems must be multiplicative and involve caregivers, educators, and mental health professionals (Subramanyam et al., 2019). Integrated treatment ensures that child mental health therapies are well-suited to the specific needs of every patient, laying the foundation for lasting improved functioning and development. But the pediatric pharmacological treatment environment is still full of challenges. Problems of long-term medication effects on developing brains need ongoing researches and close monitoring. Stigma regarding mental illness and drug treatment can deter families from seeking treatments their children need, therefore increasing the distress of psychiatric children. Moreover, evidence reviews emphasize the need for ongoing education of healthcare providers to help them deliver well-informed consultations with families over drug benefits and harms. As we better understand pediatric pharmacotherapy in pediatric psychiatry, it is imperative to support policies that foster research dollars and access to care for children with these complex mental health concerns. Enabling an open discussion that is culture-conducive between parents, clinicians, and teachers can also dismantle barriers to intervention programs that are effective as well as foemotional health in children and adolescents (Deighton et al., 2014Gausman et al., 2020) (Figure 11.10).

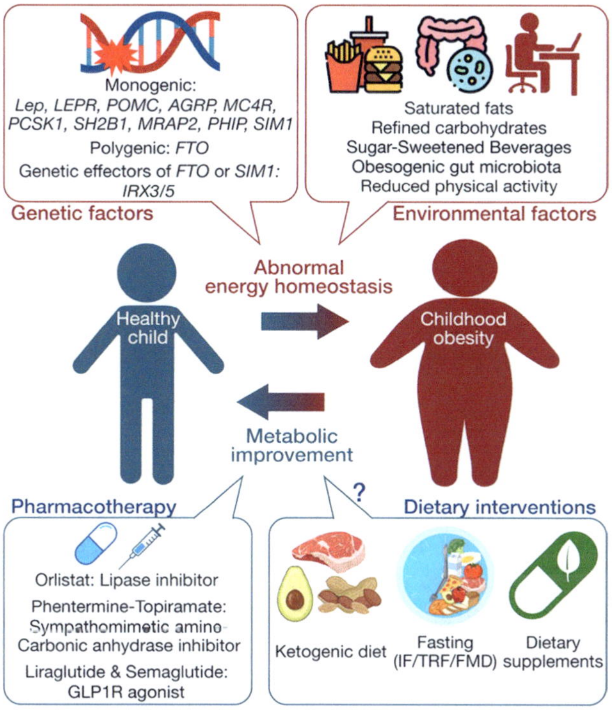

Figure 11.10. Pharmacological interventions in pediatric psychiatry and behavioral health.

Source: https://images-provider.frontierspartnerships.org/api/ipx/w=1200&f=png/https://www.frontierspartnerships.org/files/Articles/12861/jpps-27-12861-HTML/image_m/jpps-27-12861-g001.jpg.

11.4.3. Integrative and Holistic Treatment Options

In pediatric psychiatry and behavioral health practice, integrative and holistic therapies are increasingly recognized as having the capacity to complement traditional healing approaches. Such treatments prioritize the global well-being of the entire child as oposed to being obsessed with symptomatic relief. By incoporating various modalities, —e.g., psychotherapy, nutrition education, and exercise, —health professionals may address the multidimensional etiology of a child's mental health.

For instance, programs like SHINE (Self Help, Independence, Nutrition and Exercise) offer an integrated model where interventions are tailored to each child's situation. This approach, a demonstration of the stepped-care model, allows interventions to escalate in intensity as the severity of the cants, thus providing a healing and empowering atmosphere (Sharman & NoblesPowell et al., 2016). Integrating integrative healthcare models is a paradigm shift in pediatric mental health delivery. By integrating behavior health services in the primary care settings, providers are in a superior position to address the complex needs of children in one setting.

The integrated service model establishes a context where emotional and behavioral challenges are not isolated concerns but are actually components that have direct effects on physical health outcomes. Initial studies indicate that child specialists in these integrated environments report higher comprehension and efficacy while dealing with mental health problems, consequently leading to better patient satisfaction and outcomes. One-stop-shop also reduces levels of stress among healthcare providers since they are more assured of addressing whole care, the pathway to an effective health delivery system for children

(Anton et al., 2020). Further, the application of integrative and holistic modalities of treatment deals with the diverse histories and experiences of pediatric patients. The recognition of cultural, social, and personal variables in a child's life increases options for treatment and encourages greater family involvement. Practitioners are capable of tailoring interventions that resonate with the specific values and beliefs of the child and family, increasing adherence and maximizing therapeutic effect. Its attractiveness is in its flexibility; it has room to include different therapeutic approaches, community resources, and famiics and thus forms a support network that is culturally sensitive. As research ongoing in this field continues to evolve, the effectiveness of these treatments in establishing long-term health and wellness in children will become further supported, again supporting the merted models in pediatric psychiatry and behavioral health (Sharman & NoblesPowell et al., 2016).

Test Your Knowledge

1. What are the key psychotherapy and counseling techniques used in treating pediatric mental health disorders?
2. When are pharmacological interventions considered appropriate for children with mental health issues?
3. How can integrative and holistic approaches support traditional treatments in pediatric mental health care?

11.5. The Role of Pediatricians

Learning Outcome

1. Collaboration between pediatricians and psychiatrists
2. Screening for mental health issues in primary care
3. Education and training for pediatricians in mental health

Pediatricians also play a crucial gatekeeping role in child health, particularly within pediatric psychiatry and br. Their function extends beyond mere physical checkup to a comprehensive approach style that also respects the significant interrelation of a child's mental, emotional, and physical well-being. With increasing knowledge of adverse childhood experiences (ACEs) and social determinants of health (SDOH), pediatricians are now charged with identifying these factors in relation to patient care. The holistic approach is imperative not only to diagnose pediatric mental health disorders but also to provide inclusive care addressing the underlying conditions influencing a child's overall development. Through conducting thorough assessments, pediatricians can institute early intervention strategies, thereby contributing to improved outcomes in the long term (Corvini et al., 2018). These preventive measures are part and parcel of what it takes to maintain resilience and wellness among children as they navigate various issues of life. The other significant role pediatricians play is developmental monitoring and screening. Research has established that developmental delay in early childhood is not detected by primary care physicians, and this requires heightened alertness in pediatrics (Sices, 2007). Through the integration of systematic developmental screening in regular well-child visits, pediatricians can identify early signs of mental illness and behavioral disorders so that children can be provided interventions in an early manner. This proactive approach not only supports preventing long-term adverse consequences of untreatended conditions but also facilitates providing a supporting environment for families and children. Moreover, pediatricians can collaboratively work with pediatric psychiatry professionals, making referrals if necessary, and a continuum of care that is holistic and comprehensive.

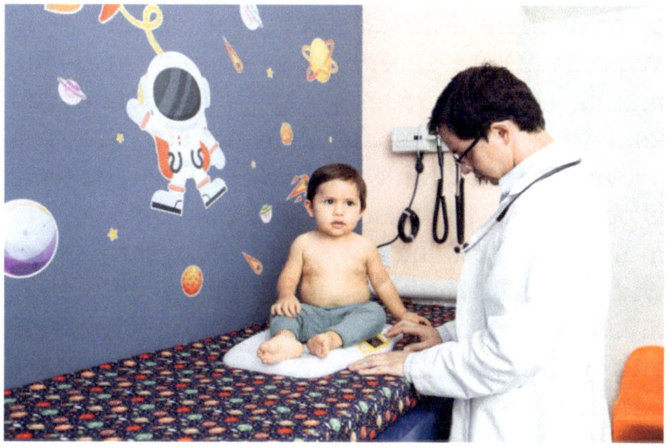

Figure 11.11. The role of pediatricians.

Source: https://pranaamhospitals.com/wp-content/uploads/2023/02/My-project.jpg.

This combined model of care exemplifies the pediatrician's central role in the world of behaviora, pediatricians also serve as educators and advocates within the community on a regular basisregularly, educating and empowering parents and caregivers to foster better mental well-being in children. Through the provision of resources, guidance, and support regarding the role of mental well-being, pediatricians can help foster a better appreciation of how early life influences development. All this advocacy is particularly crucial in the case ofealth inequities by social determinants of health (Sharman & Nobles, 2016Corvini et al., 2018). Involvement by pediatricians in community programs and partnerships can broaden the reach of mental health services, enhancing the general health environment for children. By developing awareness and open conversation around mental health, pediatricians are able to deconstruct stigma and establish a foundation for children to share their challenges openly. This complex role establishes the implicit value of pediatricians as they set the course for pediatric psychiatry and behavioral health (Figure 11.11).

11.5.1. Collaboration Between Pediatricians and Psychiatrists

The collaborative partnership of psychiatrists and pediatricians is increasingly better understood to be integral to the care of children's and adolescents' complicated mental health. From this collaborative process, the patient can be given a comprehensive diagnosis and treatment of all types of behavior and mental illness. Pediatricians are usually the first access point to the healthcare system for children and will often identify delays in development or psychiatric illness on well-child visits. By working hand-in-hand with child psychiatrists, pediatricians can coordinate on-time referrals and get patients the appropriate mental health interventions. Not only does this working together increase outcomes, but it also supports enhanced comprehensiveness in the view of a child's health, including physical and mental components of wellness, which is imperative within pediatric psychiatry and behavioral health (Ik et al., 2024). Besides, integration of services through cooperation can yield a total greancy in the care of pediatric patients. Pediatricians and psychiatrists, as one team, are able tocan coordinate treatment programs considering numerous factors affecting the mental health status of a child, including home life and school life. Multidisciplinary practices have proven particularly helpful in managing complex cases, in which behavior disorders could be superimposed on physical illnesses. Sharing information among the practitioners can also enhance thorough insight into presenting problems, which is useful for strengthening management strategies. According to recent literature, effective communication is also crucial in the application of prevention policies, which a in reducing trevalence of mental health disorders in children and adolescents (Camardellaa Moore et al., 20222011). Besides, educating parents and caregivers as to why mental health is important is also at the core of this collaborative process. ans are well-suited to provide information and advice that is empowering to families in order toto recognize early signs of emotional distress and value professional assistance from psychiatrists. Good communication practices enhance the collaborative process and empower families to be participants in care. Interdisciplinary communication between the pediatric and psychiatric communities can help families feel more at ease with mental health, becoming a more receptive population to access services when necessary. Thus, encouraging a collaborative model improves the collaboration between healthcare workers and families, ultimately leading to improved outcomes for child mental health treatment and reaffirming theof a cooperatiodel in pediatric psychiatry and behavioral health interventions (Camardellaa Moore et al., 20222011).

15.5.2. Screening for Mental Health Issues in Primary Care

The role of mental health screening in the primary care clinic, and particularly in pediatrics, cannot be overstated. As a result of the growing prevalence of mental health disorders among children and teenagers, primary care is in an ideal position to identify and manage such issues early in life. Pediatricians and other primary care physicians generally serve as the first contact for families and therefore are able to conduct mental health screenings. Early identification utine screening can lead to early referral for specialized treatment as needed, and this in turn improves outcomes for children. Studies reveal that the integration of mental health screenings in regular pediatric check-ups not only ensures that issues can be detected before they happen but also reduces the stigma of the requirement for mental health care, opening the door toward an integrated pediatric health plan (Tateno et al., 2025). There are advantages to be derived, while there are complications in the roll-out of mental health screening in primary care facilities that must be dealt with utmost caution. One of the primary challenges is a lack of equipment and training for primary care physicians, who may not be adequately prepared to identify or treat mental illness. Moreover, variations in awareness and acceptability of administering mental health screenings by pediatricians can lead to inconsistencies in practices between providers (Khadijah et al., 2025). This imbalance is particularly worrisome with the complex and multifaceted etioloental illness, often concurrent with other childhood health disorders. Systematic measures such as, such as training programs and guidelines, are warranted to facilitate empowering primary care practitioners to delial health screening, which would allow children to receive the help they require in a timely mannerpy. Furthermore, coordination between mental health professionals and primary care clinicians grows becomes more necessary as mental screening becomes more widespread. Development of strong referral networks and communication systems between child and adolescent psychiatrists and pediatricians can provide a seamless system of care that optimizes the efficiency of screening initiatives. For instance, findings from recent surveys highlight the roles pediatricians play in addressing gaming disorders, with half of responding physicians encountering gaming-related issues among their patients (Tateno et al., 2025). As gaming and internet-related problems become more prevalent, a collaborative framework that allows for shared knowledge and resources is essential.

This collaboration can also enhance the management of comorbid psychiatric disorders, in a way that children not only receive mental health treatment but also holistic treatment that caters to the areas of their overall health and well-being (Khadijah et al., 2025) (Figure 11.12).

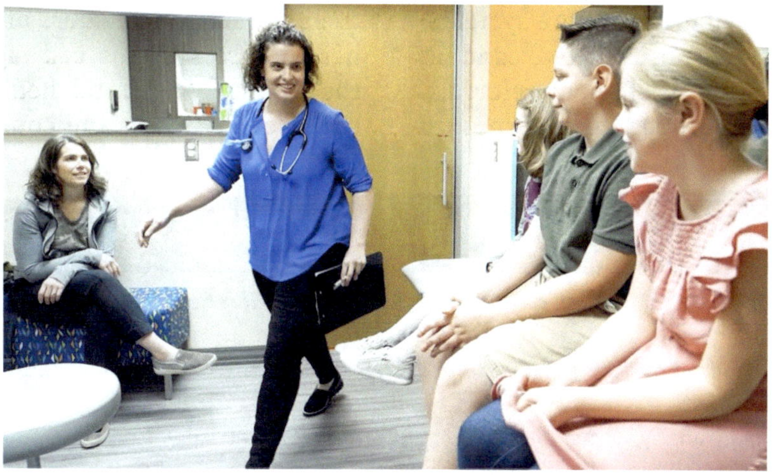

Figure 11.12. Screening for mental health issues in primary care.

Source: https://www.idahoednews.org/wp-content/uploads/2022/11/Lachiondo-e1668527437655.jpg.

11.5.3. Education and Training for Pediatricians in Mental Health

The evolving landscape of pediatric practice dictates an urgent need for more education and training of pediatricians, in particular, in the field of mental health. As disorders of mental health swell among children and adolescents, pediatricians are most likely to encounter distressed families as their first point of contact. These healthcare professionals are not, however, properly trained to identify or treat mental disorder. Current research shows that approximately 54.5% of pediatric palliative care clinicians reported no formal education in the identification and treatment of anxiety and depression in pediatric patients despite a high percentage reporting that they would like to be trained further in the topic (Vente, 2024). This edisparity carries critical consequences, as it is essential to provide early intervention in order toto maximize mental health outcomes for pediatric populations. In a bid to address such dilemmas, the American Academy of Pediatrics (AAP) has provided policy guidelines aimed at integrating mental health education into pediatric residency cuThis requires pediatricians to acquire skills in screening children for behavioral disorders, such as, such as depression and anxiety, which usually co-occur with medical illness (Yearwood, 2012). The AAP's commitment to continuous learning encourages pediatricians to update their knowledge and skills in a field of mental health so that they can provide integral care. Training must also be an integral process of interdisciplinary treatment with child psychiatrists for a comprehensive plan of care in children who are referred for behavior issues. These collaborative strategies not only increase provision of services but also promote multidisciplinary practice required in addressing the embeddedness of complexity in the nature of pediatric mental health. Additionally, increased training of mental health professionals is critical to facilitating ease of mental health provision among children and adolescents. The alarming lack of psychiatric resources is such that the majority of children only receive treatment upon crisis, thus complicating their psychiatric or behavioral needs (Yearwood, 2012). Children's mental health advocates emphasize the necessity for early prevention and intervention through primary care systems, as pediatricians are better positioned to conduct early screening and initiate efficient referrals. Thus, training programs need to incorporate systems that allow pediatricians to identify risk adolescents well and create channels to receive expert mental health treatment. With an educational system that trains pediatricians to be proactive providers of mental health care, health care systems can significantly improve the quality of mental health in children and adolescents across the country.

Test Your Knowledge

1. How do pediatricians collaborate with psychiatrists to ensure comprehensive mental health care for children?
2. What screening methods can pediatricians use to identify mental health issues during routine primary care visits?
3. Why is education and training in mental health important for pediatricians?

11.6. Impact of Social Factors

Learning Outcome

1. Influence of family dynamics on mental health
2. Socioeconomic factors and access to care
3. Cultural considerations in treatment and diagnosis

The role of social determinants in pediatric psychiatry and behavioral well-being is a fundamentalissue, particularly concerning rising rates of mental illness among youth. Social determinants, such as, such as socioeconomic status, culture, and environment, are most influential with respect to the mental well-being outcomes of youth. Poor children and those from poorer socioeconomic communities are more likely to have higher negative childhood experiences and stressors, manifesting as depression, anxiety, and behavioral issues. These inequities encompass unequal access to mental health services; studies show that children of color and low-income families have unique barriers to achieving effective treatment. Also, the aggravation of these conditions during the COVID-19 pandemic has resulted in the declaration of a national emergency, owing to thethat the necessitr specialized interventions to mitigate these inequities is a pressing need (Laura Deighton et al., 20222014). Another vital aspect of the social contribution towards children's mental health is the issue of family dynamics and caregiver stability. An affirmative and nurturing caregiving environment can be a protective factor against mental health issues. Conversely, family instability, for example, domestic violence, drug or alcohol use, or mental illness in caregivers, can cause severe emotional trauma for children. Adverse childhood experiences have been linked to increased risk for the development of psychiatric disorders in later life. Furthermore, this knowledge enables practitioners to implement holistic treatment techniques that not only address the child but the whole family. Thus, relationship-building amilies and commu networks is imperative while creating effective meth interventions (Laura Deighton et al., 20222014). Lastly, addreer issues of society, such as, such as structural racism and social disparities, is paramount in order toto improve the mental health outcome for children.

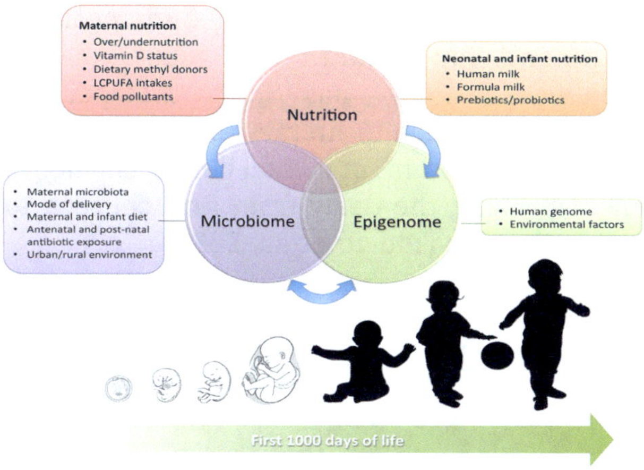

Figure 11.13. The impact of social factors on pediatric psychiatry and behavioral health.

Source: https://library.fiveable.me/_next/image?url=https%3A%2F%2Fstorage.googleapis.com%2Fstatic.prod.fiveable.me%2Fsearch-images%252F%2522Genetic_and_nutritional_influences_on_child_development_nature_vs._nurture_epigenetics_and_nutrition_impact.%2522-fped-05-00178-g001.jpg&w=750&q=75.

Structural racism causes systemic barriers that affect Indigenous and Black children disproportionately, indicating the impact of historic trauma on their mental health. Current research has illuminated the mental health crisis in these populations, highlighting the need for culturally sensitive mental health services that address and act on the specific concerns of these groups. Making available quality mental health treatment, as well as establishing programs targeting violence prevention, housing stability, and increased educational opportunity, can foster resilience and well-being. Lastly, full understanding of social influences is required fore interventions in an effort to foster healthy behavioral development among all kids (Ruth et al., 2022) (Figure 11.13).

11.6.1. Influence of Family Dynamics on Mental Health

Family relationships are crucial to assessing the mental health status of children and adolescents. Family interactions will also ascertain whether the family promotes a supportive or stressful and conflict-ridden environment. For instance, effective interaction among family members in terms of warmth, acceptance, and communication is associated with reduced instances of anxiety and depression in children. On the other hand, highly conflicted or dysfunctional families typically unknowingly contribute to a child's mental health problems. It has been proven through research that the prevalence of adverse childhood experiences (ACEs) significantly impacted the emotional lives of children, a fact that has been highlighted by efforts to diagnose and cure these experiences in pediatric centers, a case that is highlighted by New Hampshire's efforts to recognize the role of ACEs and social determinants of health towards defining a child's mental horizon (Corvini et al., 2018). In addition, the family interaction style and coding assessment yield essential data about family dynamics that can influence pediatric mental health. The Family Interaction Macro-coding System (FIMS) is a powerful tool for measuring family member interaction patterns that provides clinicians with important information about family cohesion, conflict, anng styles. It has been demonstrated by research that a number of the dimensions measured by FIMS, such as parental acceptance and family cohesion, are related to children with chronic conditions, such as, such as spina bifida and type 1 diabetes mellitus, in an emotional and behavioral adjustment manner. These findings justify the role of family functioning in the predictioild mental health, thereby making it necessary that pediatric mental health professionals include such as, such assessments within practice (Alemzadeh et al., 2010). Given that mental health challenges are faced by children, careful examination of family dynamics cannot be overlooked. With increasing focus placed on holistic therapies in pediatric psychiatry and behavioral health, it is important to consider the role of familial relationships. Improving communication within the family, decreasing conflict, and increasing overall family resilience can directly result in profound enhancements in mental health status for youth patients. Interventions focused on parents' and caregivers' parenting training in optimal parenting skills and community support networks have been promising in creating improved family environments. Ultimately, an interwoven model with the involvement of families in the process of treating mental illness is capable of leading to more effective and sustainable outcomes in pediatric mental health, ultimately growing a healthier generation (Corvini et al., 2018).

11.6.2. Socioeconomic Factors and Access to Care

The interaction between socio-economic variables and access to healthcare resources is an important concern in pediatric psychiatry and behavioral health. Reduced socioeconomic status (SES) has been found to be related to increased access barriers in the form of cost, no insurance, and location challenges. Lower SES families might fail to afford necessary treatment or lack adequate transportation to healthcare centers. This is exacerbated in children with behavioral health issues, who may potentially require ongoing therapy and care. Consequentleduled and missepointments become the norm and compound poor care and worsening mental health (Umutoni Corvini et al., 20252018). To foster equal access to psychiatric treatment, these barriers must be overcome, ultimately enhancing the overall mental health environment for pediatric populations. Apart from this, maternal health literacy is another significant determinant of access to pediatric psychiatric services. Parent and caregiver understanding of health matters plays a crucial role in enabling them to navigate complex healthcare systems and make informed decisions for the treatment of their children. Low levels of maternal health literacy may contribute to significant delays in accessing and receiving treatments for children with mental health problems. Research has shown that parents who have low health literacy are less likely to recognize symptoms of mental illness, and hence might prolong the delay from first concern to real treatment (Idowu et al., 2024).

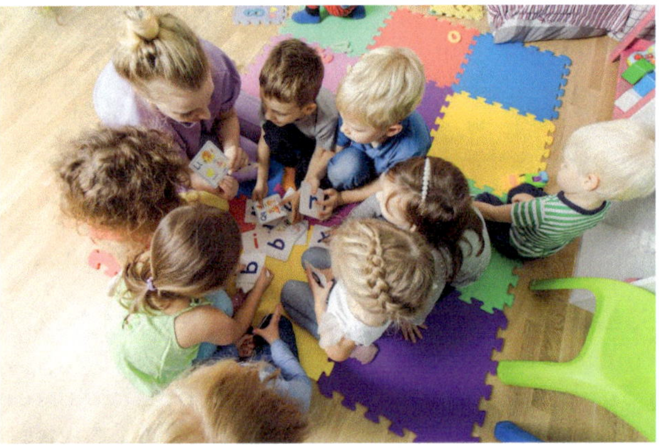

Figure 11.14. Socioeconomic factors and access to care.

Source: https://cepr.org/sites/default/files/styles/og_image/public/voxeu-cover-image/AdobeStock_415403998.jpeg?itok=0E_qYMDX.

Educating parents regarding services available to them and enhancing their ability to communicate well with medical professionals can literally make a tremendous diftimely access to care, directly impacting the effectiveness of treatment for the child patients. In order toTo reduce disparities linked to socioeconomic status and health literacy, combined efforts need to be initiated in making pediatric psychiatric services widely accessible. This includes policy actions geared towards expanding insurance coverage for behavioral health treatment, as well as programs for increasing public transportation access to mental health facilities. Community-level interventions should also target the education of families facing ecid to empower them to seek care for children in a timely mannerpromptly (Qin etal., 2021Umutoni et al., 2025). In addressing the interdependent barriers faced by families, health systems can ensure equitable access to psychiatric services, finally yielding enhanced health benefits among pediatric populations with behavioral health issues (Figure 11.14).

11.6.3. Cultural Considerations in Treatment and Diagnosis

Cultural dynamics are the critical element of diagnosis and treatment for pe illness. Determination of the different backgrounds and histories of children is essential to accommodating providing effective treatment. Children from marginalized racial or ethnic groups, for instance, will have different symptoms or stressors that depend on their background. Omission of these factors could lead to misdiagnosis or ineffective treatment strategies. As the MMWR report has highlighted, children from minoritized communities and those in poverffer high levelsdisparity in receiving care and increasing undiagnosed and untreated mental illness (Ruth Corvini et al., 20222018). Clinicians must therefore place cultural competency at the forefront through training and ongoing learning so that they are equipped to understand and integrate these cultural considerations into practice. Moreover, the impact of structural racism cannot be overstated in determining the condition of chil mental health. Those institutionalized practices intended to maintain inequity may exacerbate stressors which that lead to poor mental tcomes. In Indigenous and Black children, trauma-related experiences associated with historical trauma, such as, such as forced family disruption and institutionalheavily account for high depresicide rates among these populations (Qin etal., 2021Ruth et al., 2022). These problems are resolved by means ofthrough a multifaceted approach that not only recognizes the present-day effects of such trauma but positively seeks to undo the historical injustices involved in healthcare systems. This involves implementing policies that are designed to balance these imbalances, promoting culturally-sensitive interventions, and fostering supportive climates in families that enable caregivers and parents to be active participants in the mental health process. Lastly, successful integration of mental health care into pediatric practice requires awareness of the social determinants that have an important impact on mental health. Socioeconomic status, housing, and safety in the community are important factors in children's mental health and access to care. It has been proven that there is a positive relationship between adverse social conditions and e prevalence oftal health disorders, particularly among poor communities or vulnerable groups (RuQin etal., 2021th et al., 2022). By becoming a more inclusive model of healthcare for addressing these determinants, clinicians are able to create a fairer system for maintaining mental health. This model must highlight the need for collaborative care models, forging alliances of healthcare workers, schools, and community services to develop integrated interventions that are culturally sensitive and able to meet the needs of the pediatric patient.

Test Your Knowledge

1. How do family dynamics influence a child's mental health and emotional development?
2. Why is it important to consider cultural beliefs and values in diagnosing and treating mental health disorders in children?

SUMMARY

Paraphrasing an overview of pediatric psychiatry and behavioral health, one must appreciate the complex interplay between neurodevelopmental disorders and mental health interventions employed in this setting. The overwhelming prevalence of sleep disturbances in children with neurodevelopmental disorders highlights the pressing need for effective behavioral interventions. A systematic review identified effective practices leading to significant sleep health and related behavioral symptom improvement, supporting the effectiveness of interventions that were also tailor-made for such vulnerable children. The observation makes a case for continued research to be in a position to develop more holistic behavio can target such children directly, enabling them to receive proper support (Qin et al., 2021Kamara et al., 2025). Moreover, the analysis of emergency medical services (EMS) transport data calls for addressing the mental and behavioral health needs of children in crisis. Through focusing on the demographic profile and outcome of child and adolescent patients arriving in mental health crisis, especially those exposed to restraint interventions, tencies in current emergency care policies are brought into relief. The study indicated that some groups, such as, such as young males rounded up from schools, had grater demands for restraint transport. Such findings call for reevaluating prehospital care models and emphasizes the necessity of specialty training among EMS professionalhandling and management of behavioral emergencies in a more humane manner (Qin et al., 2021Cummings et al., 2024). The culmination of the observations implies an imperative for an integrated model in pediatric behavioral health and psychiatry that combines early intervention, tailored behavioral interventions, and enhanced emergency response procedures. Continued research and interprofessional collaboration are needed to develop evidence-based practices that can adapt to the eve-changing environment of pediatric mental health. These efforts will not only offer access to mental health care, but also responsiveness to the unique needs of children with a range of behavioral health concerns. Moving forward, developing a culture that prioritizes mental wellness will be essential in promoting healthy development in future generations.

In child psychiatry and behavioral health, it is crucial to understand the efficacy of various treatment modalities in children with anxiety disorders. A fascinating field of study would be the use of D-cycloserine (DCS) as an augmentation strategy for exposure-based cognitive behavior therapy. Research indicates that DCS has a small but significant effect in enhancing the treatment process in children undergoing treatment for anxiety disorders, obsessive-compulsive disorders, and posttraumatic stress disorder. In a systematic clinical trial review, findings indicated that patients under DCS had improved symptom severity compared to placebo, particularly after treatment. Further, the impact of the use of antidepressants concurrently proved to be minimal, suggesting that DCS could operate independently to provide improved outcomes, thus necesearch into patient factors that would maxiize response to this intervention (Qin et al., 2021Altemus et al., 2017). A further crucial field within pediatrics' behavioral health is treating trichotillomania, especially among children. Current research has emerged highlighting the use of computerized response inhibition training (RIT) as a potent intervention. This new intervention directly treats the underlying deficit in response inhibition, allowing young people to learn to suppress the impulsive urge to pull hair. In a randomized control trial, children who received RIT demonstrated a significantly higher response rate and symptom reduction than the waitlisted control group. These findings suggest not just that RIT augments clinical improvement but also functional daily functioning, as shown by lower impairment levels. The sustained therapeutic benefits observed at the one-month foup verify the potential of incorporating such evidence-based interventions into practice in pediatric psychiatry (BauerLee et al., 2018). Treatment approach-behavioral health consequence research is essential to advancing pediatric psychiatry. Both the incorporation of DCS into cognitive behavior therse of RIT for trichotillomania indicate the need for more tailored treatment approaches for managing some psychologicalpsychological states in children. These case studies indicate how tailored and research-informed approaches can lead to extreme symptom control as well as overall lifestyle improvement. Furthermore, the continued investigation into these approaches also suggests the need for continued studies looking to further enhance treatment models. Lastly, successful pediatric psychiatric care is not just dependent on the application of new treatments but eir impacts on the mental well-being of the younger population (Lee et al., 2018Altemus et al., 2017; Bauer et al., 2018).

KEY TERMS FROM THIS CHAPTER

- Adolescents
- Behavioral health
- Cognitive-behavioral therapy
- Geographic
- Mental health disorders
- Pediatric healthcare
- Pediatricians
- Social determinants of health (SDOH)
- Adverse childhood experiences (ACEs)
- Child health
- Community stakeholders
- Medication
- Parental mental health
- Pediatric Psychiatry
- Racial disparities
- Social factors

CRITICAL THINKING QUESTIONS

1. **Which of the following is a core symptom of Attention-Deficit/Hyperactivity Disorder (ADHD)?**
   a. Social withdrawal
   b. Hallucinations
   c. Inattention
   d. Compulsive behavior
2. **Autism Spectrum Disorder (ASD) typically presents with:**
   a. Sudden onset of symptoms in adolescence
   b. Impaired social interaction and repetitive behaviors
   c. Delusions and hallucinations
   d. Aggressive behavior only
3. **Which of the following is a common screening tool for autism in toddlers?**
   a. PHQ-9
   b. Vanderbilt Scale
   c. M-CHAT
   d. Conners' Rating Scale
4. **Which of the following disorders is characterized by frequent temper tantrums, defiance, and argumentative behavior?**
   a. ADHD
   b. Anxiety disorder
   c. Oppositional Defiant Disorder (ODD)
   d. Depression
5. **A 14-year-old presents with persistent low mood, fatigue, and loss of interest in activities. What is the most likely diagnosis?**
   a. Generalized anxiety disorder
   b. Conduct disorder
   c. Depression
   d. ADHD

Short Answer Questions

1. Discuss the diagnostic criteria, clinical features, and management of Attention-Deficit/Hyperactivity Disorder (ADHD) in children.
2. Describe Autism Spectrum Disorder (ASD) in terms of its core symptoms, early identification strategies, and current approaches to behavioral and educational interventions.
3. Explain the causes, symptoms, and management strategies for childhood depression.
4. Discuss the signs, risk factors, and therapeutic approaches for anxiety disorders in children, with a focus on separation anxiety and generalized anxiety disorder.
5. Outline the clinical presentation, etiology, and multidisciplinary management of conduct disorder and oppositional defiant disorder (ODD) in children.

Answer to Critical Thinking Questions

1.(c) 2.(b) 3.(c) 4.(c) 5.(c)

REFERENCES

1. Alemzadeh, R., Fitzgerald, C. J., Greenley, R. N., Holmbeck, G., et al. (2010). Use of an observational coding system with families of adolescents: Psychometric properties among pediatric and healthy populations. https://core.ac.uk/download/213077594.pdf (accessed on 16th June 2025).
2. Bashshur, R. L., Doarn, C. R., Frenk, J., Kvedar, J. C., & Woolliscroft, J. O. (2020). Telemedicine and the COVID-19 pandemic, lessons for the future. *Telemedicine Journal and e-Health, 26*, 571–573. https://doi.org/10.1089/tmj.2020.29040.rb (accessed on 16th June 2025).
3. Lee, H. J., Espil, F. M., Bauer, C. C., Siwiec, S. G., & Woods, D. W. (2018). Computerized response inhibition t). Computerized response inhiband wellbeing outcomes for children and adolescents to inform practice and policy: A review of child self-report measures. Deighton, J., Croudace, T., Fonagy, P., Brown, J., Patalay, P., & Wolpert, M. (2014). Measuring mental health and wellbeing outcomes for children and adolescents to inform practice and policy: a review of child self-report measures. *Child and adolescent psychiatry and mental health, 8*, 14. https://doi.org/10.1186/1753-2000-8-14 (accessed on 16th June 2025).
4. Cavanna, A. E., Holler-Managan, Y., Jankovic, J., Jarvie, D., et al. (2019). Practice guideline recommendations summary: Treatment of tics in people with Tourette syndrome and chronic tic disorders. https://core.ac.uk/download/322826139.pdf (accessed on 16th June 2025).
5. Chang, S. W., Dziura, J., McGuire, J. F., Peterson, A., et al. (2018). Neurocognitive correlates of treatment response in children with Tourette's disorder. https://core.ac.uk/download/213085709.pdf (accessed on 16th June 2025).
6. Corvini, Marguerite; Cox, Katherine; O'Neil, Molly; Ryer, Jeanne EdD; and Tutko, Holly Deblois, "Addressing Childhood Adversity and Social Determinants inPediatric Primary Care:Recommendations for New Hampshire" (2018). *Institute for Health Policy and Practice (IHPP)*. 1. https://scholars.unh.edu/ihpp/1
7. Daviss, W. B., House, S., Olson, A., O'Neil, M., et al. (2017). Attention deficit hyperactivity disorder (ADHD): Survey report. https://core.ac.uk/download/215540988.pdf (accessed on 16th June 2025).
8. Holt, W. (2010). The Massachusetts Child Psychiatry Access Project: re. https://core.ac.uk/download/71352967.pdf (accessed on 16 2025).
9. Lorains, J., Green, J., Hopkins, L., Fry, R., & Moore, T. G., Lorains, J., Green, J., Hopkins, L., Fry, R., & (20252011). Review of the evidence base in relation to early childhood approaches to support children in highly disadvantaged communities for the Children's Ground Project. Prepared by Community Child Health research group Murdoch Childrens Research Institute located at The Royal Children's Hospital Centre for Community Child Health in collaboration with The Royal Children's Hospital Education Institute. https://core.ac.uk/download/pdf/30672649.pdf (accessed on 16th June 2025).
10. Mani, N., & Pavuluri, S. K. (2005). Integrating pharmacotherapy and psychotherapy for pediatric bipolar disorder: Translating science to service. https://core.ac.uk/download/pdf/86380.pdf (accessed on 16th June 2025).

11. Mattingly, M. J., & Walsh, W. A. (2013). Psychotropic medicatiing a stepped-care approach to help severely obese children and young people. https://core.ac.uk/download/pdf/96564473.pdf Sharman, K and Nobles, JD (2016) *Using a stepped-care approach to help severely obese children and young people.* Primary Health Care, 26 (7). pp. 32-38. ISSN 0264-5033 (accessed on 16th June 2025).
12. Qin, H., Steenbergen, N., Glos, M., Wessel, N., Kraemer, J. F., Vaquerizo-Villar, F., & Penzel, T. (2021). The different facets of heart rate variability in obstructive sleep apnea. *Frontiers in Psychiatry, 12*. https://doi.org/10.3389/fpsyt.2021.642333 (accessed on 16th June 2025).
13. Sices, L. (2007). Developmental screening in primary care: The effectiveness of current practice and recommendations for improvement. https://core.ac.uk/download/71350769.pdf (accessed on 16th June 2025).
14. Vente, T. (2024). Antidepressant prescribing practices of pediatric palliative care providers. *Journal of Palliative Medicine*. https://www.semanticscholar.org/paper/48369cecc94ee3244d13d1fc59a0cb4cd7193d25 (accessed on 16th June 2025).
15. Wissow, L. S., Platt, R., & Sarvet, B. (2020). Policy recommendations to promote integrated mental health care for children and youth. *Academic Pediatrics, 21*, 401–407. https://doi.org/10.1016/j.acap.2020.08.014 (accessed on 16th June 2025).

PEDIATRIC PALLIATIVE AND END-OF-LIFE CARE

12

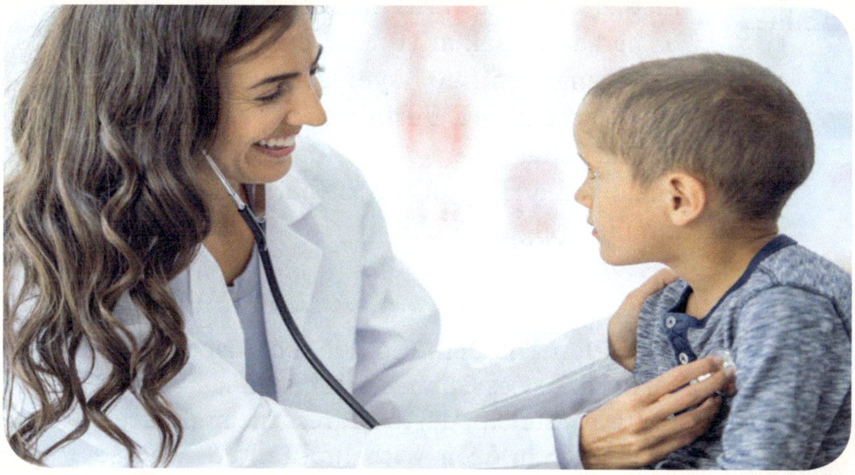

LEARNING OBJECTIVES

After studying this chapter, you will be able to:

1. Discuss the background
2. Describe the principles of pediatric palliative care
3. Point out important conditions that require palliative care
4. Appreciate communication strategies
5. Discuss the issues related to ethics
6. Point out support systems

Introduction

Children's palliative and end-of-life care is a vital nexus of medicine, ethics, and emotional support for children with life-limiting illnesses. While advancing medical technology can preserve the survival of multiple children with serious disease, so does high-quality palliative care service need to increase in parallel. Palliative care extends beyond the relief of mere symptoms to address all of the pediatric population's physical, emotional, social, or spiritual needs. Research has determined that the absence of standardized quality measures weakens the quality of these care services significantly, mirroring the gap between current trends and optimal patieHommes l.Farsi (20252021) reports that there are evolving themes across vareas such as, such as relief from unpleasant symptoms and patient and family experience that capture the necessity to institute structured frameworks for ensuring available and equitable care. The imbalance and unequal provision of pediatric palliative care services are compounded challenges, particularly in countries with diverse geograprains, such as, such as Brazil.

In Brazil, inequality is manifested in the level of access that families have to required health services, leading to the poor administration of patients end-of-life experiences. Findings of a cross-sectional study revealed that the majority of regions lack pediatric palliative care units and have resource shortages in having a specialized team of care providers and necescations, such as, such as opioidsvaro-Lozano Ang et al., 2024). These shortages not only impact the quality of care but impose hugnd psychologicalpsychological burdens on families experiencing these turning points.

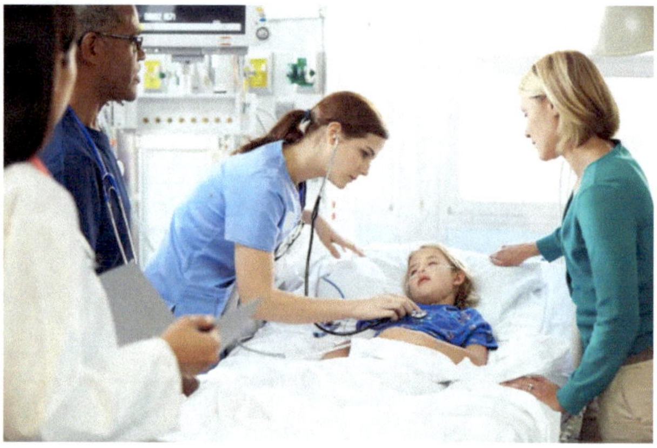

Figure 12.1. Pediatric palliative and end-of-life care represents a critical intersection of medicine.

Source: https://i0.wp.com/news.utk.edu/wp-content/uploads/sites/3/2019/03/palliative1500.jpg?fit=640%2C427&ssl=1.

Mitigating these disparities necessitates a call to action for enhancing the accessibility and delivery of services, thus facilitating an environment that provides the pediatric population with the appropriate care they deserve. In consideration of the future of end-of-life and palliative care in pediatric health settings, there is a need to facilitate ongoing education and institutional transformation of health care facilities. Medical personnel must be equipped with the necessary skills and knowledge needed to deliver quality palliative care, particularly since the delicacies of handling cases involving children evolve. Provisions that facilitate the inclusion of palliative care training in medical school curricula can significantly improve the work performance of health care providers. Besides, local managers of health services must put a high priority on the distribution of resources and employ symptom control and bereavement support approaches aimed at familiÁlvaro-Lozano Ang et al., 2024). All this will go towards the general improvement of pediatric palliative care systems that give children dignified, sympathetic, and well-coordinated care during illness and towards the terminal phase of life, thereby offering an enhanced quality of life for patients as well as families (Figure 12.1).

Definition of Pediative Care

Definition The definition of pediatric palliative care is a very essential element in understanding the integrated model to address the multifaceted needs of children with life-limited illnesses. Pediatric palliative care focuses on relief of symptoms, pain, and distress due to serious illness in the child and family. The integrated model not only considers the child's health care needs but also incorporates emotional, social, and spiritual support. It aims at enhancing the quality of life for the child and assisting families in coping with the complexities associated with serious health conditions. Starting palliative care from diagnosis, rather than delaying it for end-of-life measures, is fundamental in creating models for integrated decision-making between professionals and families, considering the unique experience and needs of each family configu(Álvaro-Lozano Cowfer et al., 2020). As a health care subspecialty, pediatric palliative care is characterized by its multidisciplinary component, consisting of a team of health professionals–physicians, nurses, social workers, and c–who collaboratetogether. With this multidisciplinary structure, there is guaranteed comprehensive care as well as intervention into the multicausal issues that gravely ill children and their families face. Family-centered care is the premise of the practice, wherein the caregivers are actively engaged in care decisions. Evidence suggests that family-centered care models help significantly improve therapeutic outcomes and general well-being for families as a whole by promoting collaboration among healthcare providers and families and ensuring that care plans consider family context and dynamics ((Álvaro-Lozano et al, 202)

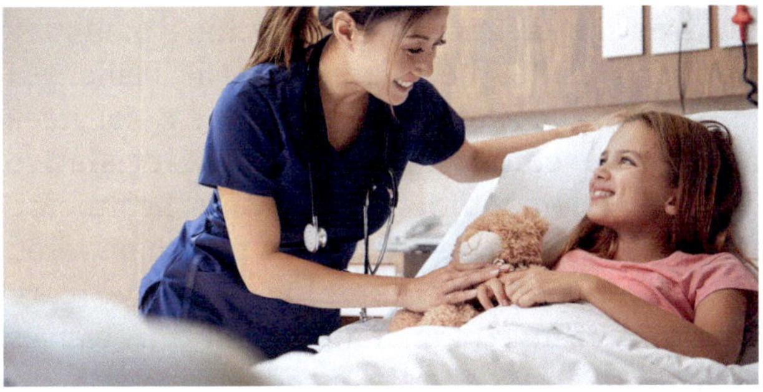

Figure 12.2. The definition of pediatric palliative care.

Source: https://www.ahdubai.com/uploads/departments/732001623128547pall.webp.

Kristina et al., 2019). Education and training in pediatric palliative care for healthcare providers also cannot be overstated. Training programs play an important role in equipping medical practitioners with the necessary competence for responding to palliative and end-of-life issues in a sensitive manner. For instance, communication and role-playing have been identified as the best means of educating students such basic skills, in facilitating enhanced competency in students in addressing difficult conversations with families ((Álvaro-Lozano et al, 22022)Cowfer et al., 2020). Hence, incorporating palliative care principles into medical education is indispensable for preparing future healthcare providers so that they will be adequately prepared to address the diverse needs of pediatric patients and families holistically, thus enhancing the quality of pediatric care offered within the clinical setting (Figure 12.2).

Importance of End-of-Life Care for Children

The user of end-of-life care in children is a key part of pediatric medicine, one that is committed not only to alleviation of physical suffering but to optimizing the quality of life at a most challenging time. This framework of care emphasizes the delivery of tailored interventions that are sensitive to the person's values, preferences, and culture. Central to good end-of-life care is the concept of shared decision-making, where there is active participation by families in discussions on treatment and palliative planning. It is observed in a study that questioning communication, transparency, and cultural issues are essential to builof care(Fisher et al., 2024). By putting these considerations first, health care practitioners can determine that provision of care is patient-specific to each child's unique needs, ultimately creating a sense of dignity and respect during the dying process. In addition, nursing roles in pediatric end-of-life and palliative care are key components of children's and families' experiences. Nurses are often in the leading role, providing not just tment but also psychologicalpsychological and emotional support amidst intense sorrow and uncertainty. A Japanese study highlights a number of areas that are crucial to successful nursing care in this specialty, including symptom control, child-centered pratice, and cultural respect ((Álvaro-Lozano et al., 2022)

Nagoya et al., 2023). These regions focus on the need to develop an overall comprehension of the needs of the child and family for nurses. Besides this, developing a culture where self-reflection about ethical issues is possible allows nurses to make shifts in their practice dynamically so that responsive care is delivered that responds to the evolving needs of the patient and family in real-time. Last but not least, access to a sensitive and compassionate end-of-life care plan for children can have a positive influence on the patients as well as their families. The care can facilitate healthy family interactions, strengthen relationships for the final days, and produce enduring memories even in the midst of bereavement. Moreover, it assures families that their child's dignity will always be assured, a witness to their love and care even during moments of looming loss. The inclusion of supportive bereavement services within this program also serves an integral role in guiding families through the complexity of bereavement following the loss of their child. The provision of these resources to families assists with the healing n combating the psychologicalpsychological impacts of losing a child, leaving a legacy that honors the life of their child and the love shared between their family and child.

12.1. Historical Context

Learning Outcome

1. Evolution of pediatric palliative care
2. Key milestones in the development of end-of-life care
3. Influence of cultural attitudes on care practices

Historical context for pediatric end-of-life and palliative care reveals a complex evolution influenced by changing societal attitudes toward childhood illness and death. Throughout history, children with serious illnesses were often regarded as solely medical issues with little concern given to holistic methods embracing emotional and social considerations. The late 20th century marked a significant shift as researchers and practitioners began advocating for pediatric palliative care (PPC) as integral to treating children with life-threatening conditions. This transition reflected broader trends in medicine towards patient-centered care, emphasizing the importance of including families in the decision-making process. As the PPC story evolved, increasingly it became clear that recognition of the unique needs of children had to occur through an interdisciplinary approach integrating medical care with psychosocial care, leading to novel paradigms of care. In most of the globe, legislatures began to create that formally there was a requirement for pediatric palliative care. For instance, Italy's Law 38/2010 represents an important step towards the creation of far-reaching palliative care services, yet there continue to be challenges in offering equal access to such services across the country. Despite this legislative action, implementation of PPC into healthcare frameworks has also oftentimes been hampered by misconceptions that blur palliative care with end-of-ife circumstances, and thus causes delay in referrals and the starting of treatment. Persistent stigma surrounding PPC has led to physician apprehension as well as family resistance, often leading to children bearing a high symptom burden with inadequate relief. This layering of misunderstanding over time serves to show the necessity of education and advocacy on the part of the medical community and families to advocate for a shift towards an integrated model in which palliative care is recognized as essential, regardless of disease course. In addition, the recent entry of telehealth has brought a new dimension to pediatric palliative care, offering innovative solutions to ancient challenges. The increased level of digitalization of healthcare, spurred by the COVID-19 pandemic, created an environment in which families became receptive to telehealth care for PPC. This shift is particularly significant since it emphasizes the necessity of adapting care solutions according to family structure and needs. Research has indicated that families desire telehealth services that preserve the humanized aspect of care but leverage digital technologies to increase accessibility and accompaniment.

The collective experience of primary caregivers reflects a strong preference for models that not only facilitate communication but also address the emotional and psychosocial demands of life-limiting children. As these technologies continue to progress, there is potential to continue developing care models that honor the past history and embrace new innovations in pediatric palliative care (Álvaro-Lozaet al., 2025; Chelazzi et al., 2025) (Figure 12.3).

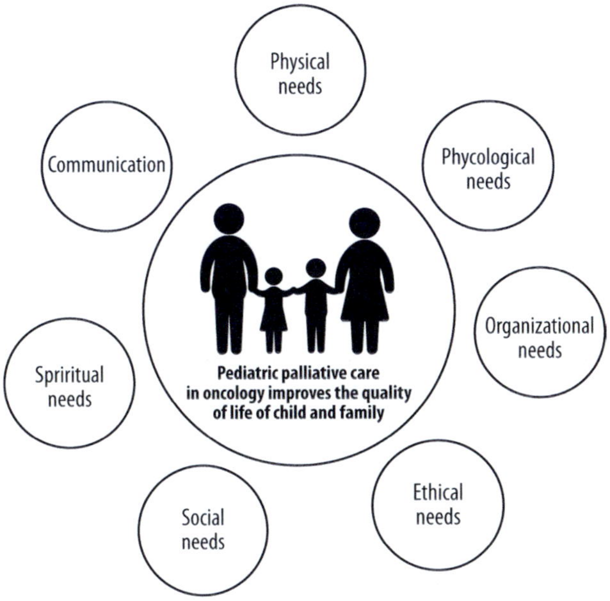

Figure 12.3. The historical context of pediatric palliative and end-of-life care.

Source: https://pub.mdpi-res.com/cancers/cancers-14-01972/article_deploy/html/images/cancers-14-01972-ag.png?1649857185.

12.1.1. Evolution of Pediatric Palliative Care

The evolution of pediatric palliative care over the last decades has seen a significant shift from traditional models focused solely on curative paradigms to a broader paradigm that focuses on quality of life. Initially, palliative care was mostly associated with adult patients, but advances in medicine have necessitated extending palliative principles to children suffering from life-limiting illnesses. With improvements in technology raising survival rates among infants and children with serious medical illnesses, there is increasing recognition of the need to deliver specialized end-of-life care that not only addre but also emotional and psychologicalpsychological needs of these patients and their families. This transition highlights a more widespread acceptance that palliative care can be initiated at any stage in the healthcare pathway, not just eginally thought(Kuchler et al., 2023). A paradigm shift of this nature promotes the necessity of intervening early in optimizing overall patient and family coping outcomes. As the specialty of pediatric palliative care has expanded, so has the recognition of the significant role played by multidisciplinary teams in providing effective care. Pediatric palliative care teams, comprising pediatricians, nurses, social workers, and spiritual care advisors, are formed to provide an individualized system of support based on the unique needs of children and families. Such a model supports collaborative practice that is essential in addressing complex medical, emotional, and social problems of children's illnesses. Further, empirical evidence has demonstrated that the integration of psychosocial care into palliative care can significantly enhance family resilience annd caregiver quality of life(N/A, 2023). This change demonstrates a stepwise progression in medicine, where steps are taken beyond symptom management to add extensive care that focuses on the experience of children and families throughout the path of illness. The global scene of children's palliative care is similarly changing with cultural, ethical, and regulatory environments that guide practice around the globe. In the majority of nations, including Bulgaria, gaps in pediatric palliative care services still persist because of inadequate regulatory standards and staff training (Kuchler et al., 2023). While some nations have implemented comprehensive guidelines and service models, others lag behind in establishing required frameworks for the delivery of quality care. With increasingly apparent growing gaps in pediatric access to palliative care, ongoing efforts should be exerted toward ensuring care both equitability and cultural competency (Álvaro-l, 2020; Buang et al., 2022)

(N/A, 2023). Developing pediatric palliative care, therefore, calls for championing stronger regulatory systems asucating health care providers in order toto ensure all children, regardless of what situation, receive the holistic and empathetic care they are entitled to.

12.1.2. Key Milestones in the Development of End-of-Life Care

The evolution of end-of-life care has itself been significantly shaped by landmark milestones that have reaffirmed the need for comprehensive models in pediatric palliative care. One such milestone was the establishment of hospice care during the late 1960s, with its combined model that addressed the entirety of dying patieith a focus on pain control, psychologicalpsychological support, and family involvement. This model laid the basis for specialty care that would be aimed at children with life-limiting disease.

It was in the early 2000s that pediatric palliative care was integrated as part of medical school education, following the mandate established by the Liaison Committee on Medical Education. This development was fueled by increasing awareness of the shortcomings in the education of health professionals regarding end-of-life discussions and managing complex medical decisions in the vicinity of pediatric patients, which recognized a premier area of teaching that still exists today (Álv; Buang et al., 2022)

(Jeffers et al., 2021). There has also been additional advancement in pediatric end-of-life care through elaborate palliative care guidelines that recognize the specificity in the needs of children. Importantly, in 2002, the inclusion of the World Health Organizations definition of palliative care emphasized ensuring quality of life and care for the patient as well as the patient's family. This complete understanding changed the language and approach to pediatric palliative care, inviting a physical, emotional, social, and spiritual approach. Within this paradigm, education specifically for medical physicians has been a key component in enhancing communication skills and training in humane bad news delivery. This cultural shift in patient care is underpinned by the movement toward a systemic commitment to changing end-of-life experiences of children thand policy revisions(Montserrat et al., 2020).

Also, recent initiatives have strived to bridge the large gaps in pediatric end-of-life care by innovative curricula and direct experience during residency training. An example of these is the Johns Hopkins University School of Medicine Transition to Residency program, Internship, and Preparation for Life Events (TRIPLE) curriculum, which uses multimodal strategies to prepare students for end-of-life discussions. This broad curriculum not only focuses on decision-making models and communication skills but also incorporates emotional elements of end-of-life conversations with families of patients. In evaluating the effectiveness of such training programs, the curriculum reflects a progressive strategy for empowering future healthcare providers and developing an encouraging environment for sensitive pediatric palliative care conversations. Lastly, such milestones portray the process of transformation towards enhancing pediatric palliative and end-of-life care through implementation of rigorous educaaradigms so that practitioners are in a place position to provide empathic, quality care (Á020; Buang et al., 2022)(Jeffers et al., 2021) (Figure 12.4).

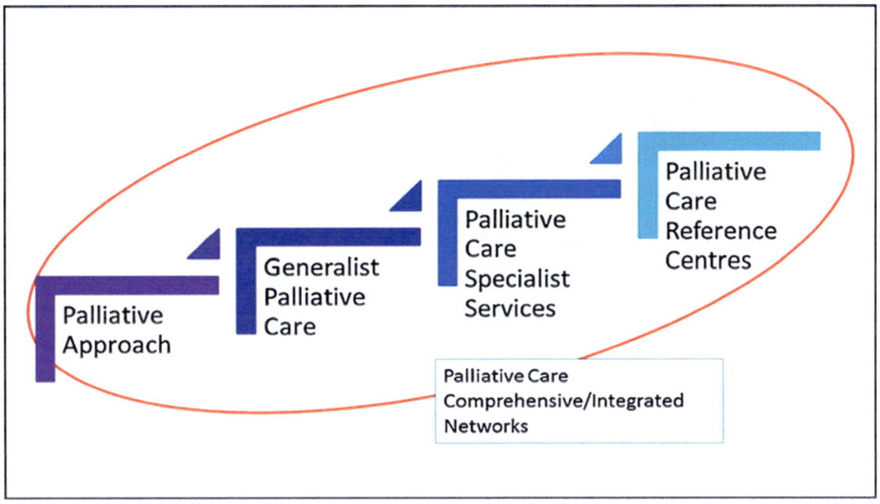

Figure 12.4. Key milestones that have underscored the need for comprehensive approaches in pediatric palliative care.

Source: https://media.springernature.com/lw685/springer-static/image/chp%3A10.1007%2F978-3-319-77740-5_2/MediaObjects/333544_1_En_2_Fig1_HTML.png.

12.1.3. Influence of Cultural Attitudes on Care Practices

Cultural perceptions have a significant impact on practice and organization of pediatric palliative and end-of-life care. Such beliefs manifest in family treatment options, caregiving roles, and the acceptance of palliative care options. For instance, in some cultures, death is strictly forbidden, and hence there's resistance to embracing palliative care, which is synonymous with giving up hope.

This cultural reluctance might interfere with the prompt referral to adequate care services. As suggested by research on cancer patients from different backgrounds, poor knowledge and negative attitudes towards palliative care can lead to poorer experiences in care, ultimately affecting patient quality of life. It is crucial that health praare aware of these cultural nuances in order toto develop mechanisms that are receptive to beliefs held by families and yet ensure the application of palliative interventions among children (Zhang et al., 2025). Secondly, the conjunction between religion and healthcare beliefs plays a pivotal role in shaping attitudes toward end-of-life care practice. Religious beliefs in the majority of cultures dictate perceptions about suffering, dying, and the acceptance of medical intervention. For example, some families would have to choose between spiritual healing or traditional forms of remedy over scientifically proven palliative care, making it difficult for healthcare professionals to fully support them. Qualitative studies on healthcare leaders have shown that moral and us convictions shape views of practices such as, such as Medical Assistance in Dying (MAiD), where cultural acceptance is largely disparate. As the medical narrative proceeds toward patient-centered practice, an understanding of these nd cultural backgrounds is required in order toto enable practitioners to navigate challenging discussions and adapt care to honor family values and utcomes in pediatric patients(Yee et al., 2025). Finally, education and awareness campaigns are a crucial element in filling the gaps created by cultural inclinations toward palliative care. There are many healthcare providers who lack the cultural competency needed to effectively engage with diverse populations, and thus, there is a mismatch between family expectations and care practice. By community outreach that is specifically focused on raising awareness regarding palliative care and its benefits, healthcare systems can strive to dispel myths and reduce stigma. Furthermore, a partnership with cultural leaders and opinion influencers in communities can encourage a more harmonized relationship between healthcare providers and families undergoing pediatric palliative care. This partnership not only respects cultural mindsets but also reinforces the functions of full care options for children on the verge of death, in the long run enhancing the care quality and assistance provided (Álvaro-Lozano et al, 2020; Buang et al., 2022).

Test Your Knowledge

1. What have been the key milestones in the development of pediatric palliative and end-of-life care?
2. How have cultural attitudes shaped the practices and acceptance of pediatric palliative care?
3. Why is understanding the historical evolution of palliative care importrent pediatric care models?

12.2. Principles of Pediatric Palliative Care

Learning Outcome

1. Holistic approach to treatment
2. Focus on quality of life
3. Family-centered care

Pediatric palliative care philosophy is grounded in a holistic and compassionate approach to caring for children with life-changing illness. The centerpiece of this specialty is the ethical principle of beneficence, which is to do what is best for the child. This bedrock principle is what guides healthcare providers to make difficult decisions regarding withholding or withdrawal of life-sustaining therapies. In neonatal and pediatric intensive care unit situations, such decisions are usually delicately resolved ethical dilemmas that require a nuance of the child's clinical status, parental wishes, and potential for significant quality of life. By focusing treatment on the best interests of the child, professionals have to make their way through the emotionally charged terrain of end-of-life care without abandoning ethical justification for the actions taken and the values of the family (Diana et al., 2025). Interdisciplinary practice is crucial to meeting the many challenges involved in the discipline. In addition to the medical team, also engaged in the palliative process is a multidisciplinary team that includes psychologists, social workers, and spiritual counselors who play equally crucial roles in assisting the family to cope through the palliative process. For instance, pediatric psts can help resolve ethical complex issues, such as, such as disagreement between families and the medical team on treatment or disclosing unfavorable prognosis (Schneider et al., 2022). These experts enh continuum by providing emotional and psychologicalpsychological support, thereby aiding families to overcome loss and bereavement. Consequently, the integration of various perspectives within this cooperative model guarantees complete and respectful care that is culturally and personally sensitive to the belief system of the family. The integration of culturally defined practice is another crucial tenet of pediatric palliative care that recognizes the profound impact of belief on culture in guiding decision-making. Families have specific belief, tradition, and values that profoundly influence their attitudes towards suffering, illness, and end-of-life care.

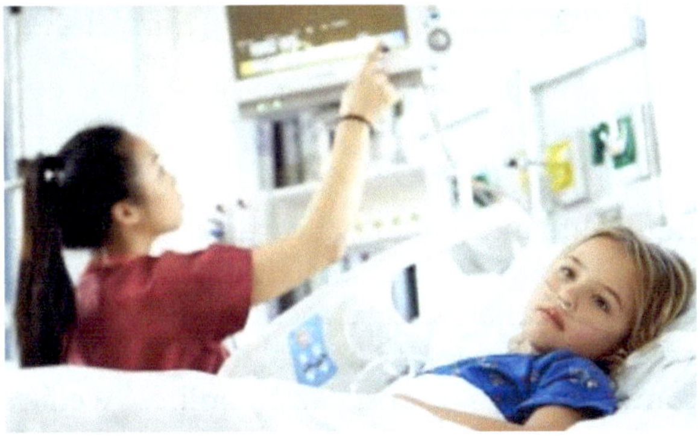

Figure 12.5. The principles of pediatric palliative care are grounded in a compassionate and holistic approach to treating children with life-limiting illnesses.

Source: https://www.rn.com/siteassets/blog/nursing-news/understanding-pediatric-palliative-care.jpg.

Understanding such cultural determinants, healthcare providers are able to modify their practice to meet the specific needs of each child and family in a more holistic care environment. In addition, recognizing tral variation might affect ethical dilemmas, such as, such as dissimilar reactions to plans of care, highlights the importance of effective communication and teamwork between the palliative care team and family (Schneider et al., 2022). In general, by keeping cultural sensitivity at center stage, pediatric palliative care providers can maximize delivery of care, affirming the principles of dignity, respect, and compassion throughout the palliative journey (Figure 12.5).

12.2.1. Holistic Approach to Treatment

In pediatric palliative and end-of-life care, the holistic treatment strategy is the imperative model of managing the multifaceted needs of children with life-threatening illnesses. This type of approach acknowledges that a child's illness experience encompasses more than the pmena; it also encompasses the emotional, psychologicalpsychological, social, and spiritual experiences. Optimal care is the convergence of a variety of therapy modalities that cumulatively have an additive effect on the general health of the child and familiesnstance, utilizing traditional healing systems such as, such as Ayurveda can have an institutional support system that not only addresses physical pain but also facilitates empowerment of families through education and shared decision-making. By establishing an environment in which mainstream and complementary approaches exist together, palliative care teams are better positioned to address the complex needs of their juvenile patients and provide a more respectful dying experience (Nariyal et al., 2025). Holistic delivery of pediatric palliative care also demands an interdisciplinary team approach, in which physicians from different specialties collaborate to formulate holistic care plans. This framework enables consideration not only of the mef the child but also of the spiritual and psychologicalpsychological care needs of the family as a whole. Good communication plays a critical role to ensure that the values and preferences of both child and family are being respected throughotreatment process. Moreover, referencing models such as, such as the WHO's Global Dementia Action Plan can provide valuable direction in building robust care continuity that includes holistic approaches. Nevertheless, though much has been accomplished to include holistic care in many healthcare settined practice gaps still need to be addressed in order toto make palliative services accessible and integrated at full capacity

(Nakanishi et al., 2024). Notably, the comprehensive care approach of pediatric palliative care is also consistent with the use of culturally sensitive practices congruent with beliefs and traditions. Integration of elements such as, such as Ayurvedic life practices can promote patient comfort and well-being through individualized care that not only aims at physical symptoms but also emotional and spiritual comfort. For instance, such practices as Dinacharya, with an emphasis on healthy daily habits, are able to ground families during the chaos of illness. By making people stronger and providing stress management techniques, these holistic practices are able to lift the psychic burden associated with end-of-life care. Overall, througg a holistic model, pediatric palliative care is able tocan offer an understanding and holistic system of support that honors each child's depth of unique journey and enables dignified care at lno et al, 2020; Buang et al., 2022)(Nariyal et al., 2025).

12.2.2. Focus on Quality of Life

Quality of life is an important concept for pediatric end-of-life and palliative care since it focuses on the overall welfare of the patients with life-limiting illnesses. Unlike the traditional medical disciplines where cure from disease is the foremost priority, palliative care focuses on relief from suffering and quality of life enhancement. Palliative care extends beyond physical health to include emotional, social, and spiritual, which significantly contribute to patients' and families' welfare. A complete appreciation of quality of life in such a setting must consider individual patient and family needs because these can have a profound impact on patient experience and outcomes.

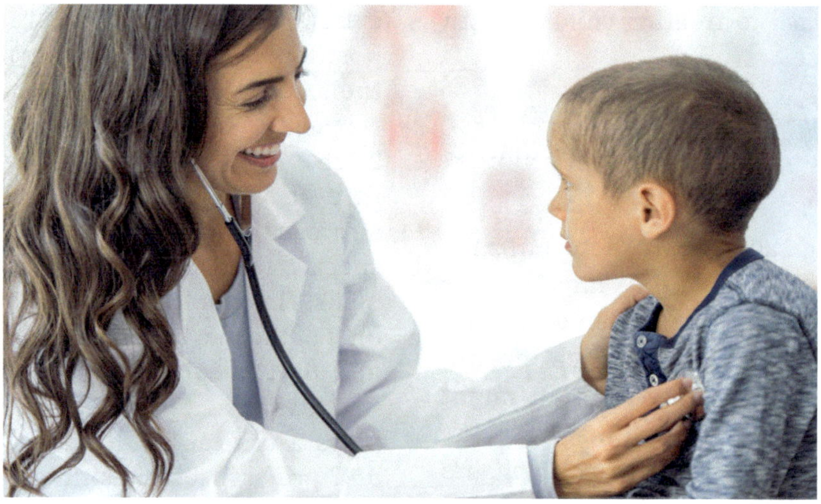

Figure 12.6. Pediatrician listening to a young patient's heartbeat during check-up.

Source: https://cancercommons.org/wp-content/uploads/2019/10/Doc-and-boy-patient-1-scaled.jpg.

The emerging literature calls for the implementation of standardized quality measures that assess several domains of pediatric palliative care to ensure that interventions are tailored to enhance comfort and dignity and opife in children with terminal illness (Hommes et al., 2025Farsi, 2021). Effective pediatric palliative care interventions strike a balance between the need for reduction of symptom distress and the psychosocial and social determinants of quality of life.

These families also report persistently high levels of emotional distress, exacerbated by the unpredictable nature of their child's illness. As a consequence, quality measures must assess family experience, identifying support systems that may act as protection from distress. It has been ted that addressing the psychosocial needs of care, such as, such as bereavement support and explicit communication about end-of-life wishes, can significantly enf life for patients and their families (Hommes et al., 2025Farsi, 2021). Cultural, ethiiderations also play a role in deciding the manner in whichhow care is delivered, necessitating a deepach family's unique values and beliefs (Hommes et al., 2025Farsi, 2021).

Additionally, the moral implications of quality-of-life measurements run into issues of respect and dignity for the individuality of the patients. The world of pediatric palliative care must move towards a knowledge of the patient's subjective experiences and how the patients' identities control their wi the end of life. For instance, neglecting variables such as, such as gender in caregiving interactions may precipitate ethical crises and impacts on the perceived dignity of the patient. Life-limited children requiring home hospice care must be aware of such concerns, ensuring that care delivery professionals receive training to appreciate the significance of personal identity in holistic care delivery. Such education not only affects the caregiver's reaction to ethical issues but also asserts the importance of placing the familys and child's welfare at the forefront, thereby contributing to improved quality of life in pediatric end-of-life care (Figure 12.6).

12.2.3. Family-Centered Care

Underlying pediatric end-of-life and palliative care is the philosophy of family-centered care, recognizing that families play a critical part in the treatment and decision-making for their critically ill children. Families are proactively involved in this process so that their experiences and wishes are used in incorporating care plans that honor the child's desires and needs. Good family-based care guarantees a partnership relationship between families and health care providers, and this includes open communication and shared decision-making. The engagement is not only important in respecting the culture and values of tfamily but also in enhancing the general quality of care to for the pediatric patients. As pediatric palliative care clinicians strive to increase patient and family outcomes, the implementation of family-centered care practices becomes essential to maximizing holistic, compassionate care along the illness trajectory ar critical transitions at the end of life(Buang et al., 2022). Incorporation of family-centered care principles into pediatric palliative settings offers families a perception of support and comprehension, thereby increasing care satisfaction. Healthcare professionals can enhance this interaction through extensive training in communication skills and methods to deal with the unique challenges of seriously ill families. An educational curriculum for the teaching of medical students and residents palliative care communication skills is essential in highlighting the importance of comprehending the family's experience as well as the determination of their goals and values. Case-based discussion and role-play educational programs have been found to greatly increase the confidence of medicng in sensitive discussions with families(Cowfer et al., 2020). Placing families at the center stage enables healthcare providers to ensure that care plans are not only patient-focused but also responsive to family problems, hence improving the quality of care. The commitment to family-centered care extends beyond caction; it addresses the long-term emotional and psychologicalpsycholos during and after the child's illness. Support for bereavemenBereavement support becomes part of this model of care since families often suffer from intense loss as a result of the death of a child. By offering ongoing care in the ways of counseling, resources, and community outreach, medical staff are provided the means to guide families through their experiences and find a path of healing. The integration of bereavement support into the offerings of pediatric palliative care demonstrates the need to consider the family as a unit rather than as a single patient. This integrated model of care has a profound effect on how families cope with loss and adjust to life post-illness, illustrating the central connection between effective family-centered care and the emotional well-being of individuals with pediatric aro-Lozano et al, 2020; Buang et al., 2022)(Buang et al., 2022).

Test Your Knowledge

1. How does a holistic approach enhance the effectiveness of pediatric palliative care?
2. Why is the focus on quality of life central to palliative care for children?

12.3. Common Conditions Requiring Palliative Care

Learning Outcome

1. Life-limiting illnesses in children
2. Chronic conditions and their impact
3. Role of palliative care in managing symptoms

Pediatric palliative care is increasingly important due to an array of long-term illnesses that necessitate ongoing management and care of symptoms. Commonly, children with complex chronic conditions (CCC) are burdened with serious health issues that tend to create life-limiting circumstances. Findings indicate that neuologic and neuromuscular diseases are prevalent among children requiring palliative care, as evidenced in one study that indicated over half of the cases presented these specific conditions (Bisen et al., 2024). Hematologic and immunologic diseases are also prevalent conditions, which form the basis of the complex symptomology that such children experience, serving to point to the need for complex and individualized care approaches. By recognizing these shared conditions, physicians can more effectively advocate for early palliative interventions, thus enhancing the quality of life for children and families affected by these conditions. In the pediatric community, the incorpo palliative care among children with varying medical needs, such as, such as those having irreversible but not progressive conditions, becomes instrumental. The ACT/RCPCH grading system identifies a high proportion of child patients falling within category 4, which encompasses children with ve disabilities that demand high support levels(Bisen et al., 2024). The children are prone to having a variety of symptoms that can impede functioning and the quality of life, and as such, a multidisciplinary care system is warranted. Care of such complexities rnly advanced medical treatment but also emotional and psychologicalpsychological treatment for the family and child, with a supportive environment to encourage utmost health and quality of life as the children face their individual circumstances.

The role of nursing experts in delivering pediatric palliative care is important since they usually find themselves in the middle of patient interaction. A narrative of nurses' experience delineates an array of emotions involved with the care of children with life-limiting illness, underscoring the requirement of proper support systems and resource facilitation.

The interplay between nurses' emotional suffering and compliance with provision of quality palliative care underscores the challenge involved with this crucial practice issue. In a bid to bring about a good death for their children, nurses must undergo ongoing education and policy development. Addressing these emotional needs will not only enhance the quality of care provided but also ensure that pediatric patients receive their entire needs effectively addressed (Álvaro-Lozano et al, 2020; Buang et al., 2022) (Figure 12.7).

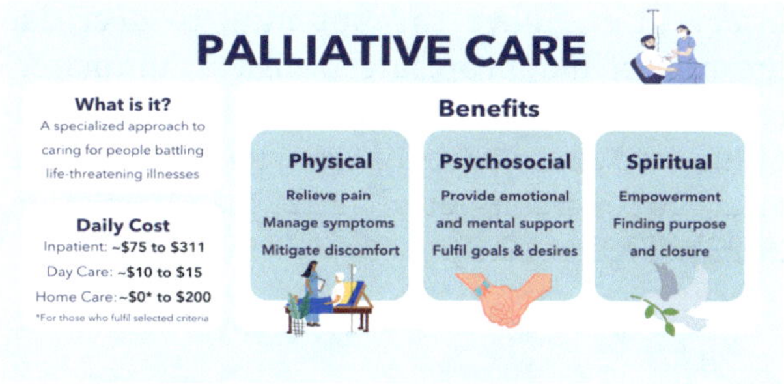

Figure 12.7. Common conditions requiring palliative care.

Source: https://www.homage.sg/wp-content/uploads/2019/12/wordpress-feature-image-49.png?v=1626167335.

12.3.1. Life-limiting Illnesses in Children

The phrase life-limiting illness in children is a general term for a variety of conditions that severely impact not just the sick child but his or her family and care-givers as well. These diseases or disorders are those that significantllife span of the patients, leading to complex medical, psychologicalpsychological, and emotional problems. Approximately 21 million children across the globe require palliative care to manage life-limiting or life-threatening illness at any given time. The enormous number underlines the urgent necessity for full-range pediatric palliative care (PPC) systems that can effectively meet the multifaceted needs of such patients. By putting alleviation of suffering and improvement of quality of life first, PPC aims to assist children and families on the illness trajectory, emphasizing interventions on time and greater communication among professionals. Pediatric end-of-life care becomes essential as health professionals face the delicate balance between curative treatment and palliative care. According to recent studies, palliative care services referral would be optimal at the time of initiating a life-threateningn waiting when curative interventions have failed(Benini et al., 2022). Such forward thinking allows families to openly discuss goals of care, aligning medical treatments with the family's desires and establishing a more compassionate environment during challenging times. Moreover, such referrals early in the course of the child's disease can have far-reaching benefits for both child and family, as it supports an integrated approach to care which addresses not only the physical but also the emotional, social, and spiritual needs of the child's life. The impact of life-limiting illness on the family overall is far-reaching and insidious. Families coping witl prognosis of a child typically go through a pattern of psychologicalpsychological loads, including grief and anticipatory loss, which are further added to by the complicated medical decision-making entailed in such chas (Álvaro-Lozano et al, 2020; Buang et al., 2022)(Benini et al., 2022). Healthcare professionals must acknowledge communication and family support dynamics present in these settings since they play an important role in influencing overall care experience. Besides, equal access to PPC services is crucial, particularly where resources are scarce. With the standards of PPC shifting at an international level, with a focus on culturally responsive models of care and education of healthcare professionals, there is the possibility for improved outcomes, with families being provided with the care that they need as they manage issues around life-limiting conditions in children.

12.3.2. Chronic Conditions and Their Impact

Chronic conditions bear a major impact on the trajectory of pediatric patients, necessitating extensive palliative and end-of-life care interventions addressing their unique needs. Chronic conditions often lead to complicated clinical cases involving intricate physical, emotional, and social concerns. Pediatric patients with chronic diseases may undergo frequent hospitalization and consultations by health care providers and multiple switches in their treatment strategies, which adversely affect their quality of life. This is compounded by the emotional stresses of the families, who have been navigating healthcare systems, making complex decisions, and advocating for their children's rights in the face of daily uncertainties. As indicated, the numerous acute and chronic medical care demands of this population often contribute to repeated hospital transfers during the final stages of life, further dilutin palliative care and exacerbating their suffering(Lanpher et al., 2025). Compounding the crisis of chronic pediatric diseases is the COVID-19 pandemic, which imposed yet another burden on affected families. Parents point to heightened fear over the health condition of their children as well as concern regarding threats from COVID-19 exposure, especially for those children with existing vulnerabilities. The COVID-19 pandemic strained healthcare resources, thus further complicating the provision of continuous and accessible palliative care. Families often ended up juggling public health protocols while tryingmaintain commitment and support towards their children at times of focifocus. Qualitative life histories of parents during this phase show that despite the fact that they went through a lot of adversity, strong support groups were key in helping them cope with their circumstance ality of life as a top priority to their children(Rapoport et al., 2023). The long-term consequences of childhood chronic disease are more than immediate medical issues; they demand redoing models clude a systems model addressing physical, emotional, and psychologicalpsychological needs. Early advance care planning must start, particularly in children who will need transfers to dying care. By allowing for discussions regarding treatment priorities and preferences, care can be individualized by healthcare professionals to address families' values and improve the quality of care delivered. In addition, creating a caring environment with sufficiently trained staff in palliative and hospice care can greatly benefit children with chronic illnesses. These interventions have the potential to decrease the risk of inappropriate transfers, ultimately resulting in a more humane and supportive end-of-life care experience for thisn ((Álvaro-Lozano et al, 2020; Buang et al., 2022)Lanpher et al., 2025) (Figure 12.8).

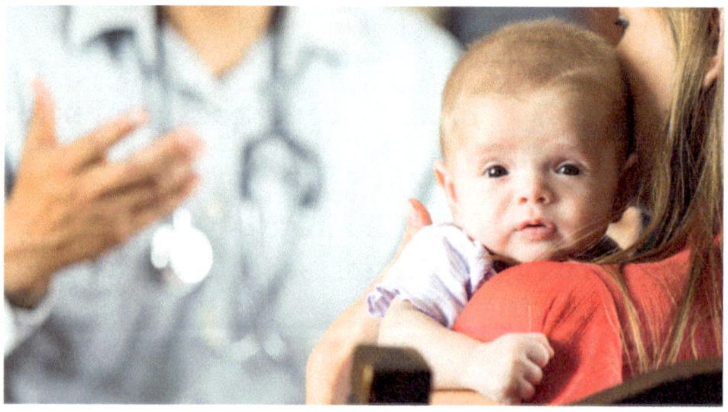

Figure 12.8. Infant held by parent during a medical consultation.

Source: https://www.apa.org/images/chronic-illness-child-title-image_tcm7-245299.jpg.

12.3.3. Role of Palliative Care in Managing Symptoms

Palliative care is instrumental in symptom management for children who are suffering from terminal illnesitizing the optimization of quality of life, palliative care is able tocan address the complex nature of symptoms that this population expptoms among children in this context can become physical, psychologicalpsychological, and social in nature, requiring an all-encompassing approach from healthcare professionals. Th comprehensive strategy of palliative care is particularly significant, in that it addresses not only pharmacological treatment but also supportive interventions developed in response to the unique needs of children and their familsing practice into the palliative care setting, Schroeder et al. (2017) Research prescribes, emphasizes the worth of holistic, person-centered care, particularly in the delivery of distressing symptoms that children may encounter throughout their course of disease. Besides, the multidisciplinary team has a significant function in pediatric care of this nature, such that numerous perspectives are considered when managing symptoms. Physicians, social workers, chaplains, and nurses typically constitute the team and leverage their respective areas of expertise and know-how in creating an effective care plan. Nurses, in particular, are in the lead in offering palliative care and possess the clinical competence to carry out sophisticated symptom evaluations and offer fused communication. The utilization of evidence-based criteria, such as, such as those presented by (Judy et al., 2016), when enacted, supports having a systematic approach to facilitate symptom management plans that are crucial in improving the quality of children patients' lives. The synergy ensures that the care is sustained and responsive, addressing the evolving needs of children as they traverse illness. Ultimately, effective palliative care can significantly enhance the overall experience of pediatric patients and families by prioritizing symptom management in a supportive and empathetic manner. Prioritizing symptom relief not only eliminates physical suffering but also alleviates emotional and spiritual suffering, resulting in an integrated model of care. This multi-dimensional modality is necessary, particularly at the end-of-life, as families are presented with highly complex decision-making regarding treatment options. Incorporating palliative care principles into children's environments emphasizes the importance of caring for families and patients across difficult journeys, indicating the necessity of quality, compassionate care to achieve optimalliative and end-of-life care. The data within (Schroeder et al., 2017) once more demonstrates the critical role nurses have in making such care possible, indicating their key position within the multidisciplinary team process.

Test Your Knowledge

1. What are some examples of life-limiting illnesses in children that may require palliative care?
2. How do chronic conditions affect the physical and emotional well-being of pediatric patients?
3. What role does palliative care play in managing symptoms and improving comfort for children with serious illnesses?

12.4. Communication Strategies

Learning Outcome

1. Importance of effective communication with famili prognosis and treatment options
2. Addressing emotional and psychologicalpsychological needs

In pediatric palliative and end-of-life care, effective communication strategies become a priority in the development of understanding and support among patients, health professionals, and families. These strategies facilitate emdialogue about complex as well as traditionally traumatic issues such as, such as emotional ramifications of future loss, end-of-life choices, and treatment options. The integration of a family model is particularly relevant in pediatric care as it allows for family members to engage in collaborative decision-making. Research has found that when healthcare professionals collaborate with families, patient and caregiver satisfaction rises, whichement of both patients' and caregivers' well-being(Jeffers et al., 2021). Understanding the varying dynamics between different types of family structurw providers must tailor conversation so that emotional and psychologicalpsychological components are adequately addressed. Training of healthcare providers in communication competencies targeted toward end-of-life discussions is a key component of pediatric palliative care education. Programs like the Transition to Residency, Internship, and Preparation for Life Events (TRIPLE) at Johns Hopkins University have instituted modules on communication skills that are specifically geared to address pediatric end-of-life issues. Such programs enhance the skill of medical graduates in having effective conversations about advanced care planning, goals of care, and the emotionalng about death and dying with children and families(Jeffers et al., 2021). This practical learning is finally locked in in an organized method where learners practice real-life scenarios, thereby becoming confident and skilled in initiating difficult conversations. Lastly, the emphasis on communication strategies remains a core pillar in facilitating the possibility of healthcare providers delivering compassionate and empathetic care throughout end-of-life scenarios. Primarily, it is imperative to realize that communication within pediatric palliative care settings also extends beyond oral communication. The non-verbal communications, including body gestures, facial expressions, and attentive listening, are essential in establishing rapport and trust with families in difficult situations.

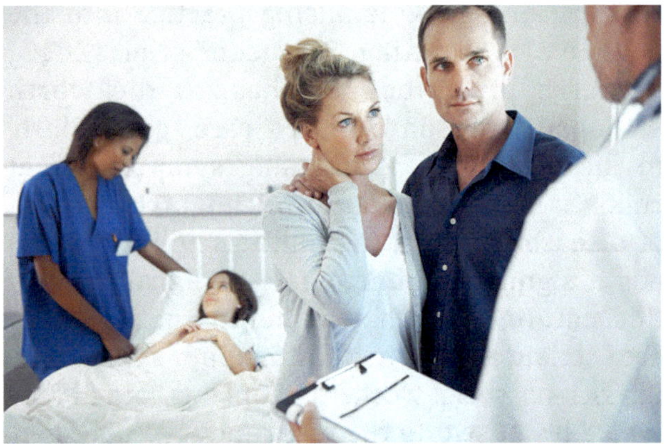

Figure 12.9. In pediatric palliative and end-of-life care, effective communication strategies are paramount in fostering understanding and support among families.

Source: https://paediatricpalliativecare.org.au/wp-content/uploads/2021/12/GettyImages-175534897-1.jpg.

Literature identifies the value of healthcare professionals possessing a sensitivity to non-verbal communication, which is likely to convey much information about a family's emotional state and readinessto address sensitive topics. Engaging multi-modal communications skills, —ranging from sympathetic listening to employing visual aid that illustrate complex medical information in a comprehensible manner, —can enhance understanding and levels of comfort among families faons (Álvaro-Lozano et al, 2020; Buang et al., 2022)(Kristina et al., 2019). The general goal of all such communication methods is to create an environment where children and their families feel heard, validated, and attended to in their care and, consequently, their experience and outcome in pediatric palliative and end-of-life care are improved (Figure 12.9).

12.4.1. Importance of Effective Communication with Families

Effective communication with families is an essential element of pediatric end-of-life and palliative care. The emotionally charged nature of end-of-life discussion necessitates more than the delivery of medical facts in aat; it demands the delivery of empathetic comprehension of the psychologicpsychological distress experienced by families during such challenging times. A trust-based relationship empowers families to feel at ease with asking questions, raising concerns, and defining their preferences regarding their child's care. Such a connection fosters a spirit of joint decision-making, which enhances the experience for the patient as well as for the family. A profound understanding of family values and dynamics allows clinicians to tailor their communication strategy such that dialogue remains attuned to the unique cultural and emotional contexts in which families are likely to operate. Furthermore, effective communication becomes a crucial tool for closing the gaps that are often present in pediatric palliative care. Families across most regions may lack adequate access to relevant information or support services, and this can lead to desperation and isolation. With proactive approaches to communication, healthcare providers can bridge this divide and ensure that families are well informed about the palliative care options available. As demonstrated through efforts like Taking Care of You in Colombia, where systematic analysis helped improve the delivery of services, good communication could increase care coordination among various medical services. Not only does this ensure that families receive holistic and comprehensive support, hem navigate complex healthcare systems more effectively(Garc et al., 2020). Ultimately, the integrated care approach for pediatric palliative care is backed by the engagement of families in decisions around end-of-life care. Placing high value on open communication, healthcare providers make sure the opinions and wishes of family members are considered in treatment plans, upholding their values and choices. This open approach dampens anxiety and uncertainty, allowing families to have open and productive discussions concerning their child's care a the future. Good communication about advance care planning is imperative – ; it can make what would otherwise be a painful process easier to tolerate for families with difficult decisions to make. Thus, prioritizing communication not only enhances the quality of care but also serves an underlying ethical requirement to treat families with dignity and respect in tmoments (Álvaro-Lozano et al, 2020; Buang et al., 2022)(Wearne et al., 2020).

12.4.2. Discussing Prognosis and Treatment Options

Talking with the child about prognosis and treatment strategies is a complex and sensitive process requiring high levels of attention to both medical data and the psychosocial context of the families. Effective communication skills are required to convey the facts about the child's condition without inducing despair or distrosis of the child has significant implications for decisions about treatmenttreatment decisions. The healthcare professionals must have this discussion with sensitivity to ensure they incorporate the values and preferences of the family. Such discussions are not only about the clinical issue but also encompass emotional support as families navigate through difficult choices concerning their child's care. Involvement of the family gives them a space to express their concerns and feelings, critical for shared decision-making and individualized care. Language of preference plays a significant role in the way families feel and interact when it comes to prognosis and treatment. The evidence indicates that families with different language backgrounds can be confronted with obstacles that influence their comprehension of palliative care interventions and end-of-life decisions. For instance, a ve study identifies disparities faced by Spanish-preferred families, such as, such as poor interpreter services and confusion rega, leading to dissatisfaction with the process of care(El-Atoum et al., 2025). Healthcare providers must observe these disparities and make a sincere effort to bridge the gap in communication. By employing culturally competent meds and ensuring interpreters are always present, clinicians may establish on trust and enable greater communication of treatment options. This approach not only serves the family's language needs but promotes a more equitable healthcare experience. The ethical implications of reporting prognosis and treatment options are important, particularly in pediatric intensive care units. As pointed out by many guidelines,ence is the primary decision-making in such a casedvance the advancement of the binterests of the child(Diana et al., 2025). Physicians are burdened with the ethical choices while making the appropriate interventions or discussing the potential for withdrawal of life-sustaining treatments. Care decisions should therefore be driven by a double concern for enhancing quality of life as well as respect for the values and wishes of the family. Additionally, as one engages in interactions with families, it becomefor one to provide an in-depth consideration of potential results in order toto enable caregivers to make informed decisions based on their ethical and moral standards about the care of their child. These integrative discussions establish a respectful environment and help families handle the emotional burden when they are facing challenging circumstances (Álvaro-Lozano et al, 2020; Buang et al., 2022) (Figure 12.10).

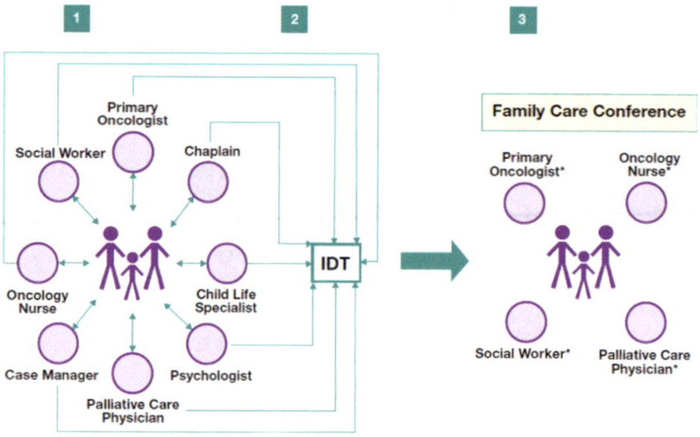

Figure 12.10. Engaging in discussions about prognosis and treatment options for pediatric patients with life-limiting conditions.

Source: https://pub.mdpi-res.com/children/children-05-00040/article_deploy/html/ima05-00040-g002.png?1569922069.

12.4.3. Addressing Emotional and PsychologicalPsychological Needs

In pediatricand palliative care, the successful address of the emotional and psychologicalpsychological needs of both the child and family is of utmost importance. The child with a life-limiting illness will experience a gamut of emotions, including fear, grief, overlaying their understanding of illness and death. Such psychological distress calls for a personalized intervention that integrates psychologicalpcal support as part of the overall model of care. Strategic treatment, such as, such as providing mental health support and promoting open communication about feelings and fears, can promote emotional resilience. In addition, the families may also go through various emotional challenges as they journey through this difficult process, which makes clinicians need to offer psychoeducation and coping strategies that promote family cohesion and emotional wellbeing during the palliative process. Given the fact that most interested parties are engaged in proper pediatric palliative care, understanding the psychosocial dynamics of family members is crucial. The needs of not only the child but also siblings, grandparents, and primary caregivers must be identified and honored. Since grandparents normally constitute an integral part of family support systems, researching their emotional experiences can help understand how to ll family dynamics. With the use of instruments that evaluate the psychologicalpsychological needs of family members, as in recent research, can substantially improve the quality of care delivered. Through evaluation of family dynamics from a perspective that incorporates grandparental views, clinicians can tailor interventions to address each member's individual emotional needs, engendering resilience and a feeling of belonging during this significe period (Nogueira et al., 2024). The application of holistic practices such as, such as those demonurveda to pediatric palliative care also serves the emotional and psychologicalpsychological needs. The holistic nature of Ayurveda, considering the interconnectedness of physical, emotional, and spiritual well-being, makes it a beneficial addition to traditional palliative practice. This approach makes possible the integration of therapeutic interventions and lifestyle modifications that promote emotional health, emphasizing the pivotal role of integrative care in enhancing the quality of life in children and their families. As reslve to make the application of such complementary methods (Nariyal et al., 2025) possible, the need for interdislaboration becomes all the more apparent so that the emotional and psychologicalpsychological needs of all are met within an integrated care framework that is attuned to the diverse cultural beliefs and practices.

Test Your Knowledge

1. Why is effective communication with families essential in pediatric palliative care?
2. How should healthcare providers approach discussions about prognosis and treatment options with parents and caregivers?
3. What communication techniques can be used to address the emotional and psychological needs of both the child and their family?

12.5. Ethical Considerations

Learning Outcome

1. Decision-making in pediatric care
2. Balancing treatment and comfort
3. Role of advance care planning

Ethics play a prominent role in the practice of pediatric palliative and end-of-life care, especially in consideration of the unique complexities surrounding the treatment of children and young people with life-limiting illnesses. Practitioners must balance an ethereal tightrope betwen humane care and observed ethical boundares. These are values of beneficence, —acting in the best interest of the child, —and respect may be most challenging in pediatric settings where children lack the capacity tocannot express wishes. Family dynamics must also be considered; family members typically serve as advocates for the child and their input can significantly impact treatment choices. Studies evidence the necessity for such knowledge of family interaction, suggesting that commu to ethical decision-making in pediatric healthcare settings (Hommes et al., 2025Farsi, 2021). Ethical child end-of-life care is also made more complex by the various perspectives on life-supportive treatments and the withdrawal of such care. Due to the diverse cultural, ethical, and legal settings where the choices are being made, health practitioners have to rely on guidelines that provide consistency in ethics and transparency. According to recent reviews, the ethical principle of beneficence remains a centrin decision-making, with the essence of ensuring that the decisions concur closelylosely concur with the child's best interests.

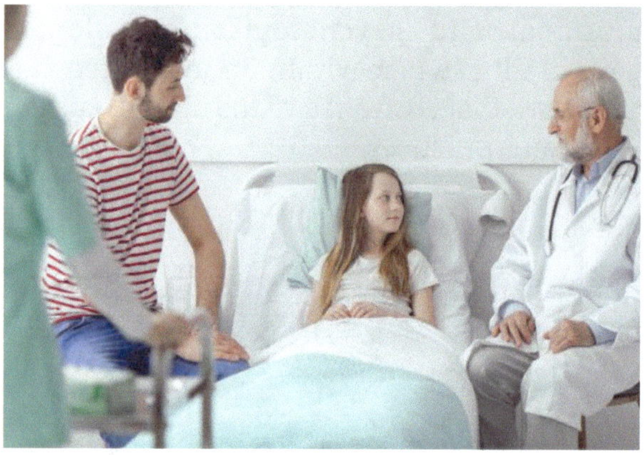

Figure 12.11. The pediatric palliative and end-of-life care, ethical considerations are paramount.

Source: https://media.istockphoto.com/id/1249594222/photo/spending-time-with-a-patient.jpg?s=612x612&w=0&k=20&c=mIELfWs2_tBeU3-QWBvcMg78hdKFa9XurcNDXktKuLU=.

It is continued in the neonatal and pediatric intensive care units with recommendations where success relies on meticulous thought by medical teams, families, and sometimes even the patients, tderstanding of the implications involved with end-of-life care(Diana et al., 2025). In addition, the fields of quality measures included in pediatric palliative care provide a model for evaluating ethical issce. These regions range from the alleviation of suffering symptoms to psychologicalpsychological and spiritual needs that cumulatively highlight the holistic approach to care and comfort at life's end. Ethical issues are most often experienced in attempting to reconcile quality of life with the realities of a child's illness. Integrating cultural as well as ethical factors into patient care practices guarantees advancing equitable and accessible care. The ongoing progress and synchronization of quality measures across these domains not only enhance patient outcomes but also entrench ethically sound practich dignity and comfort in the vulnerable end-of-life experience (Hommes et al., 2025Farsi, 2021) (Figure 12.11).

12.5.1. Decision-Making in Pediatric Care

Decision-making in pediatric end-of-life and palliative care is profoundly difficult, in which an equally sensitive balance needs to be made between family desires, medical ethics, and the specific needs of the child. Beneath this decis the ethical precept of beneficence, whereby healthcare professionals must perform act in the best interests of the child. This is most important in neonatal and pediatric intensive care units, where physicians too frequently are confronted with challenging decisions regarding withholding or withdrawing life-sustaining treatments. A systematic review of the literature concerning the subject identified 38 ethical positions that underpin decisions to withhold or withdraw such interventions, with widespding giving prior welfare of the child in the process(Diana et al., 2025). The clinicians therefore have to face both the medical realities and ethical subtleties in a manner that their decision-making represents the interest of the vulnerable pediatric patients. At the center of good decision-making in pediatric medicine is the collaborative approach known as shared decision-making. This strategy is representative of the importance of involving the family in discussion for options of treatment, deciding on medical interventions in manners that are consistent with the child's culture and values. When doctors and other healthcare providers use exploratiication, they establish an environment where families feel they are being promoted encouraged to express their beliefs, values, and concerns. A patient-centered review of shared decision-making in palliative pediatric care has illuminated key factors, including theians and families, open communication, and cultural competence(Fisher et al., 2024).

These collaborative frameworks not only enhance decision-making but also ensure that practiced care aligns with the family's definition of quality of life. Finally, the shared decision model highlights the ethical responsibility of healthcare providers to support families in making severely difficult decisions. The intersection between the ethical principles and shared decision-making processes is critical in shaping pediatric palliative and end-of-life care. Where treatment modalities may produ varying degrees of physical distress and quality of life, teams should make the utmost of open discussion concerning potential outcomes. By careful weighing of family preferences along with clinical recommendations, medical personnel can foster a climate of trust and respect. The outcome of these efforts is decision-making that enhances the dignity of the child and maximizes the role offamily throughout the care process. As the literature outlines, this practice does not only affirms the best interestf the child but also prioritizes the emotional and cultural needs of the family in atro-Lozano et al, 2020; Buang et al., 2022)(Diana et al., 2025; Fisher et al., 2024). Balancing these elements is critical in caring and morally sound care delivery in pediatric settings.

12.5.2. Balancing Treatment and Comfort

Within pediatric end-of-life and palliative care, the tension between treatment and comfort is at its greatest. Providers must navigate the intricacies of providing functional medical therapy while also ensuring that the child's quality of life is maintained. The specific needs of pediatric populations necessitate a subtle approach that typically favors symptom relief and emotional support over maximal therapy.

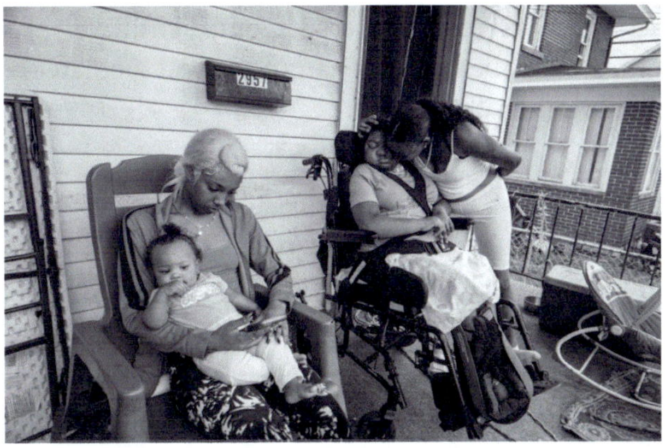

Figure 12.12. Balancing treatment and comfort.

Source: https://i.natgeofe.com/n/0b6a0126-5442-48aa-b6f8-d67642583060/MM9963_220905_03626.jpg.

Attaining such balance demands an interdisciplinary collaborative process wherein healthcare professionals, families, and even the children themselves collaborate to establish treatment goals that respect the patients values and preferences. Such a method focuses on comfort not only as the absence of pr as a multifaceted experience encompassing emotional, spiritual, and psychologicalpsychological comfort. Merging medical progresses with compassionate care is vital in achieving equilibrium in a treatment strategy. Allergen immunotherapy, for instance, demonstrates the need for tailoring medical interventions to suit the needs of the pediatric patient. When treating children against allergies, doctors and medical personnel must exercise extra caution to c their comfort levels and associated discomforts arising from interventions such as, such as subcutaneous injection or sublingual administration. This balance is critical in pediatrics, where patients may become even more anxious about receiving care. Moreover, compliance with treatment is often linked to a child's sense of comfort and trust with his or her caregivers. Thus, when children perceive that their caregivers care about their comfort as much as effective treatments, children are more likely to engage actively and positively in their healthcare.

Finally, healthcare technology and social media add new dimensions to the weighing of treatment against comfort. Internet forums offer families and healthcare professionals rich soil for information sharing and emotional release, significantly enhancing palliative care. With increasing literature emerging that recognizes the multifaceted benefits of incorporating technology into pediatric care, it is imperative that healthcare professionals embrace these tools responsibly. They must uphold the ethical principles of electronic communication while remaining committed to individual, compassionate care. Merging traditional methods of care with advances in technology is capable of providing an environment in which childrent only the necessary medical treatment but emotional sustenance as well in order toto positively cope with the complexities of pmproving their experience and quality of life (Farsi, 2021; Montserrat et al., 2020) (Figure 12.12).

12.5.3. Role of Advance Care Planning (ACP)

ACP is critical in pediatric palliative and end-of-life care because it helps families and clinicians to engage in meaningful conversations about the medical treatment preferences of children with life-limiting conditions. Early initiation of such discussions helps families articulate their values, beliefs, and care goals, which ultimately guide decision-making processes. This anticipatory planning not only enhances the quality of care but also minimizes the ethical dilemmas that may be elicited when treatment is in dispute among medical practitioners, atudy examining ethical challenges in pediatric palliative care (Megli et al., 2025). Ensuring that families and children are actively involved in those conversations enhances the likelihood of synchronizing medical interventions with the expressed wishes of families, thus ensuring dignity in the end-of-life process. Moreover, effective advance care planning is also a key factor in maximizing the emotional well-being of families navigating the challenges of pediatric palliative care. Treatment choice decisions are overwhelming, especially for families facing the reality of the child's condition. Open communication and can eliminate some of the anxiety involved with such decisions(Lucinda et al., 2025). Participants in planning report higher satisfaction with the care that they experience and are more likely to be able to make informed choices in a moment of utmost need. This ongoing discussion is not only vital to ensuring that medical care is in keeping with the family values but also to enhancing overall quality of life for the child and family, paving the way for a more compassionate care process. In addition to improving emotional outcomes, advance care planning is also instrumental in diffusing the logistically-driven issues present for families in end-of-life care. A systematic ACP process enables transparent care pathways and conveys the familys preferences to everyone on the health care team so that continuity of care can be maintained. It is particularly important in the process of transfer over a continuum of health care settings, for example, from children's hospitals to hospice or home care. The openness provided by advance care plans can significantly curtail the possibility of miscommunication, which is often a source of distress during critical jc palliative care (Álvaro-Lozano et al, 2020; Buang et al., 2022)(Megli et al., 2025). By successful implementation of ACP, healthcare professionals can provide a supportive environment that not only honors the child and family's wishes but also constructs collaboration among the interdisciplinary care team, which eventually leads to better outcomes in pediatric palliative and end-of-life care.

Test Your Knowledge

1. What ethical challenges arise when making medical decisions in pediatric palliative care?
2. How can healthcare teams balance life-prolonging treatments with the child's comfort and quality of life?
3. What is the significance of advance care planning in guiding ethical decisions for pediatric patients?

12.6. Support Systems

Learning Outcome

1. Role of healthcare professionals in palliative care
2. Importance of community and social support
3. Resources available for families

Support systems are an integral part of children's palliative and end-of-life care and are employed for families as well as children in challenging circumstances. Support systems comprise a range of emotional, social, and medical support that is specially tailored to meet the unique neen with serious illness. Good support can really help alleviate families' psychologicalpsychological distress as they navigate challenging care decisions. Here, medical professionals have to engage not only to care for patients but also to foster a sense of community and belongingness. This integrated approach is pivotal since the emotional burden of pediatric terminal illness necessarily leads to heightened experiences of isolation and helplessness on the part of caregivers, so emphasizing the need for robust support systems to facilitate supportive coping and enhance overall family resilience (Rashid et al., 2020). Moreover, the function of support systems extends beyond the confines of immediate family to community health facilities and multidisciplinary health practitioners. These professionals involve doctors, nurses, social workers, and counselors who collaborate in me compounded needs of children. Through technology and communicalatforms, such as, such as telehealth services, healthcare providers are able to avail provide timely interventions and access to resources that may otherwise be inaccessible to troubled families. For instance, telemedicine was a lifeline during the COVID-19 pandemic and allowed health workers to extend services to patients and families from distant locations, ensuring emotional care is maintained regardless of geographical distance(Downing et al., 2018). Such innovation highlights the importance of support systems that are flexible in responding to emerging healthcare needs while also maintaining child and family health. Lastly, successful support systems in pediatric palliative care design and implementation should be focused on the overall needs of families and patients.

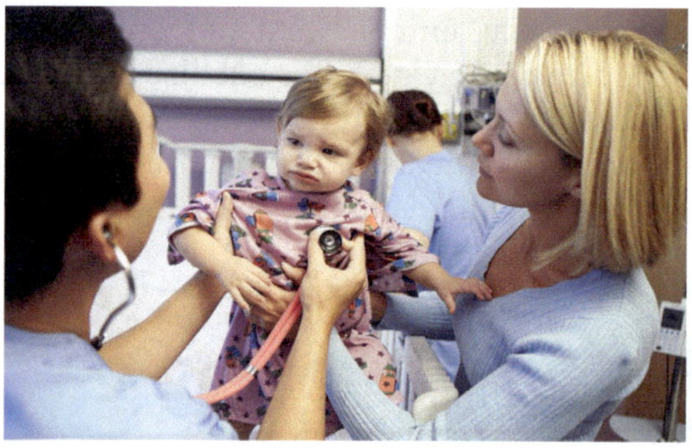

Figure 12.13. Support systems play a pivotal role in pediatric palliative and end-of-life care.

Source: https://cdn.ps.emap.com/wp-content/uploads/sites/3/2019/10/nurse-with-child-and-mother-in-hospital-.jpg.

This entails addressing physical symptoms, mental health, and emotional issues within an integrated care framework that targets all areas of patient experience. Continuing assessment and family feedback loops can provide valuable information on the effectiveness of such systems so that health care practitioners are able to modify and refine their approaches. By establishing a nurturing system in forced to feel appreciated and understood, pediatric palliative care has the ability tocan profoundly impact the quality of life during some of the most difficult moments, maintaining the indelible importance of remaining connected and com face of adversity (Álvaro-Lozano et al, 2020; Buang et al., 2022) (Rashid et al., 2020) (Figure 12.13).

12.6.1. Role of Healthcare Professionals in Palliative Care

Pediatric palliative care is very much in need of an interdisciplinary approach by healthcare professionals because the multifaceted nature of treating a child's physical and emotional needs might be too complex. The healthcare team typically consists of physicians, nurses, social workers, and psychologists who are all valuable and play highly specialized roles. Physicians are involved in medical management and symptom control and making critical treatment decisions. Nurses, most often on the frontline, provide the care and monitor the condition of the patient closely, providing essential information to child and family in difficult times. This multidisciplinary approach is not only employed to maintain medical needs but also to develop a system of support for families coping with the emotional burden of end-of-life decisions and experiences. The role of the social worker in pediatric palliative care is the key to addressing the psychosocial needs that significantly affect families. They assist in addressing the emotional needs, provide guidance on accessing healthcare services, and assist in making informed decisions while experiencing challenging circumstances. As stipulated in the study on the role of social workers in pediatric palliative care, their contribution encourages family autonomy and addresses significant psychosocial needs, which are sometimes excluded in traditional medical practice. But such specialists are faced with obstacles, structural and hierarchical as well, that could impede their co-operation as members of multidisciplinary teams. Validation and definition of the roles of the social workers by policy changes would ease their integration into pediatric palliative care and lead to a higher general quality of the services provided to the patients' families. Healthcare professionals' own quality of life is most crucial, particularly in the emotionalironment of pediatric palliative care. Nurses, for example, may be facing extreme psychologicalpsychological and physical stress attending terminally ill children anrting their families' bereavement and grief. Research shows that complementary therapies such as, such as Reiki have a buffer effect on this burden, avoiding some of the emotional burnout and increasing physiological variables in nurses. The use of self-care interventions not only improves the health practitioners but indirectly aids in providing better quality care to patients. Building a healthy work culture that prioritizes staff mental health will build a stronger, more resilient healthcare system better able to meet the comprehensive needs surrounding pediatric end-of-life care, whke everyone involved, including the children and their families, better off (Hern et al., 2025; Zucchetti et al., 2023).

12.6.2. Importance of Community and Social Support

The importance of social support and community in the area of pediatric palliative and end-of-life care cannot be overstated, as these networks provide invaluable informational, emotional, and practical assistance to the families struggling with the intricacies oess. Families involved in pediatric palliative care often have to face such a high psychologicalpsychological load, supplemented by their child's ailment and impending loss. At such trying moments, the work of community resources, viz. support groups, counseling services, and education programs, becomes crucial. Besides offering a chance for the interaction of families with similar circumstances, these resources equip individuals with coping mechanisms as well as resilience strategies and with information. The integration of social support systems produces a sense of belongingness and relieves isolation, finally enhancing the well-being of caregivers and family members at an unusually vulnerable moment. Holistic palliative care should therefore emphasize the establishment of such community networks and the provision of holistic support to families. The integration of social workers into pediatric palliative care also demonstrates the different benefits of community integration. Social workers are instrumental in bridging health care and families' psychosocial needs, providing emotional support, navigation through resources, and advocacy. According to research on the social workers' role in pediatric pa, professionals are instrumental by assisting families in dealing with emotional and psychologicalpsychological challenges, which prove more difficult at the end-of-life stages (Hern et al., 2025). Their experience with leading family conferences and taking patients through options for care guarantees not only that families are informed but also assisted in making decisions. Having trained social workers available provides families with access to valuable resources that remove some of the tension associated with palliative care, validating the need to incorporate social services into the pediatric patient's health care model. Moreover, paramedics play a significant role in community-based end-of-life and palliative care with their involvement in ensuring healthcare continuity.

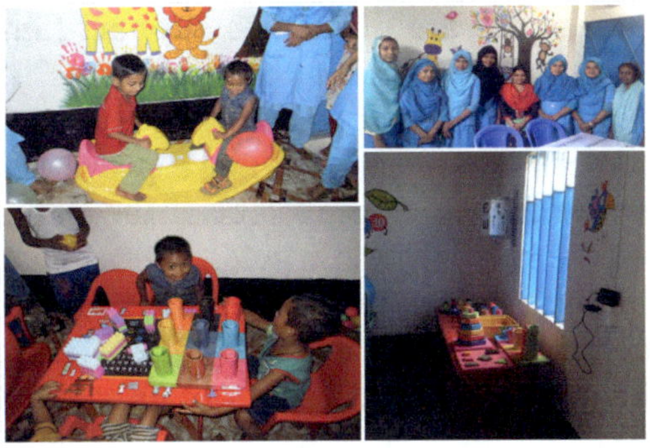

Figure 12.14. The importance of community and social support within pediatric palliative and end-of-life care.

Source: https://journals.sagepub.com/cms/10.1177/11786329231162996/asset/c8526486-8905-45e8-afb0-1c3c04e8e02d/assets/images/large/10.1177_11786329231162996-fig1.jpg.

Their expanding roles in the delivery of specialized care accentuate the impuch professionals with end-of-life communication and family dynamics training(Alanazy et al., 2025). Effective social support programs that involve paramedics can significantly influence families' perceptions of care in a way that they are heard and valued in their circumstances. By developing community support initiatives that involve paramedic services, families can get comprehensive care that entails medical treatment as well as emotional support. This coordinated response not only consolidates the provision of pediatric palliative care but also encompasses a collective societal response to end-of-life concerns, reaffirming the essential role that social support plays in alleviating the burden of families at such critical junctures (Figure 12.14).

12.6.3. Resources Available for Families

The pediatric palliative and end-of-life care process can be challenging for families emotionally and practically. There are available resources that are needed to support families through the difficult process, including informational, emotional, and practical assistance. It is becoming more prevalent for health centers to employ specialized palliative care teams comprehensive guidance on managing complex medical cases, addressing the physical and psychologicalpsychological needs of the child as well as their family. These groups can include doctors, nurses, social workers, and spiritual care professionals who collectively work to customize acute care plans that are responsive to family values and goals. Importantly, the incorporation of bereavement services within these models enhances resilience and helps families in their process of grieving, affirming the Eight Priorities developed by bereaved the importance of emotional support during and after the illness of their child(Holly et al., 2021). In addition to the assistance of medical professionals, various sites and organizations provide a multitude of resources that educate families about pediatric palliative care. Some of them include information sites and support groups that connect families with common problems. Parents may utilize workshops or webinars introducing effective coping strategies and emotional care. Also, specialty palliative care agencies have a tendency to gather collections of resources, offering literature that not only includes medical guidance but emotional preparatory materials for dying as well. Facilitating growing awareness and understanding, these resources help families become involved in care decisions, becoming integral to the discussion of their child's treatment. Strategic education and outreach work to bridge the ces and families and enable families to advocate for their child's needs effectively(Yu et al., 2020). Community-based support programs are also vital in augmenting the resources for families under pediatric palliative care. Local charities commonly fund retreats, camps, and activities specifically for parents and siblings that engender a sense of community and shared experience. These events then become unstated therapeutic communities where families can relate and exchange their current strife and triumph. Financial assistance programs are also needed to mitigate the economic burden of requiring extended care, so families can focus on emotional healing rather than economic distress. Collaboration among healthcare workers, civic groups, and policymakers is vital for maintaining such crucial resources, ultimately achieving enhanced well-being of families in end-of-life care (Álvaro-Lozano et al, 2020; Buang et al., 2022)(Holly et al., 2021; Yu et al., 2020).

Test Your Knowledge

1. How do healthcare professionals contribute to providing emotional and physical support in pediatric palliative care?
2. Why is community and social support crucial for families of children receiving palliative care?
3. What types of resources and services are available to assist families during palliative care?

SUMMARY

The pediatric palliative and end-of-life care is an increasingly important component of children's healthcare with life-limited conditions. As the needs of pediatric populations are increasingly multifaceted, it becomes imperative to adopt a comprehensive approach that includes shared decision-making, effective communication, and empathic respect for the values and wishes of children and their families. Fisher et al. (2024) puts especial emphasis on involving families in the development of purposeful goals of care that are compatible with cultural values, beliefs, and personal preferences. This not only enhances the quality of care provided but also fosters an environment of caring in which families feel empowered and more engaged in the decision-making process, fundamental to confronting the emotional challenges of serious illness. Furthermore, the heterogeneity of palliative sedation therapy practices is a reflection of the challenges faced in providing equal and quality end-of-life care to the pediatric population. Current studies are alluding to the diversity in protocols and they for moxtensive PST guidelines in pediatric settings, particularly in hospitals. Lipsitz Cuviello et al. (20222024) unmasks that while a great majority of hospitals have specialized palliative and pain management teams, end-of-life care standardization is fraught with difficulty and expectation. This variability might stimulate doubt in families at already traumatic times, representing a vital necessity for higher levels of training and education for healthcare providers who work in pediatric palliative care. Lastly, the integration of palliative care philosophy in all aspects of treatment for children ensures a holistic strategy to their care, including symptom control, emotional support, and shared decision-making. While the caregivers and healthcare providers are striving to enhance practice, it becomes vital to foster teamwork between families and professionals. The findings indicate that with the forward march of pediatric end-of-life and palliative care, ongoing research, education, and policy revision are required to bridge practice gaps, standardize interventions, and ultimately enhance the quality of life of children and families through these incredibly challenging experiences. It is only with devotion and joint efforts that the practice can proceed, offering compassionate care that truly honors the dignity and desires of young patients and their families.

The integration of palliative care in children's institutions is important in ensuring enhanced quality of life for children with life-limiting conditions. Research has established that parents of children dependent on dialysis are informed of the potential advantages of palliative care, although the majority do not hold preconceived notions regarding the necessity of the same. One such study of healthcare providers found that while a large majority of them acknowledged the benefits of palliative care, there remain impediments to its application in pediatric nephrology. Specifically, fears of healthcare providers stemming from apprehensions that the initiation of palliative care indicates a failure to pursue cure are not mirrored by the caregivers, who find the palliative consultations valuable. This conflict underscores the importance of increased education for healthcare providers regarding the role of palliative care in children's healthcare (Lipsitz et al., 2024). End-of-life care is not the only focus of pediatric palliative care; it is an integration that strives to reduce suffering through the best possible symptom control and emotional support for patients and families. In Bulgaria, inequality in palliative care services has been reported, with studies revealing insufficient set medicl standards and insufficiently trained personnel. The existing situation reflects significant barriers,uding insufficient staffing, the lack of regulations, and insufficiency of special training, which —that hamper the provision of quality palliative care. To overcome these discrepancies, there is an urgent need for more intensive training programs that place healthcare providers in the necessar der holistic care to pediatric patients with long-term diseases or disabilities (FarsiKuchler et al., 20232021). Finally, the success of end-of-life and palliative care in pediatrics depends on a solid foundation based on interdisciplinary care and family supptified by recent research, care regulation principles must conform to international standards in order toto guarantee improvements in the quality of delivery and accessibility of care. Effective care practices must also be informed by the experience of families, who undergo complex emotional and practical dilemmas. Proper training for healthcare professionals in palliative care will allow them to respond more effectively to the diverse needs of children. By building a culture that values and understands palliative care as an integral aspect of pediatric health, we can enhance the qudren and families with difficult medical courses (Farsi, 2021; Lipsitz et al., 2024; Kuchler et al., 2023).

KEY TERMS FROM THIS CHAPTER

- Communication skills
- Discomfort
- Emotional dimensions
- Healthcare
- Pediatric palliative care (PPC)
- Symptom management
- Cultural competence
- Emotional
- Family resistance
- Pediatric palliative
- Spiritual dimensions

CRITICAL THINKING QUESTIONS

1. **What is the primary goal of pediatric palliative care?**
   a. To prolong life at all costs
   b. To cure the underlying illness
   c. To improve the quality of life and relieve suffering
   d. To transition the patient to adult care
2. **Which of the following is a key principle of pediatric end-of-life care?**
   a. Avoiding all medications
   b. Maintaining life-sustaining treatments indefinitely
   c. Providing holistic support to both child and family
   d. Limiting communication with the family to avoid distress
3. **Which of the following symptoms is most commonly managed in pediatric palliative care?**
   a. Hyperactivity
   b. Fever
   c. Pain
   d. Allergic reactions
4. **What is an advance care plan in pediatric palliative care?**
   a. A vaccination schedule
   b. A legal document for guardianship
   c. A plan that outlines future medical care preferences
   d. A plan for returning to school
5. **Which professional is typically not a part of the pediatric palliative care team?**
   a. Pediatrician
   b. Social worker
   c. Nutritionist
   d. Real estate agent

Short Answer Questions

1. Define pediatric palliative care and explain its principles. How does it differ from adult palliative care, and why is early integration into the care plan important?
2. Discuss the physical, emotional, and spiritual components of "total pain" in children with life-limiting illnesses.
3. Describe the key components of an effective pediatric advance care plan. How can healthcare providers facilitate meaningful conversations with families about end-of-life decisions?
4. Explore the ethical challenges faced in pediatric end-of-life care, including decisions about Do Not Resuscitate (DNR) orders, life-sustaining treatments, and communication of prognosis.
5. Explain the approach to symptom management in pediatric palliative care, with emphasis on pain, dyspnea, nausea, and fatigue.

Answer to Critical Thinking Questions

1.(c) 2. (b) 3. (c) 4. (b) 5.(c)

REFERENCES

1. Álvaro-Lozano, M., Akdiş, C. A., Akdiş, M., Alviani, C., Angier, E., Arasi, S., Arzt-Gradwohl, L., et al. (2020). Allergen immunotherapy in children user's guide. *Pediatric Allergy and Immunology, 31*, 1–101. https://doi.org/10.1111/pai.13189 (accessed on 16th June 2025).
2. Anna, 1. 2., Cederstrom, C., et al. (2023). Exploring the gender gap in end-of-life care: Ethical considerations for dementia patients. *The European Journal of Public Health, 33*. https://www.semanticscholar.org/paper/74032f956efdb4994d4738420cd03d9ab3cc5f53 (accessed on 16th June 2025).
3. Bashshur, R. L., Doarn, C. R., Frenk, J., Kvedar, J. C., & Woolliscroft, J. O. (2020). Telemedicine and the COVID-19 pandemic, lessons for the future. *Telemedicine Journal and e-Health, 26*, 571–573. https://doi.org/10.1089/tmj.2020.29040.rb (accessed on 16th June 2025).
4. Benini, F., Papadatou, D., Bernadá, M., Craig, F., De Zen, L., Downing, J., Drake, R., et al. (2022). International standards for pediatric palliative care: From IMPaCCT to GO-PPaCS. *Journal of Pain and Symptom Management, 63*, e529–e543. https://doi.org/10.1016/j.jpainsymman.2021.12.031 (accessed on 16th June 2025).
5. Buang, S. N. H., Loh, S. W., Mok, Y. H., Lee, J. H., & Chan, Y. H. (2022). Palliative and critical care: Their convergence in the pediatric intensive care unit. *Frontiers in Pediatrics, 10*. https://doi.org/10.3389/fped.2022.907268 (accessed on 16th June 2025).
6. Davidson, J. E., Aslakson, R. A., Long, A. C., Puntillo, K., Kross, E. K., Hart, J. L., Cox, C. E., et al. (2016). Guidelines for family-centered care in the neonatal, pediatric, and adult ICU. *Critical Care Medicine, 45*, 103–128. https://doi.org/10.1097/ccm.0000000000002169 (accessed on 16th June 2025).
7. Farsi, D. (2021). Social media and health care, Part I: Literature review of social media use by health care providers. *Journal of Medical Internet Research, 23*, e23205–e23205. https://doi.org/10.2196/23205 (accessed on 16th June 2025).
8. Lipsitz, J., Beveridge, M., & Maddox, K. (2024). Palliative care for dialysis-dependent pediatric patients: A survey of providers, nurses, and caregivers. *Kidney360, 5*, 1669–1674. https://www.semanticscholar.org/paper/45d82cb7b2173fd49b956b1d28d09d7cd74fb80a (accessed on 16th June 2025).
9. Nagoya, Y., Matsuoka, M., Takenouchi, N., Hirata, M., Arita, N., Kawakatsu, K., Furuhashi, T., et al. (2023). Nursing practice and care structure for children and their families in need of pediatric palliative and end-of-life care in Japan. *Journal of Hospice and Palliative Nursing, 25*, E41–E48. https://www.semanticscholar.org/paper/17b08191ec338686124fd52bec4d196710f2e48d (accessed on 16th June 2025).
10. Nakanishi, M., Ogawa, A., & Nishida, A. (2024). Holistic dementia care continuum from the point of diagnosis to the end of life: Progress and challenges in translating national dementia policies into daily practice in Japan. *Alzheimer's & Dementia, 20*. https://www.semanticscholar.org/paper/837071fcb956692b70f8a42dded (accessed on 16th June 2025).
11. Nogueira, J., & Ribeiro, M. T. (2024). The psychologicalpsychological experience of grandparents: Proposal of a qualitative clinical assessment tool in pediatric palliative care. *Clinics and Practice, 14*, 122–131. https://www.semanticscholar.org/paper/986aa8b6dd41aa1f8431579711af262fdb034c69 (accessed on 16th June 2025).

12. Schroeder, K., & Lorenz, K. (2017). Nursing and the future of palliative care. *Asia-Pacific Journal of Oncology Nursing, 5*, 4–8. https://doi.org/10.4103/apjon.apjon_43_17 (accessed on 16th June 2025).

13. Wearne, N., Davidson, B., Motsohi, T., Mc Culloch, M., & Krause, R. (2020). Radically rethinking renal supportive and palliative care in South Africa. *Kidney International Reports, 6*, 568–573. https://doi.org/10.1016/j.ekir.2020.11.024 (accessed on 16th June 2025).

14. Yu, J., Song, I., Kim, C. H., Moon, Y., Shin, H., & Kim, M. S. (2020). Perceptions of pediatric palliative care among physicians who care for pediatric patients in South Korea. *Journal of Palliative Medicine*. https://www.semanticscholar.org/paper/a203749fe735dff38f03062faffc522cc56f04e7 (accessed on 16th June 2025).

15. Zucchetti, G., Ciappina, S., Bottigelli, C., Campione, G., Parrinello, A., Piu, P., Lijoi, S., et al. (2023). Reiki intervention for supporting healthcare professional care behaviors in pediatric palliative care: A pilot study. *Palliative & Supportive Care*. https://www.semanticscholar.org/paper/259152c1b8989c231e9cfccf7aa8adea53416521 (accessed on 16th June 2025).

INDEX

H

I

J

P

S

T

U

V

W